SKINNER'S

SCIENCE OF DENTAL MATERIALS

Eighth Edition

Ralph W. Phillips, M.S., D.Sc.

Associate Dean for Research and
Research Professor of Dental Materials
School of Dentistry
Indiana University

W. B. SAUNDERS COMPANY   Philadelphia   London   Toronto   Mexico City   Rio de Janeiro   Sydney   Tokyo

W. B. Saunders Company: West Washington Square
                           Philadelphia, PA   19105

Library of Congress Cataloging in Publication Data

Skinner, Eugene William, 1896–

Skinner's Science of dental materials.

Includes index.

1. Dental materials.   I. Phillips, Ralph W.   II. Title.
   III. Title: Science of dental materials.

RK652.5.S55 1981   617.6′95   81–51190

ISBN 0-7216-7235-3   AACR2

Listed here is the latest translated edition of this book together with
the language of the translation and the publisher.

Japanese (7th Edition)—Vol. I—Ishiyaku Publishers, Inc., Tokyo, Japan

Japanese (7th Edition)—Vol. II—Ishiyaku Publishers, Inc., Tokyo, Japan

Japanese (7th Edition)—Vol. III—Ishiyaku Publishers, Inc., Tokyo, Japan

Spanish (8th Edition)—Nueva Editorial Interamericana S.A. de C.V. Mexico 4, Mexico

Portuguese (8th Edition)—Editora Guanabara Koogan S.A., Travessa do Ouvidor—1,
                          ZC 00 Rio de Janeiro, Brazil

Skinner's Science of Dental Materials   ISBN   0-7216-7235-3

Last digit is the print number: 9   8   7   6   5

PREFACE

This revision is by far the most comprehensive of the seven that have preceded. Each chapter has been reworked to coincide with the current state of the art. Many required a complete restructuring. These sweeping alterations were dictated not only by the time interval since the last edition but also by the explosion that has occurred in dental materials science during the last few years. The investigative effort in this and related fields has resulted in the introduction of a host of newer systems and concepts, as well as marked changes in the formulations and techniques of usage for the traditional materials.

Thus the task of bringing this text abreast of these developments was decidedly more arduous than previously. Yet it was a challenge to develop a manuscript that hopefully would capture the excitement of this era and the new dimensions in dental practice that have been generated through research.

It will be noted that the title of this book still carries the name of E. W. Skinner, who was the author of the first four editions and the senior author of the fifth and sixth editions. His influence upon this discipline, and upon scholarly writing, was exemplary. Within my capabilities I have tried to maintain his basic philosophy in the organization of the text and the presentation of the subject material. That can best be summarized by quoting a paragraph from the Preface to the seventh edition.

"All of those editions were marked by certain principles about which Eugene Skinner was unyielding. One was that a textbook should be organized in an orderly fashion. The reader was not to be introduced to terminology or subject matter that was out of sequence to his level of knowledge in basic science or dentistry. Therefore, each chapter was carefully built upon the knowledge acquired by the reader in those that preceded it. Likewise, he adhered to the philosophy that it is as important to know what information should be included in a text as it is that which should be omitted. Thus, the past editions did not involve elaborate surveys of the literature. Rather, the subject matter was confined to that which was appropriately documented by research and clinical experience. Those matters which, in the view of the author, remained controversial were generally excluded. Lastly, and most important, he demanded exactness in the written word and precise accuracy in the concepts and data presented."

Thus the philosophy, organization, and objectives of this edition are those of the previous one. Emphasis continues to be placed on the *why* rather than the *how* in the selection and use of dental materials and their interaction with the oral environment. Although the manipulative parameters for attaining maximum performance are continually stressed, the reader is challenged to understand the rationale from which the technical procedures have evolved. Only with such conceptual thinking can the student appreciate the viability of the field and make the intelligent decisions that are required daily in the usage of dental materials.

It will be found that the contents of this revision reflect the major trends that have surfaced in the science of dental materials. One is the increasing attention focused on the structures of materials and their interaction with the oral environment. New illustrations, particularly SEM photomicrographs, and diagrams have been used to complement the text material in this regard.

A second area of expanded activity is concerned with the biological characteristics of restorative materials. This emphasis is appropriate, since the physical or mechanical properties of a particular material are secondary to that of the safety of the patient, the dentist, and the auxiliary staff. Furthermore, regulatory procedures are being expanded to insure biocompatibility of dental materials. Throughout the book these matters are woven into the text.

Lastly has been the growth of clinical research, much of which is designed to establish the precise relationship of a property, or group of properties, to clinical performance. The text is laced with references to such clinical investigations, especially to those that document recommendations for a particular system, and manipulative or clinical technique of use.

As noted, each chapter has been carefully edited and updated in terms of compositions, chemistry, and manipulative techniques. Selected references are included whenever it is felt that a literature annotation is pertinent to the statement or discussion. The reader who is familiar with the previous text will be readily conscious of these additions and revisions. However, it is appropriate in a Preface to cite areas of major change, and the following discussion describes those that are of special interest.

The general organization of the text remains the same. In the first three chapters a description of the structure of matter, the physical properties of materials, the phenomenon of adhesion, and biological considerations are presented. In regard to the latter, the regulatory procedures of the Food and Drug Administration have been covered. Similarly, the policies of the Council on Dental Materials, Instruments, and Equipment of the American Dental Association in respect to the Acceptance and Certification programs have been brought abreast of their current status.

The differences between mechanical bonding and true adhesive bonding are separated out and related to their specific dental applications, which are discussed later in the book. New sections on rheology and color have been added. Rheology is important to the discussions on dental cements and impression materials, for example. An explanation of the color phenomenon and its terminology is essential for an understanding of the technology used in fabricating certain restorations, such as those involving porcelain.

The classification of gypsum products has been redone so as to correlate with specification terminology. A section has been added on "special" products, e.g., mounting stones.

Chapters 8 and 9, on hydrocolloid impression materials, have been reorganized for ease in following the text. In the previous edition, the techniques for handling both the reversible and irreversible hydrocolloids were covered in Chapter 9. Now, Chapter 8 deals completely with the reversible hydrocolloids while the alginates are discussed in Chapter 9. Some subtle changes in technique have occurred, such as the "wet field" procedure for hydrocolloid, and these are included.

The chemistry of the elastomeric impression materials is now consistent with present knowledge and, of course, the addition silicones are included. The various types are compared in terms of properties and characteristics.

A discussion of polymers and their uses in denture prostheses follows. The chemistry has been adjusted to conform to current concepts, as have the technical procedures. Although the fabrication of such appliances is now generally carried out by a laboratory technician, an understanding of the scientific rationale for the basic steps involved is important in order that the dental student may properly appreciate the role of the technician and understand the problems that may occur in the clinical use of artificial dentures. Furthermore, there is no other ready reference source available for those who wish to have a further understanding of the *why* in the construction of these appliances.

A section on maxillofacial prostheses has been added. Also the discussion of other polymeric materials, such as tissue conditioners and liners, has been revised.

One of the most intriguing areas of change has been that of restorative resin, with the development of microfilled composites, light-cured systems, acid etching techniques to improve mechanical bonding, enamel bond agents, and resins for the coating of eroded gingival areas. All of these, and other, materials are covered in Chapter 14, Restorative Resins, including illustrations to clarify structure and properties. The discussion on traditional acrylic resins has been markedly condensed and is used principally as a basis for the historical presentation and for better understanding of the BIS-GMA and other composite resin matrix systems.

The chapters on metallurgy and the nature of metals and alloys now cover whiskers, lattice imperfections, and dislocations in the light of recent findings. New illustrations and text are used to simplify the interpretation of phase diagrams, as by the use of brine as a model. The same may be said for Chapter 19, Tarnish and Corrosion, in which a diagram of an electrolytic cell and an expansion of oxidation-reduction reactions are used to develop the mechanisms of corrosion.

As for restorative resins, dental amalgam alloys have gone through a tremendous transition in composition, as has our appreciation of causative factors involved in clinical deterioration. At the writing of the seventh edition, these dramatic changes had not as yet emerged. Now the evolution of the high copper alloys can be traced. Illustrations are used to show the structure and reactions of these alloys and how they relate to in vivo performance. Types of high copper systems are classified and the mechanisms for eliminating the weak, corrosion prone gamma-2 phase explained. Techniques are also consistent with present practice. The section on mercury toxicity and office hygiene conforms to modern opinion.

Chapter 24 on noble metal casting alloys is virtually rewritten, as necessitated by the avalanche of new alloys that have been introduced, such as the so-called semi-precious alloys. These various types have been classified and compared on the basis of composition, color, and usage. The history of the metal-ceramic alloys is presented, since it is the basis of reference for the discussion of that restoration which follows, particularly in Chapter 31. The role of the various components, and new metals that have been added, is elaborated upon. Much of the discussion on porosity is better associated with the technical considerations associated with the casting procedure. Thus this section has been moved to Chapter 28.

The chapters on the materials and techniques related to the cast restoration come next, with appropriate revisions. The use of wax in the direct technique has been minimized, yet additional discussion has been devoted to other waxes, i.e., baseplate and corrective.

The description of phosphate-bonded investments has been moved up to Chapter 26, owing to the increased popularity of this type of investment for the casting of small restorations. In the same vein, the discussion of these investments has been expanded.

In the two chapters devoted to casting procedures, changes and additions will be apparent. The discussion of gypsum hardeners and methods for altering the die dimensions, e.g., die spacers, has been expanded. The various types of casting machines are described and the influence of pressure gradient on efficacy has been explained. Technical considerations for phosphate-bonded investments, as they differ from those for gypsum-bonded materials, have been added. As noted earlier, the description of porosity in dental castings is now moved to this portion of the text and the subject has been subtly reclassified.

Now to the changed field of restorative and luting cements. The chapters are reorganized to better reflect usage. Luting cements are discussed in Chapter 29 and the protective agents and thermal insulating bases are placed together in Chapter 30, along with cements used for restorations. The discussion of silicate cement is minimal and is used primarily as introductory material for the glass ionomer system, which is described both as a luting agent and for the coating of eroded areas. The polycarboxylate cement is covered in greater detail, particularly in terms of technical considerations.

It was imperative that the chapter on porcelain be updated to mirror the changes that have occurred. Considerable restructuring of the subject matter will be noted, with many new illustrations to depict present usage. The compositions and properties of dental ceramics have been revised, as is information on structure and influence of technique, such as the specific effect of porosities. Particular attention is given to the metal-ceramic systems and other methods of bonding, e.g., tin oxide coatings.

The chapter on wrought alloys has been condensed, owing to the reduced usage in the construction of partial dentures. However, materials in this category, e.g., P-G-P wires, which are employed in certain other appliances, are now covered. Chapter 33 includes an expanded section on the soldering of metal-ceramic restorations.

Chapter 34, Base Metal Alloys for Dental Castings, originally Chapter 35, has been expanded to embrace the base metal alloys used for small castings as well as the traditional use in larger appliances. A comparison is made with the noble metal alloys for the metal-ceramic restoration. The matter of biological considerations, i.e., nickel and beryllium sensitivity, is faced. The subject of carbon steel is now incorporated into Chapter 37, where it fits more logically.

Much of the discussion on the basic mechanics of abrasion and polishing is still accurate and remains essentially intact. However, the sections on abrasive instruments and dentifrices are updated.

In the last chapter, the nickel-chromium alloys have been deleted from the text, since these are now seldom used in the construction of orthodontic appliances. The more common nickel-titanium and beta titanium systems are added, as are the braided and twisted wires.

This edition uses the International System of units (SI units) as the preferred system. However, since their use is not as yet universal, the English units are included. For example, temperatures are given in °C, with (°F) equivalents shown in parentheses, and stress in MPa is followed by (psi). For those who wish to convert these measurements, an Appendix has been provided. Incidentally, numerical values have frequently been rounded off to the nearest decimal unless absolute numbers are essential for precise interpretations.

RALPH W. PHILLIPS

ACKNOWLEDGMENTS

In a revision of this magnitude, an author must draw upon the expertise of many colleagues and friends. This I have done. The updating of the scientific accuracy of this text must be shared with those individuals. Without fail they constructively and enthusiastically responded to my queries.

I have long been blessed with a loyal, dedicated, and skilled faculty and technical staff. The quality of the manuscript, and the time table for completion, could never have been realized without their aid. As always, when requested, they gave unselfishly of their time, energies, and competence. In many instances, in addition to changes in the text material, it was necessary to recheck in vitro data and to provide new figures. A mere listing of their names is a most inadequate expression of my indebtedness to them.

Those faculty members are M. L. Swartz, B. K. Moore, R. J. Schnell, and J. C. Sfetcopoulos, and the technical staff: B. F. Rhodes, H. E. Clark, R. B. Doherty, and K. F. Bissonette.

A special acknowledgment is due my secretary, Edith Gladson. She typed the entire manuscript and Index, assisted in proofreading the galleys, and checked literature references. This was all done, patiently and expertly, superimposed upon a normal work load that would in itself tax the capabilities of several typical secretaries. The preciseness of the text is in no small measure due to Edith's attention to detail.

A number of other Indiana University School of Dentistry faculty members were consulted in respect to specific items, especially G. K. Stookey, A. H. Kafrawy, V. Chalian, and C. J. Goodacre.

The cooperation of R. Scott, M. Halloran, and A. Fears was essential in the meticulous preparation of new graphs and illustrations.

The science of dental materials has undergone a tremendous transition since the last edition of this book, as is elaborated upon in the Preface. Virtually every material and associated techniques have spawned a new generation of technology and body of knowledge. It is impossible for any one scientist, or even group of scientists, to remain fully informed of all these diverse developments. Thus an author has no recourse but to rely upon the skills and judgments of other scientists throughout the world. Some were consulted only on the validity of a figure, table, or statement. Others contributed advice on a broader basis. I was gratified that when the revision was initiated a number of colleagues volunteered to review areas germane to their particular area of interest.

As in the previous edition, not all of these suggestions could be heeded. Nevertheless, I hope all will feel comfortable with the end result. It is not possible to list everyone who provided useful information but the following were particularly helpful, and substantial credit is due them. Those familiar with the dental literature will recognize most of the names and the areas on which their research has focused.

These individuals are J. W. McLean, R. Neiman, C. W. Fairhurst, J. P. Nielsen, A. D. Wilson, M. M. Braden, G. A. Crim, J. P. Moffa, A. J. Goldberg, J. Cresson, J. W. Stanford, J. F. Glenn, R. M. McConnell, J. J. Tuccillo, D. D. Porteous, G. M. Brauer, C. J. Burstone, H. R. Horn, C. E. Ingersoll, E. W. Dougherty, R. L. Probst, T. Okabe, R. Mitchell, W. B. Eames, and R. L. Myerson.

The W. B. Saunders Company provided their usual careful handling of the publication and maintained their standards of excellence. I am indebted to Charles Graham for his editorial review of the manuscript, to Laura Tarves for her assistance in the composition of the book, and to Karen O'Keefe for the design of the book. Robert Reinhardt, as Dental Editor, faithfully followed the progress of the text and cooperated with me on my various requests associated with the entire production.

CONTENTS

1 INTRODUCTION

Historical Background Strange as it may seem, there is comparatively little historical background for the science of dental materials and their manipulation, in spite of the fact that the practice of dentistry itself antedates the Christian era. For example, gold bands and wires were used by the Phoenicians and Etruscans for the construction of partial dentures. Gold foil has been employed for dental restorative purposes for so long a period that its origin is not known.

Modern dentistry is said to have had its beginning during the year 1728, when Fauchard published a treatise describing many types of dental restorations, including a method for the construction of artificial dentures from ivory. Somewhat later, in 1756, Pfaff first described the method for obtaining impressions of the mouth in wax, from which he constructed a model with plaster of Paris. The year 1792 is important as the date when de Chamant patented a process for the construction of porcelain teeth; this was followed early in the next century by the introduction of the porcelain inlay.

It is evident, then, that many of the restorative and accessory materials of today have been in use for some time, yet little scientific information about them has been available until recently. Their use was entirely an art, and the only testing laboratory was the mouth of the long-suffering patient.

The first important awakening of interest was during the middle of the nineteenth century, when research studies on amalgam began. At about the same time there are also some reports in the literature of studies on porcelain and gold foil. These rather sporadic advances in knowledge finally culminated in the brilliant investigations of G. V. Black, which began in 1895. There is hardly a phase of dentistry which was not touched upon and advanced by this tireless worker.

The next great advance in the knowledge of dental materials and their manipulation began in 1919. During this year, the United States Army requested the National Bureau of Standards to set up specifications for the selection and grading of dental amalgams for use in federal service. This research was done under the leadership of Wilmer Souder, and a very excellent report was published in 1920.[1] The information contained in the report was received enthusiastically by the dental profession, and information along the same line was demanded for other dental materials.

At the time, the United States Government could not allocate sufficient funds to continue the work, so a fellowship was created and supported by the

Weinstein Research Laboratories. Under such an arrangement, the sponsor provides the salary for research associates and a certain amount of equipment and supplies. The associates then work in the National Bureau of Standards under the direction of the staff members. They are to all intents and purposes members of the staff, supported by private interests. All findings are published and become common property under such an arrangement.

R. L. Coleman, W. L. Swanger, and W. A. Poppe were the Research Associates first appointed under this arrangement. Working under Dr. Souder, they investigated the properties of dental wrought and casting golds and accessory casting materials. This phase of the work resulted in the publication of an extensive and valuable research report.[2]

In 1928, the Dental Research Fellowship at the National Bureau of Standards was assumed by the American Dental Association. The research carried on by the American Dental Association Research Associates in conjunction with the staff members of the National Bureau of Standards has been of inestimable value to the dental profession, and it has earned for this group an international reputation. The names of individuals such as Wilmer Souder, George C. Paffenbarger, and William T. Sweeney will undoubtedly live in history as the pioneer research workers whose work began a new era of intense research production in the field of dental materials. It was the enthusiasm of these men which prompted the organization of the first courses in dental materials to be taught in the dental schools of America and abroad.

American Dental Association Specifications The work at the American Dental Association Research Division is divided into a number of categories, including the determination of those physical and chemical properties of dental materials which have clinical significance and the development of new materials, instruments, and test methods. Until 1965 the primary objective of this facility was to formulate standards or specifications for dental materials and to certify the products which meet those requirements. However, when the Council on Dental Materials and Devices of the American Dental Association (now called the Council on Dental Materials, Instruments, and Equipment) was established in 1966, it assumed these responsibilities.

Such specifications are essentially standards by which the value of the particular dental materials can be gauged. They present the requirements as to the physical and chemical properties of a material which will insure that the material will be satisfactory if properly employed by the dentist. Once a specification has been formulated for a particular material, any of the various manufacturers may certify to the Council that its product meets the requirements of the particular specification. The product is then tested, and if it meets the requirements of the particular specification, its trade name and the manufacturer's name are published in *The Journal of the American Dental Association*. The manufacturer is permitted to signify on the label of the product that it has been certified by the American Dental Association by the use of a Seal of Certification.

The Council on Dental Materials, Instruments, and Equipment has the responsibility as the Administrative Sponsor of a standards formulating committee operating under the procedures of the American National Standards Institute. The American National Standards Committee MO156 is concerned with nomenclature, standards, and specifications for all dental materials and devices with the exception of drugs and x-ray films. A separate Council committee is responsible for dental x-ray, while the Council on Dental Therapeutics of the American Dental Association is accountable for the evaluation of drugs in dentistry.

Upon advice from the Council, the committee, with the aid of subcommittees, revises and formulates specifications. When a specification has been approved by the Standards Committee, it is submitted through the Council to the American National Standards Institute. Upon acceptance by that body it becomes an American National Standard. The Council on Dental Materials, Instruments, and Equipment then has the option of accepting it as an American Dental Association Specification.

Currently there are 37 American Dental Association specifications. The number of specifications is increasing rapidly, encompassing materials and devices not presently covered by a specification. Likewise, the existing specifications are periodically revised in order to reflect changes in product formulations and new knowledge in regard to behavior of materials in the oral cavity. For example, American Dental Association specification no. 1 for dental amalgam has been revised five times.

Federal Regulations and Standards   On May 28, 1976, legislation was signed into law which gave the Food and Drug Administration (FDA) of the United States the regulatory authority to protect the public from hazardous and/or ineffective medical devices. That legislation was the culmination of a series of attempts to provide safe and effective products, beginning with the passage of the Food and Drug Act of 1906, which did not include any provision to regulate medical device safety or the claims made for devices.

This newer legislation, named the Medical Device Amendments of 1976, requires the classification and regulation of all non-custom medical devices that are intended for human use. The term device includes "any instrument, apparatus, implement, machine, contrivance, implant, or in vitro reagent used in the diagnosis, cure, mitigation, treatment or prevention of disease in man or animals." Some dental products are considered drugs (e.g., fluoride products), but most products used in the operatory are considered to be devices and are thus subject to control by the FDA Bureau of Medical Devices. Also encompassed are over-the-counter (OTC) products sold to the public, such as floss and denture adhesives.

The classification of all medical and dental items is done by panels composed of non-government dental experts as well as representatives from industry and the consumer. The Dental Panel, one of 19, identifies any known hazards or problems and classifies the item into one of the following classes: Class I, II, or III. All devices are subject to general controls (Class I), which includes matters such as the registration of the manufacturer's products, adherence to good manufacturing practices, and certain record keeping requirements. If it is felt that such general controls are not in themselves adequate to ensure safety and effectiveness as claimed by the manufacturer, then the device is placed into Class II. That classification requires that it meet performance standards established by the FDA, or appropriate ones from other authoritative bodies, such as the specification program of the American Dental Association. These performance standards may relate to construction, components, ingredients, and properties of a device and may also provide that it be tested to assure that lots or individual products do conform to the regulatory requirement.

Classification into Class III, the most stringent of the three, requires that the device have approval for safety and effectiveness before being marketed. All implanted or life supporting devices are, of course, placed in this category and require data to demonstrate safety and efficacy prior to marketing. In addition, any item that does not have adequate clinical or scientific information available that would permit the formulation of a performance standard is placed in this premarket approval category. Currently, 14 types of dental-related products have been recommended by the classification panel for that category.[3]

To date 242 dental items have been classified into one of these three classes. This activity, in conjunction with the American Dental Association specification program for dental materials and devices, is providing a crucial framework for standards developments and for better assurance to the dentist and his patients that the product is safe and effective as claimed. It should be added that a number of other countries have national government agencies comparable to the FDA that, to a certain extent, include dental materials and devices under the umbrella of their regulatory authority.

International Standards   For many years there has been great interest in the establishment of specifications for dental materials on an international level. Two organizations, the *Fédération Dentaire Internationale* (FDI) and the *International Standards Organization* (ISO), are working toward that goal. Originally the FDI initiated and actively supported a program for the formulation of international specifications for dental materials. As a result of that activity, nine specifications for dental materials and devices have been adopted.

The ISO is an international, nongovernmental organization whose objective is the development of international standards. This body is composed of national standards organizations from 84 countries. The *American National Standards Institute* is the United States member. The request by the FDI to the ISO that they consider FDI specifications for dental materials as ISO standards led to the formation of an ISO committee, TC106 — Dentistry. The responsibility of this committee is to standardize terminology, test methods, and specifications for dental materials, instruments, appliances, and equipment.

There are 17 participating members and 21 observer members in the ISO committee. The nine FDI specifications have now been adopted as ISO standards. In addition 24 additional standards have been developed under ISO/TC106 since 1963, through cooperative programs with FDI. Thus, considerable progress has already been realized in achieving the ultimate goal of a broad spectrum of international specifications for dental materials and devices.

The benefit of such specifications to the dental profession has been inestimable. The dentist is provided with a criterion of selection which is impartial and reliable. In other words, if the dentist uses only those materials that meet the appropriate specifications, he can be assured that the material will be satisfactory. Probably no other single factor has contributed as much to the high level of dental practice in the United States as has this specification program. An awareness by the dentist of the requirements of these specifications is important in order that he may be able to recognize the limitations of the dental material with which he is working. As will be discussed frequently in the chapters to follow, no dental material is perfect in its restorative role any more than an artificial arm or leg can serve as well as the original body member which it replaces.

The Council also conducts another program for the evaluation of dental products, known as the Acceptance Program. This activity applies to products for which safety and effectiveness have been established by biological, laboratory and/or clinical evaluations if appropriate or where physical standards or specifications do not currently exist. Specific guidelines for acceptance for each generic area, e.g., pit and fissure sealants or powered toothbrushes, are formulated by the Council.

For this and other reasons, the research in dental materials, supervised by the Council of Dental Materials, Instruments, and Equipment of the American Dental Association, is of vital concern in the present course in dental materials. The American Dental Association specifications for dental materials are constantly referred to in the following pages, although the specific details regarding the actual test methods employed are usually omitted. For those students in foreign countries, the counterpart ISO standards, if applicable, should be used as a source reference.

Thus, the discussion in this text assumes that the student has access to a current copy of the Dentist's Desk Reference — Materials, Instruments and Equipment (formerly called Guide to Dental Materials and Devices) and to the collection of Specifications and Acceptance Programs of the American Dental Association.

The Dentist's Desk Reference can be purchased from the publisher, the American Dental Association, 211 East Chicago Avenue, Chicago, Illinois, at a nominal cost. It is revised and published every three years in order to keep the contents up to date. It reviews the recent researches in the field with an excellent bibliography, and presents the trade names of commercial products that are currently certified to meet the requirements of the particular specifications involved. Likewise, there is a listing of other brands of products available, insofar as they are known. Products classified under the Council's Acceptance Program can also be found.

Other Standards Organizations and Research Centers The work at the Bureau of Standards has stimulated comparable programs in other countries. The Australian Dental Standards Laboratory was established in 1936. H. K. Worner and A. R. Docking, as the first two directors, are recognized for their leadership in the development of the Australian specifications for dental materials. Until 1973 this facility was known as the Commonwealth Bureau of Dental Standards. Actually the oldest among the National Standards Organizations is the British Standards Institution, which was formed in 1901 as the Engineering Standards Committee.

Other countries that have comparable organizations for developing standards and certifying to standards are Canada, Japan, France, Czechoslovakia, Germany, Hungary, Israel, India, Poland, South Africa, and Sweden. Also, by agreement among the governments of Sweden, Denmark, Finland, and Norway, the Scandinavian Institute of Dental Materials (NIOM) has been formed for testing, certification, and research regarding dental materials and equipment to be used in the four countries.

An increasing number of universities in America and abroad have established laboratories for research in dental materials. In the past few years, this source of basic information on the subject has exceeded that of all other sources combined. Until very recently, dental research activities in universities were centered solely in those that had a dental school, with most of the investigation being done in the dental school itself and by the dental faculty. Now, however, research in dental materials is also being conducted in some universities that do not have dental schools. This dentally oriented research is being conducted in basic science departments, such as metallurgy, crystallography, materials science, engineering, and ceramics. These expanding perimeters of research in dental materials illustrate the interdisciplinary aspects of the science.

There have been countless contributions to this field by dental clinicians. The final criterion for the success of any material or technique is its service in the mouth of the patient. The observant clinician contributes invaluable information by his keen observations and analyses of his failures and successes. Accurate records and a well controlled practice form an excellent basis for good clinical research.

The importance of clinical documentation for claims made relative to the in vivo performance of dental materials is now readily apparent. For example, the Acceptance Program of the Council on Dental Materials, Instruments, and Equipment requires clinical data, whenever appropriate, to support the laboratory tests for physical properties. Thus, the past decade has seen an escalation in the number of clinical investigations designed to correlate specific properties to performance and to establish the precise behavior of a given material or system. In the chapters that follow frequent reference will be made to such investigations.

Another source of information is the research laboratories of the dental manufacturers. The far-seeing manufacturer recognizes the value of a research laboratory in connection with the development and production control of his products. Unbiased information from such groups is particularly valuable. As in the previous edition, the counsel of scientists from dental and nondental industry was called upon during the course of this revision. In this way the product formulations to be found in the succeeding chapters reflect more exactly the commercial materials actually used by the dentist.

This diversity of research activity is resulting in an accelerating growth in the body of knowledge related to dental materials. For example, in 1978 approximately 9 per cent of all U.S. support for dental research was focused upon restorative dental materials.[4] The percentage would no doubt be considerably higher if the monies spent by industry for the development of new materials, instruments, and appliances were included. This growing investigative effort is resulting in a marked increase in the number of new materials, instruments, and techniques being introduced to the profession. For these and other reasons, an intimate knowledge of the properties and behavior of dental materials is imperative if the modern dental practice is to remain abreast of the changing developments.

Scope of the Course   Not all of the materials used in dentistry are included in the course. For example, anesthetics and medicaments are not within the scope of this book. The science of dental materials is generally considered to comprise those materials which are employed in the mechanical procedures included in restorative dentistry, such as prosthetics, crown and bridge, and operative dentistry. Likewise, to an extent some of the materials employed in certain specialties, e.g., orthodontics and pedodontics, are included. It is one of the aims of this book to introduce the materials to the beginner, and to study their physical and chemical properties as such properties are related to their proper selection and use by the dentist. However, certain biological considerations will not be ignored. It is assumed that the reader possesses a basic knowledge of physics as well as inorganic and organic chemistry.

A relatively new science is now included in the engineering curriculum of most universities. It is called *materials science* and is concerned with the internal structure of materials and with the dependence of properties upon these internal structures. The sequence of instruction generally proceeds from atomic structure to coarser structures, from the simple to the more complex. The source of knowledge in this field draws upon various disciplines, such as physical chemistry, solid state physics, and metallurgy. Since it is these fundamentals that govern the properties of all materials, it is logical to study the finer structural characteristics before proceeding to the more gross ones.

One should remember this changing concept of relating properties of a material to its atomic or crystalline structure when reading Chapter 2, which deals with the structure of matter and certain principles of materials science that are not always included in the course in college physics. These principles are in turn related to the properties of dental materials, as discussed in Chapter 3.

The student may find that some supplementary reading in this subject, within his background knowledge, will be helpful. The author has drawn to a certain extent upon the illustrative material in *Elements of Materials Science* by Van Vlack.[5] This introductory text to the field of materials science is highly recommended as collateral reading.

The requirements placed upon dental structures and materials are excessive and unique. Unfortunately, too often the dentist and patient are unaware of the limitations involved and the rigid conditions imposed in the oral cavity. Those matters are discussed in Chapter 3. The reader thereby should be increasingly aware of the difficulties involved in producing a satisfactory dental material or in designing a technique that is usable and practical, as will be continually emphasized in the discussions that follow on specific materials.

Following these chapters on the structure of matter and the physical and biological properties of dental materials are two chapters dealing with the chemistry and manipulation of gypsum products. Impression materials are then discussed. The chemistry of synthetic resins is presented as an introduction to a study of the various types of polymeric materials used for the construction of dental restorations and appliances.

Before the metallic dental materials are described, a short discussion of the principles of metallography, physical metallurgy, and tarnish and corrosion is presented as they can be applied to dental materials and procedures. The basic science of physical metallurgy is concerned with the properties of metals and alloys, whereas the study of metallography involves the constitution and structure of metallic substances. The student will find that the subject matter in Chapter 2 is used as source information in many of these discussions.

Dental amalgam, gold foil, and their manipulation are then described. This discussion is followed by a consideration of the noble metal alloys used in dentistry, and the materials and techniques employed in dental casting procedures. The next chapter is concerned with the properties of the cements which are used in the placement of certain restorations and for other purposes. Other nonmetallic restorative materials, e.g., glass ionomer cement and porcelain, are then discussed. The final chapters deal with the techniques employed in soldering, the base metal alloys used in dentistry, and certain other technical procedures, such as abrading, polishing, and cutting with dental burs.

It will be observed that many branches of science will be drawn upon in the presentation of the information. The disciplines of materials science, physical metallurgy, and metallography have already been mentioned. Ceramics is the study dealing with the firing and properties of dental porcelain. Various specialized branches of chemistry will be utilized. Practically all the engineering applied sciences have contributed to the subject. There is also an increasing awareness of the dentist that the biological properties of dental materials cannot be divorced from their mechanical or chemical properties. Thus, interwoven throughout are discussions of the pertinent biological characteristics to be considered in the selection and use of dental materials. However, in the final analysis, the subject of dental materials is a basic science in itself, with its own cultural value and principles.

Aim of the Course   The aim of the course is to present the basic chemical and physical properties of the dental material as they are related to its manipulation by the dentist. It is intended to bridge the gap between the knowledge obtained in the basic courses in materials science, chemistry, and physics and the dental operatory. As previously noted, dental technique does not need to be an empirical process, but rather it can be based on sound, scientific principles as more information is available from further research.

In any basic science, principles should be emphasized over practice. The discussions that follow deal more with *why* the materials react as they do and *why* the manipulation variables should be observed as they are described. *How* the materials are used in the broadest sense is discussed in other dental courses. The *how* information in this course is largely limited to the material per se.

Need for the Course   One of the differences between a professional man and a tradesman is that the former possesses basic knowledge with which he can select or set up the conditions for a situation such that a prediction of eventual success of a project is reasonably assured. A riveter must be responsible for the joined beams in a bridge, but the engineer is responsible for the design of the bridge, especially where the rivets and every truss and beam are to be placed and joined, and also for the selection of the materials with which the structure is constructed. If he knew nothing about the physical and chemical properties of the steels and other metals with which the bridge is made, the structure would undoubtedly fail.

The dentist and the engineer have much in common. The dentist must analyze the stresses present in a dental bridge that he is to build, and be guided by such analyses in the design of the bridge. He should possess a sufficient knowledge of the physical and chemical properties of the different types of materials he is using so that he can exercise the best judgment possible in their selection. In other words, he must be in a position to know whether the dental operation requires the use of a gold alloy, a cement, or a synthetic resin, for example. Only if he knows the physical and chemical properties of each of these materials is he in a position to make such a judgment. In addition to the mechanical requirements of the materials, there are also certain esthetic and physiological requirements which often complicate the situation beyond the difficulties usually encountered by the engineer.

Once the dentist has selected the type of material he should use, he must choose the material made by a certain manufacturer. It is the intention of the best dental manufacturers to cooperate with the dentist in supplying him with materials of quality in an ethical manner. The competition is keen, however, and the dentist should be in a position to evaluate the claims of the respective manufacturers in an intelligent manner. Unfortunately, there are a few unprincipled dental manufacturers who make preposterous claims and who exploit the dentist for their own profit. For his own protection and for the protection of his patient, the dentist must be able to recognize spurious practices of this sort. In addition to its other aims, the course in dental materials tries to provide the dentist with certain criteria of selection which will enable him to discriminate between fact and propaganda.

Furthermore, it is hoped that the student of dental materials will be given an appreciation of the broad scientific scope of the profession which he has chosen. Since a great deal of the daily practice of dentistry involves the selection and use of dental materials, either for the treatment procedure or in the instrumentation required, it is obvious that the science of dental materials is one that cannot be ignored. In order to understand more completely the relationship of this science to clinical practice in all phases of dentistry, the student is encouraged to read the discussion of this subject in another text.[6]

The advances being made in dental materials science suggest that intriguing changes will occur in the concepts, theories, and practice of dentistry. A comparison of the current research programs in dental materials, and the clinical application of those findings, with those of less than a decade ago emphasizes the dynamic status of the field.[7,8] Within these pages will be found a challenge to identify this science with modern dental practice. Only in this way can the profession be an exciting and rewarding experience.

References

1. Souder WH and Peters CG: An investigation of the physical properties of dental materials. National Bureau of Standards Technical Paper No. 157. Washington, DC, US Government Printing Office, 1920.
2. Coleman RL: Physical properties of dental materials. National Bureau of Standards Research Paper No. 32. Washington, DC, US Government Printing Office, 1928.
3. Fise TF and Smith DC: Assessment of the impact of medical device legislation on the dental trade industry. J Am Dent Assoc 99:799, 1979.
4. National Institute of Dental Research: Dental Research in the United States and Other Countries, Fiscal Year 1978, Bethesda, Md.
5. Van Vlack LH: Elements of Materials Science, 4th ed. Reading, Mass., Addison-Wesley Publishing Co., Inc., 1980.
6. Phillips RW: Dental materials. In Shapiro, M. (ed): The Scientific Bases in Dentistry, Philadelphia, WB Saunders Co., 1966, pp. 302–304.
7. Phillips RW: The changing profile of dentistry through research. ASDC J Dent Child Jan-Feb:1, 1975.
8. Phillips RW: Future role of biomaterials in dentistry and dental education. J Dent Educ 40:752, 1976.

2 STRUCTURE OF MATTER. ADHESION

Every use of materials, however trivial, involves selection. Through understanding or experimentation it is possible to maximize any one property, but in no application is it possible to select a material for one property alone. It is precisely in the balance of one factor against another that the materials engineer finds his challenge and his satisfaction.

The study of dental materials of necessity requires a basic knowledge of matter, particularly solids, if the properties and reactions of the materials are to be understood and, often, predicted. All dental restorations, whether they be plastic or metal, are built from atoms. The collective reactions of the atoms, whether physical or chemical, determine the effectiveness of the material. A short review of atomic theory in this regard is, therefore, apropos to a basic understanding.

Change of State The first question that arises is how atoms are held together. There are, of course, attractions between molecules of a gas. When water vapor condenses to form a liquid, energy in the form of heat is released, known as the *heat of vaporization*. It is defined in this connection as the amount of heat evolved when 1 gm of vapor is condensed to the liquid state.

Conversely, the heat of vaporization may also be defined as the amount of heat required to change 1 gm of liquid to a gas. For example, 540 calories of heat are required to vaporize 1 gm of water at 100° C. One can conclude, therefore, that the gaseous state possesses more energy than does the liquid state. Although the molecules in the gaseous state exert a certain amount of mutual attraction, they can diffuse readily and generally need to be confined in order to keep the gas intact.

Although molecules may also diffuse in the liquid state, their mutual attractions are greater and energy is required for this separation as described. As is well known, if the energy of the liquid decreases sufficiently by virtue of a decrease in temperature, for example, a second transformation in state may occur and the liquid changes to a solid or freezes. Again energy is released in the form of heat. In this case the energy evolved is known as the *latent heat of fusion*.

For example, when 1 gm of water freezes, 80 calories of heat are evolved. If 1 gm of a solid is changed to a liquid, the reverse is true and an input of heat energy is required. The temperature at which this change occurs is known as the *fusion temperature*. This property will be treated further in Chapter 15.

This temperature is of considerable dental importance in casting gold alloy restorations, for example.

Inasmuch as energy is required for a change from the solid to the liquid state, one can conclude that the attraction between the atoms (or molecules) in the solid state is greater than that in either the liquid or the gaseous state. If this were not true, they would easily separate; metal would deform readily and gasify at low temperatures.

The temperature at which a liquid boils or solidifies depends, partially at least, upon the environmental pressure. A liquid can, of course, vaporize (or evaporate) at any temperature between its freezing and boiling temperatures, provided the space above the liquid is not already saturated or supersaturated with the vapor. If the latter occurs, the gaseous phase condenses to the liquid state until equilibrium is established. The force required to free the molecules from a liquid is related to the *vapor pressure* of the liquid.

Although it is possible for a solid to change directly to a gas by a process known as *sublimation,* this phenomenon is not likely to be of practical importance so far as the dental materials to be discussed are concerned. It may be of considerable theoretical importance, however.

With this short review of the theory involving change of state, the considerations involving atomic or molecular attractions will be discussed.

Primary Interatomic Bonds   Interatomic bonds may be classified as *primary bonds* or *secondary bonds*. Primary bonds are chemical in nature, whereas secondary bonds are characterized by the physical forces. Primary atomic bonds may be of different types.

IONIC BONDS   Ionic bonds are of the simple chemical type, resulting from the mutual attraction of positive and negative charges. The classic example is sodium chloride, $Na^+ \cdot Cl^-$. Since the sodium atom contains one valence electron in its outer shell and the chlorine atom has seven electrons in its outer shell, the sharing of the sodium valence electron with the chlorine atom results in the stable compound NaCl.

COVALENT BONDS   In many chemical compounds, two valence electrons are shared. The hydrogen molecule, H_2, is an example of covalent bonding. The single valence electron in each hydrogen atom is shared with that of the other combining atom and the valence shells become stable.

A very important covalent bonding is that which occurs in many organic compounds. The carbon atom has four valence electrons and can be stabilized by combining with hydrogen:

$$4\dot{H} + \ddot{\underset{\cdot\cdot}{C}} \dashrightarrow H : \overset{H}{\underset{H}{\ddot{C}}} : H$$

Methane

Such a combination is important to an understanding of the molecular structure of the dental synthetic resins and their polymerization reactions as outlined in Chapter 11.

METALLIC BONDS   A third type of primary bonding is called the *metallic bond.* This type of interatomic bond will be explained in Chapter 15.

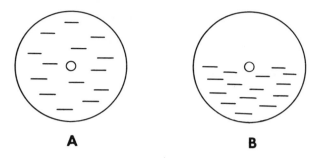

Figure 2–1 Normally the electrons surround the positive nucleus *(A)* to provide a neutral field, but momentarily the electrons may concentrate toward one side of the atom *(B)*.

Van der Waals Forces   There is, of course, attraction between atoms or molecules that is not primarily of a chemical nature. Otherwise the existence of liquids, and particularly rigid solids not chemically bonded, would be difficult to imagine. This type of bond is known as secondary bonding or *van der Waals forces*. This weaker bond may be said to be more physical than chemical in nature.

Van der Waals forces can be accounted for on the basis of a *dipole* attraction. For example, in a symmetric molecule, such as occurs in the inert gases, the electron field is pictured as constantly fluctuating. Normally, the atom appears as in Figure 2–1A; the electrons are distributed equally around the nucleus and produce an electrostatic field around the atom. However, the field may fluctuate so that it becomes momentarily plus and minus as shown in Figure 2–1B. A *fluctuating dipole* is thus created which will attract other similar dipoles. Such interatomic forces are quite weak, but nevertheless they exist.

The more important *permanent dipole* exists within asymmetric molecules. The *hydrogen bond* is a most important example of this type. The primary bond within the molecule is, of course, of the covalent type. For example, a diagrammatic representation of the electronic structure of a water molecule is shown in Figure 2–2A. Note that the two hydrogen atoms have

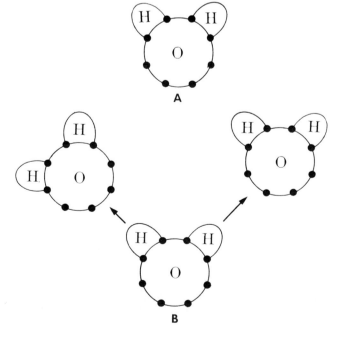

Figure 2–2 *A,* Diagrammatic structure of a water molecule. The oxygen atom and two hydrogen atoms have shared electrons. *B,* van der Waals forces result since the "exposed" hydrogen nucleus is attracted to the negative oxygen atom whose nucleus is "protected" by the unshared electrons. (Adapted from Van Vlack, Elements of Materials Science, 4th ed., Reading, Addison-Wesley Publishing Co., 1980.)

shared their valence electrons with the oxygen atom. However, the electron density around the oxygen nucleus is greater than that around the hydrogen nucleus. As a result, the hydrogen portions of the molecule are positive in relation to the oxygen. Thus, an electric dipole is formed.

When the single water molecule intermingles with other water molecules as in Figure 2–2B, the hydrogen portion (positive) of one molecule is attracted to the oxygen portion (negative) of its neighboring molecule and the intermolecular van der Waals forces are established. Such a structure is known as a *hydrogen bridge*. Polarity of this nature is important in accounting for the intermolecular reactions in many organic compounds, particularly the sorption of water by dental synthetic resins (see Chapter 13).

Interatomic Distance   Regardless of the type of structure in the solid state, there is a limiting factor that prevents the atoms or molecules from approaching each other too closely. For example, the distance between the center of an atom and that of its neighbor is limited to the diameter of the atoms involved. Although the atom, for convenience, is treated as a discrete particle with boundaries and volume, its boundaries are rather vaguely established by the electrostatic fields of the electrons. If the atoms approach too closely, they are repelled from each other by their electron charges. On the other hand, the forces of attraction tend to draw the atoms together. The position at which these forces of repulsion and attraction become equal in magnitude (but opposite in direction) is the normal or equilibrium position of the atoms as pictured in Figure 2–3.

In this position, the repelling forces are equal in magnitude to the attracting forces, and, if the two atoms are the same size, the distance between their centers is 2r, where r is the radius of the atom. Atom B can be displaced to the position B′ by some disturbing force (e.g., mechanical, thermal, or electrical). A disturbing force may also cause the atoms to move more closely together as shown at B″ (Fig. 2–3), but the disturbing force must be greater than in the case of B′ since the magnitude of the repelling force of the electrons is greater than that of the similar force of attraction for equal displacement. The distance that the atoms can be moved under compression, therefore, is much less.

This relationship can be shown graphically as in Figure 2–4. In this figure, the repulsion and attraction forces are plotted as a function of the interatomic spacing. As previously reasoned, the forces of attraction increase as the interatomic space decreases. On the other hand, the forces of repulsion remain relatively inactive until the atoms are quite close together. The sum or resultant of the two forces is indicated by the broken line (Fig. 2–4). As can be noted, the resultant becomes zero (i.e, the magnitudes of the two forces are equal) at the intersection of the broken line with the horizontal axis, labeled as the distance 0–a′. This is the interatomic distance at equilibrium as previous-

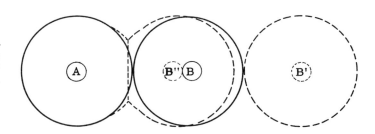

Figure 2–3 Diagrammatic representation of two atoms, A and B, in equilibrium position (solid line). B′ (dotted line) displaced away from A. B″ (dotted line) displaced toward A.

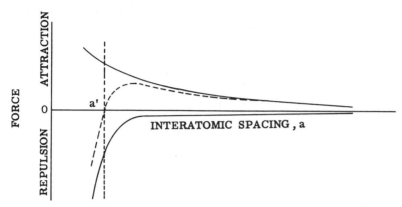

Figure 2–4 Relation of interatomic forces to interatomic spacing. (Adapted from Van Vlack, Elements of Materials Science, 4th ed., Reading, Addison-Wesley Publishing Co., 1980.)

ly discussed, and it represents the distance between the centers of the atoms involved. This force, then, is the *bonding force* between the two atoms.

Bonding Energy Since conditions of equilibrium are more nearly related to the energy factor than to interatomic forces, the relationships in Figure 2–4 are more logically portrayed in terms of interatomic energy. According to the laws of physics, energy can be measured by force times distance. If the resultant forces (F), represented by the broken line in Figure 2–4, are multiplied by their respective interatomic distances (a), the graph shown in Figure 2–5 will result.

As in Figure 2–4, the horizontal axis is the interatomic spacing, but interatomic or bonding energy is plotted on the vertical axis. As before, 0–a′ is the normal interatomic distance. In comparison with the resultant forces plotted in Figure 2–4, the energy does not change a great deal initially. Although the interatomic force of attraction is increasing (Fig. 2–4), the interatomic distance is decreasing, so that the force times the interatomic distant (F × a) remains relatively constant initially. As the resultant force approaches the horizontal axis (Fig. 2–4), the energy decreases (Fig. 2–5). It

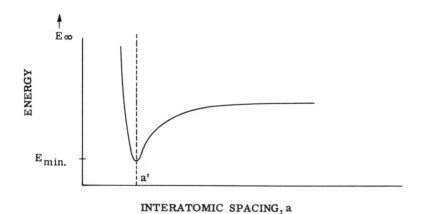

INTERATOMIC SPACING, a

Figure 2–5 Relation of interatomic potential energy to interatomic spacing. In this figure, E = ∞. If E ∞ is used in the conventional context as the energy at infinite separation of the atoms, it would lie at point 0, as in Figure 2–4.

finally reaches a minimum when the resultant force becomes zero. Thereafter, the energy increases rapidly (Fig. 2–5), since the resultant repulsive force (Fig. 2–4) increases rapidly with little change in interatomic distance. The minimal energy corresponds, of course, to the condition of equilibrium at the normal interatomic distance.

Thermal Energy   It will be recalled from previous courses in physics and chemistry that thermal energy is accounted for by the kinetic energy of the atoms or molecules at a given temperature. The atoms in a crystal, for example, at temperatures above absolute zero are in a constant state of vibration, the average amplitude of which will be dependent upon the temperature; the higher the temperature, the greater will be the amplitude and, consequently, the greater will be the kinetic or internal energy. Further consideration of Figure 2–4 and particularly Figure 2–5 can provide some interesting interpretations of these phenomena.

To recapitulate, for a given environment, the minimal energy (E_{min}) is the energy at equilibrium and is denoted by the bottom of the trough in the curve in Figure 2–5. As the temperature increases, the amplitude of the atomic (or molecular) vibration increases. It follows also that the interatomic spacing increases (Fig. 2–5), as well as the internal energy. The gross effect is, of course, an expansion known as *thermal expansion*.

If the temperature continues to increase, the interatomic spacing will increase and, eventually, a change of state will occur. The solid will change to a liquid, and the liquid will finally boil and change to a gas. It follows from Figure 2–5 that the deeper the trough in the curve, the greater will be the amount of energy required to produce melting and boiling and consequently, the higher will be the melting and boiling temperatures.

By the same reasoning, it can be argued that the deeper the energy trough, the less will be the thermal expansion per degree increase in temperature, since the interatomic spacing does not necessarily increase as the depth of the trough increases. In other words, in materials with similar atomic or molecular structures, the linear coefficient of thermal expansion (α) will tend to be inversely proportional to the melting temperatures.

Another interesting relationship that can be obtained from Figures 2–4 and 2–5 is the possible relationship between the strength and the melting temperature. The strength, or stress required to separate the atoms, can be interpreted as the maximal interatomic force, indicated by the broken line in Figure 2–4. Since the curve in Figure 2–5 represents the energy of the forces indicated by the broken line in Figure 2–4, greater fracturing forces or strengths indicate a deeper trough in the energy curve (Fig. 2–5) and, consequently, a high melting temperature, as previously shown. In other words, a high melting temperature of a material may also indicate a high degree of strength.

Thermal conductivity is concerned with interatomic spacing only to the extent that the heat is conducted from one atom or molecule to the next as adjacent basic structural units are affected by the kinetic energy of its neighbors. However, the number of "free" electrons in the material will influence its thermal conductivity. As will be shown later (Chapter 15), the metallic structure contains many "free" electrons, and most metals are good conductors of heat as well as electricity. On the other hand, nonmetallic materials do not include many "free" electrons and, consequently, they are generally poor thermal and electrical conductors in comparison.

The aforementioned principles are generalities, and exceptions do occur. Nevertheless, they are sufficiently accurate to allow one to judge the thermal properties of most of the dental materials to be discussed. The thermal properties of a dental material, particularly thermal expansion and conductivity, find many applications in dentistry, as will be described in subsequent pages.

Crystal Structure   So far we have generally assumed only two atoms or molecules. Obviously, dental materials are made up of many millions of such units. How are the units arranged in a solid, for example? How are they bound together? As early as 1665 Robert Hooke simulated the characteristic shapes of crystals by stacking musket balls in piles. It was 250 years later before anyone knew that he had exactly modeled the crystal structure of many familiar metals, with each ball representing an atom.

The atoms are, of course, bonded by either primary or secondary forces. In the solid state, they combine in the manner that will assure a minimal internal energy. For example, sodium and chlorine share one electron as previously described. In the solid state, however, they do not simply pair together, but rather all of the positively charged sodium ions attract all of the negative chlorine ions, with the result that they form a regularly spaced configuration known as a *space lattice* or *crystal*. A space lattice can be defined as any arrangement of atoms in space such that every atom is situated similarly to every other atom. Space lattices may be the result of primary, secondary, or metallic bonds.

There are 14 possible lattice types or forms, but most of the metals used in dentistry belong to the cubic system; i.e., the atoms crystallize in cubic forms. The simplest cubic space lattice is shown in Figure 2–6. The solid circles represent the positions of the atoms. Their positions are located at the points of intersection of three sets of parallel planes, each set being perpendicular to the other planes. These planes are often referred to as *crystal planes*.

In Figure 2–7A is pictured one *unit cell* of the simple cubic space lattice. The cells are repeated again and again as indicated in Figure 2–6. The simple cubic arrangements in Figures 2–6 and 2–7A are hypothetical only. Actually, the arrangements shown in Figures 2–7B and C are the cubic space lattices of practical importance. Also, Figures 2–6 and 2–7 are diagrammatic only. The atoms are actually closely packed so that the interatomic spacing is equal to

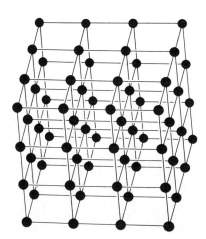

Figure 2–6 Simple cubic space lattice. (From Van Vlack: Elements of Materials Science, 4th ed. Reading, Addison-Wesley Publishing Co., 1980.)

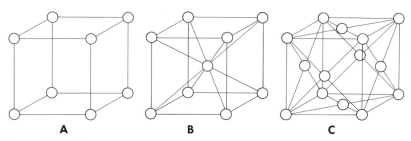

Figure 2-7 Single cells of cubic space lattices: *A*, simple cubic; *B*, body-centered cubic; *C*, face-centered cubic.

the sum of their radii. A model of a face-centered cubic structure is shown in Figure 2–8, and a similar model for a body-centered cubic lattice is pictured in Figure 2–9.

The type of space lattice is defined by the length of three of the unit cell edges (called the *axes*) and the angles between the edges. For example, the cubic space lattice is characterized by having axes which are all of equal length and meet at an angle of 90° (Fig. 2–7). Other lattice types of interest are diagrammed in Figure 2–10.

Noncrystalline Structure   There are, of course, other structures than crystalline form which can occur in the solid state. For example, some of the waxes used by the dentist may solidify as *amorphous* materials, meaning that the molecules are distributed at random. Even in this case, there is a tendency for the arrangement to be regular. It is a law of nature that any substance should approach the equilibrium condition so that the internal energy is minimal. Such a condition implies that the molecules should approach as closely together as possible in a regular pattern in the solid or liquid. Regularity of unit arrangement is most conducive to minimal energy in any given environmental condition.

For example, glass is considered to be a noncrystalline solid, yet its atoms tend to form a *short range order* lattice instead of the *long range order* lattice characteristic of crystalline solids. In other words, the ordered arrangement of the glass is more or less localized with a considerable number of disordered units between. Since such an arrangement may be considered typical of the liquid structures, such solids are sometimes called *supercooled liquids*.

Figure 2–8 Model of a face-centered cubic structure. (From Rogers, The Nature of Metals, Cleveland, American Society of Metals.)

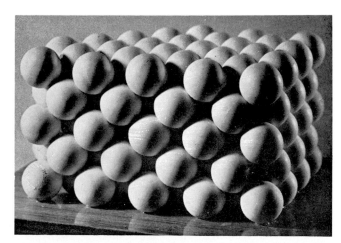

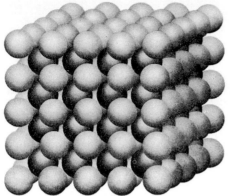

Figure 2–9 Model of a body-centered cubic structure. (Adapted from Moffat, Pearsall, and Wulff, The Structure and Properties of Materials, Vol. 1, New York, John Wiley and Sons, Inc., 1964.)

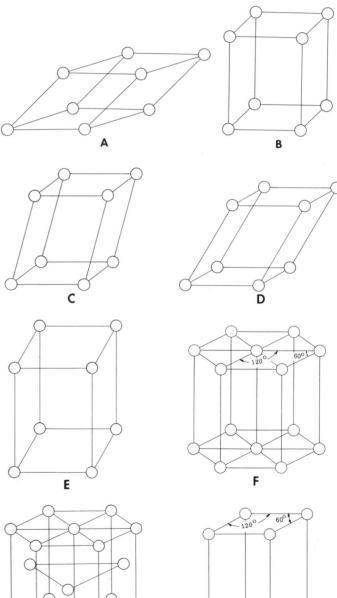

Figure 2–10 Other simple lattice types of dental interest: *A,* rhombohedral; *B,* orthorhombic; *C,* monoclinic; *D,* triclinic; *E,* tetragonal; *F,* simple hexagonal; *G,* close-packed hexagonal; *H,* rhombic.

The structural arrangements of the noncrystalline solids do not represent as low internal energies as do crystalline arrangements of even the same atoms and molecules. They do not have a definite melting temperature, but rather they gradually soften as the temperature is raised and gradually harden as they cool. The temperature at which they first form a rigid mass upon cooling, or lose hardness or brittleness upon heating, is called the *glass transition temperature* (T_g), since this effect is characteristic of glass upon heating or cooling. Occasionally, the term is shortened to *transition temperature*. The dental synthetic resins are also examples of materials that may exhibit a noncrystalline structure (Chapter 11).

Stress and Strain   It should be noted that the energy becomes greater as the interatomic spacing becomes less than a' (Fig. 2–5). It also increases initially as the interatomic spacing increases beyond a', but it later approaches zero. Although only two atoms are assumed for discussion in Figures 2–4 and 2–5, it is not difficult to assume that much the same mechanism of attraction and repulsion exists in a polyatomic arrangement, as in the space lattice shown in Figure 2–6, for example.

The normal position of the atoms (0–a') can be increased or decreased by the application of a mechanical force. For example, the interatomic distance can be increased if the atoms are displaced by a force pulling them apart. When this happens, both the resultant force (Fig. 2–4) and the energy (Fig. 2–5) initially increase. At this stage, if the acting force is released, the energy will again become minimal and the atoms will return to their equilibrium spacing (0–a').

If this conception is applied to the space lattice configuration, it is evident that many millions of atoms are thus affected. If the displacing force is measured across a given area, it is known as a *stress* and the change in dimension is called a *strain*. Theoretically, a stress and strain exist whenever the interatomic distance is changed from the equilibrium position.

If the stress exceeds the resultant force (per unit area), the energy (Fig. 2–5) or force of attraction (Fig. 2–4)* is reduced to the point at which the atoms may separate entirely and fracture or breakage will occur.

Stress can also occur under compression, but the amount of strain that can be introduced even under considerable stress is limited owing to the high repulsion of the negative electrostatic field as previously discussed. This fact is indicated by the sudden increase in energy when the interatomic distance is less than a' (Fig. 2–5).

The same reasoning can be applied to explain stress and strain in the noncrystalline structure. Further interpretations and applications concerning stress and strain will be made in succeeding chapters.

Diffusion   The diffusion of molecules in gases and liquids is well known. It is possible, however, for molecules or atoms to diffuse in the solid state as well. As previously described, the atoms in a space lattice are constantly in vibration about a center. The average kinetic energy of vibration over the entire crystal is related to the temperature. At absolute zero the vibration ceases, the energy becomes zero, and the atom occupies its center of vibration.

---

*According to Figure 2–4, as the interatomic distance (a) increases, the force (F) becomes less and eventually becomes zero when the distance (a) becomes infinitely large.

At normal temperatures, the amount of kinetic energy of the atoms may be localized and varies from atom to atom. Presumably, all of the atoms possess certain amounts of energy, but some may have more energy (i.e., greater amplitude of vibration) than others. It is possible that the atoms with greater energy may be able to displace those with lower energy levels and thereby change their location in the space lattice. The energy required for such movement or *diffusion* is known as *activation energy*.

Atoms may change position in solids even under equilibrium conditions; this is known as *self-diffusion*. However, such diffusion is generally not of practical importance since no visible or measurable dimensional changes occur.

As with any diffusion, the atoms or molecules diffuse in the solid state in an attempt to produce equilibrium. For example, a concentration of sugar molecules in solution tends to diffuse to provide equal concentration. As will be discussed later (Chapter 16), a concentration of atoms in a metal may do the same thing.

The diffusion may be in the other direction also, to produce a concentration of atoms in a solution. For example, if the sugar in the water becomes supersaturated, the molecules of sugar diffuse toward each other and the sugar crystallizes out of solution. In the same manner, too many copper atoms in a solid alloy of copper and silver may cause a supersaturation and a diffusion of the copper atoms to increase the concentration of copper, which will then precipitate.

Diffusion rates for a given substance depend mainly on the temperature. The higher the temperature, the greater will be the rate of diffusion. The diffusion rate will, however, vary with the atom size (e.g., the smaller the atom, the lower the activation energy), interatomic or intermolecular bonding, lattice imperfections, and similar phenomena. In other words, various media exhibit different diffusion rates characteristic of the particular medium. The diffusion constant, uniquely characteristic of the given element, compound, crystal, etc., is known as the *coefficient of diffusion,* usually designated as D. It can be defined as the amount of diffusion that takes place across a given unit area (e.g., 1 cm^2) through 1 unit thickness (e.g., 1 cm) of the substance in 1 unit time (e.g., 1 second). It is a physical constant and analogous to the linear coefficient of thermal expansion (α), coefficient of thermal conductivity (K), modulus of elasticity (E), etc.

The diffusion coefficients of most crystalline solids at room temperature are very low. Diffusion in metals used in dentistry is so slow at room temperature that it cannot be detected in a practical sense. Yet, at a few hundred degrees higher temperature, the properties of the metal may be changed radically by atomic diffusion. Diffusion in a noncrystalline material may occur at a more rapid rate and often may be evident with time at room or body temperature. The reason is, of course, related to the higher internal energy of the noncrystalline material. The disordered structure enables the molecules to diffuse with less activation energy.

ADHESION, BONDING

The phenomenon of adhesion is involved in many situations in dentistry. It is a principal concern in solving the problem of leakage around dental restorative materials, for example. The retention of artificial dentures is probably dependent, to some extent at least, upon adhesion both between the denture and saliva and between the saliva and soft tissue. Certainly the attachment of plaque or calculus to tooth structure is partially an adhesive mechanism. Therefore, an understanding of the fundamentals associated with the phenomenon is important to the dentist.

Adhesion is the force that causes two substances to attach when they are brought into intimate contact with each other. The molecules of one substance *adhere* or are attracted to molecules of another. This force is called *adhesion* when unlike molecules are attracted and *cohesion* when molecules of the same kind are attracted. The material or film added to produce the adhesion is known as the *adhesive,* and the material to which it is applied is called the *adherend.*

Thus, although in the broadest sense adhesion is simply a surface attachment, it is usually qualified by specifying that the phenomenon does involve some type of intermolecular attraction between the adhesive and the adherend.[1]

Mechanical Bonding   Of course, strong attachment of two substances can also be accomplished simply by *mechanical bonding* or *retention* rather than molecular attraction. Such structural retention may be somewhat gross, as by screws, bolts or undercuts. It may also involve more subtle mechanisms, as by penetration of the adhesive into microscopic or submicroscopic irregularities, e.g., crevices and pores, in the surface of the substrate. A fluid or semi-viscous liquid adhesive is best suited for such a procedure, since it readily penetrates into these surface discrepancies. Upon hardening, the multitude of adhesive projections embedded in the adherend surface provide the footholds for mechanical attachment or retention.

This mechanism has been commonly used in dentistry, in lieu of truly adhesive cements or restorative materials. As will be seen in Chapter 29, retention of cast restorations, e.g., a gold crown, is enhanced by mechanical attachment of the cementing agent into irregularities that exist on the internal surface of the casting and those that are present in the adjoining tooth structure.

Another more recent example of improving the performance of the restoration through mechanical bonding is with the resin (plastic) restorative materials. Since these resins do not have the capability of truly adhering to tooth structure, leakage around the restoration poses a major problem. As will be discussed in the next chapter, such leakage patterns contribute to marginal stain, secondary caries, and irritation to the pulp.

In order to minimize the danger of penetration by deleterious agents around the restoration, the traditional technique for placement of such materials has now been changed. Before insertion of the resin, the enamel of the adjoining tooth structure is treated with phosphoric acid for a short period of time. This is referred to as the "acid etching" technique and will be described in detail in Chapter 14. It is sufficient to note at this time that the acid produces minute pores in the enamel surface into which the resin flows when it is carried into the preparation. Upon hardening, these resin projections provide improved mechanical retention of the restoration, thereby reducing the possibility of marginal leakage.

Thus the acid etch technique is an example of how improved bonding between a dental material and tooth structure can be attained through mechanical mechanisms, not molecular adhesion. Let us now return to adhesion and the factors associated with this phenomenon.

Surface Energy   If adhesion exists, the surfaces tend to be attracted to one another at their *interface*. Such a condition may exist regardless of the phases (solid, liquid, or gas) of the two surfaces, with the exception that adhesion between two gases is not to be expected because of the lack of an interface.

The energy at the surface of a solid is greater than in its interior. For example, consider the space lattice shown in Figure 2–6. Inside the lattice, all of the atoms are equally attracted to each other. The interatomic distances are equal and the energy is minimal. At the surface of the lattice, the energy is greater because the outermost atoms are not equally attracted in all directions, as diagrammed in Figure 2–11. Atom A has a balanced array of nearest neighbors surrounding it, whereas atoms B and C each have an imbalanced number of adjacent atoms. The unsaturated bonds generate surface energies. There would be a mutual attraction between the atoms immediately under the surface layer and the surface atoms. There would also be a somewhat stronger attraction between the surface atoms themselves, thus creating the familiar phenomenon of *surface tension*. Any attraction of the atoms toward the interface would be for unlike molecules or atoms across the interface; in other words, adhesion. For example, molecules in the air may be attracted to the surface and be *adsorbed* by the material. Silver, platinum, and gold adsorb oxygen readily. With gold, the adhesive forces are of the secondary type but in

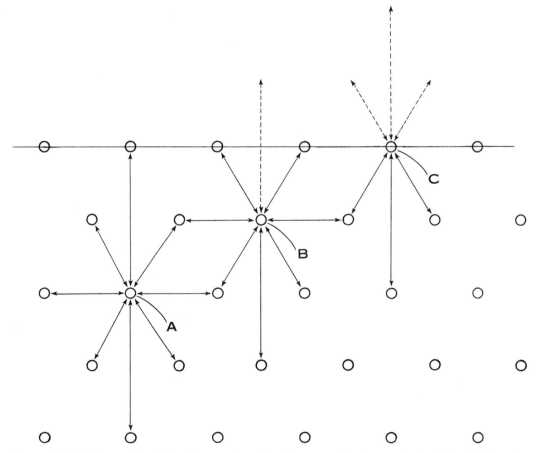

Figure 2–11 Diagram illustrating the creation of surface energies by unsaturated chemical bonds, atoms *B* and *C*. (Modified from Manko, H. H., Solders and Soldering, McGraw-Hill, 1964.)

the case of silver, the attraction may be by chemical or primary bonding, and silver oxide may form.

When primary bonding is involved, the adhesion is termed *chemisorption,* as compared with physical bonding by van der Waals forces. In chemisorption a chemical bond is actually formed between the adhesive and the adherend. As previously noted, an example of this type of adhesion is an oxide film formed on the surface of a metal. Van der Waals forces are weaker than primary bonding since they are intermolecular rather than intramolecular.

Van der Waals forces invariably precede chemisorption. Then, as the distance between the adhesive and the adherend diminishes, primary bonding may become effective. However, chemisorption is limited to the monolayer of the adhesive present on the adherend.

The surface energy and, therefore, adhesive qualities of a given solid can be reduced by any surface impurity, such as gas adsorption or oxidation as previously described. The functional chemical groups available or even the type of crystal plane of a space lattice present at the surface may affect the surface energy. In summary, the greater the surface energy, the greater will be the capacity for adhesion.

Wetting   It is very difficult to force two solid surfaces to adhere. Regardless of how smooth their surfaces may appear, they are likely to be rough when considered in atomic or molecular dimensions. Consequently, when they are placed in apposition, only the "hills" or high spots are in contact. Since these areas usually constitute only a small percentage of the total surface, no perceptible adhesion takes place. The attraction is generally negligible when the surface molecules of the attracting substances are separated by distances greater than 0.0007 micrometer (μm)*.[2]

One method of overcoming this difficulty is to use fluids that will flow into these irregularities and thus provide contact over a great part of the surface of the solid. For example, when two polished glass plates are placed one on top of the other and pressed together, they exhibit little tendency to adhere for reasons previously described. However, if a film of water is introduced between them, considerable difficulty is encountered in separating the two plates. The surface energy of the glass is sufficiently great to attract the molecules of water.

To produce adhesion in this manner, the liquid must flow easily over the entire surface and adhere to the solid. This characteristic is referred to as *wetting.* If the liquid adhesive does not wet the surface of the adherend because of its low surface energy, then the adhesion between the liquid and the adherend will be negligible or nonexistent. If there is a true wetting of the surface, adhesion failures cannot occur.[3] Failure in such cases actually occurs in the solid or in the adhesive itself, not in the area where the solid and adhesive are in contact.

The ability of an adhesive to wet the surface of the adherend is influenced by a number of factors. As previously noted, the cleanliness of the surface is of particular importance. A film of water only one molecule thick on the surface of the solid may lower the surface energy of the adherend and prevent any wetting by the adhesive. Likewise, an oxide film on a metallic surface will inhibit the contact of an adhesive.

---

*Micron.

The surface energy of some substances is so low that few, if any, liquids will wet their surfaces. For example, some organic substances are of this type. Close packing of the structural organic groups and the presence of halogens may prevent wetting. A certain synthetic resin commercially known as Teflon [poly(tetrafluoroethylene)] is often used in situations in which it is desirable to prevent the adhesion of films to a surface. Metals, on the other hand, interact vigorously with liquid adhesives because of their high surface energy.

In general, the comparatively low surface energies of organic and most inorganic liquids permit them to spread freely on solids of high surface energy. Thus, formation of a strong adhesive joint requires good wetting. In addition, the liquid adhesive must solidify and must have sufficient deformability to reduce the buildup of elastic stresses in the formation of the joint.[4]

Contact Angle   The extent to which the adhesive will wet the surface of the adherend is generally determined by measuring the *contact angle* between the adhesive and the adherend. The contact angle is the angle formed by the adhesive with the adherend at their interface. If the molecules of the adhesive are attracted to the molecules of the adherend as much as or more than they are to themselves, the liquid adhesive will spread completely over the surface of the solid and no angle will be formed (Fig. 2–12A). Stated differently, the forces of adhesion are stronger than the cohesive forces holding the molecules of the adhesive together.

However, if, for example, the energy of the surface of the adherend is

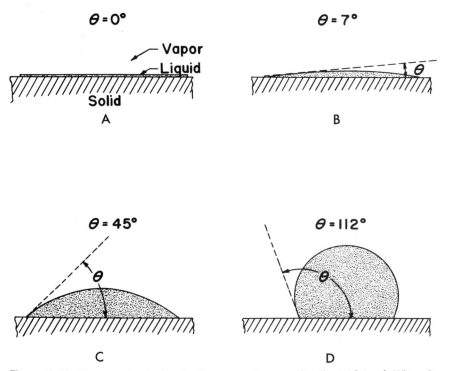

Figure 2–12   To a great extent, adhesion depends on wetting the surface. *A,* When the contact angle is 0°, the liquid contacts the surface completely and spreads freely. *B,* Small contact angle on slightly contaminated surface. *C,* Larger angle on surface contaminated with an absorbed film. *D,* Large angle formed by poor wetting of a solid which has a low surface energy.

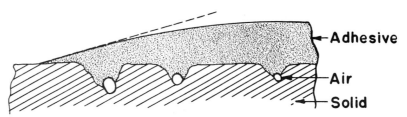

Figure 2–13 Air pockets created in a surface irregularity, even when the contact angle of the adhesive is low. Such areas contribute to propagation of adhesive failure by concentration of stress at these points.

reduced by contamination or other means, a small angle will be formed (Fig. 2–12*B*). If a monolayer film of a contaminator were present over the entire surface, a medium angle might be obtained (Fig. 2–12*C*), whereas a very high angle would result on a solid of low surface energy, such as Teflon (Fig. 2–12*D*. Either the *advancing* (θ_A) or *receding* (θ_R) angle may be measured, or both. The advancing angle is that observed when a liquid boundary advances over a clean, dry, solid surface, as just described. The receding angle is that observed when the liquid boundary recedes from a previously wetted surface. Since the tendency for the liquid to spread increases as the contact angle decreases, the contact angle is a useful measure of spreadability or wettability.

It follows, then, that the smaller the contact angle, the better able is the adhesive to fill in irregularities in the surface of the adherend. Also, the viscosity and surface tension of the adhesive influence the extent to which these voids or irregularities are filled.

Of course, solid "flat" surfaces are not actually planar. They invariably contain innumerable small hills, valleys, and crevices. Surface imperfections are always a potential hazard in attaining and maintaining an adhesive bond.[5] Air pockets may be created during the spreading of the adhesive which will prevent complete wetting of the entire surface, even if the liquid adhesive has a low contact angle (Fig. 2–13). Furthermore, such areas of discontinuity between the adhesive and solid may contribute to rupture of the adhesive joint. The adhesive joint invariably is subjected to thermal changes and mechanical stresses. Such conditions produce *stress concentrations* around these voids. The stress concentration that arises can be much higher than the mean applied stress. The stress may then become so great that it will initiate a break in the adhesive bond adjacent to the void. The crack so formed may propagate from one pocket to the next, and the joint may break as if it had a built-in "zipper."

Adhesion to Tooth Structure   Certain of the fundamentals involved in the adhesive mechanism can be readily related to dental situations. For example, contact angle measurements have been used to study the wettability of enamel and dentin.[6] It was found that the wettability of those surfaces was markedly reduced following the topical application of an aqueous fluoride solution. Carrying that information into the clinical situation, it was found that the fluoride-treated enamel surface retained less plaque over a given period of time, presumably because of lowered surface energy. Thus, it is not inconceivable that fluorides may be effective in reducing dental caries by providing a tooth surface that stays cleaner longer, in addition to the recognized mechanisms of reducing the enamel acid solubility.

In the same vein, because of the higher surface energy of many restorative materials as compared with the tooth itself, there is a greater tendency for the surface and margins of the restoration to accumulate débris. This may in part account for the relatively high incidence of marginal caries seen around dental restorations.[6]

In the following chapters, the leakage that occurs between tooth structure and dental restorations will be discussed. It will be emphasized that, in certain instances, continuing sensitivity after placement of the restoration, recurrent caries, and deterioration at the margins of the restoration can be associated with a lack of adhesion between the restoration and the tooth. A great deal of research is now in progress to develop adhesives that will adhere to tooth structure. A truly adhesive dental restorative material or cement could have a marked effect on the current practice of dentistry.

However, if one applies to dental structures the various principles that influence adhesion, it is obvious that the problems are indeed complex.[7-11] The tooth composition is inhomogeneous. Both organic and inorganic components are present and in different amounts in dentin than in enamel. A restoration that would adhere to the organic portion would not be likely to adhere to the inorganic components, and an adhesive that would bond to enamel would probably not adhere to dentin to the same extent.

After the dentist has prepared the cavity, tenacious microscopic debris covers the enamel and dentin surfaces. This surface contamination prevents wetting. In addition, the instruments used to cut the cavity leave a rough surface. These irregularities act as stress concentrators when the restoration is subjected to masticating forces and to the thermal fluctuations which are always occurring in the oral cavity.

Possibly of greatest significance is the problem of water. The inorganic phase has a strong affinity for water. In order to remove it completely, the enamel and dentin would have to be heated to a temperature unrealistic for the oral cavity. This means that a tooth cannot be safely dried at mouth temperature with the devices and agents at the disposal of the dentist. The presence of at least a monolayer of water on the surface of the prepared cavity must be accepted. That water layer reduces the surface energy and thus deters the wetting of the adhesive restorative material.

In addition, there is fluid exchange through certain components of the tooth, and the dental restoration itself is, of course, in contact with the water in the saliva. The dental adhesive must displace this water, react with it, or wet the surface better than the water that is already present in the tooth structure. Furthermore, it must maintain such adhesion in a continuously aqueous environment.

Although the obstacles are formidable, the progress of research in the field is promising. Certainly the goals are worthy of the challenges presented. A truly adhesive filling material could replace many of those now used in restorative dentistry. Likewise, the technique for placement of the material would be simplified, since the mechanical retention of the material in the cavity preparation, as now required would be unnecessary. An adhesive cement would make it possible to attach orthodontic appliances directly to the teeth without the need for placing bands on each tooth, as is already being done in selected cases by "direct bonding" of brackets.

More intriguing is the possibility of developing an adhesive film-forming material that could be topically applied to the intact enamel surface. If of low energy and durable, such a film could serve as a barrier to the formation of plaque, caries, and even the deposition of calculus. Commercial sealants have already been marketed for sealing the pits and fissures on the occlusal surface of the tooth of the child patient. These materials are discussed in Chapter 14.

Consideration will be given to some of these problems in the following chapters, particularly regarding the selection and use of restorative resins in Chapter 14 and Chapter 29 on dental cements.

References

1. Beech DR: Adhesion and adhesives in the oral environment. Roy Austral Coll Dent Surg 5:128, 1977.
2. Zisman WA: Influence of constitution on adhesion. Ind & Eng Chem 55:19, 1963.
3. Patrick RL: The Proceedings on Adhesive Restorative Dental Materials. Phillips RW and Ryge G (eds) Spencer, Ind., Owen Litho Service, 1961, p. 137.
4. Baier RE, Shafrin EG, and Zisman WA: Adhesion mechanisms that assist or impede it. Science 162:1360, 1968.
5. Zisman WA: Improving the performance in reinforced plastics. Ind & Eng Chem 57:26, 1965.
6. Glantz P: On wettability and adhesiveness. Odont Rev 20:1 (Suppl. 17), 1969.
7. Buonocore MG: Principles of adhesive restorative materials. J Am Dent Assoc 67:382, 1963.
8. Brauer GM and Huget EF: Progress Report on Adhesive and Dental Materials No. 10519, US Dept. Commerce, Dec. 13, 1970.
9. Retief DH: The intra-oral factors affecting adhesions. J Dent Assoc S Afr 25:392, 1970.
10. National Institute of Dental Research: Adhesive Restorative Dental Materials — II. Public Health Service Publication No. 1494, US Government Printing Office, Washington, 1966.
11. von Fraunhofer JA: Adhesion and Adhesives. In Scientific Aspects of Dental Materials. London, Butterworths, 1975, pp. 49–95.

3 PHYSICAL PROPERTIES OF DENTAL MATERIALS. RHEOLOGY. COLOR. THERMAL PROPERTIES. BIOLOGICAL CONSIDERATIONS

In Chapter 2, the subject of stress and strain was treated as related to individual atoms or groups of atoms. In the simplest analysis, stress is the force per unit area acting on millions of atoms in a given plane of a material. From a practical standpoint, however, such a conception is complicated in that normally the dentist is not interested directly in the relationship of the atoms, but rather in the reaction to stress over the entire structure.

For example, a dentist forms a crown on a tooth from a certain gold alloy. When the patient chews with the crown in place, although the dentist knows that the atoms in the crown will be displaced when the crown reacts to the forces of mastication, he is directly interested in the total reaction of the crown while it is in use. How much is it going to change shape when it is stressed? Can it withstand the forces of mastication without twisting out of shape or fracturing during use? These questions can be answered indirectly by subjecting the gold alloy to certain tests before it is formed into the shape of the crown. Although the atomic or molecular forces are basically important, there are other reactions that are also important.

The gross reactions to stress as tested according to the procedures to be outlined are practical manifestations of interatomic or intermolecular forces. This relationship between the practical and the theoretical should never be forgotten.

Stress and Strain In a practical sense, then, a stress is the force per unit area in a body which resists an external force. It should be noted that the two forces are equal in magnitude but differ in direction and, therefore, are not equal since they are vector quantities. In order to distinguish between them, the external force will be designated hereafter as the *load*.

As discussed in the previous chapter, whenever a stress is present, there is also deformation or strain. (An exception to this is induced thermal stress under conditions in which the strain may be prevented by restraint of the structure.) As an illustration, assume that a stretching force, or load, of 200 newtons is applied to a wire .000002 square meter in cross-sectional area. The stress, by definition, will be the force per unit area, or

$$s\ (\sigma) = \text{Stress} = \frac{200}{.000002} =$$

100 meganewtons per square meter (megapascals − MPa)*

In the English system of measurement, the stress is usually expressed in pounds per square inch.†

If the wire were 10 centimeters long, and if it stretched 0.1 centimeter under the load, the strain, by definition, would be the change in length per unit length, or

$$e\ (\epsilon) = \text{Strain} = \frac{0.1}{10} = 0.01 \text{ centimeter per centimeter.}$$

The accepted equivalent in the English system is inch per inch, foot per foot, etc.

Strain may be either *elastic* or *plastic* or a combination of the two. Elastic strain is reversible; it disappears after the stress is removed. Plastic strain is a permanent displacement of the atoms inside the material.

Types of Stresses and Strains   As previously described, a stress must be defined according to its direction and magnitude. By means of their directions, stresses can be classified under three types.

TENSILE STRESS   A *tensile stress* is any induced force that resists a deformation caused by a load that tends to stretch or elongate a body. A tensile stress is always accompanied by a *tensile strain*.

COMPRESSIVE STRESS   If a body is placed under a load that tends to compress or shorten it, the internal forces that resist such a load are called *compressive stresses*. A compressive stress is always accompanied by a *compressive strain*.

SHEAR   A stress that tends to resist a twisting motion, or a sliding of one portion of a body over another, is a *shear* or *shearing stress*. For example, if this book is closed and placed horizontally upon a table, then if it is deformed by pressing the hand on the upper cover, at the same time exerting a force parallel in direction to the cover, the pages will slip over one another and the shape of the book viewed from an end will be that of a parallelogram with two acute angles. A shear or shearing stress is thus induced in the book and is accompanied by a *shearing strain*. This stress would be present if atom B in Figure 2–3 moved vertically in reference to atom A, or tended to rotate about atom A.

Complex Stresses   It is extremely difficult to induce a pure stress of a single type in a body. For example, when a wire is stretched, the very conception of stretching connotes an internal sliding of atoms over one another. The experimentally observed stress will be predominantly tensile, but the shearing stresses and strains will also be present. Furthermore, during the deformation,

---

*1 pascal (Pa) = 1 newton/m² = 0.145 × 10⁻³ psi; 1000 psi = 6.894 MPa. In the remainder of the text, SI (Pa) units will be preferred. However, certain English and non-SI metric units are included parenthetically, as was noted in the Preface.
†Usually abbreviated as lb/sq in, lb/in², or simply psi.

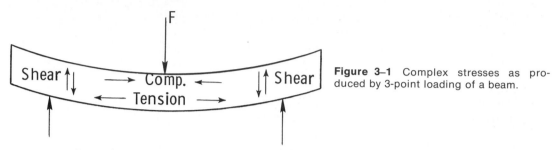

Figure 3-1 Complex stresses as produced by 3-point loading of a beam.

since the volume of the wire remains constant, it must decrease slightly in cross-sectional area, a condition which obviously indicates the presence of compressive stresses. When a tensile force is applied to an object it is observed that the increase in length (tensile strain) is accompanied by a decrease in the dimensions of the object at right angles to the tensile stress. In other words, the object becomes longer and thinner. Conversely, a compressive force acts to make an object shorter but thicker. If an axial tensile stress, σ_z, produces a tensile strain, ϵ_z, and accompanying contractions in the x and y directions, ϵ_x and ϵ_y respectively, the ratio of ϵ_x/ϵ_z or ϵ_y/ϵ_z is an engineering property of the material and is called Poisson's ratio (ν).

$$\nu = -\,\epsilon_x/\epsilon_z = -\,\epsilon_y/\epsilon_z$$

Poisson's ratio can be similarly determined in an experiment involving an axial compressive stress. Poisson's ratio is related to the nature and symmetry of the interatomic bonding forces described in Chapter 2. For an ideal, isotropic material of constant volume, the ratio is 0.5. Most engineering materials have values of approximately 0.3.

In order for a single atom or molecule to move downward and inward during deformation, a shearing stress and strain must also be present. If a cylinder of plaster of Paris, for example, is placed between the crushing heads of a testing machine so that the load is applied at its top and bottom, the load is resisted mainly by compressive stresses. However, since the sides of the cylinder are not loaded, they are free to exhibit an outward deformation. Since this deformation increases the diameter of the specimen, it is equivalent to a tensile strain and therefore tensile stresses must be present. In order for such a deformation to occur, the individual atoms or molecules must move downward and outward. Consequently, by definition, a shear stress is present. It should be noted that the compressive stress described here should be differentiated from that described in the previous chapter, a case in which the atoms were completely confined on all sides. In the latter case, compressive stress only would be present.

Another example of complex stress, as shown in Figure 3-1, is produced by bending a beam in three point loading. This situation is commonly encountered in the construction of a fixed bridge in prosthetic dentistry. As can be seen, compressive, tensile, and shear stresses are present in various parts of the structure.

Consequently, under practical conditions, although one type of stress may be predominant in a structure, the other two types are present as well.

Elastic Limit   If a small tensile stress is induced in a wire, the resulting strain may be such that the wire will return to its original length (i.e., the atoms will move into their regular positions) when the load is removed.

If the load is increased progressively in small increments, and then released after each addition of stress, a stress value finally will be found at which the wire does not return to its original length after it is unloaded. In such a case, the wire is said to have been stressed beyond its elastic limit. The *elastic limit* of a material is the greatest stress to which a material can be subjected, such that it will return to its original dimensions when the forces are released. Although tensile stress was used in the illustration, the same situation can exist with any type of stress.

Proportional Limit   If the wire discussed in the previous section is loaded in tension progressively in small increments until the wire ruptures, without a removal of the load each time, and if each stress is plotted on a vertical coordinate and the corresponding strain is plotted on the horizontal coordinate, a curve similar to that in Figure 3–2 is obtained. It can be noted that the curve starts as a straight line but gradually curves after a certain stress value is exceeded. If a ruler is laid on the straight-line portion of the curve (from O to P), and if the straight line is extended in a dotted line (b) as shown, the stress at the point P, at which the curve digresses from a straight line, is known as the *proportional limit*.

It is a fundamental law (Hooke's law) that the stress is directly proportional to the strain in elastic deformation. Since direct proportionality between two quantities is always graphically a straight line, the straight-line portion of the graph in Figure 3–2, which was plotted from actual data, is confirmation of this law. Since the proportional limit (stress P) is the greatest stress possible in accordance with this law, it may be defined as the greatest stress which may be produced in a material such that the stress is directly proportional to the

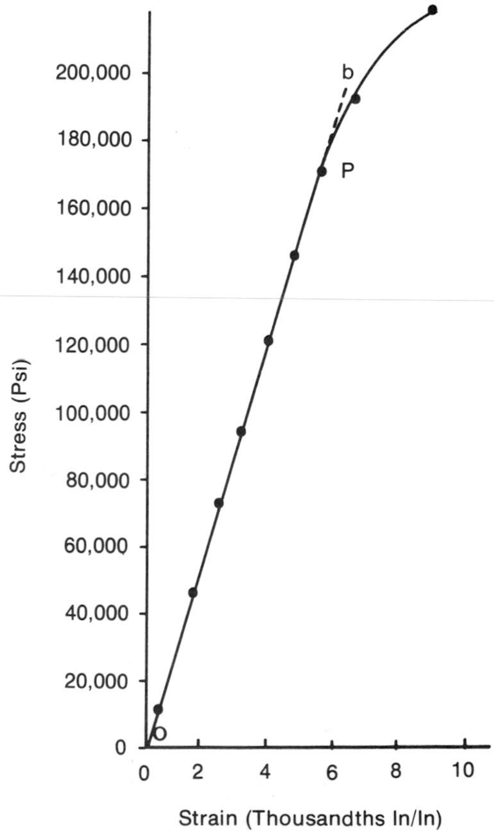

Figure 3–2 Stress-strain curve for a stainless steel orthodontic wire under tension. Proportional limit, 1150 MPa (167,000 psi); modulus of elasticity, 230,000 MPa (33,300,000 psi); modulus of resilience, 2.9 megajoules per cubic meter (420 inch-pounds per cubic inch); ultimate tensile strength, 1620 MPa (235,000 psi).

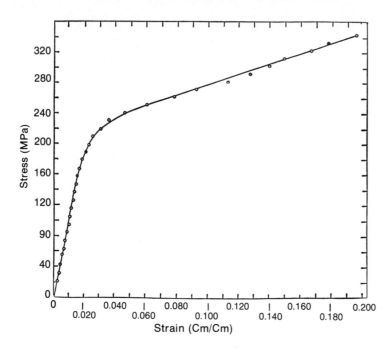

Figure 3–3 A stress-strain curve for tooth dentin under compression. (As an exercise, the student may determine the proportional limit and modulus of elasticity from the curve.)

strain. A stress-strain curve for tooth dentin under compression is shown in Figure 3–3.

Yield Strength   The conditions assumed for the definitions of elastic limit and proportional limit are not always realized under practical conditions. If the measuring instruments are sufficiently sensitive, deviations from Hooke's law, and slight permanent deformations, can be recorded at any stress when commercially processed metals and alloys are tested. Nonmetallic materials, especially, are likely to be lacking in this regard. Consequently, as an approximation, it could be assumed that the first marked deviation from a direct proportionality between stress and strain might be used as a measure of the limit of direct proportionality. For example, if the strain increases 10 per cent above previous strain increments after the addition of an equal stress increment, such a stress is indicative of the limiting stress for approximate direct proportionality between stress and strain. Such a stress is called the *yield strength* of the material. Thus, the yield strength represents a stress slightly higher than the proportional limit.

Although the three terms, elastic limit, proportional limit, and yield strength, are defined differently, their magnitudes are so nearly the same that for all practical purposes the terms can often be used interchangeably. These values are important in the evaluation of dental materials, since they represent the stress at which permanent deformation of the structure occurs. If they are exceeded by masticatory stresses, the restoration or appliance may no longer fit as originally designed. On the other hand, when fabricating an appliance, the elastic or proportional limit of the material should be relatively low in order to adjust it easily to the intended shape.

Modulus of Elasticity   In Figures 3–2 and 3–3, if any stress value equal to or less than the proportional limit is divided by its corresponding strain value, a constant of proportionality will result. This constant of proportionality is known as the *modulus of elasticity* or *Young's modulus* (E). Basically it is related to the slope of the force versus interatomic distance curve for a material, as was illustrated in Figure 2–4. It connotes *rigidity* or *stiffness*.

If, instead of unaxial stress, a shear stress predominated, the resulting shear strain could be used to define a shear modulus for the material. The shear modulus (G) can be calculated from Young's modulus and Poisson's ratio. It is determined by

$$G = \frac{E}{2\,(1 + \nu)}$$

Since a value of 0.3 for Poisson's ratio is typical, the shear modulus is usually about 40 per cent of Young's modulus.

Since the modulus of elasticity is the ratio of the stress to the strain, it follows that the less the strain for a given stress, the greater will be the value of the modulus. For example, if a wire or a similar structure is difficult to bend, considerable stress must be induced before a notable strain or deformation results. Such a material would possess a comparatively high modulus of elasticity.

The mathematical formula for the modulus of elasticity in tension, which is familiar to the student of physics, is derived as follows:

$$\text{Let } E = \text{Modulus of elasticity}$$
$$F = \text{Applied force or load}$$
$$A = \text{Cross section of the material under stress}$$
$$e = \text{Increase in length}$$
$$l = \text{Original length}$$
$$\text{By definition: Stress} = F/A = s\ (\sigma)$$
$$\text{Strain} = e/l = e\ (\epsilon)$$
$$\text{Then } E = \frac{\text{Stress}}{\text{Strain}} = \frac{\sigma}{\epsilon}$$
$$= \frac{F/A}{e/l}$$
$$= \frac{Fl}{eA} \tag{1}$$

The unit for the modulus of elasticity is force per unit area (MPa or psi). This property is only indirectly related to other mechanical properties. For example, two materials may have the same proportional limit and have elastic moduli that differ by 100 per cent.

Flexibility   In the case of dental appliances and restorations, a high value for the elastic limit is a necessary requirement for the materials from which they are fabricated, since the structure is expected to return to its original shape after it has been stressed. Usually a high modulus of elasticity is also required, since a small deformation is usually desired under considerable stress, as in the case of an inlay, for example.

There are instances, however, in which a larger strain or deformation may be needed with a moderate or slight stress. For example, in an orthodontic appliance, a spring is often bent a considerable distance with a small stress resulting. In such a case the structure is said to be *flexible*, and to possess the property of *flexibility*. The *maximal flexibility* is defined as the strain which occurs when the material is stressed to its proportional limit. The relation between the maximum flexibility, the proportional limit, and modulus of elasticity may be expressed mathematically as follows:

Let E = Modulus of elasticity

P = Proportional limit

ϵ_m = Maximal flexibility

From equation (1), $E = \dfrac{P}{\epsilon_m}$

Or $\epsilon_m = P/E$ (2)

Resilience To recapitulate, the elastic limit (or proportional limit) is the maximal stress required to separate the atoms in Figures 2–2 or 2–3 so that they will return to their original position when the load is removed. In terms of tensile strain, for example, it is the greatest interatomic distance that atoms A and B (Fig. 2–3) can be separated such that their mutual forces of attraction will be able to restore them to their original position when the disturbing external force becomes zero.

So far, we have been discussing mechanical forces which are applied constantly for a finite time, called *static* loads or stresses. The stresses in the teeth during mastication, for example, are not of this type. These stresses usually exist for only an instant; they are the result of a force created by the motion of the mandible against the maxilla. They are known as *dynamic* forces in contrast to static forces. It should be pointed out that the mechanical properties of many of the materials of dental interest are strain rate sensitive. That is, they depend upon the rate of change of the induced strain. For example, the speed at which sound travels through a solid can be readily measured. From that and the density of the material, the elastic modulus can be determined. Thus the elastic modulus can be measured by a dynamic method in place of the static technique that was previously illustrated. Such "dynamic" moduli are often found to be higher than the values obtained by static measurements.

Since the dynamic forces exist for an infinitesimally short time, the resulting deformation or strain cannot be measured. However, the *energy* imparted to the structure by the instantaneous force can be measured. For this reason, Figure 2–5 may be of more importance than Figure 2–4 in understanding this action.

As was previously pointed out, as the interatomic spacing increases, the interatomic energy increases. So long as the stress is not greater than the proportional limit, this energy is known as *resilience*.

Popularly, the term "resilience" is associated with "springiness," but basically, it connotes something more than this. On the basis of the previous discussion, *resilience* can be defined as the amount of energy absorbed by a structure when it is stressed not to exceed its proportional limit. For example, when an acrobat falls or jumps onto a trapeze net, the energy of his fall is absorbed by the resilience of the net. The net is deformed elastically by the impact, so that its energy at the time of maximal deformation is equal to the energy of the acrobat at the instant of impact. When the energy of the net is released, the acrobat is thrown into the air again, and a second impact occurs, and so on. Fortunately, part of the energy is dissipated in the form of heat; otherwise he would never stop rebounding.

As noted in the previous chapter, work is the product of the acting force and the distance through which the force moves. When work is done upon a body, energy is imparted to it. Consequently, when a dental restoration is deformed it absorbs energy. Since by definition the induced stress is not greater than the proportional limit, in order that the oral structure may not be permanently deformed, only the absorbed energy due to elastic deformation need be discussed.

When a dental restoration is deformed, the acting force is the masticating force as it acts upon the structure, and the magnitude of the deformation of the structure is determined by the induced stress. From the physical definition of work, it may be noted that either the amount of deformation may be large, and the applied force relatively small in magnitude, or the force may be large, and the deformation small. In either case, the resilience may be the same, provided that the values are chosen correctly. In most dental restorations, large strains are precluded because of the dangers of tooth displacement. For example, a proximal inlay might cause excessive movement of the adjacent tooth, if large strains developed. Hence, the restorative material should exhibit a type of resilience that allows stresses of considerable magnitude with but little strain. In other words, the material should possess a high modulus of elasticity.

The resilience of a material is usually measured in terms of its *modulus of resilience*, which is the amount of energy stored in a body, when one unit volume of a material is stressed to its proportional limit. The modulus of resilience is determined mathematically by dividing the square of the proportional limit by twice the modulus of elasticity. The mathematical proof for this statement is as follows:

$$\begin{aligned} \text{Let } R &= \text{Modulus of resilience} \\ P &= \text{Proportional limit} \\ \epsilon_m &= \text{Maximum flexibility} \\ E &= \text{Modulus of elasticity} \end{aligned}$$

Since the structure is stressed continuously from zero to P,

$$\text{the average stress} = \frac{0 + P}{2} = \frac{P}{2}$$

Then, the total work done per unit volume $= R = \dfrac{P}{2} \times \epsilon_m$ \hfill (3)

$$= \frac{P}{2} \times \frac{P}{E} \text{ [from formula (2)]}$$

$$= \frac{P^2}{2E} \hfill (4)$$

It is interesting to note that the modulus of resilience is equal to the area under the straight-line portion of the stress-strain curve, as illustrated in Figure 3–4. The area of the right angle triangle, where P is the height, is given by formula (3). The maximum flexibility is the base of the triangle.

The units for the modulus of resilience are expressed as energy per unit volume (megajoules per cubic meter or inch-pounds per cubic inch).

Formula (4) is very important as a criterion for the selection of a dental material. As previously discussed, a high modulus of elasticity (E) is imperative for a successful tooth restorative material, as is a high modulus of resilience. According to the formula, then, a high proportional limit (P) is necessary to attain a high modulus of resilience.

The mathematical interpretation of the formula is that the modulus of resilience is inversely proportional to the modulus of elasticity for a given

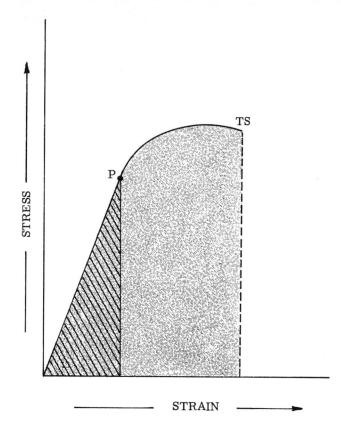

Figure 3–4 Stress-strain curve as determined by application of a tensile stress. The proportional limit is shown at P and the ultimate tensile strength at TS. The resiliency can be determined by measuring the area under the straight-line portion of the curve, i.e., that which is cross-hatched. The toughness is determined by measuring the total shaded area.

proportional limit, but directly proportional to the square of the proportional limit for a given modulus of elasticity.

Impact Force A dynamic force in its reaction during collision with a structure is called an *impact force*. The energy of impact thus becomes important during mastication. It is the energy of the impact of the teeth on the food bolus which partially determines the effectiveness of the mastication.

For example, the weight of a hammer on a table top produces no visible change in the surface of the table. Yet, if the hammer is placed in motion so that it strikes the table top, the force at impact will be much greater than the static force occasioned by the weight of the hammer alone. The magnitude of the impact force, or the stress it induced in the table, cannot be measured, but the energy received from the impact by the table can be measured. Whether or not the surface of the table will be damaged will depend upon its capacity to absorb the energy without a permanent deformation. In other words, its capacity to resist the impact elastically will be in proportion to its modulus of resilience. The analogy can, of course, be applied to a dental restoration or to any other structure. For a given material, then, the following law may be stated:

The ability of a unit volume of a material to resist an impact without permanent deformation is directly proportional to the modulus of resilience of the material.

A mathematical analysis of such a condition can be made with some interesting corollaries:

Let R = Modulus of resilience
    V = Volume
    K = Proportionality constant
Then, the ability to resist impact = KVR

$$= \frac{KVP^2}{2E} \text{ [from equation (4)]} \qquad (5)$$

The practical significance of the proportionality constant, K, in equation (5) is of especial interest. It represents the structural factors which are present in the design of the dental appliance. Although the proportional limit of the material used is the most important mechanical property, the design of the structure is also important in relation to its ability to resist impact. This factor is discussed in textbooks relating to the various branches of clinical dentistry.

According to equation (5), an increase in the volume of the material will increase its ability to resist impact without permanent deformation. The two quantities are in direct proportion to each other. It can be further concluded from the same equation that the impact resistance will be decreased with an increase in the modulus of elasticity. As previously noted, however, a high modulus of elasticity is necessary in most dental restorations to provide rigidity under stress.

Permanent Deformation   As noted in the previous chapter, when the sum of resultant force in Figure 2–4 reaches a maximum, the atoms separate permanently and a fracture occurs. It should be remembered that only two atoms are involved in this case. In a gross structure with millions of atoms, the interatomic space may become greater than that indicated at the point of maximal stress in Figure 2–4, and the atoms may be locally disarranged instead of actually fracturing, as will be described in a later chapter.

In any event, as can be noted in Figure 3–2, the stress-strain curve is no longer a straight line above P but rather curves until the structure fractures. The stress-strain curve shown in Figure 3–5 is more complete and typical. Unlike the curve at stresses below the proportional limit, the exact path of the curve above P may be unpredictable. It should also be noted that the stress is no longer proportional to the strain.

If the stress or load is removed at any time, the stress occasioned by the load becomes zero, but, as noted by the broken line extending to the horizontal coordinate (Fig. 3–5), the strain does not become zero; nor does the wire or whatever structure is being stressed return to its original dimension. It remains bent, stretched, or otherwise deformed. Although the mechanical stresses have disappeared, interatomic stresses remain as indicated by the permanently strained condition.

Strength   *Strength* is the maximal stress required to fracture a structure. It is called *tensile strength, compressive strength (crushing strength)* or *shear strength,* depending upon the predominant type of stress present.

The strength is not a measure of individual atomic attraction or repulsion, but rather it measures the interatomic forces collectively over the entire wire, cylinder, or whatever structure is stressed. Furthermore, the strength is not necessarily equal to the stress at fracture. If one assumes that the stress-strain curve shown in Figure 3–5 is tensile in character, the solid-line curve indicates

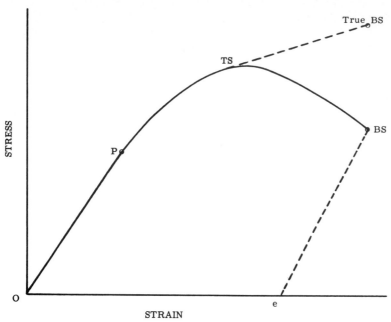

Figure 3–5   Solid line — complete stress-strain curve as determined by ordinary testing methods; P, proportional limit; TS, tensile strength; BS, breaking strength. If stress were computed according to the actual diameter of the wire, the dotted line portion of the curve would result, with the "true" breaking strength as shown.

the stress-strain relationship when the stress is calculated on the basis of the original cross-sectional area of the wire, as is the common practice.

It is evident that the cross section of the wire will decrease as it lengthens under stress. Consequently, the stress calculated for testing purposes may apparently decrease but the actual or true stress increases, as indicated by the curve in Figure 3–5. The *breaking strength* (BS) as indicated in Figure 3–5 is, then, less than the tensile strength indicated at TS.

Had the decrease in cross-sectional area of the wire been taken into consideration when the stress beyond TS (or P) was calculated, the true stress-strain curve would be indicated by the upper broken line and the breaking strength would be higher than the tensile strength as defined.

Although the true stress-strain curve represents the situation more accurately from a basic viewpoint, the stress-strain curve as indicated by the solid line is more practical in interpretation (Fig. 3–5). When we wish to know the tensile strength of a certain wire, we wish to know the maximal stress it will support in tension without regard to the small changes which may occur in cross-sectional area. The tensile strength is, therefore, defined as the maximal stress the structure will withstand before rupture.

Many brittle materials have a tensile strength that is markedly lower than the corresponding compressive strength, as was previously explained. The same is true of various dental materials, such as amalgam. It is possible that failure of certain materials in clinical usage may be associated with this particular property.

The tensile strength is generally determined by subjecting a rod, wire, or dumbbell-shaped specimen to tensile loading (a unilateral tension test). Since such a test is quite difficult to perform for many materials, another test has become popular in recent years for determining this property for many dental

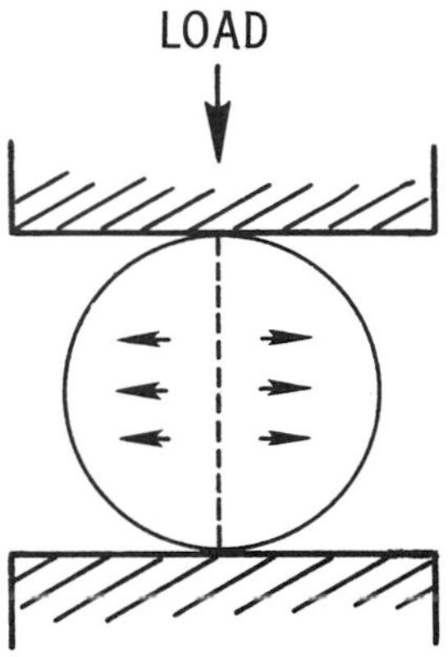

LOAD

Figure 3–6 Diametral tensile test. A compression load is applied diametrically to a cylindrical specimen. The arrows indicate the direction of the tensile stress.

materials. It is referred to as the *diametral compression* test for tension, or the *indirect tensile* test. This test is ordinarily used only for materials that exhibit very limited plastic deformation.

In this method the compressive load is placed on the diameter of a short cylindrical specimen, as diagrammed in Figure 3–6. The compressive stress introduces a tensile stress in the plane of the force application. In such a situation the tensile stress is directly proportional to the compression load applied. It is computed by the following formula:

$$\text{Tensile stress} = \frac{2P}{\pi \times D \times T}$$

Where P = Load
D = Diameter
T = Thickness

The tensile strength of many brittle dental materials now is determined by this method. The test is simple to conduct and provides excellent reproducibility of results.

Flexure Strength   Flexure strength, transverse strength, or modulus of rupture, as this property is variously called, is essentially a strength test of a beam supported at each end, under a static load (Figure 3–1). The theory involved is beyond the scope of this textbook. The mathematical formula for computing the flexure strength is as follows:

$$S = \frac{3Wl}{2bd^2}$$

Where S = Flexure strength
l = Distance between the supports
b = Width of the specimen
d = Depth or thickness of the specimen
W = Maximal load before fracture

The units are force per unit area (MPa, psi).

As previously noted, this test is, in a sense, a collective measurement of all types of stress simultaneously. When the load is applied, the specimen bends. The resulting strain is evident in that a decrease of the top linear dimensions (compressive strain) and a lengthening of the lower dimensions (tensile strain) occur. Consequently, it can be assumed that the principal stresses on the upper surface are compressive whereas those on the lower surface are tensile. Obviously, the stresses change direction somewhere between the top and the bottom, with both stress and strain being zero at the region of change. The line or plane that does not change in dimension is known as the *neutral axis*.

Fatigue   A word of caution is in order at this point. Strength values obtained from any of these "one time" measurements described may be quite misleading if used to design a structure that will be subject to repeated or cyclic loading. For example, in the aircraft industry it has been empirically demonstrated that cyclic loading at stress values well below those determined in ultimate strength measurements can produce abrupt failure of a structure. This type of failure is called *fatigue*. Normal mastication can produce thousands of stress cycles per day on a dental material.

Fatigue behavior is determined by subjecting a material to a cyclic stress of a maximum known value and determining the number of cycles that are required to produce failure. A plot of the maximum stress against the cycles to failure enables calculation of a "service lifetime" and also an endurance limit — the maximum stress value usable if an infinite fatigue lifetime is required.

Impact Strength   The *impact strength* may be defined as the energy required to fracture a material under an impact force. A Charpy-type impact tester is usually used. A pendulum is released which swings down to fracture the specimen. The energy lost by the pendulum during the fracture of the specimen can be determined by a comparison of the length of its swing after the impact with its free swing when no impact occurs. The energy units are joules, foot-pounds, inch-pounds, etc. Unlike most mechanical tests, the dimensions, shape, and design of the specimen to be tested should be identical for uniform results.

In another type of equipment, called the Izod impact tester, the specimen is clamped vertically at one end. The blow is delivered at a certain distance above the clamped end, instead of at the center of the specimen supported at both ends as for the Charpy.

Toughness   Toughness is the property of being difficult to break. It can be defined as the energy required to fracture a material. As previously noted, the modulus of resilience is the energy required to stress a structure to its proportional limit, and it can be measured as the area under the straight-line portion of the stress-strain curve. By the same token, toughness can be measured as the *total* area under the stress-strain curve from zero stress to the breaking strength (Fig. 3–4).

Although toughness is difficult to measure, it can be seen that it is generally more dependent upon the ductility (or malleability) of the material than upon its maximal flexibility or elastic modulus. Also, it can be concluded that, as a rule, a tough material is generally strong.

Brittleness   Brittleness is generally considered to be the opposite of toughness. For example, glass is brittle at room temperature; it will not bend appreciably without breaking. In other words, a brittle material is apt to fracture at or near its proportional limit.

However, a brittle material is not necessarily lacking in strength. For example, the shear strength of glass is low but its tensile strength is very high. If the glass is drawn into a fiber so that it can withstand a certain amount of shear, its tensile strength may be as high as 2800 MPa (400,000 psi). Tested in the same manner, the tensile strength of quartz may exceed 7000 MPa (1,000,000 psi).

Ductility and Malleability   When a structure is stressed beyond its proportional limit, it becomes permanently deformed. If the stresses are tensile in type, and if the material can withstand considerable permanent deformation without rupture, it is said to be ductile. *Ductility* is, therefore, the ability of a material to withstand permanent deformation under a tensile load without rupture. A metal which may be drawn readily into a wire is said to be ductile. Ductility is dependent upon plasticity and tensile strength.

The ability of a material to withstand permanent deformation without rupture under compression, as in hammering or rolling into a sheet, is termed *malleability*. It is also dependent on plasticity, but it is not as dependent upon strength as is ductility.

In general, ductility decreases with increase in temperature, whereas malleability increases with increase in temperature. Gold is the most ductile and malleable metal, and silver is second. Of the metals of interest to the dentist, platinum ranks third in ductility, and copper ranks third in malleability.

Ductility is commonly associated with the maximum allowable degree of plasticity when a material is bent or contoured at room temperature, and it is quite important from a dental standpoint. Its magnitude can be assessed by the amount of permanent deformation indicated by the stress-strain curve. For example, the strain as indicated by $\overline{0e}$ in Figure 3–5 is an estimation of the ductility of the substance. As previously noted, after fracture, the mechanical stress disappears, and the residual strain represents the amount of permanent deformation.

On the other hand, if it is assumed that the end of the curve in Figure 3–2 represents the breaking strength,* it can be concluded that the ductility of this wire is comparatively low.

MEASUREMENT OF DUCTILITY   Ductility is a quantity which is difficult to measure. There are three common methods for its measurement: percentage elongation after fracture, reduction in area at the fractured ends, and the cold bend test.

Probably the simplest and most used method of measurement is to compare the increase in length of a wire or rod after fracture in tension to its length before fracture. Two marks are placed on the wire or rod a specified distance apart which is designated as the *gauge length*. In dental testing, the standard gauge length is usually 51 mm. The wire or rod is then pulled apart under a tensile load. The fractured ends are fitted together, and the gauge length is again measured. The ratio of the increase in length after fracture to the original gauge length, expressed in per cent, is called the *elongation* or *percentage elongation*.

Another manifestation of ductility is the necking or cone-shaped constric-

---

*Note that the breaking strength and the tensile strength are presumably identical in this case.

tion which occurs at the fractured end of a ductile wire after rupture under a tensile load. The percentage decrease in cross-sectional area of the fractured end in comparison to the original area of the wire or rod is called the *reduction in area*.

A third method for the measurement of ductility is known as the *cold bend test*. The material is clamped in a vise and bent around a mandrel of a specified radius. The number of bends before fracture is counted, and the greater the number, the greater is the ductility. The first bend is counted from the vertical to the horizontal, but all subsequent bends are counted through angles of 180°.

Hardness   Surface hardness is the result of the interaction of numerous properties. Some are closely related, others are not. Among the properties that influence the hardness of a material are its strength, proportional limit, ductility, malleability, and resistance to abrasion and cutting. Because numerous factors influence hardness, the term is difficult to define. In fact, no specific definition exists. In mineralogy the relative hardness of a substance is based upon its ability to resist scratching. In metallurgy, and in most other disciplines, the concept most generally accepted is the "resistance to indentation." It is upon this precept that most modern hardness tests are designed.

Despite the lack of specificity of the term, knowledge of the hardness of materials is most useful to the engineer and furnishes valuable information to the dentist. The significance of this property is indicated by the fact that hardness tests are included in numerous American Dental Association specifications.

There are many surface hardness tests. With only a few exceptions they are based upon the ability of the surface of a material to resist penetration by a point under a specified load. One of the exceptions is the Bierbaum, which is a scratch test. The tests most frequently used in determining the hardness of dental materials are the Brinell, Rockwell, Vickers, and Knoop. The selection of the test is often determined by the material being measured. Certain tests are more applicable to one type of material than to another.

The Brinell test is one of the oldest tests employed for determining the hardness of metals. In the Brinell test a hardened steel ball is pressed into the polished surface of a material under a specified load, as diagrammed in Figure 3–7. The load is divided by the area of the surface of the indentation. Thus, the smaller the indentation, the larger is the hardness number, and the harder is the material. The quotient is referred to as the *Brinell hardness number*, usually abbreviated as BHN.

In practice the diameter of the indentation is measured accurately using a microscope with a micrometer eyepiece. The BHN is then determined from tables prepared for that purpose.

Balls of various sizes, in conjunction with specified loads, are prescribed for the Brinell test. The instrument generally employed for testing dental materials is usually referred to as the "baby Brinell." The diameter of the ball is comparatively small — 1.6 mm (¹/₁₆ inch). The standard load used in combination with this ball is 12.61 kgm (27.7 pounds).

The Brinell test has been used extensively for determining the hardness of metallic materials used in dentistry. In addition, the BHN is directly proportional to the proportional limit and the ultimate tensile strength of dental gold alloys. As the test is a relatively simple one, it may often be conveniently used as an index of properties that involve a more complicated test method.

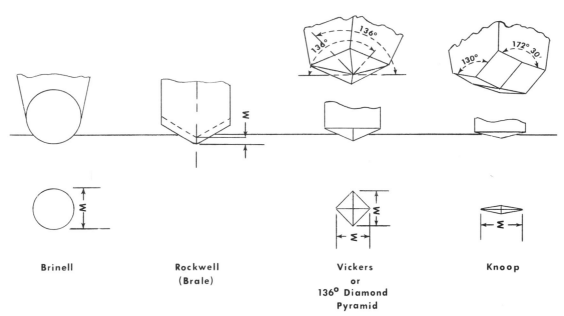

Brinell

Rockwell
(Brale)

Vickers
or
136° Diamond
Pyramid

Knoop

Figure 3–7 Diagrammatic representation of various hardness indenter points impressed into a surface. In each of the tests the dimensions of the indentation that are measured in order to determine the hardness number are designated by "M." Brinell test — a steel ball is used. The hardness is calculated from the diameter of the indentation. Rockwell — a conical diamond indenter point is shown, but the same principle would apply if the steel ball indenter were used. The dotted line represents the penetration of the indenter point upon application of the minor load, and the solid line indicates the penetration under the major load. Vickers or 136° diamond pyramid — a pyramidal point of a diamond is used. Hardness is determined from the average length of the diagonals. Knoop — the rhomboidal pyramid of a diamond is used. Hardness is determined from the length of the long axis of the indentation.

However, the application of this test to all dental materials is somewhat limited. It is not suitable for determining the hardness of brittle materials or those that exhibit elastic recovery. The steel ball tends to fracture brittle materials; thus, the indentation is not well defined. Resilient materials tend to recover upon removal of the steel ball, and the indentation is thereby inaccurate. Thus, the Brinell test is not suitable for measuring the hardness of tooth structure and cements, which are brittle materials, or the dental plastics, which exhibit elastic recovery.

The Rockwell hardness test is somewhat similar to the Brinell test in that a steel ball or, in some instances, a conical diamond point is used, as diagrammed in Figure 3–7. Instead of measuring the diameter of the impression, the depth is measured directly by a dial gauge on the instrument. Initially, the indenter is placed under a static load of a given magnitude (minor load), and the dial gauge is set at zero. The load is then increased by a given amount (major load) and maintained for a certain period. The depth of indentation is measured after the major load is again reduced to the minor load. A number of indenting points with different sizes are available for testing different types of materials. The *Rockwell hardness number* (RHN) is designated according to the particular indenter and load employed (Rockwell C, Rockwell M. etc.).

The convenience of the Rockwell test, with direct reading of the depth of the indentation, has led to wide usage in industry. As for the Brinell, it is not suitable for brittle materials, and the test procedure must be modified for materials that exhibit elastic recovery.

The Vickers hardness test employs the same principle of hardness testing as the Brinell test. However, instead of a steel ball, a diamond in the shape of a square-based pyramid is used. The angle between the faces of the pyramid is 136° (Fig. 3–7). Although the impression is square instead of round, the method for computation of the *Vickers hardness number* (VHN) is the same as that for the Brinell hardness number in that the load is divided by the area of indentation. The lengths of the diagonals of the indentation are measured and averaged. Using this value the hardness number is obtained from a table. The Vickers test is employed in the American Dental Association specification for dental casting golds. The test is suitable for determining the hardness of quite brittle materials. Therefore, it has been used for measuring the hardness of tooth structure. However, the Vickers suffers the same shortcomings as the Brinell in respect to its use with materials which exhibit elastic recovery.

The Knoop hardness test employs a diamond indenting tool that is cut in the geometrical configuration shown in Figure 3–7. The impression is diamond-shaped or rhombic in outline and the length of the largest diagonal is measured. Instead of the actual area of the indentation, the projected area is divided into the load to give the *Knoop hardness number* (KHN). Thus, as with all hardness tests, the harder the material, the higher will be the hardness number.

It will be noted that the angle of the longitudinal faces of the rhombus-shaped diamond indenting point is 172° 30′, whereas that of the transverse faces is 130°. When the indentation is made, a cutting action occurs along the major axis of the impression, and a spreading or indenting, as with the Brinell ball, takes place along the minor axis. The stresses are therefore distributed in such a manner that only the dimensions of the minor axis are subject to change by relaxation. Since the hardness number is computed on the basis of the length of the indentation, the hardness value is virtually independent of the ductility of the material tested. The hardness of tooth enamel can be compared to that of gold, porcelain, resin, and other tooth restorative materials. Also, the load may be varied over a wide range, from one gm to more than a kgm, so that values for both exceedingly hard and soft materials can be obtained by this test.

Other less sophisticated hardness tests, such as the Shore and the Barcol, are sometimes employed for assaying the hardness of dental materials, particularly rubbers and plastics. These tests use compact portable indenters of the type generally used in industry for quality control. The principle of these tests is also based on resistance to indentation. The equipment generally consists of a spring loaded metal indenter point and a gauge from which the hardness is read directly. The hardness number is based upon the depth of penetration of the indenter point into the material.

Abrasion Resistance   Hardness has often been used as an index to the ability of a material to resist abrasion. However, abrasion is an exceedingly complex mechanism, involving an interaction between numerous factors. For this reason the reliability of hardness as a predictor of abrasion resistance is limited. Often it is valid for comparing materials within a given classification, e.g., one brand of dental cement with another brand of the same type of cement. However, it may be invalid when evaluating different classes of materials, such as a metallic material with a synthetic resin, as will be discussed in Chapter 14. Abrasion resistance is an exceedingly elusive characteristic to evaluate.

The only reliable test for abrasion resistance is via a test procedure designed to simulate as closely as possible the particular type of abrasion to which the material will eventually be subjected.

Relaxation To recapitulate, whenever a substance is permanently deformed, there are internal stresses that are permanent. For example, in a crystalline substance the atoms in the space lattice are displaced and the interatomic forces are not in equilibrium. Similarly, in amorphous structures, some molecules are too close together and others too far apart after the substance has been permanently deformed.

It is understandable that such a situation is not very stable. The displaced atoms may be said to be "uncomfortable" and wish to return to their normal, regular relative positions. If given time, by diffusion they will slowly but surely move back to their proper relationship. The result is a change in the shape or contour of the solid as a gross manifestation of the rearrangement in atomic or molecular positions. The material is said to *warp* or *distort*. Such a relief of stress is known as *relaxation*.

As can be expected, the rate of relaxation will increase with an increase in temperature. For example, if a wire is bent, it may tend to straighten out if it is heated to a high temperature. At room temperature any such relaxation or diffusion may be negligible. On the other hand, there are many noncrystalline dental materials (waxes, resins, gels, etc.) that can relax during storage at room temperature after being bent or molded. Considerable attention will be given to this phenomenon in succeeding chapters, since such dimensional changes by relaxation may result in misfit of the delicate dental appliance.

RHEOLOGY

Up to this point the discussion of the physical properties of materials used in dentistry has been devoted to the behavior of solid materials subjected to various types of stress. However, many, if not most, of these materials are liquid at some stage in their dental application. Moreover, the success or failure of a given material may be as dependent on its properties in the liquid state as it is on its ultimate properties as a solid. For example, later we will study materials like cements and impression materials that undergo a liquid to solid transformation in the mouth. Gypsum products used in the fabrication of models and dies and casting alloys are materials that are shaped as liquids into structures which solidify outside the mouth. Amorphous materials such as waxes and resins appear solid but actually are super-cooled liquids that flow or plastically deform very slowly under small stresses. Finally are materials which are used as liquids, e.g., prophy pastes, dentifrices, and enamel etching solutions and gels. The ways in which these materials deform or flow when subjected to stress are quite important to their use in dentistry.

The study of the flow of matter is the subject of the science of *rheology*. Although a liquid at rest cannot support a shear stress, most liquids when placed in motion resist the forces acting to make them move. This resistance is called *viscosity* and may be viewed as due to internal frictional forces within the liquid. Different materials have different viscosities. The concept is familiar to anyone who has compared the flow properties of water with those of honey.

To put this concept on a quantitative basis, consider Figure 3–8. A fluid is

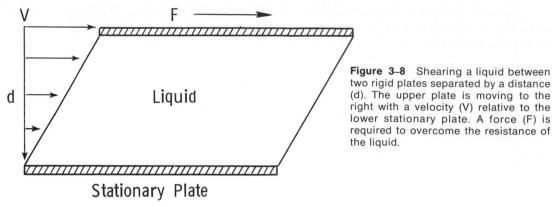

Figure 3–8 Shearing a liquid between two rigid plates separated by a distance (d). The upper plate is moving to the right with a velocity (V) relative to the lower stationary plate. A force (F) is required to overcome the resistance of the liquid.

occupying the space between two metal plates; the lower is fixed and the upper is being moved to the right with a certain velocity (V). A force (F) is required to overcome the drag produced by the friction (viscosity) of the liquid. If the plates have area A, a shear stress (σ_s) can be defined as $\sigma_s = F/A$. With a distance, d, between the two plates, strain is V/d. However, since V is a velocity, not a displacement, V/d becomes a strain rate $\dot{\epsilon}$. If we change F, we get a new value for V, and a curve can be obtained for force and velocity analogous to the load-displacement curves that were explained previously in the static-solid experiments.

Similarly, a shear stress versus strain rate curve can be plotted. Typical examples are shown in Figure 3–9. An "ideal" fluid demonstrates a shear stress that is proportional to the strain rate. Such behavior is called *newtonian*. Since the viscosity η is defined as the shear stress divided by the strain rate $\eta = \sigma_s/\dot{\epsilon}$, a newtonian fluid has a constant viscosity that does not depend on strain rate. The curve is a straight line and resembles the elastic portion of the stress-strain curve (Fig. 3–2) with viscosity the analog of the elastic modulus. Viscosity is measured in units of mPa · sec (centi-poise) and, obviously, the higher the value, the more viscous is the material. For example, pure water at 20° C has a viscosity of 1.0 mPa · sec, while the viscosity of molasses is approximately 300,000 mPa · sec. Many dental materials exhibit *pseudoplastic* behavior, as illustrated in Figure 3–9. Their viscosity decreases with increasing shear rate.

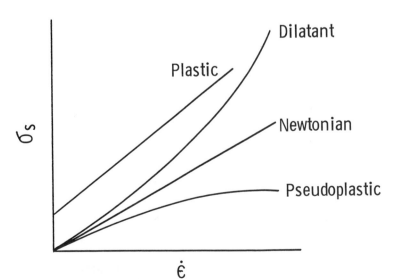

Figure 3–9 Shear stress versus shear strain rate for fluids exhibiting different types of rheological behavior.

Liquids that show the opposite tendency are called *dilatant*. These liquids become more rigid as the rate of deformation increases.

Finally, some classes of materials behave like a rigid body until some minimum value of shear stress is reached. These are referred to as *plastic*. Catsup is a familiar example — a sharp blow to the bottle is usually required in order to produce flow.

The viscosity of most liquids decreases rapidly with increasing temperature. Viscosity may also depend upon previous deformation of the liquid; such liquids are referred to as *thixotropic*. Latex paints designed for ceilings and dental prophy pastes are usually thixotropic. If these are stirred rapidly and the viscosity is measured, a lower value is obtained than that for a sample which has been left undisturbed for several hours.

The viscosity of a dental material may determine its suitability for a given application. Likewise, the nature of the shear stress-strain rate curve can be important in determining the best way in which to manipulate a material. As will be seen later, the viscosity as a function of time can also be used to measure the working time of a material which undergoes a liquid-solid transformation.

Creep, Flow   A final topic under the heading of rheological behavior is likely not to be as familiar to the student. Engineers who design structures to withstand both stress and high temperature are faced with the rheological behavior of solid materials. If a metal is held at a temperature near its melting point and subjected to a constant applied force, the resulting strain will be found to increase as a function of time. This time-dependent plastic deformation is referred to as *creep*.

Static creep is the time-dependent deformation produced in a completely set solid subjected to a constant stress. *Dynamic creep* refers to this phenomenon when the applied stress is fluctuating, such as in a fatigue-type test.

Most metals used in dentistry have melting points that are much higher than mouth temperature and thus are not susceptible to the creep phenomenon. The most important exception is dental amalgam, which has components with melting points only slightly above room temperature. Since creep produces continuing plastic deformation, the process can be very destructive to a dental restoration. The relationship of this property to the behavior of the amalgam restoration will be discussed in the chapters dealing with that material. It is sufficient to note at this point that the test is now included in specification programs designed to upgrade the clinical performance of conventional amalgam alloys.

A somewhat synonymous term is *flow*. Flow is particularly an attribute of amorphous materials, which is not surprising in consideration of their structure. Pitch is a good example of such a substance; it will fracture under a sudden blow, but if it is placed in a leaky container it will flow through the leak under its own weight. Glass tubing will bend if it is leaned against the wall or if it is laid with supports at either end.

The term flow, rather than creep, has generally been used in dentistry to describe this characteristic for amorphous materials, such as waxes. It has also been used to identify plastic deformation of amalgam under a constant load. In this case, however, the "flow" test is initiated before the amalgam has completely hardened. It would appear to be more appropriate to use the term creep to describe any deformation of the clinical restoration that might occur subsequent to the complete set.

Although creep or flow may be measured under any type of stress, compression is usually employed in the testing of dental materials. A cylinder of prescribed dimensions is subjected to a given compressive stress for a specified time and temperature. The creep or flow is measured as the percentage of shortening in length that occurs under these testing conditions.

Creep can be an important consideration for any dental material that must be held at a temperature near its melting point for an extended period of time.

COLOR

The preceding discussion of material properties has been concerned with those properties that are necessary to permit a material to restore the function of damaged or missing natural tissues. However, another important goal of modern dentistry is to restore the color and appearance of natural dentition. Thus, esthetic considerations in restorative and prosthetic dentistry have assumed an even higher priority. For example, the search for an ideal general purpose, direct filling "tooth colored" restorative material is one of the challenges of present dental materials research.

Although esthetic dentistry makes severe demands on the artistic abilities of the dentist and technician, a knowledge of the basic underlying scientific principles is equally essential. This is especially true for the increasingly popular restorations that involve ceramic materials, as will be discussed in Chapter 31. A more comprehensive and excellent treatment of the entire subject can be found in another text.[1]

Light is a form of electromagnetic radiant energy that can be detected by the human eye. The eye is sensitive to wavelengths from approximately 400 mμ (violet) to 700 mμ (dark red) as shown in Figure 3–10. The combinations of wavelengths present in a beam of light determine the property usually called *color*.

In order for an object to be visible, either it must emit light or it must reflect or transmit light incident upon it from an external source. The latter is the case for objects that are of dental interest. The incident light is usually polychromatic, i.e., some mixture of the various wavelengths, as is shown in

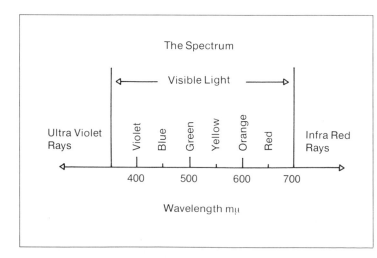

Figure 3–10 A diagram of the color bands and wavelengths of visible light. (From McLean: The Science and Art of Dental Ceramics, Chicago, Quintessence Pub. 6, 1979, p. 119.)

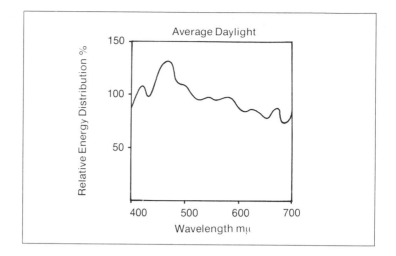

Figure 3–11 A diagram of the relative energy distribution in daylight. (From McLean: The Science and Art of Dental Ceramics. Chicago, Quintessence Pub. 6, 1979, p. 119.)

Figures 3–11 and 3–12. These figures show the intensity of the light as a function of wavelength for two common light sources. Such curves are referred to as spectral curves or distributions. The reaction of an object to the incident light is to selectively absorb and/or scatter certain wavelengths. The spectral distribution of the transmitted or reflected light will resemble that of the incident light, although certain wavelengths will be reduced in magnitude. The phenomenon of vision, and certain terminology, can be illustrated by considering the response of the human eye to light coming from an object.

Light from an object which is incident on an eye is focused onto the retina and converted into nerve impulses, which are transmitted to the brain. Cone-shaped cells in the retina are responsible for color vision. These cells have a threshold intensity required for color vision and also exhibit a response curve related to the wavelength of the incident light. Such a curve for a normal human eye is shown in Figure 3–13. As can be seen, the eye is most sensitive to light in the green-yellow region and least sensitive at either extreme, i.e., red or blue.

Since a nerve response is involved in color vision, constant stimulation by a single color may result in color fatigue and a decrease in the eye's response. The signals from the retina are processed by the brain to produce the

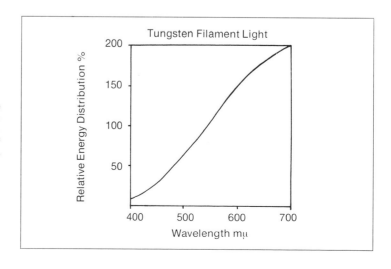

Figure 3–12 A diagram of the relative energy distribution in tungsten filament light. (From McLean: The Science and Art of Dental Ceramics. Chicago, Quintessence Pub. 6, 1979, p. 119.)

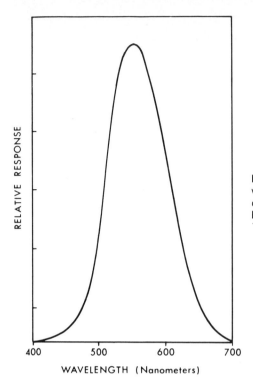

Figure 3–13 Relative response of a human eye at different wavelengths. (From O'Brien, W. J., and Ryge, G., An Outline of Dental Materials, W. B. Saunders, 1978 [Adapted from Billmeyer, F. W., Jr., and Saltzman, M., Principles of Color Technology. Interscience, New York, 1966].)

psychophysiological perception of color. Defects in certain portions of the color-sensing receptors result in the different kinds of color blindness. Thus, individuals vary greatly in their ability to distinguish colors. In a scientific sense one might liken the normal human eye to an exceptionally sensitive differential colorimeter. The eye equals or exceeds the current state of the art in instrumentation in its ability to differentiate between two colors seen side by side.

Although curves such as those shown in Figures 3–11 and 3–12 completely specify the spectral quality of light coming from a particular source or object, they do not relate well to the usual concept of color. Therefore, they are not useful in specifying the color of an object unless a spectrophotometer is available, which is not possible in dental procedures. Thus it is necessary to describe terms that are useful in communicating information about the color phenomenon; for example, the color of a tooth as seen by the dentist must be communicated to the laboratory technician.

Three Dimensions of Color   Quantitatively color has come to be described as a three-dimensional quantity specified by values for three variables, *hue, chroma,* and *value.*

Hue refers to the property commonly associated with the color of an object, whether it is red, green, blue, etc. This refers to the dominant wavelengths present in the spectral distribution and the names associated, as is shown in Figure 3–10.

Chroma refers to the strength or degree of saturation for a particular hue. In other words, the higher the chroma, the more vivid is the color.

Value is a photometric parameter associated with total reflectance or luminance, i.e., the brightness or darkness of an object. Those individuals familiar with the adjustment knobs on a color television set recognize the

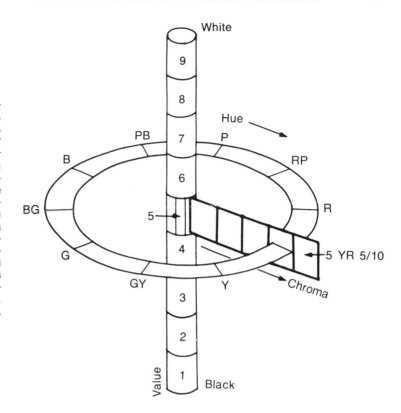

Figure 3–14   The Munsell color coordinate system. The coordinates for a specific shade are written in the form *Hue/Value/Chroma*, with a number specifying the hue subdivision preceding the hue name designation. For example, the shade shown is 5 YR 5/10. 5 YR specifies a *hue* halfway between yellow and red. 5/ specifies a *value* halfway along the axis between black and white. /10 specifies a *chroma* corresponding to complete saturation. (10 is the maximum value on the chroma scale.) (From Lemire, P. A. and Burk, B.: Color in Dentistry, J. M. Ney Co.)

functions of the hue and chroma controls. Value corresponds to the brightness control.

Measurement   Various methods have been used to define and measure color quantitatively. One of the most commonly used is the Munsell system, as illustrated in Figure 3–14. This coordinate system may be viewed as a cylinder. The hues are arrayed sequentially around the perimeter of the cylinder, while the chroma increases along a radius out from the axis. The value coordinate varies along the length of the cylinder from black at the bottom to neutral grey at the center to white at the top.

Human teeth show considerable variation in color between individuals and within individuals, and the spectrophotometric data available for large populations is quite limited. In general, Munsell data for hue range from 7.5 YR to 2.7 Y, brightness from 5.8/ to 8.5/, and chroma from 1.5 to 5.6. As can be seen, this represents only a small portion of the Munsell cylinder.

Clinically in the operatory or dental lab, color matching is usually done by the use of *shade guides* like the example shown in Figure 3–15. These are used in much the same way as paint chips are used to select the color for house paint and to specify the color to the technician who mixes the proper shade.

Although the range of hue, chroma, and value ordinarily found in human teeth represents only a very small portion of the Munsell color space, the selectivity of the human eye is sufficient to make accurate color matching very difficult by the use of a shade guide that contains only a small number of shades.

Since the spectral distribution of the light reflected from or transmitted through an object is dependent on the incident light spectral content, the appearance of an object is quite dependent on the nature of the light by which

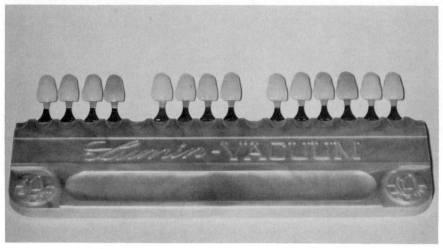

Figure 3–15   Shade guide for selection of color of a dental restorative material.

the object is viewed. Sunlight, incandescent lamps, and fluorescent lamps are all common sources of light in the dental operatory or laboratory and all these have very different spectral distributions, as seen in Figures 3–11 and 3–12. Objects that appear to be color matched under one type of light may appear very different under another light source. This phenomenon is called *metamerism*. Thus, if possible, color matching should be done under two or more different light sources, one of which should be sunlight.

In addition to the processes already discussed, natural tooth structure will absorb light at wavelengths too short to be visible to the human eye. These wavelengths between 300 and 400 mμ are referred to as the near ultra-violet. Natural sunlight, photo-flash lamps, certain types of vapor lamps, and, of course, the ultra-violet lights used in decorative lighting are all sources containing substantial amounts of near ultra-violet radiation. The energy that the tooth absorbs is converted into light with longer wavelengths, in which case the tooth actually becomes a light source. The phenomenon is called *fluorescence*. The emitted light is primarily in the 400 to 450 mμ range — a blue-white color. Fluorescence makes a definite contribution to the brightness and vital appearance of a human tooth.

Thus, the research worker developing a tooth colored restorative material and the dentist and his technician must be concerned with the color matching under light sources which contain a sufficient near ultra-violet component. Incandescent lighting contains very little if any ultra-violet. Again the dentist or laboratory technician must be aware of the importance of color matching under more than one source of light.

Additional material dealing with color and appearance will be presented in Chapter 31, on dental porcelain.

THERMAL PROPERTIES

Heat transfer through substances most commonly occurs by means of a process called conduction. The coefficient of thermal conductivity is measured by determining the quantity of heat in calories per second that passes through a specimen 1 cm thick having a cross-sectional area of 1 cm² when the temperature differential between the ends of the specimen is 1° C. The higher the value, the greater is the ability of the substance to transmit energy, and vice versa.

However, more often the temperatures are not held constant. Generally there is an unsteady state, since the thermal transfer through the material can in itself decrease the thermal gradient. Under such conditions, *thermal diffusivity* is important. The mathematical formula for calculating the thermal diffusivity *(h)* is

$$h = k/c_p \, \rho$$

where k is the thermal conductivity, c_p is the *heat capacity,* and ρ is the density. Heat capacity is numerically equal to the more commonly used term of *specific heat.* Thermal diffusivity units are cm²/sec.

For a given volume of material, the heat required to raise the temperature a given amount depends upon its heat capacity (cal/gm · °C) and the density (gm/cm³). When the product of heat capacity and density is high, the thermal diffusivity will be low, even though the thermal conductivity may also be high. In other words, more calories must be added to or removed from the material in order to change the temperature.

Therefore, both the thermal conductivity and thermal diffusivity are the important parameters in monitoring the transfer of thermal energy through a material. Since an unsteady state of heat transfer exists during the ingestion of hot or cold foods and liquids, the thermal diffusivity of a dental restorative material may be more important than its thermal conductivity.

As can be noted in Table 3–1, dentin and enamel are effective thermal insulators. Their thermal conductivity and diffusivity compare favorably with silica brick and water, in contrast to the markedly higher values for metals.

However, as for any thermal insulator, tooth structure must be present in sufficient thickness to be effective. When the layer of dentin between the bottom of the cavity floor and the pulp is too thin, then the dentist must place an additional layer of an insulating base of cement, as will be discussed in Chapter 30. The effectiveness of a material in preventing heat transfer is directly proportional to the thickness of the liner and inversely proportional to the square root of the thermal diffusivity. Thus, the thickness of the remaining dentin and the cement liner is as important as, if not more than, the thermal properties of the materials themselves.[2-4]

Since the interatomic bonding in the oral tissues is predominantly

Table 3–1. *Thermal Properties of Enamel and Dentin as Compared with Other Commonly Recognized Conductors and Insulators*

	DENSITY (gm · cm⁻³)	SPECIFIC HEAT (cal/gm · C)	CONDUCTIVITY (cal · cm/cm² · sec · C)	DIFFUSIVITY (cm² · sec⁻¹)
Enamel*	2.9	0.18	0.0022	0.0042
Dentin*	2.1	0.28	0.0015	0.0026
Silver	10.5	0.056	0.98	1.67
Copper	8.96	0.092	0.94	1.14
Silica brick	2.5	0.2	0.003	0.006
Water (20° C)	1.0	1.0	0.0014	0.0014

*Braden, M.: Heat conduction in normal human teeth. Arch Oral Biol 9:479–486, 1964.

Table 3–2. *Linear Coefficients of Thermal Expansion of Some Important Dental Materials**

MATERIAL	LINEAR COEFFICIENT OF EXPANSION $(mm/mm \cdot K) \times 10^{-6}$
Tooth (across crown)	11.4
Silicate cement	7.6
Dental amalgam	25.0
Porcelain	4.1
Dental resin [poly(methyl methacrylate)]	81.0

*From Sauder and Paffenbarger, Physical Properties of Dental Materials, National Bureau of Standards Circular C433.

primary in type, with few if any free electrons, the thermal conductivity of the oral tissues is low. Such a low thermal conductivity aids in preventing thermal shock and the resulting pain when hot or cold foods are taken into the mouth. Often sensitivity to heat or cold may indicate an abnormal or even pathological condition of the tissues involved.

However, the presence of oral restorations of any type tends to change the situation. As will be discussed later, most of the truly serviceable tooth restorative materials are metallic. Because of the free electrons present, these materials are good thermal conductors to the extent that the tooth pulp may be adversely affected by the markedly increased intensity of the thermal changes. In many cases it is necessary to insert a heat insulator between the restoration and the tooth structure. In this respect, a restorative material which exhibits a low thermal conductivity is more desirable.

On the other hand, artificial teeth are held in a *denture base,* which ordinarily is constructed of a synthetic resin, a poor thermal conductor. In the upper denture, this base may cover most of the roof of the mouth. The low thermal conductivity tends to prevent heat exchange between the bearing tissues and the mouth itself. Such a condition is not conducive to good tissue health. Furthermore, the patient partially loses the sense of heat and cold while eating and drinking. The use of a metal denture base would be more comfortable and pleasant from this standpoint.

A thermal property equally important to the dentist is the *linear coefficient of thermal expansion,* which is defined as the change in length per unit length of a material when its temperature is raised or lowered one degree. Linear coefficients of expansion of some substances of interest in dentistry are presented in Table 3–2. As an example of the importance of this property in dentistry, a tooth restoration may expand or contract more than the tooth during a change in temperature; thus, the restoration may leak or become loosened. As a specific example, according to the values in Table 3–2, a restoration made with methyl methacrylate resin will change in dimension seven times or more as much as the tooth structure for every degree change in temperature. This point will be discussed at length in Chapter 14.

PHYSICAL PROPERTIES OF TEETH

Many of the mechanical properties of human tooth structure have been measured, but the reported values vary markedly from one investigation to another. Undoubtedly the differences are due to the technical problems associated with preparing and testing such minute specimens, in some instances less than 1 mm in length.

The results reported in one study[5] are shown in Table 3–3. Inasmuch as the teeth are more subject to dynamic than static stress, as previously discussed, the modulus of resilience has been calculated.

Although the data in Table 3–3 indicate a variation in the properties of enamel and dentin from one type of tooth to another, the difference probably is more the result of variation between individual teeth than between molar and cuspid, for example. However, the properties of enamel vary somewhat with its position on the tooth. Enamel on the cusp is stronger than that on the side of the tooth. Also, the properties vary according to the histological structure. For example, enamel is stronger under compression in a direction parallel to the enamel rods than in a direction perpendicular to the rods. On the other hand, the properties of the dentin appear to be quite independent of structure, regardless of the direction of compressive stress.

It should be noted that other data[6] for enamel suggest somewhat higher values than those presented in Table 3–3. For example, the average compressive strength reported is in the range of 378 MPa (55,000 psi).

Tensile properties of tooth structure have also been measured.[7] Dentin is considerably stronger in tension than is enamel, 51.5 MPa (7500 psi) and 10.3 MPa (1500 psi), respectively.

Although the compressive strengths of the enamel and dentin are comparable, the proportional limit and modulus of elasticity of enamel are higher than the similar properties of dentin. The higher modulus of elasticity results in a lower modulus of resilience of enamel in comparison with dentin.

Stresses During Mastication   As discussed previously, because of their dynamic nature the actual biting stresses during mastication are difficult to measure. A number of studies have been made to determine the biting force. One average value reported was 77 kgm (170 pounds).[8] However, it varies markedly from one area of the mouth to another and from one individual to another. In the molar region it may range from 41 to 91 kgm (90 to 200 pounds); in the premolar area from 23 to 46 kgm (50 to 100 pounds); 14 to 34 kgm (30 to 75 pounds) on cuspids and 9 to 25 kgm (20 to 55 pounds) on incisors.[9] Although there is considerable overlapping, biting force generally is higher for males than for females and is greater in young adults than in children.[10]

It is assumed that if a force of 77 kgm (170 pounds) is applied to the apex of a cusp over an area equivalent to .039 cm^2 (0.006 in^2), the compressive stress is 193 MPa (28,000 psi). If the area is smaller, then the stress would be proportionately greater.

Undoubtedly the nearly instantaneous forces incurred during mastication are much higher than those measured in these studies. Probably the reader has had the painful experience of suddenly biting on a small hard object in food such as a shot when eating wild game. The shot may be dented, and in some cases the tooth may be injured. On the other hand, the shot cannot be dented when a conscious effect is made to apply a static force with the jaws.

Normally, of course, the energy of the bite is absorbed by the food bolus during mastication, as well as by the teeth themselves. Nevertheless, the design of the tooth is somewhat of an engineering marvel in that the tooth is generally able to absorb such impact energies. As noted in Table 3–3, the modulus of resilience of dentin is greater than that of enamel and thus is

Table 3–3. *Compressive Properties of Tooth Structure**

TOOTH	STRUCTURE	MODULUS OF ELASTICITY		PROPORTIONAL LIMIT		MODULUS OF RESILIENCE		STRENGTH	
		$MPa \times 10^4$	$psi \times 10^5$	MPa	psi	$Joules/m^3 \times 10^5$	$in\text{-}lb/in^3$	MPa	psi
Molar	Dentin	1.2	17	148	21,500	9.4	136	305	44,200
	Enamel (cusp)	4.6	67	224	32,500	5.5	79	261	37,800
Bicuspid	Dentin	1.4	20	146	21,200	7.7	112	248	36,000
	Enamel	–	–	–	–	–	–	–	–
Cuspid	Dentin	1.4	20	140	20,300	7.1	103	276	40,100
	Enamel (cusp)	4.8	69	194	28,200	4.0	58	288	41,800
Incisor	Dentin	1.3	19	125	18,000	6.0	85	232	33,700

*From Stanford, Weigel, Paffenbarger, and Sweeney, J Am Dent Assoc 60:746–756, 1960.

Table 3–4. *Compressive Properties of Some Tooth Restorative Materials**

MATERIAL	MODULUS OF ELASTICITY		PROPORTIONAL LIMIT		MODULUS OF RESILIENCE		STRENGTH	
	$MPa \times 10^4$	$psi \times 10^5$	MPa	psi	$Joules/m^3 \times 10^5$	$in\text{-}lb/in^3$	MPa	psi
Filling resin	.19	2.7	44	6400	5.2	76	76	11,000
Zinc phosphate cement	.89	13	60	8600	2.0	28	82	12,000
Amalgam	1.4	20	207	30,000	15.5	225	398	57,800
Inlay gold alloy (medium)	7.7	113	166	24,100	1.8	26		

*From Stanford, Weigel, Paffenbarger, and Sweeney, J Am Dent Assoc 60:746–756, 1960.

better able to absorb impact energy. Enamel is a brittle substance, with a comparatively high modulus of elasticity, a low proportional limit, and a low modulus of resilience. However, supported by the dentin with its ability to deform elastically, teeth seldom fracture under normal occlusion. The principle of backing a brittle substance with a plastic material, in order to increase the flexibility of the former under load, is well known by the structural engineer.

The compressive properties of the more popular restorative materials used in operative dentistry are presented in Table 3–4. Only the metallic materials (amalgam and gold alloy) approach the properties of the tooth. Although the modulus of resilience of the gold alloy is the lowest of the materials considered, it effectively resists forces of mastication because of its considerable toughness. It has a relatively high proportional limit and high ductility, both of which contribute to its toughness. When the gold alloy is subjected to high stress it tends to deform rather than fracture.

Amalgam has a higher modulus of resilience than does gold, but it is a brittle material. Thus, in instances of extreme stress it fractures rather than deforms.

Criteria of Selection   Inasmuch as most of the physical properties that have been described have been obtained on specimen shapes and sizes, and under types of stress that are in some cases dissimilar to oral conditions, the question at once arises as to how dental materials can be selected by the dentist upon the basis of these properties. The engineer employs similar criteria for the selection of materials for the construction of a bridge, for example, but he has an advantage over the dentist in this respect, inasmuch as he knows before-hand, at least approximately, what the expected stresses on his structure will be. Furthermore, he always multiplies these expected stress values by a "safety factor" in order that the structure may be able to withstand a certain amount of overstress.

Unfortunately, the magnitude of the forces of mastication is not known to the extent that the dentist can predict the stresses to which the restorative appliances will be subjected. General ideas as to the physical properties as well as rheological characteristics and color that are required for the materials employed can be obtained with experience, however. For example, if a certain gold alloy has given service in a certain type of dental restoration over a considerable period of time, it is reasonably certain that the alloy is satisfacto-ry. The physical properties of the alloy can be determined, such as its proportional limit, modulus of elasticity, and tensile strength, and these values can serve as criteria for the selection of other materials for similar use.

The physical properties can also be used as criteria for improvement of restorative appliances. For example, a dentist discovers that a certain patient has permanently deformed a dental appliance in service. Presumably, this patient exerts great stresses in the appliance during mastication. In such a case, the logical procedure is to remake the appliance with material that possesses a higher proportional limit and Brinell hardness number.

The use of such criteria has also been valuable to the manufacturer in the development of new and improved materials. With such criteria, the success or failure of the material can largely be predicted, and the patient saved much discomfort and injury to oral tissues.

It is also on such a basis that the requirements of the various dental materials specifications are determined. As discussed in a previous chapter, the most valuable criterion of selection for the dentist is whether the particular material meets the requirements of such specifications. If it does meet these requirements, the dentist can be sure that the material will be satisfactory when it is used properly.

BIOLOGICAL CONSIDERATIONS

The science of dental materials must by necessity encompass a knowledge and appreciation of certain biological considerations that are associated with the selection and use of materials designed for the oral cavity. Strength or resistance to deformation is unimportant if the material is injurious to the pulp or soft tissues. A number of factors must be considered to ensure that the health of oral tissues is preserved or restored.

Microleakage With the exception of those systems based upon polyacrylic acid (Chapter 29), none of the traditional restorative materials used in dentistry provide adhesion to tooth structure, for the reasons previously discussed. Thus, a microscopic space always exists between the restoration and the prepared cavity. The use of radioisotope tracers, dyes, the scanning electron microscope, and other techniques has clearly demonstrated that fluids and oral debris can penetrate freely along the interface between the restoration and the tooth, as diagrammed in Figure 3–16.

This phenomenon is referred to as *microleakage*. Probably microleakage can be identified with various types of dyscrasia that are commonly associated with restorative materials. Obviously gross penetration of acids and microorganisms could serve as the precursor to caries at the margins of the restoration. Accumulation of debris in that area also enhances the possibility for stain and discoloration.

If the leakage is severe, bacterial growth occurs between the restoration and the cavity wall and even into the dentinal tubules. It has been concluded that the toxic products liberated by such microorganisms might produce continuing irritation to the pulp.[11, 12] Such studies suggest, therefore, that the microleakage phenomenon may be as great a cause for pulp pathology associated with certain restorative materials as are the biological characteristics of the material itself. Further research is needed to identify the specific effects of microbial activity as associated with microleakage. However, the phenomenon has been associated with postoperative sensitivity following

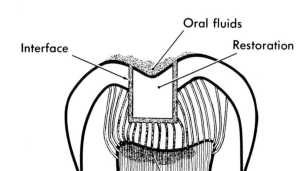

Oral fluids

Interface

Restoration

Figure 3–16 Schematic diagram of the microleakage phenomenon. In this case the penetration of possible irritants from the oral cavity has extended along the entire tooth-restoration interface, through the dentin, and into the pulp. (Modified from Massler, M.: Adhesive Restorative Materials, Spencer, Ind., Owens Litho Service.)

Penetration into pulp

placement of the restoration.[13] The superiority of certain types of materials and techniques in reducing postoperative sensitivity has been ascribed to their ability to adapt better to tooth structure and thereby minimize microleakage. These matters will be discussed in the following chapters as they relate to the proper use of various materials. Although significant progress has been made in designing materials and techniques that will lessen the problems of microleakage, further research is needed to eliminate the gap between the restoration and the tooth. A complete review of the current state of the art in this area can be found in the literature.[14]

Thermal Changes   Tooth structure and dental restorations are continually exposed to hot and cold beverages and foods. Instantaneous temperature fluctuation during the course of an average meal may be as great as 65° C (150° F). As previously noted, the thermal conductivity and coefficient of thermal expansion of restorative materials are important properties to be considered in preserving the health of the pulp and in minimizing the increased microleakage that may occur as a result of temperature cycling.

Galvanism   The presence of dissimilar metals in the oral cavity creates small currents. Thus, the irritation produced by the current generated when a gold inlay opposes an amalgam restoration, for example, may on occasion cause sensitivity. The significance of these currents and the methods for treatment of the problem will be discussed in later chapters.

Toxic Effects of Materials   Few, if any, dental materials are totally inert from a physiological standpoint. They contain a variety of potentially toxic or irritating ingredients. In addition, the chemical reactions that occur during the setting or hardening of the material may produce an undesirable effect upon the pulp.

To summarize, the dental pulp may be subjected to various types of injury before, during, and after restoration of the carious tooth. The dentist must be knowledgeable as to the cause of irritation and must take the necessary steps to eliminate or minimize them. Otherwise, degenerating pulpal reactions may continue with accompanying sensitivity.

Dental materials must also be nonirritating to soft tissues. None of the materials used in an artificial denture should produce an allergic or sensitizing effect to the underlying tissue, for example.

Recognizing the importance of the biological characteristics of dental materials, the American Dental Association has developed a series of tests that should provide acceptable methodology for screening materials for their toxicity and irritational characteristics.[15] With the advent of such a specification, the dentist is assured of a specific biological index for every material used in the oral cavity, in addition to its certification as to suitability from a mechanical standpoint.

Toxicity Evaluation of Dental Materials   Ideally, then, a dental material that is to be used in the oral cavity should be harmless to the pulp and the soft tissues. Also, it should contain no toxic diffusible substance that can be absorbed into the circulatory system to cause a systemic toxic response. The material should be free of potential sensitizing agents that could lead to an allergic response. Finally, the material should have no carcinogenic potential.

Tests are now available for evaluation of these biological aspects of dental materials. These tests can be classified into three categories.[16] Level I tests are screening tests whereby the material is evaluated for acute systemic toxicity, and for its cytotoxic, irritational, allergenic, and carcinogenic potentials. Level II tests are usage tests in which the material is evaluated in experimental animals under conditions that simulate the clinical use of the material. If the screening and the usage tests show that the material is safe, the material is then tested in humans for reactions and performance in the clinical situation (Level III tests). No longer is it morally or legally acceptable to conduct human experimentation prior to adequate testing in animals.

Acute systemic toxicity (Level I) is evaluated by oral administration, via a gastric tube, of a certain dosage of the reacted or hardened material, suspended or dissolved in a suitable vehicle to suitable laboratory animals (e.g., albino rats). The animals are examined daily for at least 2 weeks. Toxic manifestations or deaths are recorded. If more than 50 per cent of the animals survive, the material would have complied with this test.[15]

Screening for the cytotoxic and irritational potential could be done either in vitro or in vivo. In vitro tests rely mainly on cell culture techniques using established cell lines such as mouse L-929 fibroblasts and human HeLa cells. Several methods are available.[16-18] One is the monolayer agar overlay method. An overlay of agar is spread over L-cells which have grown into a monolayer in a culture plate. The material to be tested is placed over the overlay and the culture plate is incubated for a specific period. Toxic materials would show clear zones of dead cells.

In vivo tests for evaluation of the irritational potential of dental materials rely mainly on implanting the material subcutaneously in rats or intramuscularly in rabbits. One of the simplest methods for determining the primary irritational qualities of a material is to implant the test substance subdermally into rats.[19] The animals are sacrificed at various time intervals, and the sites of the implants are examined grossly and microscopically. These responses are then in turn compared with those of appropriate controls. Zinc oxide and eugenol cement is known to have a low irritational potential and is used as a negative control. Silicate cement has a high irritational potential and is used as a positive control.

The allergenic potential of the material can be tested by administration of the material intradermally into guinea pigs and then later challenging the animal with the material applied to the surface of the skin.[16] Erythema and swelling at the site of contact indicate the development of an allergic reaction.

The carcinogenic potential of a material can be tested in vivo or in vitro. In vivo tests include subcutaneous implantation of the material in suitable laboratory animals (rats, mice). The animals are sacrificed after 1 and 2 years and examined grossly and microscopically for the development of tumors. In vitro tests include the Ames test.[20] Mutant strains of a particular bacterium have been developed that are histidine dependent. The microorganisms are inoculated in a histidine-free culture medium in the presence of the material to be tested, and microsomal fractions are obtained from the liver. The latter contains the enzymes needed for activating indirectly acting carcinogens. If the material tested has a mutagenic potential, reverse mutation of the microorganism would occur, with growth in the histidine-free medium. There is a strong positive correlation between the mutagenic and the carcinogenic potential of chemicals.

At Level II, the material is tested in animals under conditions that simulate the clinical use of the material.[21, 22] For evaluation of pulp reactions, Class V cavities are prepared in sound teeth of subhuman primates. The cavities are then restored with the material under test. The teeth are extracted at different time intervals, and histologic sections are made through the cavity and the underlying pulp. The sections are examined microscopically for the presence and intensity of pulp inflammation and evidence of repair. The reactions are compared with those produced by zinc oxide and eugenol cement (negative controls) and silicate cement (positive controls).

Having passed the screening tests and the usage tests in animals, the material is then ready for evaluation in humans for reactions and performance in the clinical situation (Level III).

As was noted in the Introduction, the FDA in the United States and counterpart national agencies in other countries also monitor the biocompatibility of dental materials and devices. The end result of such programs has been a greater awareness by the dentist of the importance of the biological characteristics of the materials he uses and an improvement of commercial products in those properties.

References

1. McLean J W: The Science and Art of Dental Ceramics. Volume 1: The Nature of Dental Ceramics and their Clinical Use. Amador City, Calif., Quintessence Publishing Co., Inc., 1979.
2. Braden M: Heat conduction in teeth and the effect of lining materials. J Dent Res 43:315, 1964.
3. Tibbetts V R, Schnell R J, Swartz M L, and Phillips R W: Thermal diffusion through amalgam and cement bases: Comparison of in vitro and in vivo measurements. J Dent Res 55:441, 1976.
4. Harper R H, Schnell R J, Swartz M L, and Phillips R W: In vivo measurements of thermal diffusion through restorations of various materials. J Prosthet Dent 43:180, 1980.
5. Stanford J W, Weigel K V, Paffenbarger G C, and Sweeney W T: Compressive properties of hard tooth tissue. J Am Dent Assoc 60:746, 1960.
6. Craig R G, Peyton F A, and Johnson D W: Compressive properties of enamel, dental cements and gold. J Dent Res 40:936, 1961.
7. Bowen R W and Rodriguez M S: Tensile strength and modulus of elasticity of tooth structure and several restorative materials. J Am Dent Assoc 64:378, 1962.
8. Black G V: Practical utility of accurate studies of the physical properties of teeth and of filling materials. Dent Cos 38:302, 1896.
9. Howell A H, and Manly R S: An electronic strain gauge for measuring oral forces. J Dent Res 27:705, 1948.
10. Manly R S and Shiere F R: Effect of dental deficiency on mastication and food preference. Oral Surg 3:674, 1950.
11. Brannstrom M and Nyborg H: The presence of bacteria in cavities filled with silicate cement and composite resin materials. Swed Dent J 64:149, 1971.
12. Brannstrom M and Vojinovic O: Response of the dental pulp to invasion of bacteria around three filling materials. J Dent Child 43:83, 1976.
13. Dachi S F and Stigers R W: Reduction of pulpal inflammation and thermal sensitivity in amalgam-restored teeth treated with copal varnish. J Am Dent Assoc 74:1281, 1967.
14. Going R E: Reducing marginal leakage: A review of materials and techniques. J Am Dent Assoc 99:646, 1979.
15. Council on Dental Materials and Devices: Recommended standard practices for biological evaluation of dental materials. J Am Dent Assoc 84:382, 1972.
16. Autian J: General toxicity and screening tests for dental materials. Int Dent J 24:235, 1974.

17. Spangberg L: Kinetic and quantitative evaluation of material cytotoxicity in vitro. Oral Surg 35:389, 1973.
18. Tronstad L, Wennberg A and Hasselgren G: Screening tests for dental materials. J Endo 4:304, 1978.
19. Mitchell, D F: Irritational qualities of dental materials. J Am Dent Assoc 59:954, 1959.
20. Ames B N, McCann J and Yamasaki E: Method for detection of mutagens and carcinogens with salmonella/mammalian microsome mutagenicity test. Mutat Res 31:347, 1975.
21. Langeland K: Criteria for biologic evaluation of anterior tooth filling materials. Int Dent J 17:405, 1967.
22. Stanley H R: Design for a human pulp study. Oral Surg 25:633, 1968.

4 GYPSUM PRODUCTS: CHEMISTRY OF SETTING. BASIC PRINCIPLES

A number of gypsum products are used in dentistry as important adjuncts to dental operations. Various types of plaster are used to form molds and casts on which dental prostheses and restorations are constructed. When the plaster is mixed with silica, it is known as *dental investment*. Such dental investments are used to form molds for the casting of dental restorations in metal; they will be discussed at length in Chapter 26. The present discussion will be confined to the essentially pure gypsum products, such as plaster, which will harden when they are mixed with water.

An excellent illustration of the importance of plaster in dentistry is its use in the preparation of a cast for an artificial denture. A mixture of plaster of Paris and water is placed in an *impression tray* and seated against the tissues of the jaw, for example. The plaster is allowed to harden, or *set*, and then the impression is withdrawn. The dentist now has a *negative* form of those tissues of the oral cavity. If another variety of plaster known as "dental stone" is now mixed with water, poured into the impression, and allowed to set, the hardened plaster impression serves as a mold to form a *positive* model, or *cast* master. It is on this cast that the denture is constructed, without the patient being present.

GYPSUM AND GYPSUM PRODUCTS

Gypsum Gypsum is a mineral mined in various parts of the world. Chemically, the mineral as used for dental purposes is nearly pure calcium sulfate dihydrate ($CaSO_4 \cdot 2H_2O$).

Different forms of gypsum have been used for many centuries for construction purposes. It is supposed that the alabaster used in the building of King Solomon's temple of Biblical fame was a form of gypsum. Products made from gypsum are widely used in industry, and practically every home and building has walls of plaster.

Dental Plaster and Stone These materials are the results of the calcining of gypsum. Commercially, the gypsum is ground and subjected to temperatures of 110 to 120° C (230 to 250° F) to drive off part of the water of crystallization. This corresponds to the first step in reaction (1). As the temperature is further raised, the remaining water of crystallization is removed, and products are formed as indicated.

$$CaSO_4 \cdot 2H_2O \xrightarrow[110-130° C]{} (CaSO_4)_2 \cdot H_2O \xrightarrow[130-200° C]{} CaSO_4 \xrightarrow[200-1000° C]{} CaSO_4 \tag{1}$$

| Gypsum (calcium sulfate dihydrate) | Plaster or stone (calcium sulfate hemihydrate) | Hexagonal anhydrite | Orthorhombic anhydrite |

The principal constituent of the dental *plasters* and *stones* is the calcium sulfate hemihydrate, $(CaSO_4)_2 \cdot H_2O$ (or $CaSO_4 \cdot \frac{1}{2} H_2O$). Depending upon the method of calcination, different forms of the hemihydrate can be obtained. These forms will be referred to as α- or β-hemihydrate.*

If gypsum is heated to the temperatures indicated in the first part of reaction (1) in a kettle, vat, or rotary kiln open to the air, a crystalline form of the hemihydrate results known as β-hemihydrate, or more popularly, as plaster of Paris. As can be seen in Figure 4–1, the β-hemihydrate crystals are characterized by their sponginess and irregular shape in contrast to the

---

*Current knowledge[1] suggests that the use of the α and β prefixes should be discontinued as they indicate the presence of two phases, from the point of view of the phase rule, but this is not the case. There is a trend toward using the adjective that describes the process by which the materials are made, i.e., autoclaved hemihydrate and dry calcined hemihydrate. The α and β designations will be continued in this edition because of tradition and convenience. However, it should not be inferred that there are any mineralographic distinctions between them. The differences between the α- and β-hemihydrates are a result of differences in crystallite size, surface area, and lattice perfection. In reality, the beta form is a fibrous aggregate of fine crystals with capillary pores, whereas the alpha form consists of cleavage fragments and crystals in the form of rods or prisms.

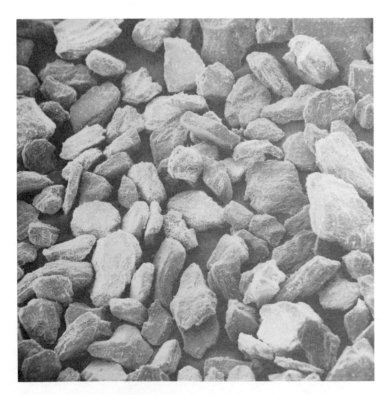

Figure 4–1 Powder particles of plaster of Paris. Crystals are irregular in shape and spongy. × 400. (Courtesy of B. Giammara and R. Neiman.)

α-hemihydrate (stone) crystals, which are more dense and which have a prismatic shape. Powder particles of dental stone are shown in Figure 4–2.

Different procedures can be employed to obtain α-hemihydrate.[2] The gypsum can be (1) calcined under steam pressure in an autoclave at a temperature of 120 to 130° C (250 to 265° F); (2) dehydrated in an autoclave in the presence of sodium succinate (0.5 per cent or less); or (3) dehydrated in a boiling solution of 30 per cent calcium chloride in a kettle. The product of these processes is the principal constituent of the dental stones with which casts and models are made.

When the α-hemihydrate is mixed with water, reaction (1) is reversed, as described in the next section, and the product obtained is one much stronger and harder than that resulting from β-hemihydrate. The chief reason for this difference is that the α-hemihydrate powder requires much less gauging water when it is mixed than does the β-hemihydrate. The β-hemihydrate requires more water to float its powder particles so that they can be stirred, because the crystals are more irregular in shape and are porous in character.

Although particle size is one of the chief factors in determining the amount of gauging water required, the particle size distribution also plays an important role. The grinding of the particles after the preparation of the hemihydrate can eliminate needle-like crystals and will provide better packing characteristics, hence lowering the amount of mixing or gauging water required.

Adhesion between the particles of hemihydrate is also a factor in determining the amount of water required to produce a product which can be poured. Small amounts of some surface active materials, such as gum arabic plus lime, added to the hemihydrate can reduce markedly the water requirements of both plaster and dental stone.

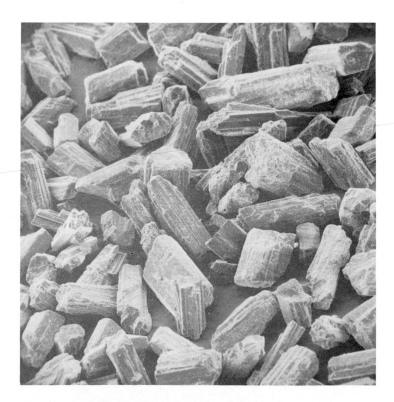

Figure 4–2 Powder particles of dental stone. Crystals are prismatic and more regular in shape than those of plaster. The very fine particles that are normally present have been removed, as was done for the plaster particles in Figure 4–1. × 400. (Courtesy of B. Giammara and R. Neiman.)

From the above, it is clear that various gypsum products will require different amounts of gauging water and that these differences are accounted for principally by shape and compactness of the crystals. These factors are regulated by the manufacturer and are dependent on the type of process used, dehydration temperatures, particle size of the gypsum to be calcined, length of time of calcination, finished product grinding, and addition of surface active ingredients to the final product.

Commercial Gypsum Products The various plasters and stone that are available commercially consist essentially of one of the forms of hemihydrate. Since they are process products, however, they contain additional small amounts of impurities, unconverted hexagonal or orthorhombic anhydrites. Additional gypsum and other salts may also be added to control the setting time and expansion, as will be discussed.

SETTING OF GYPSUM PRODUCTS

Reaction (1) can be reversed as follows:

$$(CaSO_4)_2 \cdot H_2O + 3H_2O \longrightarrow 2CaSO_4 \cdot 2H_2O + Heat \qquad (2)$$

The product of the reaction is, of course, gypsum, and the heat evolved in the exothermic reaction is equivalent to the heat used originally in calcination.

The different products formed during calcination all react with water to form gypsum but at different rates. For example, hexagonal anhydrite reacts very rapidly, whereas the reaction may require hours when the orthorhombic anhydrite is mixed with water. This is due to the fact that the orthorhombic anhydrite has a more stable and closely packed crystal lattice. In any event, the hemihydrate phase is formed before the gypsum during hydration.

Setting Reactions Nature has provided us with a unique material in gypsum. The various hydrates have a relatively low solubility with a distinct difference in the solubility of the hemihydrate and the dihydrate. The dihydrate is too soluble for use in structures exposed to the atmosphere, which is probably fortunate, since such usage would long ago have exhausted our natural supply of gypsum.

In Table 4–1 it can be seen that the hemihydrate is three times more soluble in water than is the dihydrate. Thus the setting reactions can be understood as follows:

1. When the hemihydrate is mixed with water, a suspension is formed that is fluid and workable.

2. The hemihydrate dissolves until it forms a saturated solution.

Table 4–1. *Solubility of Gypsum and Gypsum Products (20° C)**

TYPE	FORMULA	SOLUBILITY, GM/100 ML
Dihydrate	$CaSO_4 \cdot 2H_2O$	0.2
Hemihydrate	$(CaSO_4)_2 \cdot H_2O$	0.9
Anhydrite	$CaSO_4$	0.3

*From Worner, Aust Dent J, 46 (1942).

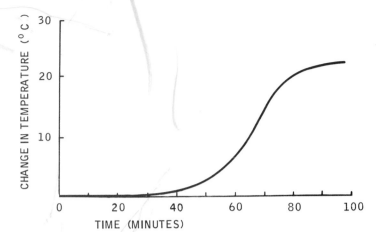

Figure 4–3 Temperature increase during the setting of plaster of Paris. (Courtesy of A. R. Docking.)

3. This saturated solution of the hemihydrate is supersaturated with respect to the dihydrate, so the latter precipitates out.

4. As the dihydrate precipitates, the solution is no longer saturated with the hemihydrate, so it continues to dissolve. Thus the process continues, solution of the hemihydrate and precipitation of the dihydrate as either new crystals or further growth on those already present.

Thus the reaction is continuous and repetitious until exhausted. Also, it is actually quite simple.

The reaction rate can be followed by the exothermic heat evolved (temperature rise), as shown in Figure 4–3. Initially there is very little reaction and thus little or no rise in temperature. That time is referred to as the *induction period.* This is accompanied by a slight thickening of the mass, which permits the mix to be poured into an impression or tray. As the amount of gypsum forming increases, the mass thickens and then hardens into needle-like clusters called *spherulites,* as shown in Figure 4–4. Finally the intermeshing and entangling of crystals of gypsum lead to a strong, solid structure (Fig. 4–5).

W/P Ratio The amounts of water and hemihydrate should be gauged accurately by weight. The ratio of the water to the hemihydrate powder is

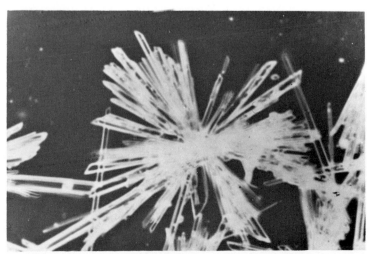

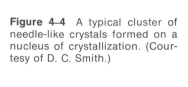

Figure 4–4 A typical cluster of needle-like crystals formed on a nucleus of crystallization. (Courtesy of D. C. Smith.)

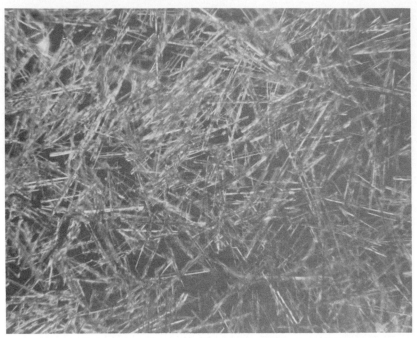

Figure 4–5 Dark field photomicrograph of set plaster mixed with excess water to prevent the field from becoming opaque. × 200. (Courtesy of R. Neiman.)

usually expressed as the water/powder ratio or the quotient obtained when the weight (or volume) of the water is divided by the weight of the powder. The ratio is usually abbreviated as W/P.

For example, if 100 gm of plaster are mixed with 60 ml of water, the W/P ratio will be 0.6; if 100 gm of dental stone are mixed with 28 ml of water, the W/P ratio will be 0.28.

The W/P ratio is a very important factor in determining the physical and chemical properties of the final gypsum product. For example, the higher the W/P ratio, the longer will be the setting time and the weaker will be the gypsum product. Although the W/P ratio will vary for the particular brand of plaster or stone, the following are some typical recommended ranges: plaster, 0.45 to 0.55; Type III stone, 0.30 to 0.35; Type IV stone, 0.20 to 0.25.

Setting Time Reaction (2) requires a definite time for completion. The powder is mixed with the water, and the time elapsing from the beginning of mixing until the material hardens is known as the *setting time*.

It is important that the dentist be able to control the time during which reaction (2) takes place so that the product becomes hard at a convenient time after mixing. For example, in the taking of an impression, the plaster should have a short setting time so that the patient will not be unduly inconvenienced by holding the plaster in his mouth for too long a time. On the other hand, if the plaster sets too fast, the dentist will not have sufficient time to mix it with water, to place it in the impression tray, and to carry it to the patient's mouth.

The setting time is generally measured by some type of penetration test. The most common method is by means of the Vicat needle, seen in Figure 4–6. The rod holding the needle weighs 300 gm; the needle is 1 mm in diameter and

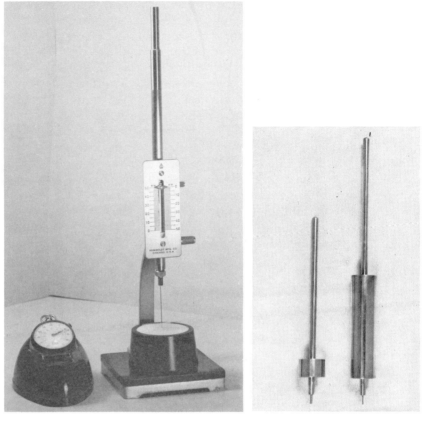

Figure 4–6   Vicat needle, *left,* being used to measure the setting time of a gypsum product. The setting time is the elapsed time from start of mix until needle no longer penetrates to the bottom. *Right,* set of Gillmore needles. (Photograph of Vicat needle courtesy of R. Neiman.)

5 cm long. The rod is supported so that the needle can be lowered onto the surface of the plaster contained in the truncated cone container. The time that elapses from the start of the mix until the needle no longer penetrates to the bottom of the plaster is known as the setting time.

Another instrument, the Gillmore needle (Fig. 4–6), may also be employed for this purpose, although it is more commonly used for determining the setting time of dental cements. The smaller 113.4 gm (¼ pound) needle has a 2.13 mm point; the other needle weighs 453.6 gm (1 pound) and has a 1.06 mm diameter point. The water and plaster are gauged in a certain W/P ratio and mixed for a specified time. The mixture is spread out in a shallow container and the surface impressed with the point of the 113.4 gm needle. The elapsed time from start of the mix until the needle no longer penetrates the surface is known as the *initial setting time.* For all practical purposes, the initial setting time obtained with this Gillmore needle is the same as the time obtained with the Vicat needle. When the other needle is used in the same manner, the elapsed time until the point no longer penetrates the surface of the set plaster is known as the *final setting time.*

A third method for the determination of the setting time is to note the time at which the gloss disappears from the surface of the plaster and water mixture.[3] As in the previous tests, the *loss of gloss* is measured in minutes from the time the mixing begins. The loss of gloss precedes the setting time obtained with the Vicat needle by several minutes. There are other methods for measuring setting time, but they are not generally used in dentistry.

In actuality, all of the methods for assessing setting time are measurements of the progress of the crystallization. When the interstices in the skeleton framework formed by the growing crystals are sufficiently developed, they withdraw the surface water film by capillary action to replace the water of hydration. At this point, the loss of gloss occurs. Later, when the rigidity of the intermeshed crystals is sufficient to prevent full penetration of the Vicat needle, the initial set occurs. Finally, when the crystalline framework will support the needle, the final setting time is determined. The crystallization sometimes continues for a considerable period after the observed setting time is measured.

From a practical standpoint, none of these tests of setting time are truly reliable for determining the working time or when the material is ready to use. The measurements are indicative of the stages of setting that are occurring in this continuous process and will vary with the W/P ratio, method, and time of mixing. The tests are useful in ensuring batch control and uniformity of the product.

Control of the Setting Time As previously noted, it is necessary for the dentist to control the setting time. Theoretically, there are at least three methods by which such control can be effected.[4, 5]

1. The solubility of the hemihydrate can be increased or decreased. For example, if the solubility of the hemihydrate is increased, supersaturation of the calcium sulfate will be greater. The rate of crystalline deposition will thus be increased.

2. The number of nuclei of crystallization can be increased or decreased. The greater the number of nuclei of crystallization, the faster the gypsum crystals will form and the sooner the hardening of the mass will occur because of crystalline intermeshing.

3. If the rate of crystal growth can be increased or decreased, the setting time can be accelerated or retarded respectively.

Practically, the control can be effected either by the physical or chemical composition of the gypsum product or by the method of manipulation used by the dentist.

IMPURITIES If the calcination is not complete so that gypsum particles remain, or if the manufacturer adds gypsum, the setting time will be shortened because of the increase in potential nuclei of crystallization.

If orthorhombic anhydrite is present, the induction period will be increased; it will be decreased if hexagonal anhydrite is present.

FINENESS The finer the particle size of the hemihydrate, the faster the mix will harden, particularly if the product has been ground during manufacture. Not only will the rate of the solution of the hemihydrate be increased but also the gypsum nuclei will be more numerous and, therefore, a more rapid rate of crystallization will occur.

W/P RATIO The more water used for mixing, the fewer nuclei there will be per unit volume. Consequently, the setting time will be prolonged. This effect is evidenced by the results presented in Table 4–2.

MIXING Within practical limits, the longer and the more rapidly the plaster

Table 4–2. *Effect of the W/P Ratio and the Mixing Time on the Setting Time of Plaster of Paris**

W/P Ratio	Mixing Time (min)	Setting Time (min)
0.45	0.5	5.25
0.45	1.0	3.25
0.60	1.0	7.25
0.60	2.0	4.50
0.80	1.0	10.50
0.80	2.0	7.75
0.80	3.0	5.75

*From Gibson and Johnson, J Soc Chem Ind, 51:25T (1932).

is mixed, the shorter the setting time will be. Some gypsum crystals form immediately when the plaster or stone is brought into contact with the water. As the mixing begins, the formation of these crystals increases; at the same time the crystals are broken up by the mixing spatula and are distributed throughout the mixture, with the resulting formation of more nuclei of crystallization. Thus, the setting time is decreased, as indicated in Table 4–2.

TEMPERATURE Although the effect of temperature on the setting time is likely to be erratic and may vary from one plaster (or stone) to another, little change occurs between 0° C (32° F) and 50° C (120° F); but if the temperature of the plaster-water mixture exceeds approximately 50° C (120° F) a gradually increasing retardation occurs. As the temperature approaches 100° C (212° F), no reaction takes place. At the higher temperatures, reaction (2) is reversed, with the tendency for any gypsum crystals formed to be changed to the hemihydrate form.

RETARDERS AND ACCELERATORS Probably the most effective and practical method for the control of the setting time is the addition of certain chemical modifiers to the mixture of plaster or dental stone. If the chemical added decreases the setting time, it is known as an *accelerator*; if it increases the setting time, it is known as a *retarder*.

Retarders generally act by forming an absorbed layer on the hemihydrate to reduce its solubility and upon the gypsum crystals present to inhibit growth. Organic materials, such as glue, gelatin, and some gums, behave in this manner. Another type of retarder consists of salts which form a layer of a calcium salt that is less soluble than is the sulfate. In small concentrations many inorganic salts act as accelerators, but when the concentration is increased they can become retarders.

Since the action of these chemical additions also affects other properties, such as setting expansion, the behavior of accelerators and retarders will be discussed at greater length in a subsequent section.

Setting Expansion Regardless of the type of gypsum product employed, an expansion of the mass can be detected during the change from the hemihydrate to the dihydrate. Depending upon the composition of the gypsum product, this observed expansion may be as low as 0.06 per cent linear to as high as 0.5 per cent.

On the other hand, if the equivalent volumes of the hemihydrate, water, and the reaction product (dihydrate) are compared, the volume of the dihydrate formed will be found to be less than the equivalent volumes of the hemihydrate and the water required.

The calculations are as follows:

$$(CaSO_4)_2 \cdot H_2O + 3H_2O \longrightarrow 2CaSO_4 \cdot 2H_2O$$

Mol. mass	290.284	54.048	344.332
Density (gm/cm^3)	2.75	0.997	2.32
Equiv. vol.	105.556 +	54.211 $\longrightarrow$	148.405
		159.767 $\longrightarrow$	148.405

$$\text{Change in volume} = \left(\frac{148.405 - 159.767}{159.767} \right) 100 = -7.11 \text{ per cent}$$

It follows, therefore, that actually a volume contraction occurs during the setting.

This seemingly anomalous situation that, although a contraction can be calculated, an expansion is actually observed, can be rationalized on the basis of the mechanism of the crystallization.

As previously noted, the crystallization process is pictured as an outgrowth of crystals from nuclei of crystallization. On the basis of the entanglement of the dihydrate crystals, as indicated in Figures 4–4 and 4–5, it is not difficult to imagine that crystals growing from the nuclei not only intermesh but may also intercept each other during growth. If the growth of one crystal is interrupted by another, a stress is present at this point in the direction of the growth of the impinging crystal.

If this process is repeated by thousands of the crystals during growth, it is possible that this outward stress or thrust could produce an expansion of the entire mass; thus, an *apparent* or observed expansion could take place even though the *true volume* of the crystals alone may be less as calculated. This crystal impingement and movement results in the production of micropores.[6]

Since the product of reaction (2) (gypsum) in practice is greater in *external* volume but less in *crystalline* volume, it follows that the set material must be porous.

The final structure immediately after setting is, therefore, composed of interlocking crystals between which are the micropores and pores containing the excess water required for mixing, as previously described. On drying, the excess water is lost, and the total empty space is greatly increased.

The porosity of the set product for various W/P ratios of hemihydrate can be calculated,[7] as indicated in Table 4–3. As can be noted, the greater the W/P ratio, the greater is the porosity. Such a consideration is to be expected on the basis that there are fewer nuclei of crystallization as the W/P ratio is increased. Consequently, there is less intermeshing of the crystals of gypsum.

As far as the dentist is concerned, only that part of the setting expansion which occurs after the initial set is of interest. Any expansion or contraction that occurs before this time can be overcome by friction between the mold surface onto which the plaster is poured and the fluid plaster. At the time of initial set, the crystalline framework is sufficiently rigid that it can overcome, for the most part, such frictional retention. However, it cannot always

Table 4–3. *Porosity of Set Gypsum as Affected by the W/P Ratio**

W/P RATIO	POROSITY *(per cent)*
0.25	10.3
0.30	15.3
0.35	20.3
0.40	25.3
0.50	35.3
0.60	45.3
1.00	85.3

*From Jørgensen, Odont T (1953).

overcome any confinement by the mold boundaries. Furthermore, any initial contraction that occurs during the induction period will not affect the accuracy, since the mix is fluid at this stage and it occurs at the free surface.

For example, if a mix of plaster and water is spread on a glass surface, the distance between any two surface reference points will not change appreciably during the induction period. The adhesion of the water-powder mix to the glass can prevent the linear contraction theoretically expected. Only when the crystalline framework is sufficiently rigid (after the initial set) will a visible setting expansion be evident.

On the other hand, if the frictional factor is reduced by spreading the mix on the surface of mercury,[8] for example, the setting expansion curve shown in Figure 4–7 might result. The initial contraction is evident. When sufficient crystals form to produce the outward thrust by impingement, the setting expansion follows. The initial setting time occurs approximately at the minimal point of the curve, the point at which the expansion begins. According to the graph, the stone actually shrank during setting and never recovered its original dimensions. On the other hand, in the previous experiment on the glass plate, a setting expansion of approximately 0.12 per cent would have been reported.

Control of Setting Expansion As will be discussed in subsequent chapters, sometimes a setting expansion is advantageous in a dental operation and sometimes it is disadvantageous, since it may be a source of error. Consequent-

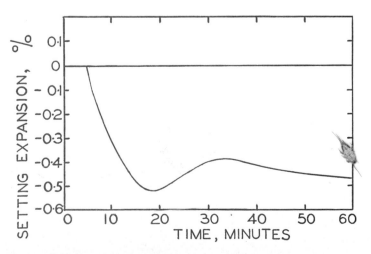

Figure 4–7 Dimensional changes which occur during the setting of a gypsum product. (Courtesy of A. R. Docking.)

Table 4–4. *Effect of the W/P Ratio and Mixing Time on the*
Setting Expansion of Plaster of Paris*

W/P	MIXING TIME (min)	SETTING EXPANSION (per cent)
0.45	0.5	0.41
0.45	1.0	0.51
0.60	1.0	0.29
0.60	2.0	0.41
0.80	1.0	0.24

*From Gibson and Johnson, J Soc Chem Ind, 51:25T (1932).

ly, it is necessary to control it to obtain the desired accuracy in dental applications.

As can be noted from the experimental results presented in Table 4–4, the less the W/P ratio and the longer the mixing time within practical limits, the greater is the setting expansion.

The effect of the W/P ratio on the setting expansion is to be expected on theoretical grounds. Since, with the higher W/P ratios, fewer nuclei of crystallization per unit volume are present than with the thicker mixes, and since it can be assumed that the space between the nuclei will be greater in such a case, it follows that there will be less growth interaction of the dihydrate crystals with less outward thrust resulting.

The most effective method for the control of the setting expansion is the addition of chemicals.

Theory of Accelerators and Retarders   Not only do the chemical accelerators and retarders regulate the setting time of the gypsum products but also they generally reduce the setting expansion. The theory of such effects is still obscure in many areas. One study confirms that accelerators increase the rate of gypsum formation, whereas retarders have a reverse effect.[9]

The concentration of the chemical additive is a very potent factor in its effect on the setting time. For example, sodium chloride in concentrations of less than 20 per cent is an accelerator of the setting reaction. In higher concentrations, the setting time is increased; in concentrations of 20 per cent or more, sodium chloride acts as a retarder.[5]

The explanation of this effect is that, in low concentrations, the sodium chloride increases the rate at which the hemihydrate goes into solution. Thus, the saturation of the solution [reaction (2)] occurs more rapidly. The result is a shorter induction period and a more rapid rate of growth of the dihydrate crystals. As the dihydrate forms, the concentration of the sodium chloride increases so that the remaining water finally becomes supersaturated. The sodium chloride crystals that form may deposit on the nuclei of crystallization* so that further crystallization is retarded.

Solutions of sodium sulfate act similarly. In concentrations lower than approximately 12 per cent, the chemical acts as an accelerator, but in higher concentrations the setting time is slower. The maximum accelerator effect occurs at approximately 3.4 per cent.

The most commonly used accelerator is potassium sulfate, which appears to accelerate the setting time in any concentration. In low concentrations its

*A process known as nuclei "poisoning."

accelerating action is the same as that of sodium chloride, but in concentrations of 2 to 3 per cent or above, the reaction product is syngenite [$K_2Ca(SO_4)_2 \cdot H_2O$], which crystallizes very rapidly. The setting time becomes so short that the effect of higher concentrations is impossible to study.

One of the most effective retarders is borax. It increases the setting time in any concentration because insoluble calcium borate is a product of its reaction with calcium sulfate. The calcium borate deposits on the nuclei of crystallization and thus effectively reduces the rate of crystallization.

The reduction of the setting expansion is effected by either a change in the crystalline form of the dihydrate or an initial rate of crystallization so rapid that subsequent growth is resisted.

For example, if the concentrations of sodium chloride and sodium sulfate are low, the dihydrate crystals are spherulitic, but they are shorter and thicker than the normal gypsum crystals. Consequently, the setting expansion is reduced. In higher concentrations, the gypsum crystals are fewer, flat, and tabular in shape. Consequently, a low setting expansion results, since with this crystalline form there is less crystal interaction during growth. A similar tabular crystalline form occurs when borax and similar retarders are used, with a consequent reduction in setting expansion for the same reason.

When the setting expansion of a gypsum product accelerated with a solution of potassium sulfate is measured on a mercury bath, it is found to be greater than normal.[8] The spherulitic gypsum crystals formed in this environment are thicker and longer than usual. Consequently, a greater setting expansion is to be expected. However, the crystals begin to form copiously very early in the reaction period, even before the end of the induction period. Consequently, the plastic mass may appear to expand before the initial set when floated on the mercury. Such an expansion is not, of course, evident in practice when the time between the induction period and the initial set is very short. The longer needles enmesh with each other so rapidly that a rigid framework is formed before the crystallization is complete and the setting expansion is reduced thereby.

"Poisoning" of nuclei also occurs in the presence of many colloids. Dried blood, most colloidal gels, and similar colloidal forms are excellent retarders for gypsum products for this reason.

Most soluble sulfates in the proper concentration accelerate the setting rate. Powdered gypsum accelerates the setting rate when added to the hemihydrate powder, since the particles act as nuclei of crystallization. It does not affect the setting expansion to any extent, however.

The citrates, acetates, and borates generally retard the reaction. For a given anion, the particular cation employed appears to affect the retardation markedly. For example, with the acetates, the order of retardation[10] in terms of the cation employed appears to be $Ca^{+2} < K^+ < H^+$, whereas potassium tartrate has a marked accelerating effect in contrast to the calcium salt, which has little effect on setting.[11] The behavior of citrates is more complex.[12]

Hygroscopic Setting Expansion It has been assumed in the discussion thus far that the plaster or stone is allowed to set in air. If the setting process is allowed to occur under water, the setting expansion may be more than doubled in magnitude.

The reason for the increased expansion when the hemihydrate is allowed to react under water is related to the additional crystal growth permitted and not to any differences in chemical reaction (2).

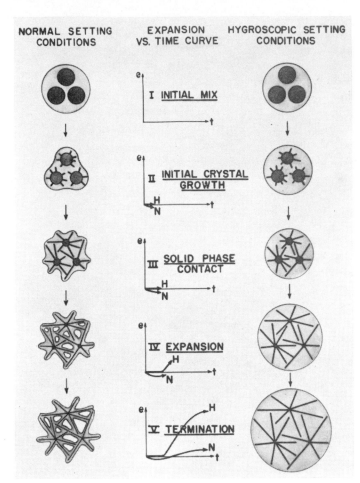

Figure 4–8 Diagrammatic representation of the setting expansion of plaster. Left: the crystal growth is inhibited by the lack of excess water. Right: water added during setting provides more room for longer crystal growth. (From Mahler and Ady, J Dent Res May–June, 1960.)

The theory is illustrated diagrammatically in Figure 4–8. In stage I, shown at the top of the figure, the initial mix is represented by the three round particles of hemihydrate surrounded by water.

In stage II, the reaction has started and the crystals of the dihydrate are beginning to form. In the diagram on the left, the water around the particles is reduced by the hydration and the particles are drawn more closely together by the surface tension action of the water. In the right diagram, because the setting is taking place under water, the water of hydration is replaced and the distance between the particles remains the same.

As the crystals of dihydrate grow, they contact each other and the setting expansion begins. As indicated in stage III, the water around the particles is again decreased in the example on the left. The particles with their attached crystals tend to be drawn together as before but the contraction is opposed by the outward thrust of the growing crystals. On the other hand, the crystals in the right diagram are not so inhibited, since the water is again replenished from the outside. In fact, the original particles are now separated further as the crystals grow, and the setting expansion is definitely evident.

In stages IV and V the effect becomes more marked. The crystals being inhibited on the left become intermeshed and entangled much sooner than those on the right, which grow much more freely during the early stages before the intermeshing finally prevents further expansion. Consequently, the observed setting expansion that occurs when the gypsum product set under water may be greater than that which occurs during the setting in air.

It follows, therefore, that the basic mechanism of crystal growth is the same in both instances, and both phenomena are true setting expansions. In order to distinguish between them, the setting expansion without water immersion is often termed the *normal setting expansion* (N in Figure 4–8), whereas the expansion that occurs under water is known as *hygroscopic setting expansion* (H in Figure 4–8).

Again, it should be emphasized that the hygroscopic setting expansion is physical and not due to chemical reaction any more than is the normal setting expansion. The reduction in the W/P ratio increases the hygroscopic setting expansion and the normal setting expansion in the same manner. Increased spatulation results in increased hygroscopic expansion as well.

As might be expected from the theory, if insufficient water is added during setting, the hygroscopic setting expansion will be reduced. Also, if the addition of water is delayed, the hygroscopic expansion will be reduced, since the crystal framework formed before the water is added will inhibit further setting expansion, as previously discussed.

The hygroscopic expansion obtained during the setting of dental stone or plaster is generally small in magnitude. For example, a dental stone used in making casts may exhibit a normal linear setting expansion of 0.15 per cent, with a maximal hygroscopic expansion of not more than 0.30 per cent. Nevertheless, the error may be sufficient to cause the misfit of a denture or similar device made on the cast.

On the other hand, as will be explained in a subsequent chapter, the hygroscopic setting expansion of hemihydrate-bonded investments is sometimes utilized in the fabrication of accurate dental cast restorations.

Strength The strength of gypsum products is generally expressed in terms of compressive strength, although tensile strength should also be considered if one is to secure a satisfactory guide to the total strength characteristics.[13]

As might be expected from the theory of setting, the strength of a plaster or stone increases rapidly as the material hardens after the initial setting time. However, the free water content of the set product definitely affects its strength. For this reason, two strengths of the gypsum product are recognized, the *wet strength** and the *dry strength.* The wet strength is the strength when the water in excess of that required for the hydration of the hemihydrate is left in the test specimen. When the specimen has been dried free of the excess water, the strength obtained is the dry strength. The dry strength may be two or more times the wet strength.[14] Consequently, the distinction between the two is of considerable importance.

The effect of drying on the compressive strength of set plaster is shown in Table 4–5. It is interesting to note that relatively slight gains in strength occurred until after the sixteenth hour. Between the 8-hour period and the 24-hour period, only 0.6 per cent of the excess water was lost, yet the strength doubled. A somewhat similar change in surface hardness takes place during the drying process.[15]

A good explanation of this effect is the fact that as the last traces of water leave, fine crystals of gypsum precipitate. These anchor the larger crystals.

---

*Often referred to as the "green" strength.

Table 4–5. *Effect of Drying on the Strength of Plaster of Paris**

DRYING PERIOD (hrs)	COMPRESSIVE STRENGTH (MPa)	(psi)	LOSS IN WEIGHT (per cent)
2	9.6	1400	5.1
4	11.7	1700	11.9
8	11.7	1700	17.4
16	13.0	1900	......
24	23.3	3400	18.0
48	23.3	3400	18.0
72	23.3	3400	......

*From Gibson and Johnson, J Soc Chem Ind, 51:25T (1932).

Then if water is added, or if excess water is present, these small crystals are the first to dissolve and thus the reinforcing anchors are lost.[14]

As previously noted, the set plaster or stone is porous in nature, and the greater the W/P ratio, the greater will be the porosity (Table 4–3). As might be expected on such a basis, the greater the W/P ratio, the less is the dry strength of the set material, as shown by the data in Table 4–6, since the greater the porosity, the fewer crystals there will be per unit volume for a given weight of hemihydrate.

The tensile strength of plaster or stone is less affected by variations in the W/P ratio than is the compressive strength.[13] However, the materials mixed at a high W/P ratio have tensile strengths as high as 25 per cent of the corresponding compressive strength. When mixed at low W/P ratios the tensile strength is less than 10 per cent of the corresponding compressive strength.

It is particularly interesting to note from Table 4–6 that the spatulation time also affects the strength of the plaster. In general, with an increase in mixing time, the strength will be increased to a limit that is approximately equivalent to that of a normal hand mixing for one minute. If the mixture is overmixed, the gypsum crystals formed are broken up, and less crystalline interlocking results in the final product.

The incorporation of an accelerator or retarder lowers both the wet and dry strengths of the gypsum product. Such a decrease in strength can be partially attributed to the salt added as an adulterant and to the reduction in intercrystalline cohesion.

When relatively pure raw hemihydrate is mixed with minimal amounts of water, as used in dentistry, the working time is short and the setting expansion is unduly high. However, as just noted, dental gypsum products contain additives that reduce the setting expansion, increase the working time, and provide a rapid final set. The addition of more chemicals can upset

Table 4–6. *Effect of W/P Ratio and Mixing Time on the Strength of Plaster of Paris**

W/P	MIXING TIME (min)	COMPRESSIVE STRENGTH (DRY) (MPa)	(psi)
0.45	0.5	23.4	3400
0.45	1.0	26.2	3800
0.60	1.0	17.9	2600
0.60	2.0	13.8	2000
0.80	1.0	11.0	1600

*From Gibson and Johnson, J Soc Chem Ind, 51:25T (1932).

the delicate balance of these properties. Thus, if a change is desired in the setting time it should be done by modest alterations in the W/P ratio and/or spatulation time.

References

1. Goto M, Molony B, Ridge MJ, and West GW: Forms of calcium sulfate hemihydrate. Aust J Chem 19:313, 1966.
2. Combe EG and Smith DC: Some properties of gypsum plasters. Br Dent J 117:237, 1964.
3. Earnshaw R and Marks BI: The measurement of setting time of gypsum products. Aust Dent J 9:17, 1964.
4. Smith DC: The setting of plaster. Dent Pract 13:473, 1963.
5. Sunoo YG, Smith DC, and Skinner EW: The effect of accelerators and retarders on the setting and crystal structure of plaster. IADR Program and Abstracts, No. M–7, 1961.
6. Lautzenschlager EP and Corbin F: Investigation on the expansion of dental stones. J Dent Res 48:206, 1969.
7. Jørgensen KD: Studies on the setting of plaster of Paris. Odont T 61:305, 1953.
8. Docking AR, Chong MD, and Donnison JA: The hygroscopic setting expansion of dental casting investments. Part 2. Aust Dent J 52:160, 1948.
9. Harcourt JK and Lautzenschlager EP: Accelerated and retarded dental plaster setting investigated by x-ray diffraction. J Dent Res 49:502, 1970.
10. Combe EC and Smith DC: The effects of some organic acids and salts on the setting of gypsum plaster. I. Acetates. J Appl Chem 14:553, 1964.
11. Combe EC and Smith DC: The effects of some organic acids and salts on the setting of gypsum plaster. II. Tartrates. J Appl Chem 15:367, 1965.
12. Combe EC and Smith DC: The effects of some organic acids and salts on the setting of gypsum plaster. III. Citrates. J Appl Chem 16:73, 1966.
13. Earnshaw R and Smith DC: The tensile and compressive strength of plaster and stone. Aust Dent J 11:415, 1966.
14. Fairhurst CW: Compressive properties of dental gypsum. J Dent Res 39:812, 1960.
15. Mahler DB: Hardness and flow properties of gypsum materials. J Prosthet Dent 1:188, 1951.

5 GYPSUM PRODUCTS: TECHNICAL CONSIDERATIONS

As described in the preceding chapter, gypsum products have many uses in dentistry. The criteria for selection of any particular gypsum product depend upon its use and the physical properties necessary for that particular use. For example, a dental stone is a poor material for use as an impression material because if teeth are present it would be impossible to remove the impression over the undercuts in the teeth without injury because of the high strength of the stone (α-hemihydrate).

On the other hand, if a strong cast is required on which to build a denture, one would not choose to employ a weak plaster (β-hemihydrate) containing considerable amounts of modifiers. In other words, there is no "all purpose" dental gypsum product.

Impression Plasters Impression plasters are plaster of Paris to which modifiers have been added. The purpose of the modifiers is twofold: to regulate the setting time and to control the setting expansion.

It is important from the standpoint of both the patient and the dentist that the setting time be under accurate control. The dentist should have sufficient time to mix the plaster and water, to place the mixture in the impression tray, to carry the loaded impression tray to the patient's mouth, and to place it in position against the oral tissues. However, once the plaster is in position against the surface to be reproduced, it should harden promptly so that the discomfort to the patient is not prolonged unduly. The setting time for a given W/P ratio is determined by the addition of the proper amount of accelerator.

The setting expansion of an impression plaster should be kept as low as possible because of the danger of warping the impression, as illustrated in Figure 5–1. The impression shown diagrammatically is for the maxilla. The flanges of the metal tray are shown at A and B. If the plaster expands against these flanges, the expansion will be confined, and the resulting stress will cause a warpage at C. As a result, the depth of the palate portion will be changed and the denture or other appliance will not fit. It should be noted that the only dimensional change of practical interest occurs after the initial set; any changes in dimension that occur before the material hardens are compensated immediately by the flow of the fluid mix.

The use of an accelerator is indicated to reduce the setting expansion as well as the setting time. If the setting time is unduly shortened to obtain a

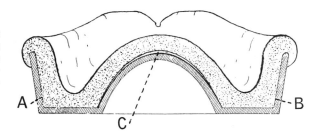

Figure 5–1 Warped impression due to tray flanges. The impression warps at C because the flanges A and B are fixed and do not allow lateral setting expansion. (Adapted from Prothero: Prosthetic Dentistry. Medico-Dental Publishing Co.)

minimal setting expansion, a retarder can be used to counteract the accelerator, and at the same time to decrease the setting expansion further. A setting expansion of approximately 0.06 per cent is the lowest that can be expected. The setting time is usually established at 3 to 5 minutes, depending upon the desired W/P ratio.

The modifiers are usually included in the plaster, ready to be dissolved in the water when the powder and water are mixed. If desired, however, solutions containing the proper amount of modifiers can be used for mixing without changing the composition of the plaster.

When teeth are present, the plaster impression must be fractured and re-assembled; otherwise, the unyielding plaster impression cannot be removed over the undercuts caused by the heights of contour of the teeth and the spaces between the teeth. Consequently, a high degree of strength is an undesirable property for an impression plaster; rather, it should be brittle and relatively easy to fracture. The use of a high W/P ratio in mixing aids in this respect, and at the same time it prevents the formation of excessive exothermic heat during the setting reaction.

Some of the impression plasters are colored and flavored to make them more palatable to the patient. The color also helps the dentist or technician to distinguish between the cast material and the impression plaster when the impression is separated from the cast.

Before the stone is poured into the impression to form the cast, the pores in the plaster impression must be sealed. Otherwise, the water and dissolved α-hemihydrate will soak into the impression, and crystals will form so that the cast and impression cannot be separated. The impression should always be coated first with a separating medium, such as varnish or lacquer, to render it impervious to water. The film formed by the separating medium should be very thin to avoid inaccuracies from this cause.

Impression plasters sometimes contain potato starch to render them "soluble." In such a case, after the cast has thoroughly hardened, the impression and cast are placed in water and heated; the starch swells, the impression disintegrates, and its removal from the cast is facilitated. If a starch modifier is not used, a careful and tedious dissection of the impression from the cast is often necessary to avoid injury to the latter.

Dental Stone   Modern dental stones are composed chiefly of α-hemihydrate. Modifiers constitute only 2 to 3 per cent of the total composition. Coloring matter is generally added so that the dental stone can be readily distinguished from the dental plaster. Both α- and β-hemihydrate are white and cannot be distinguished from each other.

The modifiers are generally potassium sulfate, which is used as an accelerator, and sodium citrate, which is used as a retarder. As described for impression plaster, the setting expansion is reduced by both chemicals.

However, the setting time is determined by the addition of proper quantities of both the accelerator and the retarder. A stone with a setting time established by this method is said to be "balanced." The setting expansion is not affected by the method of mixing when a "balanced" stone is used nor is its setting time affected. Both properties are, however, affected by the W/P ratio in the usual manner.

In addition to the modifiers, some commercial dental stones may contain a small amount of β-hemihydrate to provide a mix of smoother consistency.

It is important that a dental stone possess a low setting expansion, particularly when it is used for the construction of a cast in a plaster impression. The reason for this becomes apparent from Figure 5–2, which represents a cross section of the impression shown in Figure 5–1 after the cast material has been poured. The discrepancy caused by the setting expansion of the impression plaster is shown at C. If the dental stone possesses a large setting expansion, its expansion will be inhibited by the impression and the cast will warp as shown at D. The total warpage is, therefore, cumulative and the vault portion of the cast will be too high. For this reason, the setting expansion of the stone is usually limited to 0.06 to 0.12 per cent, a value which should be negligible so far as any error of practical significance is concerned.

Modern dental stones can be classified according to their particle shape and compactness as *Type III* or *Type IV.* The classification used in the American Dental Association specification for dental gypsum products is seen in Table 5–1. The table also includes the older designations and traditional names that are still occasionally used to describe the respective materials. The particles of a Type III stone were shown in Figure 4–2; those of the Type IV are seen in Figure 5–3. The particles of the two types of stone are quite similar in shape. The main difference is that the Type IV stone is characterized by more compact and smoother particles, resulting in a lower surface area. Therefore, less water can be used in mixing, and the dry strengths are generally greater than those of the Type III stones.

Cast and Die Materials   One of the principal requisites for a cast or die material is great strength and hardness. A lower W/P ratio can be used with the dental stones than with plaster of Paris; therefore, the former are used almost exclusively for this purpose.

Some of the physical properties of gypsum cast and die materials are presented in Table 5–2. All of the materials are commercial dental stones. Materials A through C are presumably Type III stones; materials D through H are Type IV.

The W/P ratios that provide a mixing consistency which enables the material to be poured easily, without being too fluid or too viscous, are shown

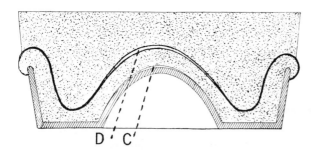

Figure 5–2 Warped cast due to restricted lateral setting expansion. The warpage of the impression in Figure 5–1 may be seen at C. After the cast was formed, further warpage occurred at D. (Adapted from Prothero: Prosthetic Dentistry. Medico-Dental Publishing Co.)

Table 5–1. *Classification of Dental Gypsum Products*

	ADA SPECIFICATION	TRADITIONAL TERMINOLOGY
Type I	Plaster, impression	Impression plaster
Type II	Plaster, model	Model or lab plaster
Type III	Dental stone	Class I stone or Hydrocal
Type IV	Dental stone, high strength	Class II stone, Densite or improved stone

in column 2. As predicted, the cuboidal particles of the Type IV stones allow a lower W/P ratio to be employed than do the Type III stones. However, there is very little difference in the setting times of any of the stones (column 3). Presumably, all have been "balanced" to provide a setting time of 5 to 8 minutes, which is sufficiently long to allow the dentist to complete the required manipulation of the material before set.

As previously noted, a low setting expansion is desirable for a cast or die material. Unfortunately, when the setting expansion of a gypsum product is reduced below about 0.1 per cent, it may gradually increase during storage. However, the Type IV stones are apt to be more stable than the Type III stones and plaster in this respect.

As will be noted later, the use of a *cast* is generally restricted to the construction of dentures to fit the soft tissues of the mouth; stone *dies* are generally reproductions of teeth with prepared cavities used in constructing restorations. Although a low setting expansion is always desirable in these instances, an error occasioned by a slight setting expansion can be tolerated by the soft tissues, but not when a tooth is involved. Type III stones are preferred for preparing casts upon which dentures are to be processed because they are easier to remove after processing, yet have adequate strength. The Type III

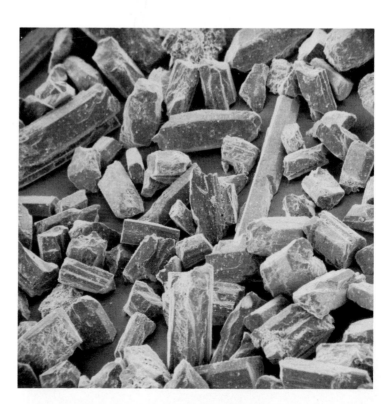

Figure 5–3 Powder particles of Type IV stone. × 400. (Courtesy of B. Giammara and R. Neiman.)

stones are generally used for such casts and the Type IV stones for dies (called "die stones").

The hygroscopic setting expansion obtained when the stone is allowed to set under water is given in column 5 (Table 5–2). If possible, the cast or die should be allowed to set in air to avoid the error produced by hygroscopic expansion. However, as will be discussed later, sometimes the stone die must be allowed to set in a water environment and the unavoidable error incurred may be considerable.

It is very likely that the lower wet compressive strengths noted in column 6 may be due to a small amount of β-hemihydrate in some of the stones. Otherwise, there is apparently not much difference in the strengths of the stones at the end of one hour. The 7-day dry strength of the Type IV stones is somewhat greater than that of the Type III materials, however. Here again, the composition is a factor. For example, stones E and F are significantly stronger when dry than the other stones listed.

Another requisite for a dental stone is that it exhibit a high degree of surface hardness, particularly when used as a die material. The die usually contains a prepared cavity to receive a cast gold alloy inlay or crown. Part of the technique is to mold the restoration in wax on the die. Such a procedure requires that the wax be carved flush with the die, using a sharp instrument. In such a case, the die material must be hard and smooth in order not to be abraded by the carving instrument. Gypsum hardening solutions are often used to increase the surface hardness of the die. These agents are discussed in Chapter 27.

Probably the most effective method for producing a hard surface on a cast is to employ as little water as possible in mixing the stone. Inasmuch as the α-hemihydrate crystals are not porous and are relatively smooth, a water-powder mixture of a putty-like consistency can be vibrated into very small areas with ease.

The surface hardness of a cast made from a dental model plaster can be increased by immersing it in a 2 per cent solution of borax for several hours.[2] The more concentrated and the higher the temperature of the solution (within limits), the more borax will be taken up. Presumably a thin layer of calcium

Table 5–2. *Some Physical Properties of Dental Stone*

MATERIAL	W/P RATIO	SETTING TIME* (min)	SETTING EXPANSION NORMAL (per cent)	SETTING EXPANSION HYGROSCOPIC (per cent)	COMPRESSIVE STRENGTH WET† MPa	psi	COMPRESSIVE STRENGTH DRY‡ MPa	psi
Type III								
A	0.30	5.5	0.16	0.27	25	3,600	71	10,200
B	0.30	7.0	0.09	0.19	24	3,400	66	9,500
C	0.28	8.0	0.18	0.27	32	4,700	70	10,100
Type IV								
D	0.23	6.5	0.08	0.13	32	4,700	71	10,300
E	0.24	5.5	0.09	0.15	29	4,300	89	13,000
F	0.24	7.0	0.10	0.14	34	4,900	85	12,400
G	0.24	6.5	0.09	0.13	22	3,200	72	10,400
H	0.23	7.5	0.08	0.16	32	4,500	73	10,500

*Gillmore initial.
†After one hour.
‡After seven days.

tetraborate deposited on the surface is the cause for the increase in hardness. Unfortunately, such a treatment is not effective with dental stone.

The surface hardness increases more rapidly after setting than does the compressive strength, because of the more rapid drying of the surface in comparison to the interior of the cast.[3]

The average dry surface hardness of the Type IV stones ("die stones") is approximately 92 (RHN)[1]; that of the Type III stone is 82. Even though the surface of the stone die is harder, care should be observed when carving the pattern.

In any event, it is most important that the stone powder be weighed and that the water be gauged accurately. The stone is usually employed instead of plaster in order to provide strength and hardness. It is definitely possible to obtain a stone cast that is weaker than one made with plaster if too much water is used in mixing the former.

Proportioning As previously noted, if a high strength is desired, as low a W/P ratio should be used as possible. However, decreasing the amount of water increases the viscosity of the mix, and care must be taken to insure that the thick mixture flows into every detail when it is poured or vibrated into the impression.

Since a high strength is not only unimportant but also undesirable in plaster impressions, a relatively high W/P ratio can be used to provide a creamy consistency in the mix, which will flow into every detail when the impression is obtained. The lowest limit of the viscosity permissible is governed by the ability of the water-plaster mixture to remain in position in the tray while the impression is being taken. The proper W/P ratio for an impression plaster is approximately 0.6 to 0.7, depending upon the plaster.

Some dental stones (Type IV) can be used successfully with a W/P ratio as low as 0.20. As previously noted, it is important that the water and powder be measured — preferably weighed. It is impossible to gauge a powder accurately by volume because of the packing effect. The packing effect of different commercial products of the same type may vary considerably from one product to another. Furthermore, the bulk of the mixed or set product may be entirely independent of the bulk of the original powder. Consequently, the use of volume measurement for proportioning purposes is unreliable.

Mixing The plaster or stone is usually mixed in a flexible rubber or plastic bowl, using a stiff-bladed spatula. The mid-cross section of the interior of the bowl should preferably be parabolic in shape, so there will be no corners or other discontinuities in which the plaster or stone can collect and stagnate during the mixing procedure. The walls of the bowl should be smooth and resistant to abrasion. Any scratches or creases are likely to retain set plaster after the bowl has been washed. As a result, the setting time and other properties of subsequent mixes will be altered by the nuclei of crystallization unintentionally added.

The spatula should have a stiff blade. A flexible blade "drags" when it is forced through a thick mixture of stone and water, and as a result the mixing is seldom thorough. The end of the spatula blade should be rounded to conform to the shape of the mixing bowl, so that the surface of the bowl can be wiped readily by the blade of the spatula during mixing. The handle of the spatula should be of a design that can be readily grasped by the hand.

One great disadvantage to be avoided during the mixing of a gypsum product with water is the incorporation of air. Air bubbles in the completed cast are unsightly, weaken the cast, and produce surface inaccuracies (Fig. 5–4).

An automatic vibrator is of considerable aid in removing air bubbles during mixing, provided that the vibrations are of a high frequency and of a limited amplitude. A churning effect by the vibrator is decidedly undesirable, since violent agitation whips air into the mixture.

The water should be placed in the plaster bowl, and the powder should be sifted into the water. When the powder sinks into the water without an agglomeration of the particles, less air is carried down.

The mixture should then be held on the automatic vibrator for a few seconds to remove any large air bubbles which might have been incorporated inadvertently. The actual spatulation is carried on by stirring the mixture vigorously, and at the same time wiping all of the inside surfaces of the bowl with the spatula to be sure that all of the powder is wet and mixed uniformly with the water. The mixing is continued until all of the mixture is smooth and homogeneous in texture. Further mixing is likely to break up the crystals of gypsum formed, and thus weaken the final product. The time for hand mixing is approximately 1 to 2 minutes.

The mix is then vibrated until no more air bubbles come to the surface. Some dental offices and laboratories are equipped so that the final vibration of the mix is accomplished in a vacuum to eliminate the air bubbles more completely.

The use of a mechanical spatulator* for mixing gypsum products offers considerable advantage. The rapidly moving blades of such a device tend to break up any air bubbles into fine voids and the strength of plaster and Type III stones is increased. One report noted that mechanical spatulation of Type IV stones did not produce a significant improvement in either the compressive or the tensile strength.[4] However, another investigation found mechanical

---

*Described in Chapter 27.

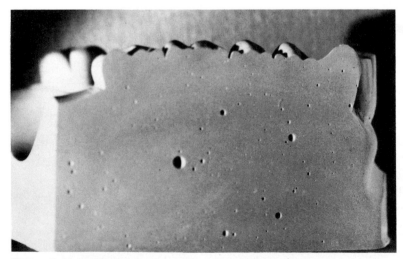

Figure 5–4 Section through a cast of a set stone which was improperly mixed. Air voids weaken the stone and impair its appearance.

spatulation, with or without vacuum, increased the strength of Type IV stones, and that in only 10 seconds of mechanical mixing the strength was equal to that of stone prepared by a full minute of hand mixing.[5] Possibly the differences reported may be attributed to the type of spatulators or brands of stone used. Certainly, mechanical spatulation does reduce the possibility of a void occurring in the die at some critical part of the cavity preparation.

If the maximal strength is desired, the W/P ratio should not be changed during mixing. If the proportions are estimated by guesswork, the addition of more powder to a mix that is judged to be too thin provides essentially two mixes of plaster setting at different times, and a weakened product always results. In the same manner, the addition of water to a too-thick mixture probably causes a disarrangement of crystalline growth and a lack of inter-crystalline cohesion. The very fact that the mix was judged to be too thick may indicate that the setting reaction has started. As repeatedly stated, in order to obtain the maximal strength, the proportions of water and powder should be measured. Preweighed packages of stones are available.

Construction of the Cast   There are at least two methods for the construction of the cast. In one case, a mold for the cast is constructed. Briefly, strips of soft wax are wrapped around the impression, so that they extend approximately 12 mm (½ inch) beyond the tissue side of the impression. A base for the cast is formed in this manner. The process is called "boxing." The mixture of stone and water is then poured into the impression under vibration. The mixture is allowed to run down the side of the impression, so that it pushes the air ahead of itself as it fills all tooth impressions and other irregularities.

Another method is to fill the impression first as described. The remainder of the stone-water mixture is then piled on a glass plate. The filled impression is then inverted over the pile of stone, and the base is shaped with the spatula before the stone sets. Such a procedure is not indicated, however, if an impression material that is easily deformed has been used.

The cast should not be separated from the impression until it has thoroughly hardened. The minimal time to be allowed for setting will vary from 30 to 60 minutes, depending on the rate of setting of the stone or plaster, and the type of impression material. The completed cast should be smooth, neat, and accurate in every detail, as that seen in Figure 5–5.

Care of the Cast   If the surface of the cast is not hard and smooth when it is removed from the impression, its accuracy is questionable. The cast is supposedly an accurate reproduction of the mouth tissues, and any departure from the expected accuracy will probably result in a poorly fitting appliance. The cast should, therefore, be handled carefully and with intelligence.

Once the setting reactions in the cast have been completed, its dimensions will be relatively constant thereafter under ordinary conditions of room temperature and humidity. As later outlined, however, it is sometimes necessary to soak the gypsum cast in water, in preparation for other techniques. It should be remembered that the gypsum of which the cast is composed is slightly soluble in water. When a dry cast is immersed in water, there may be a negligible expansion, provided that the water is saturated with calcium sulfate. If it is not so saturated, gypsum may be dissolved in sufficient amount to cause a measurable reduction in its dimensions. If the stone cast is immersed in running water, its linear dimension may decrease approximately 0.1 per cent for every 20 minutes of such immersion.

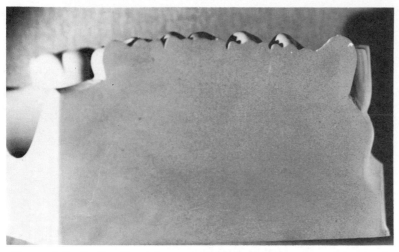

Figure 5–5   Section through a cast of set stone that was properly mixed.

The safest method for soaking the cast is to place it in a water bath made for the purpose, in which plaster debris is allowed to remain constantly on the bottom of the container to provide a saturated solution of calcium sulfate at all times.

As previously noted, storage of either set plaster or stone at room temperature produces no significant dimensional change. However, if the storage temperature is raised to 90 to 110° C (194 to 230° F) a shrinkage occurs as the water of crystallization is removed and the dihydrate reverts to the hemihydrate.[6] The contraction of the plaster at high temperature is greater than that of the stone; it will also lose strength.

Such contractions may occur during storage in air at temperatures above that of the room, as when a stone cast is dried. Probably it is not safe dimensionally to store a stone cast in air at a temperature higher than 55° C (130° F) for any length of time.

Special Gypsum Products   In addition to the more standardized gypsum materials just described, there are some that have been characterized for special purposes. For example, the orthodontist prefers an unusually white stone or plaster for his study models and may even treat the surface with soap for an added sheen. These products generally have a longer working time for ease in trimming.

The use of an articulator makes it necessary to mount the casts with a gypsum product, as is shown in Figure 5–6. These materials are referred to as "mounting" stones or plasters. They are fast setting and have low setting expansion.[7] In the case of the mounting plaster, it has low strength to permit easy trimming and so that the cast can be readily separated from the articulator mounting plates.

Care of Gypsum Products   Gypsum products are somewhat sensitive to changes in the relative humidity of their environment. Even the surface hardness of plaster and stone casts may fluctuate slightly with the relative humidity of the atmosphere. Gypsum surfaces made with thinner mixes appear to be affected more than those with a low W/P ratio. Although the effect is small, it is worthy of note.

The hemihydrate of gypsum takes up water from the air quite readily. For

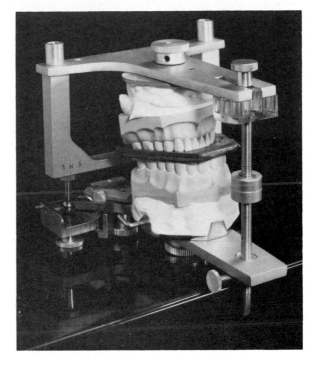

Figure 5–6 A dental articulator, a device that incorporates artificial temporomandibular joints. This permits orientation of casts in a manner simulating various positions of the mandible. In this figure, showing the inverted position of the articulator, the casts have been attached to the mounting plates with a quick-setting gypsum product. The dark wafer between the two casts is a wax interocclusal record. (Courtesy of Whip-Mix Co.)

example, if the relative humidity exceeds approximately 70 per cent, the plaster takes up sufficient water vapor to start a setting reaction. The first hydration probably produces a few crystals of gypsum on the surface of the hemihydrate crystal. These crystals act as nuclei of crystallization, and the first manifestation of the deterioration of the plaster is a decrease in the setting time.

As the hygroscopic action continues, more crystals of gypsum form until the entire hemihydrate crystal is covered. Under these conditions, the water penetrates the dihydrate coating with difficulty and the setting time is unduly prolonged. It is, therefore, important that all types of gypsum products be stored in a dry atmosphere. The best means of storage is to seal the product in a moistureproof metal container. When gypsum products are stored in closed containers, generally the setting time is retarded slightly, approximately 1 to 2 minutes per year. This may be counteracted by a slight increase in the mixing time if necessary.

References

1. Storer R and Skinner EW: Evaluation of gypsum cast and die materials. IADR Program and Abstracts, No. M19, 1962.
2. Buchanan AS and Worner KH: A study of the action of borax in retarding the setting of plaster of Paris. J Soc Chem Ind 65:23, 1946.
3. Mahler DB: Hardness and flow properties of gypsum materials. J Prosthet Dent 1:188, 1951.
4. Earnshaw R and Smith DC: The tensile and compressive strength of plaster and stone. Aust Dent J 11:415, 1966.
5. Neiman R: Personal communication, 1980.
6. Sweeney WT and Taylor DF: Dimensional changes in dental stone and plaster. J Dent Res 29:749, 1950.
7. Dilts WE, Duncanson MG Jr, and Collard EW: Comparative stability of cast mounting materials. J Okla Dent Assoc 68:11, 1978.

6 IMPRESSION COMPOUND

The use of plaster of Paris as an impression material was described in the preceding chapter. Plaster is, however, only one of several materials that can be used to obtain an impression.

Classification of Impression Materials   There are several ways by which impression materials can be classified. One way is according to the manner in which they harden. For example, plaster of Paris hardens by chemical action, as do the impression pastes and the alginate and rubber impression materials to be discussed in subsequent chapters.

On the other hand, the impression compounds soften under heat and solidify when they are cooled, with no chemical change taking place. Such materials are, therefore, classified as *thermoplastic* substances. Although the reversible hydrocolloid materials to be described in Chapter 8 may not be classified strictly as thermoplastic materials, they are liquefied by heat, and they solidify, or gel, when they are cooled. In Table 6–1 can be seen a classification of the various dental impression materials based upon the mode of hardening and thermal behavior.

Another way to classify the dental impression materials is according to their uses in dentistry. As previously noted, an impression made with plaster of Paris cannot be removed over undercuts without the impression being fractured. If an impression of teeth is made with impression compound, the compound flows when the impression is withdrawn over the undercuts, and the tooth form is not preserved with accuracy. The same is true of an impression made with the impression pastes. Although these three types of materials can be used with certain limitations for all types of impressions, they are best suited for obtaining impressions of edentulous mouths. Therefore, they may be classified as impression materials for use in complete denture prosthesis.

On the other hand, the elastic hydrocolloid impression materials are best used for obtaining an accurate reproduction of tooth form, including the undercuts and interproximal spaces. Although these materials can be employed for edentulous impressions, they are used most extensively in crown and bridge, partial denture, and operative dentistry when impressions of teeth are included.

Uses of Impression Compound   When the compound is used for edentulous impressions, it is softened by heat, inserted in an impression tray, and pressed

Table 6–1. *Classification of Dental Impression Materials*

	RIGID OR INELASTIC	ELASTIC
Set by chemical reaction (Irreversible)	Plaster Zinc oxide-eugenol	Alginate hydrocolloid Non-aqueous elastomers Polysulfide polymer Polyether Silicone
Set by temperature change (Reversible)	Compound Wax	Agar hydrocolloid

against the tissues before it hardens. The bottom of the tray is cooled with water until the compound hardens, after which procedure the impression is withdrawn. Such material is true *impression compound,* and is referred to as Type I compound in the American Dental Association specification.

Impression compound is also used in operative dentistry to obtain an impression of a single tooth in which a cavity has been prepared. In this case, a cylindrical copper band (called a *matrix band*) is filled with the softened compound. The filled band is then passed over the tooth, and the compound flows into the prepared cavity. Such an impression is sometimes referred to as a "tube" impression. After the compound has been cooled, the impression is withdrawn, and a cast, or die, is constructed in the impression. As previously related, the contour of the entire tooth may not be reproduced accurately because of the flow or fracture of the compound when it is withdrawn from the tooth. However, the form of the prepared cavity will be accurately recorded.

Another type of compound, called *tray compound,* is used in the construction of dentures to form a tray which can then be employed with other types of impression materials for reproducing the mouth tissues. Tray compound is referred to as a Type II compound in the American Dental Association specification. An impression is obtained with tray compound, as was described. This impression is referred to as the *primary* impression. The rigid primary compound impression may then be used as a tray on which other types of impression materials may be carried to be placed against the tissues. For example, a mix of impression plasters may be placed in such a tray, and a final impression then obtained with the plaster, which is spread over the compound. The thin layer of plaster reproduces the fine detail of the denture area and, when used in this manner, is referred to as a *corrective impression material.* This impression is known as the *secondary* impression. Secondary impressions may also be taken with the zinc oxide and eugenol pastes and the hydrocolloids.

There are several other ways in which such corrective impressions may be made. Generally, this basic procedure has been further refined in that an intermediate cast is prepared from which is produced an individual plastic tray for making the secondary impression. A primary impression is taken with impression compound (Fig. 6–1A). A cast, made from plaster or stone, is formed in this impression (Fig. 6–1B). Now a tray, of a dental plastic, is contoured over this cast (Fig. 6–1C). After the plastic has hardened, it is removed from the cast and filled with another type of impression material, such as a zinc oxide and eugenol paste to be discussed in the next chapter. The secondary impression is then made (Fig. 6–1D).

In contrast to impression compound, the tray compound is somewhat more viscous when it is softened and more rigid when it is hardened. Since

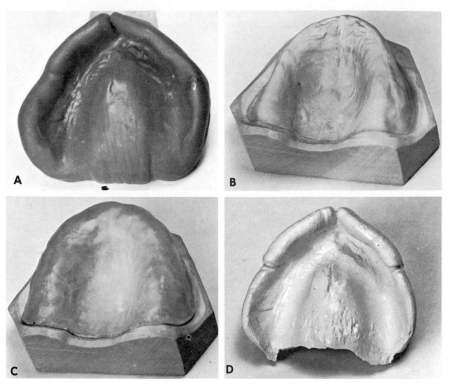

Figure 6–1 Steps involved in preparing secondary impressions in the construction of a denture; *A,* primary compound impression; *B,* cast made from the primary compound impression; *C,* plastic tray fabricated over the cast; *D,* secondary impression of zinc oxide–eugenol paste obtained in the plastic tray.

reproduction of fine detail is not essential for tray compound, it is generally stiffer and has less flow than the regular impression compound.

Composition   Because the formulas of modern impression compounds are trade secrets, any discussion of composition cannot be very specific. In general, compounds are a mixture of waxes, thermoplastic resins, a filler, and a coloring agent.

One of the first substances used as an impression material was beeswax, and it may still be one of the ingredients in some modern products. Since such waxes are brittle, compounds such as shellac, stearic acid, and gutta-percha can be added to improve the plasticity and workability. When used in this manner, these substances are referred to as *plasticizers*.

Synthetic resins are being used in increasing amounts, usually in conjunction with the natural resins, providing more stable production from batch to batch and being more readily plasticized.

Fillers   Many materials are strengthened or otherwise changed in physical properties by the addition of small particles of usually inert materials, known as *fillers*, which are chemically distinct from the principal ingredient or ingredients. In such a case, the filler particles are sometimes referred to as the *core* and the surrounding ingredients as the *matrix*.

For example, the waxes or resins in the impression compound are the principal ingredients. The mixture is mostly noncrystalline in character in order that the desirable thermoplastic properties of the compound can be realized. However, such a structure alone is likely to result in a relatively high flow of the compound and a low strength even at room temperature. Consequently, a filler is added. The filler particles can reduce the plasticity of the matrix material by frictional action. Therefore, both the viscosity at temperatures above that of the mouth and the rigidity of the compound at lower temperatures will be enhanced. A filler agent, such as French chalk, is usually added for such a purpose.

The structure of this compound is somewhat like that of a *composite*. Technically the term composite refers to a materials system composed of a mixture of two or more macro constituents that differ in form and are essentially insoluble in each other.[1]

The influence of the addition of fillers to a matrix will be discussed in greater detail in relation to composite restorative resins (Chapter 14). At this time it is sufficient to mention that if factors such as particle size and concentration are controlled, then the filler can substantially alter many of the properties of the matrix material itself.

Fusion Temperature   A typical time-temperature cooling curve for impression compound is shown in Figure 6–2. As can be noted, the "plateau" or horizontal straight-line portion of the curve characteristic of a pure crystalline material is ill-defined. Furthermore, the indication of a fusion temperature of approximately 43.5° C (110.3° F) is not a solidification temperature, since the glass transition temperature for this particular compound is approximately 39° C (102° F).

The fusion temperature indicated in Figure 6–2 is probably the temperature at which the crystalline fatty acids solidified. The noncrystalline components solidify more slowly and at a lower temperature.

The practical significance of the fusion temperature is that it indicates a definite reduction in plasticity during cooling. Above this temperature, the

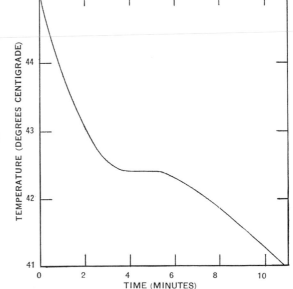

Figure 6–2 A typical time-temperature cooling curve for impression compound.

fatty acids are liquid and probably plasticize or lubricate the softened material to form a smooth, plastic mass while the impression is being obtained. Thus, every detail of the mouth tissues is more likely to be reproduced. Once the impression tray is seated, it should be held firmly in position until the fusion temperature is reached. Below this temperature an accurate and detailed impression cannot be expected. Under no circumstances should the impression be disturbed or removed until mouth temperature is reached.

Miscellaneous Thermal Properties   As might be expected theoretically from their composition, the thermal conductivity of these materials is very low. This property should be taken into consideration particularly during heating and cooling. During the softening of the material, the outside always softens first and the inside last. It is important that the material be uniformly soft at the time it is placed in the tray. To obtain a uniform softening, time must be allowed for the material to be heated uniformly throughout its mass.

It is even more important to cool the material thoroughly in the tray before the impression is withdrawn from the mouth. Usually cold water is sprayed on the tray while it is in the mouth. Such a procedure should be continued until the compound is thoroughly hardened throughout, before the impression is withdrawn. Failure to attain a complete hardening of the material before the impression is withdrawn may result in a serious distortion of the impression by relaxation.

The coefficient of linear thermal expansion of impression compound is considerable in comparison to many other substances. For example, the average linear contraction of impression compound from mouth temperature to room temperature of 25° C (77° F) may vary between 0.3 and 0.4 per cent. The volume expansion over the same temperature range may be as great as 1.38 to 2.29 per cent.[2] Depending on the room temperature, then, the dimensions of the impression may be measurably different from the original dimensions in the mouth. Such an error is unavoidable and it is inherent in the technique.

However, the lower the temperature of the compound at the time the impression is obtained, the less will be the error from this source. One way to reduce the error due to thermal contraction is first to obtain an impression as usual. Then pass the impression through a flame until the surface is softened, and obtain a second impression. During the second impression, the shrinkage is relatively slight, since only the surface layer has been softened completely. Another modification of this technique is to spray cold water on the metal tray just before it is inserted in the mouth. Thus the portion of the material adjacent to the tray will be hardened, while the surface layer is still soft. When either of these techniques is employed, the impression will likely be stressed considerably, and the stone cast should be constructed before the relaxation becomes appreciable.

Flow   The flow of impression compound can be beneficial or it can be a source of error. After the compound has softened and during the period it is impressed against the tissues, a continuous flow is desired; as previously described, the material should flow easily to conform to the tissues so that every detail and landmark are reproduced accurately. No subsequent relaxation should occur. The viscosity or flow of the material at this stage is a function of the temperature and of the composition of the compound.

Once the compound has solidified, any deformation should be completely elastic, so that the impression can be withdrawn without distortion or flow. Actually, such a condition cannot be realized with this type of nonelastic material.

In the American Dental Association Specification no. 3 for dental impression compound, certain tests are described to indicate the flow of the compound at various temperatures. A cylinder of the material, 10 mm in diameter and 6 mm in height, is loaded at a definite temperature with a weight of 2 Kgm (4.4 pounds) for 10 minutes. The flow is designated as the shortening in length of such specimens during the test. According to the specification for the Type I compound, a maximum flow of 6 per cent is allowable at mouth temperature. It is presumed that this amount of flow would be negligible in respect to any distortion occurring in the impression when it is withdrawn from the mouth.

However, the specification states further that the flow should not be less than 85 per cent when the temperature of the impression compound is 45° C (113° F). This requirement is most important, since 45° C is the approximate temperature of the compound when it is placed against the tissues. The amount of flow at this temperature determines the type of impression that is obtained. The flow characteristics of a typical impression compound that complies with this specification are shown in Figure 6–3. It is obvious that these materials are unusual in that they possess entirely different viscosities, or flow characteristics, at relatively small differences in temperature.

The specification requires that the flow of the tray compound (Type II) shall not be more than 2 per cent at 37° C (98.6° F) and not less than 70 per cent nor more than 85 per cent at 45° C (113° F). As can be noted, the tray compound is not as plastic as the impression compound when it is softened. As a result, it can be expected that it will not record detail as readily as does the impression compound.

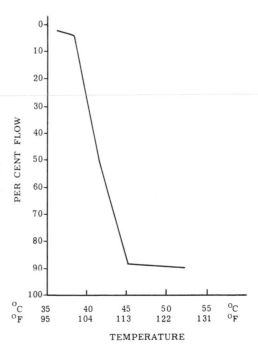

Figure 6–3 Flow of a typical impression compound at different temperatures. This material meets the American Dental Association Specification no. 3 for Dental Impression Compound.

Distortion   In a generally noncrystalline structure such as occurs in impression compound, a stressed condition can occur more readily than in a crystalline material because of the lower activation energy of the latter. Relaxation can occur quite readily either during a comparatively short lapse of time or with an increase in temperature. The result is a warpage or distortion of the impression.

Inasmuch as it is practically impossible to avoid stressing the impression compound at some point in the operation, the safest procedure is to construct the cast or die as soon as possible after the impression has been obtained — at least within the first hour. If a longer period elapses, a warpage may occur.

Once the impression is chilled and removed from the mouth, it should not be subjected to a change in temperature before the stone cast has hardened.

In any event, there are certain causes of warpage that can be avoided. One avoidable cause of warpage is the removal of the impression from the mouth before it is thoroughly cooled. If the surface of the compound is hard, but the inside is soft, a relaxation will occur immediately after the impression is withdrawn. This condition can be demonstrated easily. A piece of compound is softened, and then plunged into cold water for a few seconds. The outside will be reasonably firm, but the inside will be soft so that the piece of compound can be bent slowly into the shape of a horseshoe. When it is released, its tendency to straighten can be observed readily, but it will not recover its original dimensions. When such a condition is present in an impression at the time it is removed from the mouth, one cause of the warpage of the impression is evident. Such a condition is especially likely to be present if the impression is disturbed in any manner in or slightly below the fusion temperature range indicated in Figure 6–2, and above the glass transition temperature of the compound.

Softening of Impression Compound   Whenever possible, compound should be softened with "dry" heat as in an oven or similar device. Often small amounts of compound are softened over a gas flame. When a direct flame is used, the compound should not be allowed to boil or ignite so that important constituents are volatilized.

When a large amount of compound is to be softened, as when an impression is to be obtained of an entire arch, it is difficult to heat the compound uniformly. The softening is better accomplished in a water bath.

After the compound is removed from the water bath, it is usually worked, or kneaded, with the fingers in order to obtain uniform plasticity throughout the mass. Prolonged immersion or overheating in the water bath is not indicated; the compound may become brittle and grainy because some of the low molecular weight ingredients may be leached out. Likewise, undue kneading of the compound in order to produce uniform plasticity can incorporate water into the material, and the flow after hardening will be increased.

The student is referred to a textbook on prosthetic dentistry for the details of preparing the tray and obtaining the impression.

Construction of the Cast   The gypsum cast material is mixed and poured in the same manner as described for the plaster impressions. The same precautions should be observed to avoid air bubbles.

The vault portion of the cast will not warp because of the setting expansion of the stone or plaster as shown in Figure 5–2 in the preceding chapter. The cast material usually generates sufficient exothermic heat to soften the compound so that any setting expansion can occur unimpeded.

In fact, the compound may become sufficiently soft at this stage to allow the removal of the impression from the cast, although such a procedure should be done cautiously, so that the tooth forms, if present, will not be fractured. The safest method for the removal of the impression is to immerse it in *warm* water until the compound softens sufficiently to allow it to be separated easily from the cast. If the compound is overheated at this stage, it may adhere to the cast and cause a discoloration of the stone.

References

1. Materials in Engineering Design: The promise of composites. M/DE Special Report #210, September 1963, pp 79–126.
2. Combe EC and Smith DC: Further studies on impression compounds. Dent Pract 15:292, 1965.

7 ZINC OXIDE–EUGENOL IMPRESSION PASTES

One of the dentally useful chemical reactions is that between zinc oxide and eugenol. Under the proper conditions a relatively hard mass is formed which possesses certain medicinal advantages as well as a mechanical usefulness in certain dental operations. This type of material has been applied to a wide range of uses in dentistry as a cementing medium, surgical dressing, temporary filling material and root canal filling, bite registration paste, temporary relining material for dentures, and as an impression material for edentulous mouths.

The basic composition of all of these materials is the same: mainly, zinc oxide, eugenol, and rosin. Plasticizers, fillers, accelerators, and other additives are incorporated as necessary to provide the desired properties for the particular use of the product.

Impression Pastes Impression pastes are used as a corrective lining in a preliminary impression. For example, a preliminary impression may be taken with tray compound, as described in the previous chapter. The paste is then spread over the compound, and a second impression is obtained.

The paste may be mixed from a powder containing the zinc oxide, rosin, and a liquid containing the eugenol. However, most of the commercial products are dispensed as pastes in tubes. One tube is filled with a paste containing the active ingredient, zinc oxide, and the other tube contains the eugenol and rosin in a paste form. The two pastes are mixed together in the proper proportions, and the mixture is spread over the preliminary impression as described. The impression is removed after the paste has hardened.

Impression pastes for edentulous mouths should be classified as rigid or inelastic impression materials that harden by chemical action (see Table 6–1).

Chemistry Before the impression pastes can be studied, it is necessary to discuss the reaction between zinc oxide and eugenol.* Admittedly, the reaction has never been completely defined. It is undoubtedly very complex.

---

*Often referred to as the ZOE reaction.

98

The structural formula for eugenol is

$$\underset{\begin{array}{c}\\ CH_2-CH\!=\!CH_2\end{array}}{\overset{\begin{array}{c}OH \quad OCH_3\end{array}}{\bigcirc}}$$

Presumably, one of the conditions necessary to such a reaction is that the organic reactor has a methoxy group, ortho to the hydroxyl group in the benzene ring, as in the case of eugenol. Among other organic compounds that possess such a structural formulation are guaiacol and methyl guaiacol, both of which react with zinc oxide in a manner similar to eugenol.

It is fairly well established that the first reaction may consist of the hydrolysis of the zinc oxide to its hydroxide,[1] thus indicating that water is essential to the reaction. Dehydrated zinc oxide will not react with dehydrated eugenol. Water is probably one of the products of the reaction. Consequently, the reaction is autocatalytic.

The setting reaction then occurs as a typical acid-base reaction to form a chelate:[2]

$$ZnO + H_2O \rightleftharpoons Zn\,(OH)_2$$

$$\underset{Base}{Zn(OH)_2} \; + \; \underset{\substack{Acid \\ (Eugenol)}}{2HE} \; \rightleftharpoons \; \underset{\substack{The\ Salt \\ (Zinc\ eugenolate)}}{ZnE_2 + 2H_2O}$$

The reaction can take place either in solution or at the surface of the zinc oxide particles.

The chelate is thought to form as an amorphous gel that tends to crystallize, imparting increased strength to the set mass. Formation of the crystalline zinc eugenolate is greatly enhanced when the setting reaction is accelerated by zinc acetate dihydrate, which is more soluble than $Zn(OH)_2$ and can supply zinc ions more rapidly. The incorporation of rosin, a characteristic component of a ZOE impression material, into the mix reduces crystallization of the chelate gel.[3]

The structure of a set mass resulting from a mixture of zinc oxide powder and eugenol is shown in Figure 7–1.

An acid, such as acetic, is a more active accelerator for the setting reaction than is water, since it increases the speed of formation of the zinc hydroxide.[2] High atmospheric temperature and humidity are also very effective accelerators of the setting reaction.[4]

The water that is formed in the setting reaction probably aids in binding the individual chelate units together, possibly in a chain or in an octahedral structure;[2, 5, 6] or the water may be merely absorbed by the excess zinc oxide. The stoichiometric ratio of zinc oxide to eugenol is approximately 0.25 gm/ml, whereas a common P/L ratio in a dental zinc oxide–eugenol cement would be 4.2 gm/ml.

The free eugenol content of the set cement is probably very low. It may appear to be much higher than it actually is, since the chelate hydrolyzes readily, forming free eugenol and zinc ions.

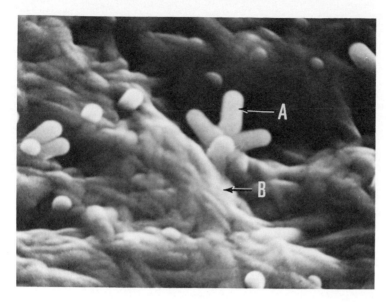

Figure 7–1 Bulk structure of set zinc oxide–eugenol cement. A, particles of zinc oxide powder embedded in B, a matrix of particles of zinc eugenolate.

Accelerators   There are many soluble salts that may act as accelerators, but certain zinc salts, such as zinc acetate, are very efficient in this respect.

The chemical action of the accelerators is not clear. It is suggested that the rate of the hydration of the zinc oxide may be increased by these chemicals,[1] which would be a catalytic effect. It has been shown that, although the hardening time is decreased by the accelerator, the time at which the free eugenol becomes minimal is not affected.[7]

Although the addition of water undoubtedly decreases the setting time of the ZOE product, it should not be classified as an accelerator in the strict sense of the term. Furthermore, if too much water is present, the reaction may be retarded.

Composition   As previously noted, most modern impression materials are dispensed as two separate pastes. A typical formula is shown in Table 7–1. One of the tubes contains the eugenol and rosin, and the other contains zinc oxide and fixed vegetable or mineral oil.

The type of zinc oxide used may be critical. It should be finely divided, French processed, and it should contain a very slight amount of water.

Table 7–1.   *Composition of a Zinc Oxide–Eugenol Impression Paste**

COMPONENTS	PER CENT
Tube No. 1	
Zinc oxide (French processed or U.S.P.)	87
Fixed vegetable or mineral oil	13
Tube No. 2	
Oil of cloves or eugenol	12
Gum or polymerized rosin	50
Filler (silica type)	20
Lanolin	3
Resinous balsam	10
Accelerator solution ($CaCl_2$) and color	5

*Courtesy of E. J. Molnar.

The addition of rosin to the paste in tube 2 apparently facilitates the speed of the reaction, and a smoother, more homogeneous product results. It is possible that the rosin enters the reaction in some way because it reinforces the final product. Its chemical reaction, if any, must be dependent upon the presence of both eugenol and zinc oxide. The use of a hydrogenated, polymerized, or gum rosin provides greater stability than that obtained with the natural rosin, as they prevent crystallization of the paste. However, natural rosin may be used if it is first oxidized in the presence of moisture. This treatment prevents the crystallization of rosin–eugenol paste mixtures.

The calcium chloride (Table 7–1) acts as an accelerator of the setting time. Other chemicals commonly used commercially as accelerators are zinc acetate, primary alcohols, and glacial acetic acid. The accelerator can be incorporated in either one or both pastes.

Oil of cloves contains 70 to 85 per cent eugenol. It is sometimes used in preference to eugenol because it reduces the burning sensation in the soft tissues of the mouth when the mixed paste is first placed in contact with them. The American Dental Association specification for these pastes requires that the eugenol content be specified on the package by the manufacturer.

The fixed vegetable or mineral oil in tube 1 acts as a plasticizer, and it also aids in masking the action of the eugenol as an irritant.

Canada balsam and Peru balsam are often used to increase flow and improve mixing properties. If the mixed paste is too thin or lacks body before it sets, a filler, such as a wax or an inert powder (kaolin, talc, diatomaceous earth, etc.), may be added to one or both of the original pastes.

The variations in composition that can be used are many, and such differences may influence the choice of the dentist considerably in the selection of an impression paste.

Setting Time   Setting time is important, since there must be sufficient time for mixing, filling the tray, and seating the impression. Once the material, in a plastic condition, has been carried to the mouth, only a minimal time should elapse before the impression hardens. Prolonged setting may result in inaccuracy due to unavoidable movement of the tray while the paste is still soft. The composition of the paste influences the setting time. For example, within practical limits, the greater the ratio of the zinc oxide to the eugenol, the shorter will be the setting time. Also the smaller the particle size of the zinc oxide, or if it is acid coated, as from acetic acid, the shorter will be the setting time.

The accelerating effect of the rosin on the setting time has been mentioned. It is effective in this regard provided that the rosin is in the correct proportion to the eugenol.

The type and amount of accelerator used are by far the most important composition factors in the control of the setting time. The setting time is often affected considerably by very small changes in the amount of the accelerator and moisture present.

Two setting times, initial and final, are recognized by the American Dental Association Specification no. 16 for dental impression pastes. Also, two types of paste are designated — Type I (hard) and Type II (soft). The difference between the two types is related to their hardness after setting.

The initial setting time is the period from the beginning of mixing until the material ceases to pull away or string out when its surface is touched with a metal rod of specified dimensions. The impression should be seated in the mouth before the initial set. The final set occurs when a needle of specified dimensions fails to penetrate the surface of the specimen more than 0.2 mm under a load of 50 gm. The initial set may vary between three and six minutes, whereas the final set should occur within 10 minutes for Type I pastes and 15 minutes for Type II pastes. When the final set occurs, the impression can be withdrawn from the mouth. The setting times noted in this specification are determined at 23 ± 2° C and at 50 per cent relative humidity. Thus, the time is considerably shorter when the material is carried to the mouth.

The setting time generally decreases with an increase in temperature and humidity. As a matter of fact, on a hot day with high humidity, some pastes may set while they are being mixed.

Control of the Setting Time   The setting time of these materials is not as easily controlled by the operator as is the setting time of plaster, for example. A number of factors such as the method of manufacturing the zinc oxide, such as its coating and particle size, are solely under the control of the manufacturer. He may also add accelerators and usually controls the initial water content. There are, however, a number of methods by which the operator may control the setting time:

1. If the paste sets too slowly, a small amount of zinc acetate or other accelerators may be added. Also, a small drop of water may be mixed into the paste containing the eugenol before blending the two pastes. Water should be added cautiously, however. It should be mixed uniformly into the paste, otherwise its effect may be unpredictable, depending on the composition of the product.

2. When the setting time is too short, the cause is usually high humidity and/or temperature. Cooling the spatula and mixing slab may help to increase the setting time, provided the temperature is not below the dew point. The most effective means for retardation under such circumstances is to include a small amount of boroglycerin, which is an effective retarder, in the mix.

3. The setting time can also be prolonged by the addition of certain inert oils and waxes during the mixing, such as olive oil, mineral oil, and petrolatum. The dilution effected in this manner decreases the ratio of the accelerator to the total volume of paste, and thereby the setting time is prolonged. However, such a practice is not entirely satisfactory, since it tends to reduce the rigidity of the hardened material and, unless used with discretion, it may result in an inhomogeneous mix.

4. The setting time can be controlled in most instances by a change in the ratio of the zinc oxide paste to the eugenol paste. Whether retardation or acceleration will be obtained depends upon which paste contains the accelerator. If the accelerator is contained in the eugenol paste, a decrease in the amount of zinc oxide paste should accelerate the setting and, conversely, an increase should retard it, since the total amount of accelerator will be reduced percentagewise.

It is possible, in consideration of the rosin content of each paste, and particularly in the cases in which both pastes contain an accelerator, that the change in ratio of the two pastes may not be predictable in its control of the setting time.

5. The time of mixing affects the setting time to a very limited extent.[8] With most pastes, the longer the mixing time (within limits), the shorter will be the setting time.

Consistency and Flow   The consistency and flow of the freshly mixed paste when it is impressed against the tissues may be of considerable clinical importance. A paste of a thick consistency or high viscosity can compress the tissues, whereas a thin, fluid material results in an impression which copies the tissues in a relaxed condition with little or no compression. The explanation of the clinical significance of these differences is not within the scope of this book except to state that different impression techniques require different paste consistencies.

In any event, the impression paste should be homogeneous and it should flow uniformly against the tissues while the impression is being obtained. Otherwise, a tissue displacement instead of a uniform compression may occur. Pastes of varying consistencies are commercially available from which the dentist may choose.

The American Dental Association Specification no. 16 previously quoted contains a requirement for consistency as tested by the amount of spreading of a given quantity of material under a specified load when placed between two glass plates immediately after mixing. According to the requirements, the spread of Type I pastes should be between 30 and 50 mm and that of Type II pastes between 20 and 45 mm. It is evident that the Type I pastes are likely to be more fluid than the Type II pastes and may not be suitable for those impression techniques for which the Type II variety is required, as previously discussed. (A thick or heavy consistency corresponds to a low consistency spread, i.e., a small disk diameter.)

The consistency spread is inversely related to the shear strength of the material being tested. Radial flow of the paste between the glass plates will continue until the disk diameter becomes large enough that the stress induced by the load falls to a level equal to the shear strength of the paste.[4]

There is no flow test in American Dental Association Specification no. 16 for zinc oxide–eugenol impression paste analogous to the flow test for impression compound. For the non-aqueous elastomeric impression materials there is a consistency test for the uncured material and a flow test for the cured material.

Not only is there a wide range of consistencies in the various commercial products, but also the flow of the freshly mixed paste varies as it is related to the time before setting. This relation is indicated by the graphs in Figure 7–2.

The results in Figure 7–2 were obtained by subjecting a freshly mixed disk of each product to a specified load at various intervals after mixing in a manner similar to that described in the specification.[9] The flow of the particular paste in a specified time is expressed in terms of the spread of the disk in mm or increase in diameter at the various times of load application.

Possibly the better pastes (A and B) are those in which the diameter decreased the least over the period indicated. These materials are quite thin and their working time is apparently satisfactory.

An entirely different behavior is exhibited by pastes C and D. Although their initial consistencies are comparable, decrease in flow occurred approximately three minutes after spatulation. Thus, their working time would be limited and, if a specific consistency or fluidity is desired, the time between mixing and insertion of the tray is critical. On the other hand, the reduction in flow, provided the tray was seated, might be advantageous in reducing the possibility of distortion while the impression hardens in the mouth.

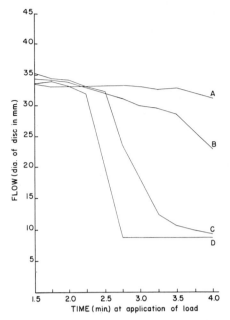

Figure 7–2 Flow of four commercial zinc oxide–eugenol impression pastes at various periods after mixing.

Generally, there is a correlation between flow and setting time. Those materials that show a decrease in flow at various time intervals also have shorter setting times and a shorter time interval between the initial and final set.

Rigidity and Strength As is the case with impressions obtained with compound, the paste impression should be unyielding when it is removed from the mouth and should resist fracture. Impression pastes can be compounded that will exhibit a resistance to flow at mouth temperature which is equal or superior to the similar properties of compound.[10]

The compressive strength of hardened ZOE impression pastes may be as great as 7MPa (1000 psi) two hours after mixing.[11]

Dimensional Stability The dimensional stability of most of the impression pastes is quite satisfactory. A negligible shrinkage (less than 0.1 per cent) may occur during hardening.

No significant dimensional change subsequent to hardening is to be expected with the better commercial products. The impressions can be preserved indefinitely without a change in shape due to relaxation or other causes of warpage. Such a statement assumes that the tray material is dimensionally stable.

Tray Material As previously noted, a preliminary impression is often obtained with tray compound, which can be used as a tray for the paste impression. Such a technique is subject to the general errors of the compound impression, such as thermal changes and warpage due to relaxation. Certainly, the dimensional stability of the paste impression can be no better than that of the tray material on which it rests.

To obtain greater accuracy, many prosthodontists obtain the preliminary impression and then construct a stone cast. A tray of acrylic resin or similar material is constructed on the cast. This tray is then used for obtaining the zinc oxide–eugenol paste impression. The technique was illustrated in Figure 6–1.

Reproduction of Tissue Detail   One of the prime requisites of any impression material is the ability to reproduce accurately the minute detail of the oral tissues. Differences have been noted in the sharpness of detail reproduced by the various pastes commercially available.[11]

Although most pastes are readily separated, there is a tendency for some to adhere to the stone cast. Any film of paste left on the cast will naturally reduce the accuracy of reproduction. The American Dental Association specification for this material requires that examination of a poured stone cast show no visible evidence of adherence of the paste to the cast or of the stone to the impression.

Mixing Technique   The mixing of the two pastes is generally accomplished on an oil-impervious paper, although a glass mixing slab can be used as well.

The proper proportion of the two pastes is generally obtained by squeezing two ropes of paste of the same length, one from each tube, onto the mixing slab. The orifices of the two tubes are regulated to deliver the proper amount from each tube when the lengths of the ropes are the same.

A flexible stainless steel spatula is satisfactory for the mixing. The two ropes are combined with the first sweep of the spatula, and the mixing is continued for approximately one minute, or as directed by the manufacturer, until a uniform color is observed.

General Considerations   The mixture is spread over the preliminary impression, and the tray is carried into the mouth in the usual manner.

The impression should be held firmly in position until it has thoroughly hardened. The accelerating action of the heat of the mouth and the saliva on the surface of the tissues may cause the adjacent surface of the impression to harden first. Any disturbance of the impression at this stage will result in a warpage. Only when the material has hardened completely should the impression be removed from the mouth.

The cast can be constructed in the usual manner. As with impression compound, no separating medium is necessary.

Surgical Pastes   The ZOE pastes have other uses than for edentulous impressions. For example, after a gingivectomy (i.e., surgical removal of diseased gingival tissues), a zinc oxide–eugenol paste may be placed over the wound to aid in the retention of a medicament and to promote healing.

The basic ingredients of the surgical pastes are essentially the same as those of the impression pastes. However, these pastes are generally less brittle and weaker after hardening. Furthermore, their setting time is considerably longer.

In practice, the dentist mixes the paste as usual, but after mixing, it should be capable of being formed into a rope which is packed into the gingival wounds and the interproximal spaces to provide retention of the dressing. The final product should be sufficiently strong that it will not be readily displaced by the patient during mastication, but it should not be so brittle that it will shear readily under localized stresses.

The properties described are attained chiefly by the use of the proper filler, both as to amount and particle size and shape. These pastes may also contain more eugenol than do the impression pastes. The accelerator content is less, if it is present at all.

ZOE compounds of similar composition may also be used as temporary crown and bridge cements, for stabilizing base plates, and as temporary denture relining materials following oral surgery.

Bite Registration Pastes   The materials that are used for recording the occlusal relationships between natural or artificial teeth include impression plaster, compound, wax, resin, and metallic oxide paste. Zinc oxide–eugenol pastes are often used as such recording materials in the construction of complete dentures and fixed or removable partial dentures. One such product is a noneugenol type. Plasticizers such as petrolatum are often added, as is silicone, in order to reduce the tendency of the paste to stick to the mouth tissues. In general, though, bite pastes follow conventional zinc oxide–eugenol–resin formulations.

In contrast to wax, the ZOE impression paste offers almost no resistance to closing of the mandible, thus allowing a more accurate interocclusal relationship record to be formed. Also, the ZOE interocclusal record is more stable than one made in wax.

Noneugenol Pastes   One of the chief disadvantages of the ZOE pastes is the possible stinging or burning sensation caused by the eugenol when it contacts the soft tissues. Furthermore, as previously noted, the ZOE reaction is never completed, with the result that the free eugenol may be leached out into the mouth. Some patients find the taste of the eugenol extremely disagreeable and, in cases in which a surgical pack is worn for several weeks, a chronic gastric disturbance may result.

It has been found that a material similar to the ZOE reaction product can be formed by a saponification reaction to produce an insoluble "soap" if the zinc oxide is reacted with a carboxylic acid.[12, 13] The reaction is:

$$ZnO + 2RCOOH \rightarrow (RCOO)_2Zn + H_2O$$

Almost any carboxylic acid will react with zinc oxide, but only a few such acids provide compounds of dental interest. Ortho-ethoxybenzoic acid, commonly abbreviated as EBA, has been found to be valuable in this connection, for example. The carboxylic acid is not necessarily a liquid. Powdered acids can be dissolved or dispersed in a liquid carrying agent, such as ethyl alcohol, and then reacted with the zinc oxide. The reaction is well understood and it is not greatly affected by temperature or humidity. Bactericides and other medicaments can be incorporated without interfering with the reaction.

Presumably this reaction can be substituted for the ZOE reaction to form any type of dental paste.

References

1. Smith DC: The setting of zinc oxide/eugenol mixtures. Br Dent J 105:313, 1958.
2. Crisp S, Ambersley M, and Wilson AD: Zinc oxide–eugenol cements. V. Instrumental studies of the catalysis and acceleration of the setting reaction. J Dent Res 59:44, 1980.

3. El-Tahawi HM and Craig RG: Thermal analysis of zinc oxide–eugenol cements during setting. J Dent Res 50:430, 1971.
4. Batchelor RF and Wilson AD: Zinc oxide–eugenol cements. I. The effect of atmospheric conditions on rheological properties. J Dent Res 48:883, 1969.
5. Braden M and Clark RL: Dielectric properties of zinc oxide–eugenol type cements. J Dent Res 53:1263, 1974.
6. Wilson AD and Mesley RJ : Zinc oxide–eugenol cements. III. Infrared spectroscopic studies. J Dent Res 51:1581, 1972.
7. Molnar EJ: Residual eugenol from zinc oxide–eugenol compounds. J Dent Res 46:645, 1967.
8. Vieira DF: Factors affecting the setting of zinc oxide–eugenol impression pastes. J Prosthet Dent 9:70, 1959.
9. Clark RJ and Phillips RW: Flow studies of certain dental impression materials. J Prosthet Dent 7:259, 1957.
10. Skinner EW, Cooper EN, and Ziehm HW: Some physical properties of zinc oxide–eugenol impression pastes. J Am Dent Assoc 41:449, 1950.
11. Asgar K and Peyton FA: Physical properties of corrective impression pastes. J Prosthet Dent 4:555, 1954.
12. Molnar EJ: Dental composition and process of making same. U. S. Patent No. 3,028,247, 1962.
13. Smith DC: A materialistic look at periodontal packs. Dent Pract 20:263, 1970.

8 HYDROCOLLOID IMPRESSION MATERIALS: REVERSIBLE HYDROCOLLOID

The impression materials described in the previous chapters are best suited for use in edentulous mouths, in which there are no severe undercuts. Any undercuts prevent the removal of such impressions without distortion or fracture. In the case of the plaster impression, the set plaster is fractured intentionally to remove the impression in pieces, which are reassembled. When compound or an impression paste is used for an impression of teeth, the material distorts, or flows, upon removal over the height of contour of the tooth, and the result is an inaccurate reproduction of the part.

A substance that will deform elastically when it is removed over an undercut, so that it will spring back to its original position, will produce an accurate impression of a tooth. Such a material can be obtained by using a flexible *gel*. The problem is to introduce a viscous fluid into the mouth on an impression tray, and to allow it to gel in position. The impression can then be removed intact, since the flexibility of the gel is sufficient to allow the impression to be withdrawn over extremely sharp undercuts, with no perceptible permanent distortion. The stone cast can be poured in the usual manner.

The ideal impression material, then, for accurately reproducing tooth form and relationship would be some substance which would be sufficiently elastic to be withdrawn from the undercut area and would return to its original shape without distortion.

The first material that might come to mind is soft rubber. In the earlier days, the difficulty with rubber was that it could not be placed in an impression tray in a plastic condition from which the elastic rubber would form after the tray was in position in the mouth. Rubber impression materials are now available and they will be discussed in Chapter 10.

The first elastic impression materials to be used were composed of colloidal gels, jelly-like substances which can be formed in the mouth in an impression tray and removed over the undercuts readily.

THE COLLOIDAL STATE

Owing to their differences in structure, constitution, and reactions, colloids are often classed as a fourth state of matter known as the *colloidal state*. The

108

principles and laws pertaining to this subject are many and very complex. Only the principles and theories directly related to the materials employed in dentistry, particularly the hydrocolloid impression materials, will be briefly described.

Colloids   Colloids represent a particle distribution qualitatively similar to the molecular distribution in a solution of sugar in water, for example. In such a case, the sugar molecules (or solute) are assumed to be dispersed uniformly in the water (or solvent). There is a mutual attraction between the sugar molecules and the water molecules. The former can diffuse at will.

If the particles are large and can be seen by the naked eye or through a microscope, the system is termed a *suspension* or *emulsion*. Solids distributed in liquids are suspensions; liquids distributed in liquids are emulsions. These suspended particles do not readily diffuse and tend to fall out of the suspending medium unless some type of bonding is employed to maintain the suspension or emulsion.

Somewhere between the extremes of the very small molecules in solution and the very large particles in suspension is the colloidal solution or colloidal *sol*. However, there is no clear line of demarcation among these systems. For example, some colloids consist of particle sizes normally thought to be molecular; the particles in other colloids are large enough to be seen with the electron microscope. Generally, though, the sizes of the colloid particles are considered to be in the range of 1 to 200 nanometers.*

True solutions exist as a single phase. There is no separation between the molecule (solute) and the solvent. However, both the colloid and the suspension have two phases, the *dispersed phase* or *dispersed particle* and the *dispersion phase* or *dispersion medium*.

In the colloid, the particles in the dispersed phase consist of molecules that are held together by either primary or secondary forces. Often the molecular attraction is the result of dipoles.

The two phases will be either compatible or incompatible. That is, the dispersed phase will or will not stay suspended in the dispersion medium. In addition to particle size, factors common to any two-phase system (surface energy, surface charge, and wettability) will determine the stability of the colloid.

Types of Colloids   With the exception of the gaseous state (two gases), colloidal sols may be composed of combinations of any other states of matter: e.g., liquid or solid in air (aerosol); gas, liquids, or solids in liquid (lyosol); gas, liquid, or solid in solid. All colloids are termed sols, and not just those in which a liquid is the dispersion medium. Since the hydrocolloid impression materials are solids suspended in liquids, they are *lyophilic* (liquid loving) sols. In general, organic colloids are lyophilic, whereas the metallic dispersions tend to be *lyophobic* (liquid hating).

If gelation or agar is dissolved in water, the gelatin particles attract the water molecules and swell in size, thus forming a *hydrocolloid*.

Gels   If the concentration of the dispersed phase in the hydrocolloid is of the proper amount, the sol may be changed to a semi-solid material known as a gel or jelly when the temperature is decreased. The temperature at which this

---

*1 nm (nanometer) = 10^{-9} m.

change occcurs is known as the *gelation temperature*. A gelatin sol, for example, will gel at a temperature of 18 to 20° C (65 to 68° F). The dispersed phase agglomerates to form chains or fibrils (sometimes called *micelles*). An agar sol gels at a somewhat higher temperature of approximately 37° C (99° F) or slightly above.

The fibrils may branch and intermesh to form a brush heap structure, which can be imagined to resemble the intermeshing of twigs in a brush pile. The dispersion medium is held in the interstices between the fibrils by capillary attraction or adhesion.

In the case of gelatin or agar, the fibrils are held together by secondary molecular forces. As will be described later, the fibrils can also be formed by chemical action. Since gelation by a physical reaction involves a simpler theory, the gelatin-like gels will be discussed first.

Reversible Hydrocolloids   The gelation of a hydrocolloid is, in a sense, a solidification process. The internal energy of the gel is less than that of the sol.

On the other hand, unlike ice for example, the hydrocolloid gel does not return to the sol at the same temperature that it solidified. The gel must be heated to a higher temperature, known as the *liquefaction temperature*, to return it to the sol condition. The temperature lag between the gelation temperature and the liquefaction temperature of the gel is known as *hysteresis*.

However, the process is reversible in that the gelatin can be gelled at the gelation temperature and liquefied at the liquefaction temperature at will. For this reason, it is called a *reversible hydrocolloid*. The reaction can be expressed as

$$sol \rightleftarrows gel$$

Thus the change from the sol to gel, and vice versa, is essentially a physical effect induced by a temperature change.

Parenthetically, it is the phenomenon of hysteresis which makes it possible to use agar as the base for dental impression material. The dentist can liquefy the gel, place it in the impression tray, and carry it to the oral cavity at a temperature the patient can tolerate. The material can then be cooled in the mouth to the gelation temperature and removed as gel.

In practical usage such agar-based materials are simply referred to as hydrocolloids. That abbreviated terminology will be used generally in the following discussion.

Irreversible Hydrocolloids   A gel can be formed from a sol by a chemical reaction rather than a physical effect based on a temperature sensitivity of the colloid. The gel formed from a hydrocolloid sol of sodium alginate to be described in the next chapter, for example, is of this type and it is the base for one of the most widely used impression materials.

Although the final structures of the two types of gel are similar, the fibrils of the gels formed chemically are primary bonded and, therefore, are not affected by temperature changes. They can be returned to the sol only by a reversal of the original chemical reaction and not by heat. For this reason they are known as *irreversible hydrocolloids*. The reaction can be diagrammed as

$$sol \rightarrow gel$$

Again, in usage the terminology has been simplified and such hydrocolloids are usually called *alginate* impression materials.

Gel Strength The gel can support considerable stress, particularly shear, without flow, provided the stress is applied rapidly. It is very likely that the fibrils resist such stresses successfully, but if the stresses are sustained, a flow results, possibly as a result of disturbing the network relation between the dispersion medium and the fibrillar structure.

The stiffness and strength of the gel are directly related to the brush heap density or concentration. For example, in a reversible gel, the greater the concentration of the dispersed phase in the sol, the greater will be the number of fibrils formed upon gelation.

Another factor is the temperature of the reversible gel. The lower the temperature, the stronger the gel will be, and vice versa. When the gel is heated, the kinetic energy of the fibrils increases, with the result that the interfibrillar distances will become greater and their cohesion less. Also, as the temperature increases, more of the fibrils may revert to the sol. Presumably, part of the fibrils can be pictured as constantly reverting to the sol while others are being re-formed. As the temperature rises, more of the fibrils revert until finally more fibrils are reverting than are forming, at which temperature the liquefaction to the sol occurs.

On the other hand, the strength of the irreversible gel is not as greatly affected by normal temperature changes, since the fibrils are formed by chemical action and do not revert to the sol condition upon heating.

The strength of the gel can be increased by the addition of certain modifiers such as fillers and chemicals. The fillers usually consist of fine powders of an inert substance. The powder particles may be imagined to be "caught" in the micelle network in such a manner that the brush heap is rendered more rigid with less flexibility.

Imbibition and Syneresis As might be expected from the structure of the hydrocolloids, a great part of the volume of the gel is occupied by the water. If the water content of the gel is reduced, the gel will shrink, and if the gel then takes up water, the gel will expand or swell. Such possible changes in dimension are of considerable importance in dentistry. If these materials are used for obtaining impressions, any change in dimension of the impression after it has been removed from the mouth is a source of error.

The gel may lose water by evaporation from its surface, or by the exuding of fluid by a process known as *syneresis*. This is one of the characteristic properties of a gel. The exudate that appears on the surface of the gel during and after syneresis is not pure water, as is shown by the fact that it may be either alkaline or acid, depending upon the composition of the gel. In any event, whenever water or fluid is removed from the micelles of the gel by syneresis or otherwise, a shrinkage of the gel occurs.

If a gel is lacking in water content, a sorption of water will occur by a process known as *imbibition* if it is placed in contact with water. A swelling of the gel occurs during imbibition, until the original water content is restored. Gels appear to exhibit a "memory" in this respect; if a certain amount of water is removed from a gel of a given concentration, imbibition will occur only to the extent that the lost water is restored. The minimal concentration of the gel at a given temperature is, therefore, established by the concentration of the sol before gelation. Thus, it follows that when a hydrocolloid impression material gels around the teeth, the specific water content is then established for that particular impression at that specific temperature.

As will be seen later, the properties of syneresis and imbibition are very important in the control of the proper dimensions of the impression.

REVERSIBLE HYDROCOLLOID IMPRESSION MATERIALS

As implied in the previous discussion, the reversible hydrocolloid impression materials are manipulated by changing the gel to a sol with heat. The material is placed in an impression tray in the sol condition and impressed against the mouth tissues, which are in turn to be reproduced in dental stone. The tray is held rigidly in place, and water is circulated through the cooling tubes attached to the outside surface of the tray. When the material has gelled, the tray is removed and the impression is prepared for the pouring of the dental stone. The complete technique will be discussed shortly.

The gelation temperature of the impression material must be at, or slightly above, oral temperature. On the other hand, in order to flow and to reproduce all the detail desired, it must be a fluid sol at a temperature compatible with the oral tissues. It is evident that agar provides a base for the reversible hydrocolloid impression materials that satisfy these requirements.

Agar   Agar is an organic hydrophilic colloid (polysaccharide) extracted from certain types of seaweed. It is a sulfuric ester of a linear polymer of galactose. The generally accepted structural formula for agar is:

The gelation temperature of agar is approximately 37° C (99° F). The exact gelation temperature depends upon several factors, including the molecular weight, the ratio of agar to other ingredients, and the purity of the agar. The temperature at which the gel changes to the sol is 60 to 70° C (108 to 126° F) higher than the gelation temperature.

There are many species of agar and each has somewhat different properties. Often impurities and constituents of low molecular weight are washed from the agar in running water before it is used for a dental impression material. Commercial dental hydrocolloids are usually blends of several species. Although the manufacturers try to maintain constant gel characteristics by this blending, variations in individual batches of agar may make it necessary on occasion for the dentist to alter his manipulative procedures.

Composition   The basic constituent of the hydrocolloid impression materials is agar, but it is by no means a main constituent by weight. It is present in a concentration of 8 to 15 per cent, depending upon the desired properties of the material both in the sol and in the gel condition. The principal ingredient by weight is water. However, some of the modifiers present in minor amounts by weight exert a considerable influence on the properties of the material, and they may be the deciding factor in the success or failure of the material.

The composition presented in Table 8–1 is typical of the present commercial materials.

The function of the agar and the water in the impression material has already been discussed. The borax is added to increase the strength of the gel. It is very likely that the reaction by which this is accomplished is that a borate is formed which increases the strength or density of the micelle framework in some manner. Almost any soluble borate, either organic or inorganic, will produce the same effect. The borate not only increases the strength of the gel but it also can increase the viscosity of the sol so that a filler is unnecessary.

As noted in a previous chapter, a borate, particularly borax, is an excellent retarder of the setting of gypsum products. For this reason, its use in hydrocolloid impression materials is detrimental in that it retards the setting of the plaster or stone cast when the gypsum product is poured into the finished impression. As a matter of fact, the setting of the stone is inhibited whenever it is in contact with a gel, regardless of whether the borate is present. Consequently, the incorporation of the borax aggravates a disadvantage already present.

It has been shown that the surface of a gypsum cast prepared from a hydrocolloid impression exhibits a high concentration of residual hemihydrate and of syngenite as compared with a surface allowed to harden against glass.[1] This results in a soft surface on the gypsum cast.

This disadvantage can be overcome in two ways: (1) The impression can be immersed in a solution containing an accelerator for the setting of the gypsum product, prior to filling the impression with the dental stone and water mixture, or (2) a "plaster hardener" or accelerator can be incorporated in the material by the manufacturer. The sulfates in the formula given in Table 8–1 serve such a purpose. The problem of the hardness of the gypsum cast will be discussed later in this chapter.

Some commercial products contain a certain amount of filler for the control of strength, viscosity, and rigidity, as previously discussed. Some of the fillers used are diatomaceous earth, clay, silica, wax, rubber, and similar inert powders.

Table 8–1.   *Composition of a Commercial Reversible Hydrocolloid Impression Material**

INGREDIENT	COMPOSITION (PER CENT)
Agar	13–17
Borates	0.2–0.5
Sulfates	1.0–2.0
Wax, hard	0.5–1.0
Thixotropic materials	0.3–0.5
Water	Balance

*Courtesy of K. H. Strader.

Other ingredients, such as thymol and glycerine, may also be added as a bactericide and plasticizer respectively. Pigments and flavors are usually present.

Viscosity of the Sol   The viscosity of the sol is of considerable importance in the successful manipulation of the material. After the material has been liquefied, it must be sufficiently viscous so that it will not flow out of the tray, even though the tray is inverted when it is placed in the mouth. On the other hand, its viscosity must not be so great that it will not readily penetrate every detail of the teeth and soft tissues to be impressed.

The agar sol by itself is likely to be too fluid for this purpose, and the use of fillers and other modifiers is employed as previously described. As noted in the previous section, the incorporation of a borate definitely increases the viscosity of the sol.

The viscosity of five commercial hydrocolloid impression materials in the sol condition as influenced by the temperature is shown in Figure 8–1. All of the materials increase in viscosity as the gelation temperature is approached. The beginning of the molecular cohesion to form the micelle structure can be noted by the rather abrupt change in the slope of the curves toward the horizontal, as the temperature decreases.

The greater viscosity and its slow increase with decrease in temperature in the case of materials C, D, and E are probably due to the fact that these materials contain some type of borate compound. Presumably the viscosity of the sol in materials A and B is regulated by fillers or thermoplastic substances, or both, which may be effective only near the gelation temperature. Since the material in the impression tray is usually at a temperature slightly above the gelation temperature at the time it is impressed against the tissues, the viscosity of the material at such temperatures may be an important consideration.

Gelation Temperature   The temperature at which the hydrocolloid impression material sets to a gel is of importance to the dentist. If the material gels at too high a temperature, it is possible that injury may result to the oral tissues

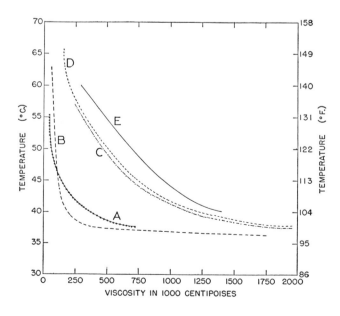

Figure 8–1 Viscosity of the sols of five reversible hydrocolloid impression materials as influenced by temperature. (Courtesy of Coe Laboratories, Inc.)

involved, or if the surface of the sol gels when it contacts the tissues, a severe surface stress may develop. If the gelation temperature is too far below the oral temperature, it will be difficult or even impossible to chill the material to a temperature sufficiently low to obtain a firm gel adjacent to the oral tissues.

The temperature of gel formation is best determined for dental purposes by determining the temperature at which a hollow cylindrical object, such as a metal tube, can be imprinted into the material and withdrawn so that a clean, clear-cut hole is left in the gel. A metal tube with a 10 mm bore and a wall thickness of approximately 1 mm is prescribed for this purpose in the American Dental Association Specification no. 11. According to this specification, the gelation temperature must not be less than 37° C (98.6° F) nor more than 45° C (113° F). Most modern hydrocolloid impression materials exhibit a gelation temperature between 36° C (97° F) and 42° C (108° F).

Gelation Time   Gelation of reversible hydrocolloid is, of course, a function of both temperature and time. As indicated, the lower the ambient temperature, the more rapid will be gelation. Also, the longer the sol is held at a given temperature, the greater will be the viscosity of the sol. The importance of leaving the tray in the mouth until the gelation has proceeded to a point at which the gel strength is sufficient to resist deformation or fracture is well known.

Mechanical Properties   According to the American Dental Association Specification no. 11 for dental agar impression material, the compressive strength should not be less than 0.245 MPa (35.6 psi). In other words, if the material exhibits a compressive strength of at least 0.245 MPa under the test conditions, it will be satisfactory. Presumably, the material will not fracture upon removal if it meets this requirement.

The stress-strain relationships of the hydrocolloid impression materials are not linear over any portion of their stress-strain curve. Although the slope of the curve is a general indication of their stiffness under static loading, it is doubtful that true values for the modulus of elasticity and proportional limit can be obtained. The greater the rate of loading the specimen, the closer the stress-strain curve approaches a straight line. In other words, when a low rate of loading of the specimen is employed in testing, the amount of flow or permanent deformation is relatively great, and vice versa.

Translated into practical terms, this fact has considerable clinical importance. It demonstrates the necessity of deforming the impression rapidly when it is removed from the mouth if the original dimensions are to be preserved. The impression should never be removed by a teasing or weaving method, but rather it should be removed suddenly in a direction as nearly as possible parallel to the long axes of the teeth. A slow removal of the impression is a common cause of inaccuracy.

The amount of deformation these materials can withstand is not primarily dependent on their comparatively high strength. Actually the strain at the point of rupture more truly measures the ability of the material to resist rupture than does compressive strength.[2]

For testing purposes, the permanent deformation of the material after stressing is measured as the percentage deformation, or *set*, that occurs in a cylindrical specimen after a 10 per cent linear strain in compression is applied for 30 seconds. According to the current American Dental Association Specification no. 11, this set should not exceed 1.5 per cent.

Repeated stressing and unstressing of a gel apparently increases its stiffness, as determined by experiments involving repeated loading and unloading. In other words, when a hydrocolloid impression is removed from the mouth and thereby subjected to considerable stress as it is withdrawn over the undercuts, for the most accurate results it should be stressed suddenly and only once.

Since repeated stressing increases the stiffness, it follows that the gel becomes more brittle and the likelihood of fracture increases. This may be the reason for fracture when the subsequent stone cast or die is removed from the impression. Even though the gel may not be fractured during such deformation, it will probably be deformed permanently to a greater extent than the equivalent of the 1.5 per cent set limit included in the specification. Consequently, a distortion may be introduced that will likely increase with subsequent deformation. This is one of the reasons why a second or third stone die prepared in the same hydrocolloid impression may be less accurate than the first.

Regardless of the type of loading, the relaxation of the gel is never complete, and it does not return entirely to its original dimension after deformation. The permanent deformation remaining should, of course, be as small as possible. Although these materials are classified as elastic, they are not perfectly so. However, the amount of permanent deformation is clinically negligible provided the material is adequately gelled, is removed with a sharp thrust, and undercuts present in the cavity preparation are minimal.

MANIPULATION

Accuracy   In the preceding discussion, the accuracy of the impressions, and the effect of certain characteristics on the accuracy of hydrocolloid, has been emphasized. In the last analysis, the dental appliance must fit satisfactorily in the mouth. Consequently, studies concerned with the accuracy of fit of the final dental appliance are necessary for the proper evaluation of the particular dental materials involved.

For such evaluations of the usefulness of the materials in connection with the fabrication of gold inlays and crowns, the steel master dies shown in Figure 8–2 are often used. An accurately fitting gold casting is cast to fit the respective steel die. Then, for example, an impression of the master die is obtained with a hydrocolloid impression material. A stone die is prepared in the impression. The master casting can then be refitted on the stone die, and the accuracy of fit can be compared with that of the casting when placed on the master die.

In such a test, any dimensional change of the stone during setting or subsequently is ignored in estimating the accuracy of the impression material itself. Such an assumption is possibly justified if a Type IV stone is employed with a definite W/P ratio and technique. It can be recalled that the setting expansion of such stones is slight and consistently uniform with a standardized technique.

Granted that it is much more difficult to fabricate gold alloy castings to fit the dies shown in Figure 8–2 than conventional clinical cavity preparations; however, any procedures that are sufficiently accurate for these dies will undoubtedly more than satisfy the clinical requirements. These dies may also be used to evaluate the various techniques employed in the fabrication of dental castings.

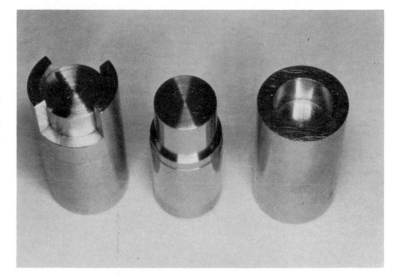

Figure 8–2 Steel dies used for determining accuracy in techniques which involve impression materials and castings. They represent an MOD *(left)*, full-crown *(center)*, and one-surface inlay *(right)*.

Impressions of Prepared Cavities   Cavities are prepared in carious teeth for the reception of artificial restorations of some sort, such as inlays, onlays, or crowns. Generally, either hydrocolloid or the elastomeric impression materials to be described in Chapter 10 are used for this purpose.

No attempt will be made to outline the indirect technique in detail; only the fundamental steps involved will be presented. Although the following discussion is concerned principally with the indirect techniques, much of it is also applicable to the use of these materials in prosthetics and other applications.

Preparation of Material   Proper equipment for preparing and storing the hydrocolloid is essential, and the dental office must be organized for this work. Various types of conditioners for preparation and storage of the hydrocolloid are available, such as the one shown in Figure 8–3.

The hydrocolloid is usually supplied in two forms. Small sticks or cartridges are available for use in the syringes shown in Figure 8–4. By means of the syringe the fluid material can be injected in and around the prepared cavity. Water cooled trays (Fig. 8–4) are used for carrying the hydrocolloid into the mouth to form the bulk of the impression.

The hydrocolloid that is used to fill the tray itself is liquefied in the metal or plastic tubes in which it is supplied. The only difference between the two types is a difference in color and a greater fluidity in the syringe material.

The first step is to reverse the hydrocolloid gel to the sol state. Boiling water is a convenient way of liquefying the material. A *minimum* of 10 minutes of boiling is essential, and there is no evidence that longer periods are harmful.

If the dental office is located in a city of high altitude, e.g., Denver, then other methods must be used, since the boiling point of water is too low to liquefy the gel. A pressure cooker can be used or an agent such as propylene glycol can be added to the water until a temperature of 100° C is attained.

Whenever the material is re-liquefied after a previous use, it is more difficult to break down the agar brush-heap structure, so approximately three minutes should be added each time the material is re-liquefied.

After it has been liquefied, the material may be stored in the sol condition

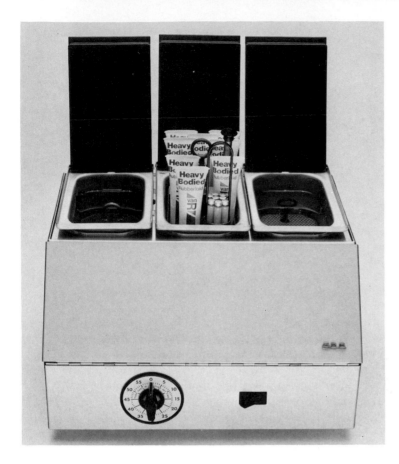

Figure 8–3 A conditioner for the hydrocolloid technique. The various components are used for liquefying the material, for storage after boiling, and for conditioning the tray hydrocolloid. (Courtesy of Van R Dental Products, Inc.)

until it is needed for injection into the cavity preparation or for filling the tray. One of the advantages of the hydrocolloid technique is that in the morning the dental auxiliary can prepare a sufficient number of tubes and syringes for use throughout the day. The material can then be held ready for quick use when

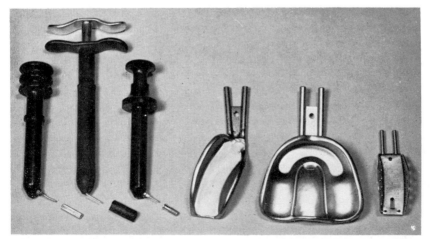

Figure 8–4 Armamentarium for use in obtaining impressions with hydrocolloid impression material. At the left, three types of syringes are shown which can be used for injection of the sol into prepared cavities. On the right are two water-cooled unperforated trays with overhanging rims for retention of the gel. At the extreme right is a sectional tray.

needed. Here again, suitable equipment permits safe storage of the prepared material until it is needed. A storage temperature of 66° C (151° F) or 68° C (155° F) is usually ideal. Lower temperatures may result in some gelation and inaccurate reproduction of fine detail. Since temperatures required in the various steps of preparing the hydrocolloid are critical, those in the different compartments of the conditioner should be checked each week.

Conditioning   The material that is used to fill the tray must be cooled or "tempered." The purpose of this *conditioning* is to increase the viscosity of the hydrocolloid so that it will not flow out of the tray, and to reduce the temperature enough so that the material will not be uncomfortable to the patient. Therefore, the tray is filled and placed in the conditioning section of the equipment.

Since the rate of gelation is influenced by the temperature at which the hydrocolloid is held, various combinations of temperatures and times may be employed. A satisfactory one is to gel the material for approximately 10 minutes at a temperature of 46° C (115° F). The time may be varied for the particular batch or brand of hydrocolloid and for the fluidity preferred by the dentist. For example, impressions for partial dentures require less body. Therefore, a shorter conditioning time is indicated. At any rate, the lower the temperature, the shorter should be the storage time in the conditioning compartment. In any case, the loaded tray should never be stored in this bath for more than 15 minutes, since gelation may have proceeded too far.

The Impression   After the tray material has been conditioned, the prepared cavities are filled with hydrocolloid sol, using one of the syringes shown in Figure 8–4.

The sol, taken directly from the storage compartment, is first ejected at the base of the preparation and then the remainder of the prepared tooth is covered, as shown in Figure 8–5. The needle is held close to the tooth, beneath the surface of the ejected material, in order to prevent a trapping of air bubbles.

When the entire technique is properly standardized, by the time the cavity preparations and adjoining teeth have been covered, the tray material has

Figure 8–5 A hydrocolloid impression sol being ejected (arrow) onto a full-crown cavity preparation. The impression material can be seen covering the preparation on the tooth at the right.

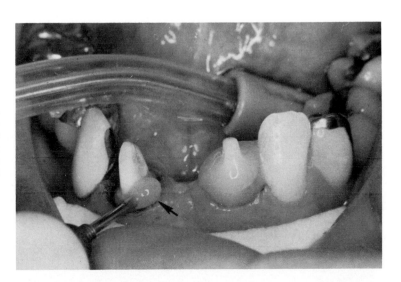

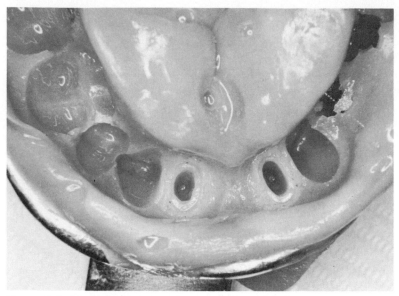

Figure 8–6 The final hydrocolloid impression taken of the cavity preparations and teeth shown in Figure 8–5.

properly conditioned and is ready to be placed immediately in the mouth to form the bulk of the impression. The water-soaked outer layer of tray hydrocolloid is first blotted with a dry gauze sponge before placing it in the mouth. Failure to do so may prevent a firm union between the tray material and the syringe hydrocolloid.

The tray is immediately brought into position and seated with passive pressure. The sol in the tooth bonds to the hydrocolloid in the tray to form a homogeneous impression.

Gelation is accomplished by circulating cool water, approximately 18 to 21° C (64 to 70° F), through the tray for not less than 5 minutes. *Care must be exercised to prevent any movement of the tray during the time the gel is forming.* After gelation, the impression is withdrawn in one piece. Properly done, the resulting impression (Fig. 8–6) is an accurate reproduction of the hard and soft tissues.

Wet Field Technique   A recent technique has become popular for taking impressions in a wet field. It differs somewhat from what has just been described in that the tooth surfaces and tissue are purposely left wet. The areas are actually flooded with warm water. Then the syringe material is introduced quickly and liberally to cover the occlusal and/or incisal areas only. While the syringe material is still liquid, the tray material is seated. The hydraulic pressure of the viscous tray material forces the fluid syringe hydrocolloid down into the areas to be restored.

Distortion During Gelation   Certain stresses are always introduced during gelation. The hydrocolloid materials contract initially after gelation. If the material is held rigidly by the retention in the impression tray, such a contraction of the material may be manifested by an expansion of the space or area surrounded by the impression. It is conceivable that portions of the impression near the tray may be enlarged.

In the case of hydrocolloid, the gelation begins adjacent to the cool tray and continues to the warmer oral tissues. Since the sol is a poor thermal conductor, rapid cooling may cause a concentration of stress near the tray when the gelation first takes place. Consequently, water at approximately 20° C (68° F) is more suitable for cooling the impression than is ice water, for example.

Distortion During Removal   The brush-heap structure of the gel is of such a nature that a sudden force is always more successfully resisted without distortion or fracture than is a force that is applied slowly. Consequently, when the impression is removed, it is necessary to remove it suddenly, with a jerk, rather than to tease it out, as might be done with an impression in compound or plaster. The scientific rationale for this was discussed in the section on Mechanical Properties. Also it was noted that the removal is accomplished in a direction as nearly as possible parallel to the long axes of the teeth.

Dimensional Stability   As previously noted, gels are invariably subject to changes in dimension by syneresis and imbibition, depending on their environment. Once the impression is removed from the mouth and carried into the air at room temperature, syneresis usually starts immediately, with a resulting shrinkage of the gel. Since the impression must be exposed to the air for sufficient time to construct the cast, some shrinkage is bound to occur. Furthermore, if the impression is immersed in water to replenish the lost water, the swelling by imbibition does not restore the original dimension.

A typical example of the dimensional change that can occur during syneresis and imbibition of a hydrocolloid impression material is shown in Figure 8–7.

As can be noted, the material shrank in air. During the subsequent imbibition, the original dimension was almost regained but there was a slight over-expansion. It is very likely that the gel lost water and dimension before the measurements began, with the result that the swelling by imbibition was greater than the observed shrinkage.

Unfortunately, however, the gels are notably subject to stresses in localized areas. These stresses may be relieved and cause distortions which are not included in the linear measurements quoted.[3] One cause for production of such stresses is exertion of pressure on the tray during the gelation period. As noted, this is one of the reasons why the tray should be held firmly but under

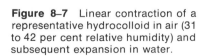

Figure 8–7   Linear contraction of a representative hydrocolloid in air (31 to 42 per cent relative humidity) and subsequent expansion in water.

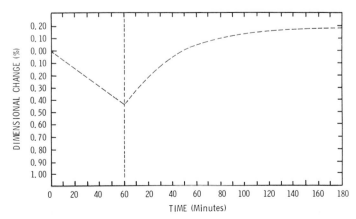

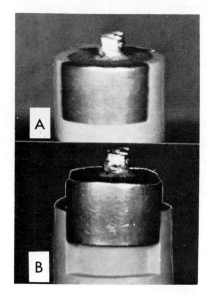

Figure 8–8 *A*, Fit of a master casting on a stone die constructed immediately after the hydrocolloid impression was removed from a master steel die. *B*, Fit of same casting when the stone die was constructed one hour after the impression was removed.

passive pressure. It is clear that the impression should be exposed to the air for as short a time as possible if the best results are to be obtained. The importance of constructing the stone cast immediately is clearly illustrated in Figure 8–8.

Various storage media, such as 2 per cent potassium sulfate or 100 per cent relative humidity, have often been suggested to prevent dimensional change. Results obtained for one dental hydrocolloid by storing impressions in these and two other media may be seen in Figure 8–9. These results are typical, and they indicate that a relative humidity of 100 per cent best preserves the normal water content.[4] Unfortunately, however, there is some alteration in the water content and contraction even when the impression is stored in this environment. Furthermore, even if it were possible to preserve

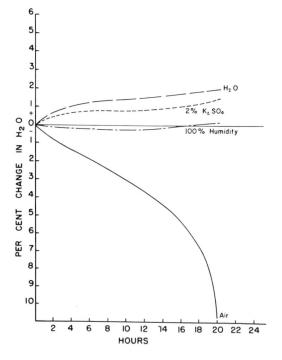

Figure 8–9 Percentage change in water content by weight of a hydrocolloid impression material in various storage media.

the water equilibrium, distortion would still likely occur during storage because of the relaxation of the internal stress that is always present in the impression, as noted. Thus, it is evident that there is no satisfactory method for storing a hydrocolloid impression.

However, there are situations that prevent the die from being poured promptly. Therefore, not recommended but as an alternative, the impression should be rinsed in tap water and wrapped in a surgical paper towel, saturated with water, and placed in a closed container. The container, e.g., a plastic bag or a humidor, should be kept closed until time is available to pour the die.

Surface Hardness of the Die   Some form of gypsum will ordinarily be used as the cast or die material in a hydrocolloid impression. Every precaution must be taken to insure maximum surface hardness. The slightest porosity or chalkiness on the die will result in inaccuracy and lack of sharp detail. One of the factors involved in this regard is the compatibility of the impression material and the gypsum die material.

A properly formulated reversible hydrocolloid, as it is now available, will have little deleterious effect upon the hardness of a Type II or III gypsum cast (Table 8–2). However, the hardness of a Type IV gypsum may be reduced by approximately one third from contact with a reversible hydrocolloid.[5] In general, though, the surface character, including hardness, of any type of gypsum properly proportioned and mixed should be satisfactory after setting in contact with the present commercial reversible hydrocolloids.

The use of so-called "hardening solutions" has often been advocated as an aid to increasing further the surface hardness of the stone. The impression is immersed in the hardening solution prior to pouring the stone. Various chemicals have been employed, such as potassium sulfate, zinc sulfate, manganese sulfate, and potash alum. The most effective, however, is a 2 per cent potassium sulfate solution.

The hardening solution may increase the hardness of the stone in a number of ways. It may act as an accelerator for the set of the gypsum product to overcome the retarding action of the gel surface on the setting of the dental stone. Also, it may react with the gel to produce a surface layer that will reduce or prevent syneresis and therefore eliminate the retarding action of the gel. The effect of the potassium sulfate solution on the surface hardness of the die is apparently dependent upon the particular compatibility of the hydrocolloid and the gypsum product used. In fact certain combinations may result in a reduction in surface hardness of a Type IV gypsum.[6]

Improvements in some reversible hydrocolloid materials now make it possible to obtain a satisfactory surface on stone casts without using a

Table 8–2.   *Effect of a Hydrocolloid Impression Material on the Surface Hardness of Three Gypsum Products*

Gypsum Product	Control* (KHN)	In Contact with Reversible Hydrocolloid (KHN)
Type II gypsum	7.0	8.1
Type III gypsum	24.6	23.9
Type IV gypsum	51.8	32.4

*Gypsum product allowed to set in contact with a glass surface.

hardening solution. If it is found that a smooth, hard stone surface is obtained with a particular hydrocolloid-stone combination without the use of a hardening solution, the treatment can be eliminated. The manufacturer's directions can probably be relied upon in this regard.

As was noted in Figure 8–9, such solutions may affect the dimensions of the impression. For this reason, if a hardening solution is used, the impression should not be immersed in it for more than 10 to 15 minutes, since only the surface layer of the gel need be saturated with the solution. Usually, a period of 5 minutes is sufficient to provide such a saturation. This treatment may be done while the stone mix is being prepared. The hardening solution may be reused until it becomes unduly contaminated.

The use of hardening agents that are added to the stone mixture itself, e.g., colloidal silica, will be discussed in Chapter 27.

Other Factors   A rough stone surface will result if excess water has collected on the surface of the impression at the time the stone mixture is poured. However, the surface of the impression should not be dried completely, or the gel will adhere to the surface of the cast upon its removal. Undue dehydration will also result in syneresis and a distortion of the impression. The surface of the impression should be shiny but with no visible water film or droplets at the time the cast is constructed.

After the impression has been filled with stone, it may be placed in either a humidor or a 2 per cent potassium sulfate solution while the stone hardens. For some reason, somewhat superior stone surfaces are obtained if the stone hardens in an atmosphere of approximately 100 per cent relative humidity. In any event, the filled impression should never be immersed in water while the stone sets.

The stone cast, or die, should be kept in contact with the impression for at least 30 minutes or, preferably, 60 minutes before the impression is separated from the cast. The setting time of the stone in contact with the impression material will probably be increased, and sufficient time should be allowed for the stone to set.

It is possible, however, to allow the stone to remain in contact with the hydrocolloidal gel for too long a time. On occasion, if the cast is allowed to remain in contact with the hydrocolloid impression overnight, a chalky stone surface may be evidenced. For this reason it is wise to separate the cast within a reasonable period of time.

Types of Failure   Common causes for failures encountered with the reversible hydrocolloid impression materials are summarized in the following list.

Type	*Cause*
1. Grainy material	a. Inadequate boiling
	b. Conditioning or storage temperature too low
	c. Conditioning or storage time too long
2. Separation of tray and syringe material	a. Water-soaked layer of tray material not removed
	b. Undue gelation of either syringe or tray material
3. Tearing	a. Inadequate bulk
	b. Moisture contamination at gingiva
	c. Premature removal from mouth
	d. Syringe material partially gelled when tray seated

4. External bubbles	a. Undue gelation, preventing flow
5. Irregularly shaped voids	a. Moisture or debris on tissue
	b. Material too cool or grainy
6. Rough or chalky stone cast	a. Inadequate cleansing of impression
	b. Excess water or potassium sulfate solution left in impression
	c. Premature removal of die
	d. Improper manipulation of stone
7. Distortion	a. Impression not poured immediately
	b. Movement of tray during gelation
	c. Premature removal from mouth
	d. Improper removal from mouth
	e. Use of ice water during initial stages of gelation

References

1. Smith DC and Fairhurst CW: Effect of hydrocolloid impression materials on the surface of dental stone. J Dent Res 41:1103, 1962.
2. Cresson J: Suggested revisions for testing dental elastic impression materials. J Dent Res 28:573, 1949.
3. Gilmore HW, Phillips RW, and Swartz ML: The effect of residual stress and water change on the deformation of hydrocolloid impression materials. J Dent Res 37:816, 1958.
4. Swartz ML, Norman RD, Gilmore HW, and Phillips RW: Studies on syneresis and imbibition in reversible hydrocolloid. J Dent Res 36:472, 1957.
5. Skinner EW and Gordon C: Some experiments on the surface hardness of dental stones. J Prosthet Dent 6:94, 1956.
6. Eames WB, Rogers LB, Wallace SW, and Suway NB: Compatibility of gypsum products with hydrocolloid impression materials. Oper Dent 3:108, 1978.

9 ALGINATE (IRREVERSIBLE HYDROCOLLOID)

At the end of the last century a chemist from Scotland noticed that certain brown seaweed (algae) yielded a peculiar mucous extraction. He named it "algin" and it was used for many purposes.

In England 40 years later another chemist, S. William Wilding, received a basic patent for the use of algin as a dental impression material.[1]

When the popular agar impression material became scarce because of World War II (Japan was a prime source of agar), research was accelerated to find a suitable substitute. The result was, of course, the present irreversible hydrocolloid, or *alginate* impression materials. Their general use far exceeds that of the reversible hydrocolloid type.

The major chemical and physical properties of alginate are described in this chapter. The principal factors responsible for the success of this type of impression material are: (a) it is easy to manipulate; (b) it is comfortable for the patient; and (c) it is relatively inexpensive and does not require elaborate equipment.

Chemistry The chief ingredient of the irreversible hydrocolloid impression materials is one of the soluble alginates. It is generally conceded to be a linear polymer of the sodium salt of anhydro-beta-*d*-mannuronic acid with the structural formula shown in Figure 9–1.

Alginic acid is insoluble in water, but some of its salts are not. The acid can be changed to an ester salt very readily, since the polar carboxyl groups are free to react. Most of the inorganic salts are insoluble, but the salts obtained with sodium, potassium, and ammonium are soluble in water. Sodium, potassium, and triethanol amine alginate are used in dental impression materials.

When mixed with water the soluble alginates form a sol similar to the agar sol. The sols are quite viscous even in low concentrations, but the soluble alginates, useful in dentistry, form sols quite readily if the alginate powder and water are mixed vigorously. The molecular weight of the alginate compounds may vary widely, depending on the manufacturing treatment. The greater the molecular weight, the more viscous is the sol.

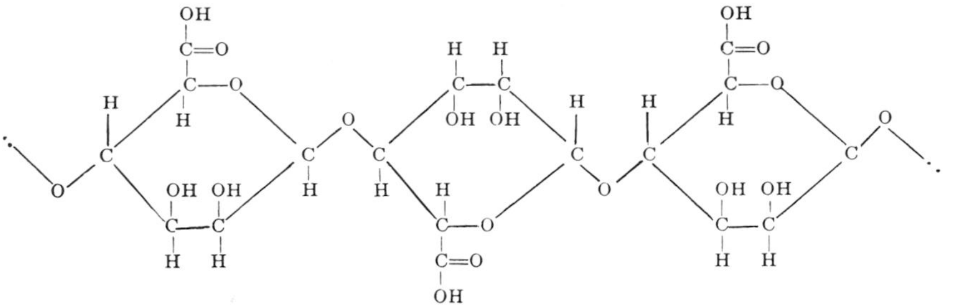

Figure 9-1 Structural formula of alginic acid.

The manufacturer supplies the dentist with the alginate powder, containing the added ingredients to be discussed. The dentist prepares the alginate sol of the proper viscosity and places it in the mouth in an impression tray. Gelation occurs by chemical reaction and the impression is then removed. The procedure differs essentially from that employed with the reversible hydrocolloid materials in that the dentist prepares the sol himself and the temperature is not an active factor in gelation.

There are a number of methods for the production of this chemical change, but the simplest and best understood method is to react the soluble alginate with calcium sulfate to produce insoluble calcium alginate as a gel. Practically, such a reaction must take place in the mouth; therefore, it must be delayed while the impression material is mixed with water, placed in the impression tray, and carried to the mouth. The reactions are best illustrated by a typical example.

Calcium sulfate is an excellent compound for the production of an insoluble calcium alginate when it reacts with potassium or sodium alginate in an aqueous solution. In practice, the production of the calcium alginate is delayed by the addition of a third soluble salt to the solution, with which the calcium sulfate will react in preference to the soluble alginate to form an insoluble calcium salt. Thus, the reaction between the calcium sulfate and the soluble alginate is prevented so long as any of the added salt is left.

The added salt is known as a *retarder.* There are a number of soluble salts which can be used, such as sodium or potassium phosphate, oxalate, or carbonate. Trisodium phosphate, sodium tripolyphosphate, and tetrasodium pyrophosphate have been employed, but the latter two are now most common. The calcium sulfate, or whatever chemical is used to produce the gel, is known as the *reactor.*

For example, if suitable amounts of calcium sulfate, potassium alginate, and trisodium phosphate are mixed together in proper proportions in water, after they become partially or totally dissolved the following reaction will take place:

$$2Na_3PO_4 + 3CaSO_4 \longrightarrow Ca_3(PO_4)_2 + 3Na_2SO_4 \qquad (1)$$

When the supply of trisodium phosphate is exhausted, the calcium ions begin to react with the potassium alginate to produce calcium alginate as follows:

$$K_nAlg + \frac{n}{2} CaSO_4 \longrightarrow \frac{n}{2} K_2SO_4 + Ca \frac{n}{2} Alg \qquad (2)$$

Composition A formula* for an alginate impression material based upon the reactions shown is as follows (per cent by weight):

Potassium alginate	15%
Calcium sulfate	16%
Zinc oxide	4%
Potassium titanium fluoride	3%
Diatomaceous earth	60%
Sodium phosphate	2%

The exact proportion of each chemical to be used varies with the type of raw material. Particularly the amount of retarder (sodium phosphate) must be adjusted carefully to provide the proper gelation time. In general, if approximately 15 gm of the powder is mixed with 40 ml of water, gelation will occur in about 3 to 4 minutes at normal room temperature.

The purpose of the diatomaceous earth is to act as a filler. The filler, if added in proper amounts, can increase the strength and stiffness of the alginate gel, produce a smooth texture, and insure a firm gel surface that is not tacky. It also aids in forming the sol by dispersing the alginate powder particles in the water. Without a filler, the gel formed lacks firmness and exhibits a sticky surface covered with a syneretical exudate. The zinc oxide also acts as a filler and has some influence on the physical properties and setting time of the gel.

Any type of calcium sulfate can be used as the reactor. The dihydrate form is generally used, but under certain circumstances the hemihydrate is said to produce an increased shelf life of the powder, and a more satisfactory dimensional stability of the gel.

A fluoride, such as potassium titanium fluoride, is added to ensure a hard, dense stone cast surface. In proper concentrations, fluoride salts are accelerators for the setting gypsum products.

One impression material, which originated in Japan, uses triethanol amine alginate, soluble and insoluble carbonate (instead of a phosphate), and calcium sulfate.[2] So far as is known, all of the commercial formulas include calcium sulfate as the reactor.

Shelf Life Alginate impression materials deteriorate rapidly at elevated temperatures. Materials that were stored for one month at 65° C (149° F) proved to be unsuitable for dental use, either failing to set at all or setting much too rapidly.[3] Even at 54° C (129° F) there was evidence of deterioration, probably due to depolymerization of the alginate constituent.

The American Dental Association Specification no. 18 for alginate impression materials specifies that, after storage in the original container for one week at 60° C (140°F) in a relative humidity of 100 per cent, the deterioration of the material should not be so great that the compressive strength of the gel is less than .255 MPa (37 psi). In any event, it is better not to stock more than 1 year's supply in the dental office, and to store the material in a cool, dry environment.

The alginate impression material is dispensed to the dentist in individually sealed pouches, with sufficient powder pre-weighed for an individual impression, or in bulk form in a can. The individual pouches are preferred,

---

*Courtesy of J. Cresson, 1980.

since there is less chance for contamination during storage, and the correct water-powder ratio is ensured, since plastic cups are provided for the measurement of the water. However, the bulk form of packing is by far the most popular.

If the bulk package is employed, the lid should be firmly replaced on the container as soon as possible after each use so that a minimal amount of moisture contamination occurs.

Furthermore, ideally the powder should be weighed and not measured by volume by means of a scoop, as many manufacturers direct. However, unless one uses a grossly incorrect method of scooping the powder, it is unlikely that the variation in powder weight per scoop is greater than a few tenths of a gram. Such variations in individual mixes would have no measurable effect on the physical properties.

Nonetheless, if reasonable care is not exerted in following the manufacturer's directions precisely, the handling characteristics of the alginate mix will be influenced. For example, a variation of only 15 per cent from the recommended liquid/powder ratio will markedly affect the setting time and consistency.[4]

If the powder in the can is fluffed before measurement, it is important to avoid breathing the dust, which will rise from the can when the lid is removed. Some of the silica particles in the dust are of such a size and shape to be a possible health hazard.

Gel Structure   As described in the preceding chapter, the fibrils in an alginate gel are assumed to be held together by primary bonds rather than by intermolecular forces, as in the case of reversible hydrocolloids. When the alginic acid is changed to a soluble salt, such as sodium alginate, the cation is attached at a carboxyl group to form an ester or salt. When the insoluble salt is formed by the reaction of the sodium alginate in solution with a calcium salt, for example, the calcium ion may replace the sodium ions in two adjacent molecules to produce a cross-linking between the two molecules. As the reaction progresses, a cross-linked molecular complex or polymer network forms. Such a network can constitute the brush heap structure of the gel.

The cross-linking can be envisioned as diagrammed in Figure 9–2. The base molecules can be recognized as the sodium salt of alginic acid (Fig. 9–1). With the exception of the polar groups, all of the side chains have been omitted for simplification. Some of the sodium ions have not reacted as yet, but may be replaced by a calcium ion as indicated in the other polar groups. Thus, the individual sodium alginate molecules may be linked to form larger molecules or, theoretically, one large molecule. Actually, cross-linking may be classified as a form of polymerization. It can be recognized that this cross-linking is the product of reaction (2).

It is necessary, however, to control the amount of cross-linking.* For example, if a soluble salt such as calcium chloride is used as the reactor, the cross-linkage is virtually complete in a few seconds, and the entire sol is converted to insoluble calcium alginate, a formless mass resembling fresh egg albumin. Such a material would be entirely useless as an impression material.

Calcium sulfate, being more insoluble than calcium chloride, supplies calcium ions at a slower rate so that only part of the alginate molecules become

---

*Cross-linking will be explained at more length in Chapters 11 and 12.

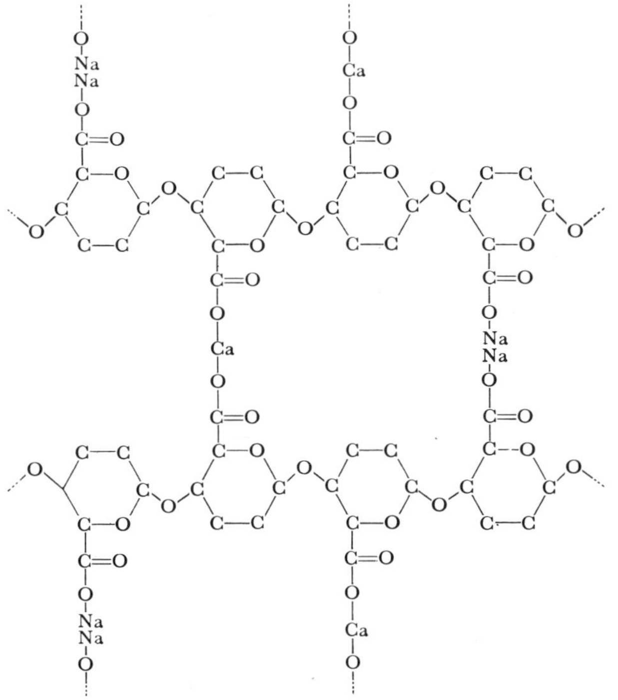

Figure 9–2 A schematic representation of the cross-linking of sodium alginate molecules to form calcium alginate. Note that only some of the molecules have been cross-linked.

cross-linked. The remaining sol becomes encapsulated in a sheath of the insoluble calcium alginate. As a result, the reaction does not continue to completion.

The final structure, then, can be envisioned as a brush heap of a calcium alginate fibril network enclosing unreacted sodium alginate sol, excess water, filler particles, and reaction by-products. Syneresis and imbibition can occur by the loss or gain of water by the entrapped sol. It can be seen that the final structures of the two types of gel, irreversible and reversible, are similar, and that they share the same relationship to environment, strength, and other properties.

Control of Gelation Time   The gelation time, measured from the beginning of mixing until the gelation occurs, is of interest, since sufficient time must be allowed for the dentist to mix the material, to load the tray, and to place it in the patient's mouth. A prolonged gelation time is tedious for both the patient and the dentist. On the other hand, a premature gelation, which begins before the filled impression tray is placed in position in the mouth, will result in a distorted and generally useless impression. Once the gelation starts, it must not be disturbed because any fracturing of the fibrils will be permanent. A fractured gel cannot be joined again unless it is re-gelled. Probably the optimal gelation time is between 3 and 4 minutes at a room temperature of 20° C (68° F).

There are several methods for the measurement of gelation time, but probably the best method for the dental practitioner is to observe the time from the start of mixing until the material is no longer tacky or adhesive when it is touched with a clean, dry finger.

On the basis of a similar test, two types of alginate hydrocolloids are described in the American Dental Association Specification no. 18. Type I (fast setting) must gel in not less than 60 seconds nor more than 120 seconds. Type II (normal setting) must gel between 2 and 4.5 minutes.

As previously related, the gelation time is best regulated by the amount of retarder added. However, such a method of control is not feasible for use by the dentist, since the action of the retarder is critical, and its addition is better regulated by the manufacturer. The gelation time of some commercial products can be altered by changing the W/P ratio and the mixing time, but such changes are likely to impair certain characteristics of the gel.

The best method for the dental practitioner to control the gelation time is to alter the temperature of the water for mixing the alginate material.

The effect of the temperature of the water on the gelation time of an alginate impression material is shown in Figure 9–3. It is evident that the higher the temperature, the shorter is the gelation time. The importance of having the water at the proper temperature is evident. In hot weather, special precautions should be taken to provide cool water for mixing so that a premature gelation will not be obtained. It may even be necessary to pre-cool the mixing bowl and spatula, especially when small amounts of impression material are to be mixed. In any event, it is better to err by having the mix too cool, rather than too warm.

Some materials exhibit greater sensitivity to temperature changes than do others. The change in gelation time per degree Celsius between 20 and 30° C (68 and 86° F) in the material used for obtaining the data in Figure 9–3 is 0.1 minute, or 6 sec/°C (3 sec/°F). Some commercial materials have been found to exhibit as much as 20 second change in gelation time for every degree Celsius change in temperature. In such a case, the temperature of the mixing water should be regulated carefully within a degree or two of a standard temperature, usually 20° C (68° F) so that a constant and reliable gelation time can be obtained. Obviously, the manufacturer should inhibit the effect of temperature on his product as much as possible. If the desired setting time cannot be achieved by varying the water temperature within reasonable limits, it is better to select another product having the desired setting time rather than to resort to other modifications in the manipulative technique.

Strength   As noted in the preceding chapter, the compressive strength of a reversible hydrocolloid impression material should be at least .245 MPa (35.6 psi). With proper manipulation, the strength of the alginate impression materials may be greater than that of the agar materials. In fact, the American Dental Association specification for alginate type hydrocolloid

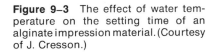
Figure 9–3 The effect of water temperature on the setting time of an alginate impression material. (Courtesy of J. Cresson.)

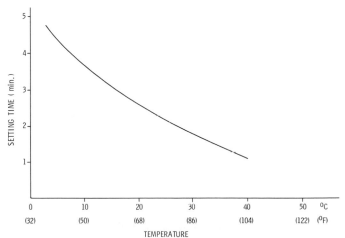

requires a minimal strength of .343 MPa (49.8 psi) and some products may double this value.

The composition of the alginate material can radically affect its gel strength. As previously noted, the type of reactor used can influence the strength. The type and amount of the soluble alginate used are of considerable importance, as are the nature and proportions of the other ingredients.

All of the manipulative factors affect the gel strength, and these factors are under the control of the dentist. For example, if too much or too little water is used in mixing, the final gel will be weakened. The proper W/P ratio should be employed as specified by the manufacturer.

The strength of the final gel can be radically reduced if the mixing is not thorough. Insufficient spatulation results in failure of the ingredients to dissolve sufficiently so that the chemical reactions can proceed uniformly throughout the mass. Overmixing gives equally poor results, since any calcium alginate gel formed during prolonged spatulation will be broken up, and the strength will, therefore, be impaired. The directions supplied with the product should be adhered to in all respects.

Even after thorough spatulation, the smoothness of the final material will differ with various brands of alginate. However, a smooth, creamy mixture should be expected when the better commercial products are employed.

Although the stress-strain relationships of the alginate impression materials are approximately the same as those specified for the reversible hydrocolloid materials, the set of the alginate materials is always slightly higher than that found with the other type.

MANIPULATION

Preparing the Mix Although special plastic spatulas and bowls are available for the mixing, generally a plastic bowl and metal spatula are employed. It may appear to the reader that undue emphasis is constantly being placed upon the use of clean equipment. However, many of the problems, and the related failures, attributed to various materials are in fact associated with dirty or contaminated mixing or handling devices. Contamination during mixing may result in too rapid a set, inadequate fluidity, or even rupture of the impression upon removal from the mouth. For example, small amounts of gypsum left in the bowl from a previous mix of plaster or stone contaminate the impression material and accelerate the set. It is probably desirable to use separate bowls for mixing the alginate and stone.

Maximum gel strength is required in order to prevent fracture and to ensure elastic recovery of the impression upon its removal from the mouth. All the manipulative factors affect the gel strength, as discussed earlier. For example, the proper W/P ratio as specified by the manufacturer should be employed.

The mixing time is particularly important. For example, the strength of the gel can be reduced as much as 50 per cent if the mixing is not complete. Insufficient spatulation results in failure of the ingredients to dissolve sufficiently so that the chemical reactions can proceed uniformly throughout the mass. On the other hand, if the mixing time is unduly prolonged, the gel will be broken up as it is forming, and the strength will be decreased. The directions supplied with the product should be adhered to in all respects.

The weighed powder is placed into the water and incorporated by careful

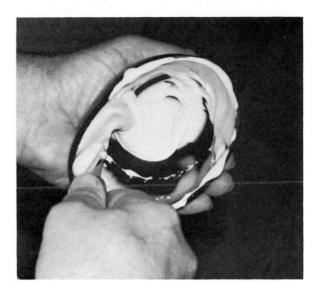

Figure 9–4 The mix of an alginate impression material is made by a vigorous "stropping" of the material against the sides of the mixing bowl.

spatulation. As for gypsum products, care should be taken to avoid whipping air into the mix. Improper mixing of alginate impression materials is all too common. A vigorous figure-eight motion is used, with the mix being swiped or stropped against the sides of the rubber mixing bowl, as demonstrated in Figure 9–4. This is effective in working out most of the air bubbles and also wipes dissolved algin from the surface of the yet undissolved algin, thereby promoting complete dissolution. It is important to get all of the algin dissolved. If it is not, a good gel cannot form and the properties suffer accordingly.

A mixing time of 45 seconds or 1 minute is generally sufficient, depending upon the brand and type of alginate. The result should be a smooth, creamy mixture that does not drip off of the spatula when it is raised from the bowl. With the better commercial products, a smooth creamy mixture can be expected. A variety of mechanical devices are also available for spatulating the alginate materials. Their principal merit is convenience, speed, and elimination of the human variable.

Taking the Impression   The mixture is placed in a suitable tray, which is carried into place in the mouth. It is imperative that the impression tray be one in which the gel will be locked mechanically so that the impression can be withdrawn from around the teeth. Therefore, a perforated tray is generally used. The thickness of the gel between the tray and the tissues for either hydrocolloid or alginate should always be at least 3 mm (⅛ inch).

The strength of the alginate gel increases for several minutes after the initial gelation. As can be noted from Table 9–1, the gel strength of the

Table 9–1. *Increase in Compressive Strength of an Alginate Gel from the Time of Gelation*

TIME FROM GELATION (min)	COMPRESSIVE STRENGTH (MPa)
0	.33
4	.77
8	.81
12	.71
16	.74

particular impression material investigated actually doubled during the first 4 minutes after gelation, but it did not increase appreciably after the first 4 minute period. Most alginate materials improve in elasticity with time, thus permitting superior reproduction of undercut areas. Such data clearly indicate that the alginate impression should not be removed from the mouth for at least 2 to 3 minutes after the gelation has occurred, which is approximately the time at which the material loses its tackiness.

Although the tendency is to remove the tray prematurely, it is possible to leave an alginate impression in the mouth too long. Recall that in the previous chapter it was pointed out that reversible hydrocolloids show no deleterious effect even when held in the mouth for as long as 10 minutes. However, with certain alginates it has been shown that if the impression is held for 6 to 7 minutes, rather than 2 or 3 after gelation, a definite distortion results.[5, 6]

Surface Reproduction   The accuracy of any model produced from an impression material is obviously a function of its inherent accuracy. This accuracy of reproduction is dependent not only on the dimensional behavior of the materials involved but also on the surface condition of both the impression and the model. Surface accuracy involves the duplication of surface detail and is governed by the intersurface relationship between the impression material and the cast material.

The American Dental Association specifications for both the reversible and the irreversible hydrocolloid impression materials require a surface reproduction test. The impression material is placed against a stainless steel block which is marked with a series of ruled lines of graduated widths. A gypsum cast is made from the impression. The cast poured from either type of impression material must reproduce the line that is 0.075 mm in width. The gypsum itself must be capable of reproducing the 0.050 mm line when it is allowed to harden against the block.

However, casts made in alginate impression materials may not reproduce the finer lines as well as do the reversible hydrocolloid materials.[7] Likewise, the surface of the gypsum cast may sometimes be inferior to the surface obtained with the reversible type. Reproduction of surface detail may also vary, depending upon the particular impression material–stone combination used. Some combinations are more compatible than others, particularly when evaluated by test methods more critical than the one just described.[8]

This is one of the principal reasons that alginate impression materials are not used to any extent in fixed prostheses. Such restorations (e.g., a crown) require precise reproduction of detail. The hydrocolloids and the elastomers (to be discussed next) are markedly superior in this respect.

Dimensional Stability.   The phenomena of imbibition and syneresis, discussed in Chapter 8, Reversible Hydrocolloid, are also applicable to the alginate materials (see Fig. 8–7). Fluctuations in water content, and thus dimensional changes, occur upon storage in any medium. As is the case with the reversible hydrocolloids, these materials are most stable when stored in a humidor at 100 per cent humidity. However, for accurate results the cast should be constructed immediately after the impression is obtained. There is no adequate method for storage of any of the hydrocolloid impression materials.

Construction of the Cast   Immediately after being removed from the mouth, the impression is thoroughly rinsed under running water. In the past, most alginate impressions required immersion in a hardening solution before the stone cast was constructed. However, the formulas have now been adjusted so that gypsum hardening solutions are not required unless their use is specifically indicated by the manufacturer.

The method of preparing the mix of stone and filling the impression is the same as that described for the reversible hydrocolloid materials. The stone cast should not be separated for 30, or preferably 60, minutes. For the alginate, it is generally advisable to remove the cast from the impression at approximately 1 hour if maximum density of the stone surface is to be achieved.

Types of Failure   Many of the causes for the common difficulties experienced with the alginates are the same as those encountered with the reversible hydrocolloids. For example, inaccuracy in the alginate impression can often be attributed to failure to construct the cast immediately after removal of the impression from the mouth, to premature or improper removal, or to movement of the tray during the gelation period. However, since the two types of materials are prepared differently, the causes of stiffness or granular consistency are obviously different. Common types of difficulties and the potential causes are summarized below.

Type	Cause
1. Grainy material	a. Improper mixing b. Prolonged mixing c. Undue gelatin d. Water/powder ratio too low
2. Tearing	a. Inadequate bulk b. Moisture contamination c. Premature removal from mouth d. Prolonged mixing
3. Bubbles	a. Undue gelation, preventing flow b. Air incorporated during mixing
4. Irregularly shaped voids	a. Moisture or debris on tissue
5. Rough or chalky stone cast	a. Inadequate cleaning of impression b. Excess water left in impression c. Premature removal of cast d. Leaving cast in impression too long e. Improper manipulation of stone
6. Distortion	a. Impression not poured immediately b. Movement of tray during gelation c. Premature removal from mouth d. Improper removal from mouth e. Tray held in mouth too long (only with certain brands)

Duplicating Materials   Both types of hydrocolloid are used in the dental laboratory to duplicate dental casts or models. The duplicated cast is used in the construction of prosthetic appliances and for orthodontic models. Reversible hydrocolloid is the most popular because it can be used many times. Also, with intermittent stirring it can be kept in liquid form for one or two weeks at a constant pouring temperature, and its price is reasonable.

The hydrocolloid-type duplicating materials basically have the same composition as the impression materials, but their water content is higher. Consequently, the agar or alginate content is lower, which influences their compressive strength and per cent set.[9] These materials are encompassed in American Dental Association Specification no. 20.

Resinous duplicating materials are also available, e.g., a highly plasticized vinyl chloride type resin.

References

1. Wilding SW: Material for taking impression for dental or other purposes. US Patent No. 2,249,694, 1941.
2. Higashi S et al: Impression material. US Patent No. 3,246,998, 1969.
3. Pfeiffer KR, Harvey JL, and Brauer GM: Deterioration during storage of alginate hydrocolloidal dental impression material. US Armed Forces Med J 5:1315, 1954.
4. Personal communication, J. Cresson, 1980.
5. Phillips RW, Price RR, and Reinking RH: Use of alginate for indirect restorations. J Am Dent Assoc 46:393, 1953.
6. Khaknegar B and Ettinger RL: Removal time: A factor in the accuracy of irreversible hydrocolloid impressions. J Oral Rehabil 4:369, 1977.
7. Ayers HD, Phillips RW, Dell A, and Henry RW: Detail duplication test used to evaluate elastic impression materials. J Prosthet Dent 1:374, 1960.
8. Morrow RM, Brown CE, Stansbury BE, deLorimier JA, Powell JM, and Rudd KD: Compatibility of alginate impression materials and dental stone. J Prosthet Dent 25:554, 1971.
9. Craig RG and Peyton FA: Physical properties of elastic duplicating materials. J Dent Res 39:391, 1960.

10 ELASTOMERIC IMPRESSION MATERIALS

In addition to the hydrocolloid gels discussed in the last two chapters, there is another group of elastic impression materials, which are rubber-like in nature, known technically as *elastomers*. They are identified in American Dental Association Specification no. 19 as Non-Aqueous Elastomeric Dental Impression Materials. An elastomeric material must contain large molecules with weak interaction among them, tied together at certain points to form a three-dimensional network. On stretching, the chains uncoil. Upon removal of the stress, they snap back to their relaxed entangled state. Elastomer polymers are discussed further in the next chapter. These materials are also classified as synthetic rubbers, in contrast to natural rubber. Although these rubbers are often classified as colloid gels, in contrast to the hydrocolloid gels, they are hydrophobic in character. Since these materials are generally called "rubber impression materials," that terminology is used in the following discussion.

These materials are usually two component systems. Polymerization and/or cross-linking occurs by either a condensation reaction or an addition reaction.

Chemically there are four kinds of such elastomers used as dental impression materials: *polysulfide, condensation polymerizing silicone, addition polymerizing silicone,* and *polyether.* Representative products are seen in Figure 10–1.

The current American Dental Association specification recognizes three types of these rubber-like impression materials. The type classification is based upon selected elastic properties and dimensional change of the set materials rather than upon their chemistry. However, each type is further divided into four viscosity classes, as determined by a consistency test similar to that described for zinc oxide–eugenol impression pastes.

Chemistry (Polysulfide) The process of changing the rubber base product, or liquid polymer, to a rubber-like material is generally known in industry as *vulcanization* or *curing.* Both terms originated in connection with the production of rubber by heating the natural rubber gum, or latex, with sulfur. By analogy, the two terms have been carried over into the synthesis of the rubber-like molecule even though in some cases no sulfur is present. More properly, the process is termed *cross-linking* and will be discussed in greater detail in the next chapter.

137

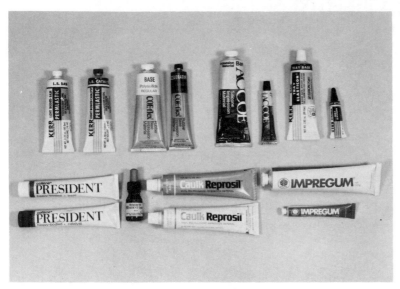

Figure 10–1 The four kinds of non-aqueous elastomeric impression materials. Two polysulfides at upper left and two condensation silicones at upper right. Two addition silicone products, lower left and center, and a polyether at lower right.

The basic ingredient of the liquid polymer is a polyfunctional mercaptan or polysulfide polymer with the general structural formula:

$$HS\ (R{-}S{-}S)_{23}{-}R{-}SH$$

where R is:

$$C_2H_4{-}O{-}CH_2{-}O{-}C_2H_4$$

In addition, this linear polymer contains approximately 2 moles per cent of branching to give pendant mercaptan groups as cross-linking sites. A representative commercial product is LP-2 made by the Thiokol Corporation, and its technology is well known.[1] Dental polysulfide polymers utilize this technology with modifications appropriate for dental usage. This polymer is usually cross-linked with oxidizing agents, lead dioxide being most commonly used.

Addition of lead dioxide to the polysulfide polymer causes both lengthening of the polymer chain by oxidation of terminal — SH groups and cross-linking by oxidation of pendant — SH groups:

$$
\begin{array}{l}
HS\;{\sim}\!{\sim}\!{\sim}\;S\;\boxed{H\;H}\;S\;{\sim}\!{\sim}\!{\sim}\;S\;\boxed{H\;H}\;S\;{\sim}\!{\sim}\!{\sim}\qquad \leftarrow(\textit{Chain lengthening})\\[2pt]
\qquad\qquad\qquad O\qquad\qquad\qquad\ \ O
\end{array}
$$

$$
\begin{array}{l}
S\,\boxed{H}\\
\quad\ \ \boxed{\ }\ O\leftarrow(\textit{Cross-linking})\\
S\,\boxed{H}
\end{array}
$$

$$\downarrow {-}H_2O$$

$$
\begin{array}{l}
HS\;{\sim}\!{\sim}\!{\sim}\;S{-}S\;{\sim}\!{\sim}\!{\sim}\;S{-}S\;{\sim}\!{\sim}\!{\sim}\\[4pt]
\qquad\quad S\\
\qquad\quad |\\
\qquad\quad S\\[4pt]
\qquad {\sim}\!{\sim}\!{\sim}
\end{array}
$$

Because the pendant groups compose only about 1 mole per cent of the available — SH groups, chain lengthening will predominate at first. This will principally increase viscosity. It is the subsequent cross-linking reaction that links all the chains together in a three-dimensional network which confers elastic properties to the material.[2] (The initial increase in viscosity before the material sets is familiar to the dentist accustomed to handling this type of material.) This reaction is much more effective if a small amount of sulfur is present.

As an alternative to lead dioxide, an organic hydroperoxide can be used, e.g., t-butyl hydroperoxide. Unfortunately such compounds used in dentistry have poor dimensional stability owing to the volatility of the hydroperoxide used. The other cross-linking system successfully used in dental polysulfides consists of certain complex inorganic hydroxides, e.g., copper. However, their chemical mechanism is obscure.

The polymerization reaction of polysulfide polymers is exothermic; the amount of heat generated depends on the amount of total material and the concentration of initiators. Moisture and temperature exert a significant effect on the course of reaction.

The mixing is done on a sheet of plastic-lined paper or a glass slab. The curing reaction starts at the beginning of mixing and reaches its maximum rate soon after the spatulation is complete, at which stage a resilient network has started to build. During the final set a material of adequate elasticity and strength is formed which can be removed over undercuts quite readily.

Chemistry (Silicone-Condensation Type)   The polymer consists of an α-ω hydroxy terminated poly(dimethyl siloxane):

$$\text{HO}-(\underset{\underset{\text{CH}_3}{|}}{\overset{\overset{\text{CH}_3}{|}}{\text{Si}}}-\text{O}-\underset{\underset{\text{CH}_3}{|}}{\overset{\overset{\text{CH}_3}{|}}{\text{Si}}}-\text{O})_{\overline{n}}\text{H}$$

Cross-linking occurs through a reaction with tri- and tetrafunctional alkyl silicates, commonly tetraethyl orthosilicate in the presence of stannous octoate [$Sn(C_7H_{15}COO)_2$]. These reactions are effected at ambient temperatures and the materials are therefore called RTV (room temperature vulcanization) silicones in the technical literature. The average RTV polymer consists of

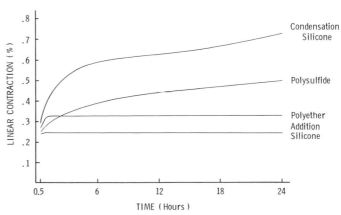

Figure 10–2   Contraction of four elastomeric impression materials.

about 1000 units. The base material is supplied as a paste similar in consistency to polysulfide elastomers, while the catalyst is dispensed as a fluid of low viscosity or, less often, as a paste.

The formation of the elastomer occurs through a cross-linkage between terminal groups of the silicone polymers and the alkyl silicate to form a three-dimensional network as follows:[3]

$$
\begin{array}{c}
\text{CH}_3 \\
| \\
\text{\textbackslash\textbackslash Si} \quad - \text{O} \quad \boxed{\text{H} \quad \text{C}_2\text{H}_5\text{O}} \quad \text{OC}_2\text{H}_5 \\
| \\
\text{CH}_3 \\[8pt]
\text{CH}_3 \qquad\qquad\qquad\qquad\qquad \text{Si} \\
| \\
\text{\textbackslash\textbackslash Si} \quad - \text{O} \quad \boxed{\text{H} \quad \text{C}_2\text{H}_5\text{O}} \quad \text{OC}_2\text{H}_5 \\
| \\
\text{CH}_3
\end{array}
$$

↓ Stannous Octoate

$$
\begin{array}{c}
\text{CH}_3 \\
| \\
\text{\textbackslash\textbackslash Si} \quad - \text{O} \qquad \text{OC}_2\text{H}_5 \\
| \\
\text{CH}_3 \\
\qquad\qquad\qquad \text{Si} \qquad\qquad + \ 2\text{C}_2\text{H}_5\text{OH} \\
\text{CH}_3 \\
| \\
\text{\textbackslash\textbackslash Si} \quad - \text{O} \qquad \text{OC}_2\text{H}_5 \\
| \\
\text{CH}_3
\end{array}
$$

It will be noted that ethyl alcohol is a by-product of the setting reaction. Its subsequent evaporation probably accounts for much of the contraction that takes place in a set silicone rubber, as shown in Figure 10–2.

The alkyl silicates are slightly unstable, particularly if mixed with the organo-tin compound to form a single catalyst liquid. Thus, a limited shelf life may result because of oxidation of the tin component within the catalyst. Shelf life failure may also occur as a result of degradation of the base or cross-linkage of the base during storage.

As with the polysulfides, the supplier is trying to achieve a compromise in the conflicting requirements, i.e., long shelf life stability, rapid rate of cure, and high performance in physical properties.

Chemistry (Silicone-Addition Type) In this case the polymer is terminated with vinyl groups and is cross-linked with silane groups activated by a platinum salt catalyst, by an addition reaction, as follows:[4]

$$
\begin{array}{c}
\text{CH}_3 \\
| \\
\text{\textbackslash\textbackslash O} - \text{Si} - \text{CH}{=}\text{CH}_2 \ + \ \text{H} - \overset{|}{\underset{|}{\text{Si}}} - \text{CH}_3 \\
| \\
\text{CH}_3 \qquad\qquad\qquad\qquad \text{O} \qquad\qquad\qquad\qquad \text{CH}_3 \\
\\
\text{Base polymer} \qquad\qquad \text{CH}_3 - \overset{|}{\underset{|}{\text{Si}}} - \text{H} \ + \ \text{CH}_2{=}\text{CH} - \overset{|}{\underset{|}{\text{Si}}} - \text{O}\text{\textbackslash\textbackslash} \\
\qquad\qquad\qquad\qquad\qquad \text{O} \qquad\qquad\qquad\qquad \text{CH}_3 \\
\text{CH}_3 \\
| \\
\text{\textbackslash\textbackslash O} - \text{Si} - \text{CH}{=}\text{CH}_2 \ + \ \text{H} - \overset{|}{\underset{|}{\text{Si}}} - \text{CH}_3 \\
| \\
\text{CH}_3
\end{array}
$$

↓ Pt Salt

$$
\begin{array}{c}
\quad\quad CH_3 \\
\quad\quad | \\
\text{\large\leftwavy}O-Si-CH_2-CH_2-Si-CH_3 \\
\quad\quad | \quad\quad\quad\quad\quad\quad | \\
\quad\quad CH_3 \quad\quad\quad\quad O \quad\quad\quad\quad CH_3 \\
\quad\quad\quad\quad\quad\quad\quad\quad | \quad\quad\quad\quad | \\
\quad\quad\quad\quad\quad CH_3-Si-CH_2-CH_2-Si-O\text{\large\rightwavy} \\
\quad CH_3 \quad\quad\quad\quad | \quad\quad\quad\quad | \\
\quad | \quad\quad\quad\quad\quad O \quad\quad\quad\quad CH_3 \\
\text{\large\leftwavy}O-Si-CH_2-CH_2-Si-CH_3 \\
\quad | \\
\quad CH_3
\end{array}
$$

Note that there are no reaction by-products; hence the dimensional stability of these materials is greatly superior to condensation silicones, and even to the polysulfides.

The addition silicone is also frequently called *poly (vinyl siloxane)*.

Chemistry (Polyether)   There is another type of elastomeric impression material that was introduced in Germany in the late 1960's. It is a polyether base polymer that is cured by the reaction between aziridine rings,

$$
\begin{array}{c}
R_2C \text{———} CH' \\
\searrow \quad\quad \swarrow \\
NH
\end{array}
$$

which are at the end of branched polyether molecules:[3, 5]

$$
\begin{array}{c}
\quad\quad\quad\quad\quad\quad\quad\quad\quad R \quad\quad\quad\quad\quad\quad R \\
\quad\quad\quad\quad\quad\quad\quad\quad\quad | \quad\quad\quad\quad\quad\quad | \\
CH_3-CH-CH_2-CO_2-\Big[CH-(CH_2)_n-O\Big]_n-CH-(CH_2)_n-CO_2-CH_2-CH-CH_3 \\
\quad\quad | \quad\quad\quad\quad\quad\quad\quad\quad\quad\quad\quad\quad\quad\quad\quad\quad\quad\quad\quad | \\
\quad\quad N \quad\quad\quad\quad\quad\quad\quad\quad\quad\quad\quad\quad\quad\quad\quad\quad\quad\quad N \\
\quad \swarrow \searrow \quad\quad\quad\quad\quad\quad\quad\quad\quad\quad\quad\quad\quad\quad\quad \swarrow \searrow \\
CH_2\text{——}CH_2 \quad\quad\quad\quad\quad\quad\quad\quad\quad\quad\quad CH_2\text{——}CH_2
\end{array}
$$

The main chain is probably a copolymer of ethylene oxide and tetrahydrofuran. Cross-linking, and thus setting, is brought about by an aromatic sulfonate ester of the type:

$$
\begin{array}{c}
\bigcirc \quad\longrightarrow\quad R^+ + \quad \bigcirc \\
| \quad\quad\quad\quad\quad\quad\quad\quad\quad\quad | \\
SO_3R \quad\quad\quad\quad\quad\quad\quad\quad SO_3^-
\end{array}
$$

where R is an alkyl group. This produces cross-linking by cationic polymerization via the imine end groups, viz:

$$
\begin{array}{c}
\quad\quad\quad | \quad\quad\quad\quad\quad\quad\quad\quad\quad\quad\quad\quad | \\
R^+ + N \quad\quad\longrightarrow\quad\quad R-N(+) \\
\swarrow \searrow \quad\quad\quad\quad\quad\quad\quad\quad\quad \swarrow \searrow \\
CH_2\text{——}CH_2 \quad\quad\quad\quad\quad\quad CH_2\text{——}CH_2
\end{array}
$$

$$
\begin{array}{c}
\quad | \quad\quad\quad\quad\quad\quad\quad | \quad\quad\quad\quad\quad\quad\quad\quad\quad\quad | \\
R-N(+) \quad\quad\quad N \rightarrow R\text{--}N\text{--}CH_2-CH_2-N(+), \quad \text{etc.} \\
\swarrow \searrow \quad + \quad \swarrow \searrow \quad\quad\quad\quad \swarrow \searrow \\
CH_2\text{——}CH_2 \quad CH_2\text{——}CH_2 \quad\quad\quad CH_2\text{——}CH_2
\end{array}
$$

Composition (Polysulfide)   The polysulfide polymer, an amber fluid of viscosity 35–45 Pa-s,[3] is compounded with a suitable filler (e.g., lithopone, titanium dioxide) to provide the required strength, and a plasticizer such as dibutyl phthalate to confer the appropriate viscosity to the paste. A small quantity of sulfur, approximately 0.5 per cent, is also added. This is termed the "base paste." The so-called "catalyst" or "accelerator paste" contains the lead dioxide which gives the characteristic dark brown color. (The terms *catalyst* and *accelerator* are really misnomers, however. The term *reactor* is more appropriate.) The same plasticizer as is used in the base paste constitutes the liquid vehicle, as well as a quantity of the same filler. Oleic or stearic acid, both retarders, are often added to control the rate of set.

Each paste is dispensed in a tube, with nozzles such that equal lengths of each paste give the appropriate polymer/cross-linking reagent ratio.

Composition (Condensation Silicone)   The condensation silicone rubbers are usually supplied as a base paste and a liquid catalyst. Since the silicone polymer is a liquid, colloidal silica or microsized metal oxide is added as a filler to prepare a paste. The selection and pretreatment of the filler are of extreme importance, since silicones possess a low cohesive energy density and, therefore, weaker intermolecular interaction.

The influence of the filler on the strength of silicone elastomer is much more critical than when it is added to polysulfide rubbers. The particle size should be very close to the optimum, between 5 and 10 μm. Smaller particles tend to aggregate, but larger ones do not contribute to reinforcement. The particles are often surface-treated to provide better compatibility with, and reinforcement of, the silicone rubber.

As for the polysulfide rubbers, the American Dental Association Specification no. 19 provides for four viscosities of silicone impression materials, depending on the consistency. One of these materials is of very heavy viscosity and is commonly referred to as a "putty" silicone. These putties are highly filled and because of their viscous nature are supplied in a jar. They are used as a tray material, in conjunction with a low viscosity silicone. The technique of use and the properties of these elastomers will be discussed later in this chapter.

Colorants are commonly used as an aid in obtaining a homogeneous mix. They may be organic dyes or pigments; the choice depends upon the system, the properties desired, and the manufacturer's skills.

In some cases two catalyst liquids are supplied in order to keep the alkyl silicate and organo-tin compounds separate until the time of mixing. This prolongs the shelf life of the catalyst system, as previously noted.

Composition (Addition Silicone)   The base paste, which contains poly(methyl hydrogen siloxane), as well as other silane prepolymers, is compounded in a manner similar to the method used for the condensation polymers. However, the "catalyst" is dispensed not as a liquid but as a paste containing divinyl poly(dimethyl siloxane) and poly(dimethyl siloxane), filler, and the platinum salt activator.

Composition (Polyether)   The polyether rubbers are also supplied as two pastes. The base contains the polyether polymer, a colloidal silica as a filler, and a plasticizer such as a glycolether or phthalate. The accelerator paste contains the alkyl-aromatic sulfonate in addition to the aforementioned filler and plasticizer.

Spatulation   The polysulfide elastomers are mixed as described for the zinc oxide–eugenol pastes. The proper lengths of the two pastes are squeezed onto a mixing pad. Since the composition of the tube of the rubber base material is balanced with that of the accelerator, the same matched tubes originally supplied by the manufacturer should always be used. For certain products some flexibility in working and setting time can be obtained by changing proportions. This must be done with caution, since physical properties may be adversely affected.[6]

The catalyst paste is first collected on a stainless steel spatual, then distributed over the base, and the mixture is spread out over the mixing pad. The mass is then scraped up with the spatula blade and again smoothed out. The process is continued until the mixed paste is of uniform color, with no streaks of the base or catalyst appearing in the combined paste. If the mixture is not homogeneous, curing will not be uniform, and a distorted impression will result. Adherence to the manufacturer's instructions is always advisable. Similar considerations apply to the polyether and addition silicone rubbers.

If both the base and the accelerator for the condensation silicone rubber impression materials are supplied in paste form, the mixing procedure is the same as for the polysulfide rubber material. As previously noted, however, the reactor is usually supplied in the form of a colored oily liquid. When the base paste is dispensed from the tube, a certain length is extruded onto the mixing pad and the liquid is placed beside the rope of paste with a stated number of drops per unit length of paste, according to the directions supplied by the manufacturer of the product. If the mixing pad absorbs the oily liquid accelerator, a less permeable pad or a glass slab should be used. The absorption of the accelerator by the pad can also be reduced by placing the drops of liquid on the spatula rather than on the pad.

As mentioned, the putty silicones are supplied in a jar, and the proper quantity is measured by volume in a measuring cup. The accelerator is dispensed by drops according to the volume of the paste.

In any case, the paste is picked up with the spatula and smoothed into the liquid and the mixing is continued as previously described. The process is continued as before until a complete blending is attained, as indicated by an even color throughout the mass.

Regardless of the type of the rubber, whether polysulfide, silicone, or polyether, it should again be emphasized that a homogeneous mix is essential for accuracy.

Setting Time   The setting time can be defined as the time elapsing from the beginning of mixing until the curing has advanced sufficiently that the impression can be removed from the mouth with a minimum of distortion. It should be noted that the setting time does not correspond to the curing time. Actually, the curing may continue for a considerable time after setting. Particularly the condensation silicone rubber impression materials may continue to polymerize for two or more weeks after mixing.[7]

Another related property is *working time*. The measurement of working time also begins with the start of mixing and ends just before the impression material has developed elastic properties. The working time of an acceptable material must exceed the time required for mixing, filling the syringe and/or tray, injecting the preparations, and seating the tray.

Ordinarily working time is measured at room temperature, while setting time, following mixing at room temperature, is measured at mouth temperature.

Penetrometer tests have been used to assess both working and setting time. For example, working time might be considered to have ended when a certain diameter and weight of needle fails to penetrate a volume of impression material to a specified depth. Setting time would not have been reached until another flat ended needle or other blunt instrument fails to permanently indent the set impression material.

In the British Standards Test a reciprocating rheometer is used to measure both setting and working times.[8] The property being recorded is more closely related to viscosity and shear properties than it is to elasticity.

In American Dental Association Specification no. 19, working time is determined from an indirect measurement of viscosity. Working time as determined by that method, or by a clinical type test such as prodding the material in the mouth with a blunt instrument, tends to be somewhat shorter than that recorded by a rheometer.[9]

Working and setting times for the various kinds of elastomeric materials, as measured by an oscillating rheometer, are shown in Table 10–1.[10]

An increase in temperature accelerates the curing rate of all of these elastomeric impression materials, and thus decreases both setting and working time, and vice versa. The decrease in setting time as effected by an increase in temperature is also shown in Table 10–1. This is fortunate, since working time can be prolonged by a low room temperature or by mixing on a chilled, dry glass slab. Then, when the impression material is carried to the mouth, setting time is shortened by the higher temperature.

The user can control the curing rate of most of these elastomers. This might be done either to shorten the setting time or to increase the working time. The effect of temperature has just been illustrated. Cooling is a practical method of increasing the working time of most polysulfide impression materials.

Oleic acid is also an effective retarder for the lead dioxide cured polysulfide materials. The copper hydroxide cured materials may be purchased as "fast" or "regular" setting. Moisture, as by the addition of a drop of water, accelerates the curing rate.

The curing rate of some, but not all, of the polysulfide impression materials is sensitive to alterations in the base/accelerator ratio. However, mechanical properties can be adversely affected if marked changes in the base/accelerator ratio are employed.

On the other hand, alteration in the base/accelerator ratio is an effective and practical method of changing the curing rate of the condensation silicones. However, the retardation obtained by a reduction of the accelerator may be

Table 10–1. *Working and Setting Time of*
Non-Aqueous Elastomeric Impression Materials

MATERIAL	MEAN WORKING TIME (MINUTES)		% DECREASE IN WORKING TIME WHEN TEMPERATURE INCREASED (Mean)*	MEAN SETTING TIME (MINUTES)		% DECREASE IN SETTING TIME WHEN TEMPERATURE INCREASED (Mean)*
	23°C	37°C		23°C	37°C	
Polysulfide	6.0	4.3	30	16.0	12.5	23
Condensation Silicone	3.3	2.5	16	11.0	8.9	15.5
Addition Silicone	3.1	1.8	38	8.9	5.9	31
Polyether	3.3	2.3	31	9.0	8.3	8.5

*Based on data for individual materials.
From Harcourt, J. K.: A Review of Modern Impression Materials. Aust Dent J 23:178, 1978.

more marked than is the acceleration obtained by increasing the accelerator beyond a certain limit.

In contrast to the condensation silicones, the curing rate of the addition silicones appears to be even more sensitive to temperature change than are the polysulfides (Table 10–1). In addition to cooling the mixing slab, working and setting times can be extended (up to 100 per cent) by the addition of a retarder as supplied by the respective manufacturer. Alteration in base/accelerator ratio as a means of changing working or setting time is not economical, as a portion of the paste will be unused.[11]

The curing rate of the polyethers is less sensitive to temperature change than is that of the addition silicones. Some modification in base/accelerator ratio can be used to extend working time. Use of the thinner will also extend working time with only a slight increase in setting time. It will also reduce the viscosity of the mixed but unset material and the elastic modulus or stiffness of the set material without increasing contraction, permanent deformation, or flow.[12]

Elasticity As might be expected, the elastic properties of these rubber impression materials improve with curing time. In other words, the longer the impression can remain in the mouth before removal, the more accurate it will be. Setting time as stated by a manufacturer, or as determined by a rheometer, is not always adequate for the development of sufficient elasticity to prevent permanent deformation upon removal of the impression, especially with the polysulfide and addition silicones. For example, the setting times as measured by a rheometer are 1 or 2 minutes less than those required to produce an acceptable level of elasticity before removal of the impression.[13]

In Specification no. 19 the Types I and II elastomers are allowed 2.5 per cent permanent deformation after 12 per cent strain is held for 30 seconds. Type III materials are permitted 5.5 per cent under the same test. With the exception of the putty rubbers, strain in compression should fall between 2 and 20 per cent when the stress is increased from .0098 to .098 MPa (1.42 to 14.2 psi).

The rank order for permanent deformation following strain in compression, in increasing order, for the four kinds of non-aqueous elastomeric impression materials is: 1) addition silicone, 2) condensation silicone, 3) polyether, and 4) polysulfide.[13]

Recovery of elastic deformation following strain is less rapid for the polysulfides than for the other three kinds of materials. However, even when strain is prolonged, as when an impression is removed slowly rather than rapidly from the prepared teeth, recovery is sufficiently rapid. Therefore, pouring of the impression need not be delayed on the concept that some time must be permitted for elastic recovery to take place.[14, 15]

Since these impression materials are visco-elastic, fairly rapid, repeated straining, as when teasing an impression out of the mouth, will increase permanent deformation.[10] Permanent deformation correlates positively with both the amount and duration of strain.[16]

Excluding the very high viscosity putty class of rubbers, stiffness of the various kinds increases in the following order: polysulfide, condensation silicone, addition silicone, polyether.

Rheological Properties The rheological properties of the elastomeric impression materials play a major role in their successful application as high accuracy impression materials. As will be seen, these materials are introduced into the mouth as a viscous liquid with carefully adjusted flow properties. The setting reaction then converts them into a visco-elastic solid. The flow behavior of the solid form is also quite important if an accurate impression is to be obtained. Even the viscosity and flow behavior of the unmixed components are important, since these control ease of mixing, the amount of air trapped during mixing, and the tendency for the trapped air to escape before the impression is taken.

Complete characterization of the flow properties requires measurement of viscosity as a function or shear rate over a wide range of values. Estimates indicate that shear rates up to 1600 sec^{-1} may be encountered during mixing, and rates up to 1000 sec^{-1} during extrusion from the syringe. These rates are considerably higher than those employed in many of the measurements of viscosity that have been reported.

Future studies of these materials will likely pay close attention to these details, and specifications for these materials may likely include quantitative ranges for viscosity and a characterization of the rheological behavior for the elastomeric impression materials.

Dimensional Stability   There are a number of sources of dimensional change: (1) All rubbers contract slightly during curing as a result of a reduction in volume on cross-linking. (2) As has been seen, during setting the condensation silicone rubbers lose alcohol. This is accompanied by a shrinkage. Similarly, the loss of volatile accelerator components causes a marked contraction in hydroperoxide polysulfide rubbers.[17] (3) Although both silicone and polysulfide rubbers are water-repellent, the polyether polymer absorbs water, a process complicated further by the simultaneous extraction of the water-soluble plasticizer. This results in dimensional changes if such materials are exposed to water or high humidity for a period of time.[18] (4) There is incomplete recovery after deformation because of the visco-elastic nature of rubbers.

Dimensional changes during curing have been measured directly and indirectly, using confined and free standing specimens of the elastomers in various geometrical shapes. In the American Dental Association Specification no. 19 for elastomeric impression materials, a disk of the impression material is placed on a talc covered glass plate. At the end of 24 hours the contraction should not exceed 0.50 per cent for Types I and III materials or 1.00 per cent for a Type II elastomer. Thus the measurement includes contraction due to thermal change (32° C to 23° C), polymerization shrinkage, and loss of volatile components. For example, the linear coefficients of thermal expansion for the elastomeric impression materials range from 150×10^{-6} to 220×10^{-6} per ° C.[5, 19, 20]

Mean values for linear contraction for a number of non-aqueous elastomers, using the method just described, are shown in Figure 10–2. As noted in the discussion on working and setting time, there is considerable variation between brands for the condensation silicone and polysulfide materials, occasionally resulting in overlapping of contraction values between these two groups.

It can certainly be stated from the results presented in Figure 10–2 that the rubber materials are much more stable dimensionally when stored in air than are the hydrocolloid impression materials. However, it is evident that all of the materials change dimensionally with time, and that such a change is

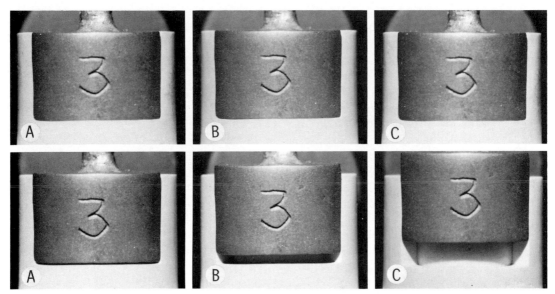

Figure 10–3 Fit of a master casting placed on stone dies constructed from an addition silicone, upper row, and a condensation silicone, bottom row. Stone poured at: *A*, 30 minutes; *B*, 6 hours; and *C*, 24 hours.

greater in magnitude for the condensation silicone impression materials and the polysulfide rubber materials than for the polyether and addition polymerizing silicone elastomers. Likewise, some of the condensation silicones take much longer to reach a maximum contraction than either the polysulfide, addition silicone, or polyether materials.[13]

If maximal accuracy is to be maintained, the stone die or cast should be constructed within the first 30 minutes after the removal of the impression from the mouth whenever a polysulfide or condensation silicone rubber material is employed. This is illustrated in Figure 10–3. A master casting made to fit the master MOD steel die is seated under the same force on Type IV gypsum dies made from condensation and addition silicone impressions poured at various time intervals. The greater distortion of the condensation silicone impression, as compared to the more stable addition silicone, is obvious, correlating with the dimensional change previously seen in Figure 10–2. Similar results may be anticipated with a polysulfide impression (as compared to the condensation silicone impression) that has been stored for longer than 30 minutes before the die is formed.

The time interval is not nearly as critical for the addition silicones and polyethers (Fig. 10–2).

Shelf Life A properly compounded polysulfide or polyether impression material does not deteriorate appreciably in the tubes when stored under normal environmental conditions. Such is not always the case, however, with the silicone impression materials. Although the situation is greatly improved over what it was a few years ago, occasionally the silicone gum may stiffen in the tube if the material is stored for too long a time. Also, the liquid reactor may deteriorate with age, but a proper stabilization can be effected that virtually eliminates such deterioration, as already discussed. On the other hand, the manufacturers of the addition polymerizing silicones claim a 2 year shelf life. However, that claim is not always valid for some batches.

Continuous exposure of either the silicone paste or the reactor to the air hastens deterioration. For this reason, the containers should be kept tightly closed when not in use. Also, storage in a cool environment is advisable. American Dental Association Specification no. 19 requires that after storage of the base and accelerator for seven days at $60 \pm 2°$ C $(140 \pm 3.6°$ F) the material still meet the test for permanent deformation. If the rubber has inferior shelf life, the poor elastic behavior will show up as high "set" values.

Miscellaneous Matters   The storage medium for a rubber impression is not critical, except that with polyether and some silicones a high humidity environment should not be used.[18] As previously stated, a long storage time is not indicated because of the distortion occasioned by a continued curing. If the tray material is of a plastic type that may imbibe water and change in dimension, the impression should not be stored in a moist environment.

Spherical indentations sometimes appear on the surface of an impression obtained with a polysulfide rubber material. Such indentations appear on the surface of the stone die as convexities, or nodules. Presumably, this effect is due to the collapse of a void near the surface. Such voids are probably the result of air bubbles trapped during mixing. However, since such imperfections usually do not appear for a number of hours after the impression is removed from the mouth, they should not be troublesome if the stone die is constructed within the first half-hour, as previously suggested.

Unlike the hydrocolloid impression materials, the rubber impression materials do not materially affect the hardness of the stone surface. A smooth, hard stone surface on the die can be expected when the rubber impression materials are used properly. It is true that the stone mix does not wet the surface of polysulfide and silicone impression materials very well.[21, 22] However, entrapment of air between the gypsum and impression material may be alleviated by proper use of a wetting agent. Only a minimal amount should be used or a soft, porous stone surface will result.

With some batches of addition silicone impression materials, small crater-like pits may appear on the surface of the stone die if the impression is poured immediately. It is postulated that the pitting is a result of escaping hydrogen gas but not necessarily associated with the setting reaction. The problem can be eliminated by waiting 15 to 30 minutes before pouring such an elastomer.

The choice of a rubber impression material is governed by the particular characteristics preferred by the operator. In general, it may be said that the silicone and polyether materials have the advantage of superior color, odor, and similar esthetic properties. They are also cleaner to handle. On the other hand, in general the silicones are inferior to the polysulfide and the polyether rubbers from the standpoint of shelf life. Impressions of similar accuracy, as with hydrocolloid, can be secured with all materials with the proper technique. Some of the characteristics of the four kinds of elastomers can be seen in Table 10–2. The table is intended only to serve as a general guideline. There is a noticeable variation among individual products. Likewise, dentists differ greatly in their working habits and skills in mixing a given type of material and taking impressions.

Biological Properties   It is clear that in the Western World more stringent legislation is now being applied to dental materials, and this is not limited to those materials that are to be retained permanently in the mouth. There is already in existence an American Dental Association specification for testing

Table 10–2. *Comparison of Certain Characteristics of Elastomeric Dental Impression Materials*

	POLYSULFIDE	CONDENSATION SILICONE	POLYETHER	ADDITION SILICONE
Mixing	Fair to easy	Fair to easy	Easy	Easy
Flow	Variable	Good	Good	Good
Stack	Fair to good	Fair	Good	Fair to good
Elastic recovery	Fair	Very good	Very good	Excellent
Reproduction of detail	Excellent	Excellent	Excellent	Excellent
Odor and taste	Unpleasant	Acceptable	Acceptable	Acceptable
Clean up	Difficult	Easy	Easy	Easy

biocompatibility, including that of impression materials. These tests were discussed in Chapter 3.

Such legislation is not pointless, as hypersensitivity of the catalyst system for the polyether impression materials has already been reported.[23]

TECHNICAL CONSIDERATIONS

The rubber impression materials can be described as a universal type of impression material. They can be employed for any type of dental impression required by the dentist. However, they are primarily intended for impressions of the hard tissue in which elasticity is a necessary prerequisite.

Preparation of the Tray   The methods for proportioning and mixing the rubber impression materials have already been discussed.

As can be concluded from the fit of the master castings shown in Figure 10–4 on the stone dies constructed from rubber impressions with different bulk, the less the distance between the impression tray and the master die, the more accurate is the impression (Fig. 10–4A). It will be recalled that the accuracy of impression materials can be readily determined by the use of master castings constructed on critical steel dies (Fig. 8–2). The better the fit of the casting when placed back on the stone dies, the more accurate is the impression material and technique.

It should be noted that this finding is directly opposite to that recommended for the hydrocolloid impression, in which a greater bulk of material produced better accuracy than did the smaller bulk. The bulk should not only be less with the rubber impression materials but it should also be evenly distributed. In general, the optimal thickness of the impression is 2 to 4 mm.[17]

Although stock impression trays are available that can be contoured closely to the oral tissues, a better method is to construct a tray with a plastic material, such as a self-curing resin which will be described in a subsequent chapter. An impression is obtained of the mouth using any convenient impression material. A stone cast is constructed. The important parts of the cast, such as the prepared cavities, are covered with one or two thicknesses of base plate wax and tin foil, which is later overlaid with the uncured resin. After the resin has cured, the resin tray is separated from the cast and the wax and tin foil is removed. It can then be used as a tray. The impression material occupies the space left by the base plate wax. Thus, a uniform bulk of impression material with a minimal thickness is provided.

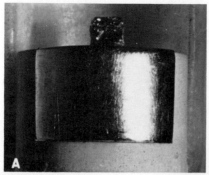

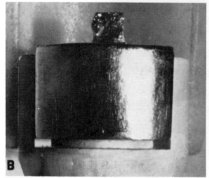
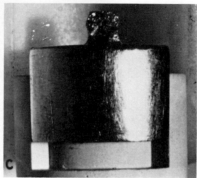

Figure 10–4 The greater the thickness of the wall of the rubber impression from which the above stone dies were constructed, the poorer is the fit of the casting. Wall thickness: *A*, 0.5 mm; *B*, 2.0 mm; *C*, 4.5 mm.

Adhesion to the Tray   The next problem concerns the adhesion of the rubber impression material to the tray. As with the hydrocolloid impression materials, complete adhesion to the tray is imperative when the impression is removed from the mouth. Otherwise, a distorted impression will result.

Although perforated trays, similar to those used for hydrocolloid impressions, would be satisfactory from this standpoint, they are not as convenient or practical as the custom-built resin tray just described. Adhesion can be obtained by the application of adhesive to the plastic tray, previous to the insertion of the impression material. The adhesive then forms a tenacious bond between the rubber material and the tray.

The adhesive cements furnished with the various types of rubber impression materials are not interchangeable. Adhesives employed with the polysulfide rubber impression materials include butyl rubber or styrene/acrylonitrile dissolved in a suitable volatile solvent such as chloroform or a ketone. The base for the adhesive employed with the silicone rubber materials may contain poly(dimethyl siloxane), or a similar reactive silicone, and ethyl silicate. The poly(dimethyl siloxane) acts as an adhesive for the rubber, and hydrated silica forms from the ethyl silicate to create a physical bond with the impression tray. In either case, a slightly roughened surface on the tray will increase the adhesion.

In general, the adhesives for polysulfide, polyether, and condensation silicones are quite satisfactory. Those used with the addition silicones are less effective. Some of the putty class condensation silicones require mechanical retention in the tray, since the adhesive is ineffective.

Multiple Mix Technique   As with the hydrocolloid impression materials, an impression of a number of teeth can be obtained at one time with the use of a syringe.

The problem is somewhat different with the rubber impression materials than with the reversible hydrocolloid impression materials. In the latter case, the sol will remain fluid as long as the temperature is held above the gelation point. In the case of the rubber materials, a thickening of the mix occurs as the curing proceeds. Although the consistency may be such that an impression with the tray can be effected, the rubber may be too thick to be extruded from the syringe. The working time may be satisfactory with the polysulfide rubber materials, but it may be too short when the silicone rubbers are employed and not altered, as by varying the base-accelerator ratio or adding a retarder.

In order to provide a less viscous material for use with the syringe, most manufacturers have provided rubber materials with at least two consistencies: one consistency for use with the tray, and a thinner one for use with the syringe. The syringe type also usually has a longer working and setting time, as well as greater polymerization and thermal contraction. For this reason, the syringe material alone is not used.

The method of using both the syringe and tray types of rubber materials is often referred to as the *multiple mix* technique because two separate mixtures are required with two separate mixing pads and spatulas. When the tray material is mixed first, the tray is filled with a uniform thickness of material and set aside, or the manufacturer may have adjusted the setting time of the two materials so that the syringe material should be mixed first or at the same time as the tray material. The material is injected from the filled syringe into the prepared cavities, as described for the hydrocolloid impression materials. The filled tray is then carried to place.

The procedure should be timed so that neither the tray nor the syringe material cure to a point at which they will not cohere when they are brought together.

The stiffness of the material at the time the impression is seated influences the accuracy, particularly in the case of the silicone materials. If the material has cured to a point that elastic properties have developed, elastic deformation will occur when the impression is seated. Upon removal from the mouth, that deformation will recover and a smaller die will result. Ideally, each commercial product has an optimal time at which it should be carried to the mouth.

Reline Technique   As discussed previously, a very heavy-bodied silicone impression material has become popular.[24] The rapid-curing putty or dough-like material is placed in a stock tray and a preliminary impression is taken. This results in what is essentially an intraoral custom-made tray formed by the silicone rubber. Relief for the final or "wash" impression is provided either by cutting away some of the "tray" silicone or by using a thin resin, rubber, or wax sheet as a spacer between the silicone and the prepared teeth. This area is then filled with a thinner consistency silicone, and the tray is reseated into the mouth.

For reliable reproduction of sharp angles in cavity preparations, it is often still necessary to inject this material with a syringe. With certain products the silicone used for the wash or final impression is the manufacturer's light-bodied or syringe material. Whether or not a syringe is required depends upon the design of the cavity preparation.

The mixing of the base and accelerator for the putty consistency material may seem strange at first. Although the liquid accelerator is incorporated into the dough consistency condensation silicone in the conventional way on a mixing pad, the mix is completed by kneading with the fingers. When the putty impression material is a polysulfide or an addition silicone, the viscous base and accelerator pastes are combined entirely by kneading.

A conventional tray silicone or polysulfide may be used in the same way, but the putty-like elastomers have several advantages, the principal one being rapid curing. The preliminary impression needs to be held in the mouth only for a minute or two. Likewise, the relatively high stiffness of the putty material reduces the possibility of the impression distorting due to elastic deformation of the tray material when it is reseated. Regardless of the material used, it should be held under pressure only during seating of the tray and not while the wash material is curing. The putty elastomer, and the associated technique, supplements but does not replace the older, less viscous tray material and the techniques previously described for use with them.

Properly used, the putty-wash technique can produce impressions with accuracy comparable to that of the homologous multiple mix procedure. Theoretically, the procedure is more convenient and the bulk of the impression is formed by the highly filled putty material, which has relatively low polymerization and thermal contraction. However, in practice, the putty-wash system can, and not infrequently does, lead to a grossly inaccurate impression if a critical portion of the primary impression is held under pressure while the wash material is setting. This leads to elastic deformation. Inadequate relief may be a principal cause of distorted putty-wash impressions. Whenever the putty material is visible in an area of the impression that is in contact with a prepared tooth, the accuracy is highly suspect.

The popularity of a stock, rather than a custom, tray may be associated with the increased use of the silicone putty reline technique.[24] Here the primary putty impression actually serves as a custom tray for the wash or reline material.

Removal of the Impression   Under no circumstance should the impression be removed until the curing has progressed sufficiently to provide adequate elasticity so that distortion will not occur. One method for determining the time of removal is to inject some of the syringe material into an interproximal space not in the area of operation. As previously noted, this material can be prodded with a blunt instrument from time to time, and when it is firm and returns completely to its original contour, the impression can be removed. When a multiple mix technique is used, it is advisable to test both the syringe and the tray materials in this manner. The curing times may vary for the two different consistencies.

From a practical standpoint, the curing rate of the rubber impression material should not be so slow that the time before removal from the mouth is unduly long. It is estimated that with a satisfactory rubber material the impression should be ready to be removed within at least 10 minutes from the time of mixing, allowing 6 to 8 minutes for the impression to remain in the mouth.

For the same reasons presented in the discussion of the hydrocolloid impression materials, the rubber impression should be removed suddenly.

Single Impressions   The technique for single tooth impressions is similar to that for multiple teeth impressions except that only one tooth is involved.

The "tray" employed is usually a copper matrix band, which is a short copper tube, approximately 30 gauge (Brown and Sharpe) in thickness, with a length and diameter suitable for encompassing the particular tooth involved. The band material should be stiff — not a soft, flexible metal.

The band should be fitted to the tooth and then reinforced with compound or self-curing resin. Otherwise, the impression will be squeezed with the fingers when it is removed from the tooth and a distortion will occur. The reinforcement can be obviated if a copper "shell" is employed, which is essentially a copper band of the same gauge of copper metal, with one end closed to form a cup-shaped receptacle.

The adhesive is applied to the band and the band is filled with the previously mixed rubber material. If the band is cleaned of oxide, e.g., by a rotating stone, and if a polysulfide impression material is used, no adhesive is required.[25] The prepared cavity is injected as usual with the syringe, and the filled band is pressed into place. The same precautions are observed in removal as previously described for the multiple impressions. Either a syringe or a tray type material can be used, but usually only one type is employed.

Stone Die   As previously noted, the stone die should be constructed shortly after the impression has been removed from the mouth to prevent distortion of the impression when the rubber is a polysulfide or condensation silicone.

Die materials other than conventional gypsum products will be discussed in Chapter 27.

Miscellaneous Techniques   Under no circumstance should the rubber impression material be allowed to develop elastic properties before the tray or band is seated. Owing to the compressive stresses induced in the partially set material, the impression will "spring back" or relax upon removal, and the dies will be too small.

For much the same reason, it is difficult to repair a rubber impression by adding more material and then reseating the impression. The added material is cushioned by the induction of compressive stress in the already cured rubber. When the impression is removed, the stresses are released. Therefore, a small die or cast results. If such a repair is attempted, it is essential to relieve the first impression. This is usually done by cutting away the interproximal and gingival areas of the impression. Even with proper relief of the initial impression, reseating the tray is difficult. The safest method is to obtain a new impression when bubbles or similar defects appear.

It is possible to construct successive stone dies or casts from impressions obtained with these elastomers when duplicate stone dies are needed. The successive dies will be slightly less accurate than the first die constructed if the material is a polysulfide or a condensation silicone.[26] The distortion that does occur appears to be related primarily to the normal dimensional change that takes place with the rubber impression material, not to the process of pouring or removing the stone dies.[27, 28] However, since the condensation silicone and polysulfide materials are not as dimensionally stable as the addition silicone or polyethers, the time interval between pours should not be greater than 30 minutes with such materials.

There are other problems that can arise with multiple pours when intracoronal preparations involving sharp margins and bell-shaped crowns are involved. The stiff impression materials may be abraded at proximal margins when the die is pulled from undercut areas. Also, in the case of polyether materials, moisture sorption from the gypsum may result in a detectable distortion if multiple pours are made in rapid succession.[26, 29]

Reproduction of Oral Detail   The necessity for the impression material to reproduce the finest detail of the oral cavity is, of course, self-evident. Various tests have been employed by investigators to evaluate the ability of impression materials to reproduce surface detail.[30] Likewise, a surface reproduction test is a part of the specification for the elastic impression materials, as has been noted. There is no doubt that these elastomers and the reversible hydrocolloids record detail to a fine degree. However, the irreversible hydrocolloids do not compare favorably to these other materials in this regard.

When dental stone is formed over such test impressions, the finest detail is not always reproduced. In other words, the rubber impression materials are able to reproduce detail more accurately than can be transferred to the stone die or cast.

The clinical significance of such tests is not entirely evident. First, it is possible that the surface interaction between the impression materials and the laboratory specimen may not be the same as between the material and oral tissue. This difference is probably of particular importance in alginate impression materials, and it might account for their inadequacy in this respect. Furthermore, it is possible that the detail obtained with the rubber impression materials on the in vitro test specimen might be greater than that obtained in the mouth because of the property of water repellence exhibited by these materials.

Types of Failure   Some common failures that occur with the use of the non-aqueous elastomeric impression materials are summarized in the following list, along with their causes.

Type	*Cause*
1. Rough or uneven surface on impression	a. Incomplete polymerization caused by premature removal from the mouth, improper ratio or mixing of components, or oil or other organic material on the teeth b. Too rapid polymerization from high humidity or temperature c. Excessively high accelerator/base ratio with condensation silicone
2. Bubbles	a. Too rapid polymerization, preventing flow b. Air incorporated during mixing
3. Irregularly shaped voids	a. Moisture or debris on surface of teeth
4. Rough or chalky stone cast	a. Inadequate cleaning of impression b. Excess water left on surface of the impression c. Excess wetting agent left on impression d. Premature removal of cast e. Improper manipulation of stone f. Not delaying for 20 minutes pouring of an addition silicone
5. Distortion	a. Resin tray not aged sufficiently and still undergoing polymerization shrinkage b. Lack of adhesion of rubber to the tray caused by not enough coats of adhesive, filling tray with material

Type	Cause
	too soon after applying adhesive, or using wrong adhesive
	c. Lack of mechanical retention for those materials where adhesive is ineffective
	d. Development of elastic properties in the material before tray is seated
	f. Excessive bulk of material
	g. Insufficient relief for the reline material if such technique is used
	h. Continued pressure against impression material that has developed elastic properties
	i. Movement of tray during polymerization
	j. Premature removal from mouth
	k. Improper removal from mouth
	l. Delayed pouring of the polysulfide or condensation silicone impression
6. Faulty electroplating	See Chapter 27

References

1. Jorczak JS and Fettes EM: Polysulfide polymers.Ind Eng Chem 43:324, 1951.
2. Braden M: Characterization of the setting process in dental polysulfide rubbers. J Dent Res 45:1066, 1966.
3. Braden M: Personal Communication.
4. Braden M: The quest for a new impression rubber. J Dent 4:1, 1976.
5. Braden M, Causton B, and Clarke RL: A polyether impression rubber. J Dent Res 51:889, 1972.
6. Skinner EW and Cooper EN: Desirable properties and use of rubber impression materials. J Am Dent Assoc 51:523, 1955.
7. Watt JAC: Silicone liquid rubbers, Chem Brit 19:519, 1970.
8. Wilson, HJ: Elastomeric impression materials. Part I. The setting material. Br Dent J 121: 277, 1966.
9. Nayyar A, Tomlins CD, Fairhurst CW, and Okabe T: Comparison of some properties of polyether and polysulfide materials. J Prosthet Dent 42:163, 1979.
10. Harcourt JK: A review of modern impression materials. Aust Dent J 23:178, 1978.
11. Stannard JC and Craig RG: Modifying the setting rate of an addition-type silicone impression material. IADR Program and Abstracts, No. 197, 1979.
12. Craig RG: A review of properties of rubber impression materials. J Mich Dent Assoc 59:254, 1977.
13. Jones DW and Sutow EJ: Setting characteristics and elastic recovery of elastomeric impression materials. IADR Program and Abstracts, No. 193, 1979.
14. Lautenschlager EP, Miyamoto P, and Hilton R: Elastic recovery of polysulfide base impressions. J Dent Res 51:773, 1972.
15. Inoue K and Wilson HJ: Viscoelastic properties of elastomeric impression materials. III. The elastic recovery after removal of strains applied at the setting time. J Oral Rehabil 5:323, 1978.
16. Mansfield MA and Wilson HJ: A new method for the determination of the tension set of elastomeric impression materials. Br Dent J 135:101, 1973.
17. Brown D: Factors affecting the dimensional stability of elastic impression materials. J Dent 1:265, 1973.
18. Bell JW, Davies EH, and von Fraunhofer JA: The dimensional changes of elastomeric impression materials under various conditions of humidity. J Dent 4:73, 1976.
19. Jørgensen KD: Thiokol as a dental impression material. Acta Odontol Scand 14:313, 1956.
20. Anderson JN: The dimensional stability of three silicone-base impression materials. Dent Pract and Dent Rec 8:368, 1958.

21. Lorren RA, Salter DJ, and Fairhurst CW: The contact angles of die stone on impression materials. J Prosthet Dent 36:176, 1976.
22. Norling BK and Reisbick MH: The effect of nonionic surfactants on bubble entrapment in elastomeric impression materials. J Prosthet Dent 42:342, 1979.
23. Nally FF and Storrs J: Hypersensitivity to a dental impression material. Br Dent J 134:244, 1973.
24. Shillingburg HJ Jr, Hatch RA, Keenan MP, and Hemphill MW: Impression materials and techniques used for cast restorations in eight states. J Am Dent Assoc 100:696, 1980.
25. Shigeto N, Kawazoe Y, Hamada T, and Yamada S: Adhesion between copperplated acrylic tray resin and a polysulfide rubber impression material. J Prosthet Dent 42:228, 1979.
26. Locht AA: MSD Thesis: Dimensional accuracy of three consecutively poured stone dies using a single elastomeric impression. Indiana University School of Dentistry, 1978.
27. Schnell RJ and Phillips RW: Dimensional stability of rubber base impressions and certain other factors affecting accuracy. J Am Dent Assoc 57:39, 1958.
28. Luebke RJ, Scandrett FR, and Kerber PE: The effect of delayed and second pours on elastomeric impression material accuracy. J Prosthet Dent 41:517, 1979.
29. Rosenstiel S: MSD Thesis: The marginal reproduction of two elastomeric impression materials. Indiana University School of Dentistry, 1977.
30. Ayers HD, Phillips RW, Dell A, and Henry RW: Detail duplication test used to evaluate elastic impression materials. J Prosthet Dent 10:374, 1960.

11 CHEMISTRY OF THE SYNTHETIC RESINS

There is probably no other single class of substances that has influenced modern living during the present century more than the synthetic plastics. By definition, synthetic plastics are nonmetallic compounds, synthetically produced (usually from organic compounds), which can be molded into various forms and then hardened for commercial use. Clothing, building materials, household appliances, electronic equipment, and almost every line of human endeavor have some items or parts constructed of a plastic of some form. The term "plastic" includes fibrous, rubber-like, and resinous or hard, rigid substances. All of these materials have certain chemical similarities in that they are composed of polymers, or complex molecules of high molecular weight. The particular form and morphology of the molecule determine to a large extent whether the plastic is a fiber, a rubber-like product, or a resin.

The field of the giant molecules, or the high polymers as the chemist calls them, is one of the most exciting of all areas in science. Their discovery and historical development is one of the most fascinating stories in chemistry. Originally they were literally laboratory nuisances — the waxy, sticky residues left after certain organic reactions. It was only during the last 40 or 50 years that these resinous materials, composed of giant molecules, attracted the attention of the chemist; thus, the field of plastics was born. The impact on dentistry of current research in this field is difficult to envision, but probably nowhere else may one anticipate as far-reaching or significant effects as upon dental practice.

Classification of Resins   A rigorous system of nomenclature for classifying resins appears impractical because of their heterogeneous and complex nature. Not only is it difficult to describe the nature of a resin, but often the quantitative determination of its composition and structure is not possible by the analytical methods now available.

One classification can be made on the basis of the thermal behavior of the resin. Synthetic resins are usually molded in some manner under heat and pressure into useful articles. If the resin is molded without chemical change, for example, by softening it under heat and pressure and by cooling it after it has been molded, the resin is classified as *thermoplastic*, as was previously described in relation to impression compound (Chapter 6). Thermoplastic resins are fusible, and they are usually soluble in organic solvents. On the other hand, if a chemical reaction takes place during the molding process, so

157

that the final product is chemically different from the original substance, the resin is classified as *thermoset*. Thermoset resins are generally insoluble and infusible.

A more exact means for classifying a resin is in terms of its structural units. Such a classification will be used in the following discussion.

Dental Resins   The dentist uses many forms of synthetic plastics in one way or another. The elastomeric impression materials discussed in the previous chapter are examples of synthetic resins. Other types of synthetic resins are employed for the restoration of missing teeth and missing tooth structures. The denture base (the part of the denture that rests on the soft tissues of the mouth) is customarily made of a resin; often the denture teeth are also made of it. The optical and color properties of the resins thus employed are so excellent that the restoration will often escape detection.

The particular synthetic resin most used currently in dentistry is that based on an acrylic resin, poly(methyl methacrylate). Consequently, the properties and use of this particular resin will be stressed.

However, there are so many different types of synthetic resins, and more types are being developed constantly, that the dentist cannot afford to limit his knowledge to one specific resin.[1] Rather, he should possess some knowledge of the basic concepts of resin chemistry, so that he can better evaluate new developments in this field as they occur. For this reason, the present chapter is devoted largely to a brief review of the fundamentals of resin chemistry.

Requisites for Dental Resin   The reason the present-day dental resins are more or less limited to poly(methyl methacrylate) and other methacrylate polymers is that these are the only resins so far developed that will provide routinely, with relatively simple techniques, the essential properties for use in the mouth.

Ideal requisites for a dental resin are as follows:

1. The material should exhibit a translucence or transparency such that it can be made to duplicate esthetically the oral tissues it is to replace. It should be capable of being tinted or pigmented to this end.

2. There should be no change in color or appearance of the material subsequent to its fabrication, whether this is accomplished in or out of the mouth.

3. It should neither expand, contract, nor warp during processing nor during subsequent normal use by the patient. In other words, it should be dimensionally stable under all conditions of service.

4. It should possess adequate strength, resilience, and abrasion resistance to withstand all normal usage.

5. It should be impermeable to the oral fluids to the extent that it will not become unsanitary or disagreeable in taste or odor. If used as a filling material or cement, it should chemically bond to the tooth itself.

6. It should be completely insoluble in the oral fluids or in any substances taken into the mouth, with no evidence of corrosive attack. It should not sorb such fluids.

7. The resin should be tasteless, odorless, nontoxic and nonirritating to the oral tissues.

8. It should have a low specific gravity.

9. Its softening temperature should be well above the temperature of any hot foods or liquids taken into the mouth.

10. In case of unavoidable breakage, it should be possible to repair the resin easily and efficiently.

11. The fabrication of the resin into a dental appliance should be easily effected with simple equipment.

No resin has yet been found that will meet all of the above requirements. As was discussed in Chapter 3, the conditions in the mouth are most rigorous; only the most chemically stable and inert materials can withstand such conditions without deterioration.

POLYMERIZATION

The composition of a polymeric substance is customarily described in terms of its structural units, as is implied by the etymology of the term *polymer* (i.e., "many parts"). Polymerization occurs through a series of chemical reactions by which the macromolecule, or *polymer,* is formed from large numbers of single molecules known as *monomers* (monomer meaning one molecule or one *mer*). In other words, a large number of low molecular weight molecules (mers) of one or more species react to form a single large molecule of high molecular weight.

The most significant features of polymers are that they consist of very large molecules, that almost invariably the molecular weight of the individual macromolecules varies over a wide range, and that their molecular structure is capable of virtually limitless configurations and conformations.

Basically, the polymer is made up of a particular recurring, simple structural unit, which is essentially related to the monomer structure. The structural units are usually connected to each other in the polymer molecule by covalent bonds. In some cases, the molecular weight of the polymer molecule may be as high as 50,000,000. Any chemical compound possessing a molecular weight in excess of 5000 is considered to be a macromolecule. In general then, polymerization is a repetitive intermolecular reaction that is functionally capable of proceeding indefinitely.

The macromolecule may be an inorganic polymer, such as graphite or clay. However, at present mainly organic polymers are used in dentistry. Therefore, the discussion in these chapters will be limited to organic polymers.

The molecules within the polymer invariably consist of molecular species which vary in degree of polymerization, generally over a considerable range. However, the *average degree of polymerization* may be found by dividing the total number of structural units by the total number of molecules. Another method of expressing the degree of polymerization is by the *number average molecular weight,* which represents the weight of the sample divided by the number of mols it contains. The number average molecular weight for various commercial dental polymer powders varies from 3500 to 36,000, while the same products after curing show average molecular weights from 8000 to 39,000.[2] Molecular weights as high as 600,000 have been reported for polymerized denture base.[3] Cross-linked resin denture teeth may have an even higher molecular weight.

Polymerization is never entirely complete and the percentage of residual monomer has a pronounced effect on the molecular weight. For example, with 0.9 per cent residual monomer in a sample of resin polymer having an original number average molecular weight of 22,400, the molecular weight of the resultant cured resin was approximately 7300.

Physical Properties   The physical properties of the polymer are greatly influenced by almost any changes in temperature, environment, composition, or molecular weight and structure. In general, the higher the temperature, the softer and weaker the polymer becomes. When a thermoplastic resin becomes sufficiently soft to mold, it is said to have reached its *softening temperature* or *molding temperature*. The lower the molecular weight of the polymer, the lower will be the softening temperature.

As macromolecules are formed, the secondary bonding or intermolecular force holding them together increases. The result is that properties related to these forces, such as softening temperature and tensile strength, tend to increase. Polymers show no appreciable mechanical strength until an apparent minimal average degree of polymerization is reached. Although dependent upon its type, generally a resin possesses mechanical strength only when its degree of polymerization is relatively high, in the general range of approximately 150 to 200 recurring units. The strength of the resin increases quite rapidly with increase in degree of polymerization until a certain molecular weight is attained that is characteristic for the given polymer. Above this molecular weight, there is not a great change in strength with further polymerization. The number average molecular weight is indicative of the strength of the resin. The value for the number average molecular weight is lowered markedly by the presence of a relatively few molecules with a low degree of polymerization, which weaken the resin considerably.

Likewise, the molecular weight distribution of the polymer plays an important role in determining physical properties. In general, a narrow molecular weight distribution gives the most useful polymers. However, most polymers include a wide range of molecular weights.

Complex side chains on the monomer molecule generally produce a weaker resin with a lower softening temperature in comparison to the similar properties of a polymer that possesses a straight chain structure. If the chains are cross-linked, however, the strength is increased, and the resin is generally infusible.

Polymerization can be effected either by a series of condensation reactions or by simple addition reactions.[4-6] If the polymerization occurs by condensation reactions, the process is known as a *condensation polymerization*. If the polymerization is brought about by an addition reaction, an *addition polymerization* takes place. It will be recalled that these terms were used in the previous chapter in conjunction with the curing of the elastomeric impression materials. They will now be discussed in greater detail.

Condensation Polymerization   The reactions producing condensation polymerization progress by the same mechanism as similar chemical reactions between two or more simple molecules. The primary compounds react with the formation of by-products such as water, halogen acids, and ammonia. The structure of the monomers is such that the process can repeat itself and build macromolecules. However, the mers (repeating units) contain fewer atoms than the original monomer.

In the past, several condensation resins have been used in dentistry for the construction of denture bases. The principal resin so employed was a phenol-formaldehyde resin known popularly as "Bakelite," named after its inventor, L. H. Baekeland.

The reactions of this resin are very complicated, and the exact nature of the final structure is not known. The first reactions are between phenol and formaldehyde to form an alcohol of some type. The alcohols can then react by condensation to form the macromolecules.

When the molecular weight is relatively low, the material is known as a *resole*. At this stage it is thermoplastic and alcohol-soluble. It can be molded at this stage and reacted further under heat to a *resite*, which is its final form. In the resite stage it is both insoluble and infusible.

Although the product as used for denture bases was translucent and strong, it proved to be chemically unstable in the mouth. It gradually discolored, possibly by oxidation.

As resin science has progressed, the classification of condensation resins has been broadened. Polymers whose repeating units are joined by functional groups (such as amide, urethane, ester, or sulfide linkages), even without the formation of a by-product, are also classified as condensation resins. *Polyurethane* is an example of a polymer of this type which to date has had relatively limited application in dentistry. It can be formed by reacting a diol with diisocyanate. The urethane linkage (OCONH) is repeated throughout the chain.

Thus, condensation resins are those in which (1) polymerization is accompanied by repeated elimination of small molecules or (2) functional groups are repeated in the polymer chain.

The formation of polymers by the condensation method is rather slow and tends to stop before the molecules have reached a truly giant size because, as the chains grow, they become less mobile and less numerous. Products such as nylon have acquired their valuable properties when they reach a molecular weight of 10,000 to 20,000. However, to build molecules with molecular weights in the hundreds of thousands or millions by condensation is very difficult.

At present, condensation resins are not employed extensively in dental restorations or prosthetic appliances. However, the advances in polymer chemistry could rapidly alter such a situation. Therefore, the dentist should be familiar with the basic concepts involved in this particular type of polymerization. An example of one condensation polymerization reaction that is widely used in dentistry is the polysulfide rubber impression material. The low molecular weight polysulfide paste is converted to a high molecular weight material by a condensation reaction (Chapter 10).

Addition Polymerization   All of the resins employed extensively in dental procedures at the present time are produced by *addition polymerization.* As a matter of fact, this type of polymerization is so common that often the term "polymerization," when used alone, is generally understood to indicate addition polymerization.

Unlike condensation polymerization, there is no change in composition during addition polymerization; the macromolecules are formed from smaller units, or monomers, without change in composition, since the monomer and the polymer have the same empirical formulas. In other words, the structure of the monomer is repeated many times in the polymer. This process proceeds without the formation of by-products.

As opposed to condensation polymerization, the addition method can readily produce giant molecules of almost unlimited size. Starting from an active center, it adds one monomer at a time and rapidly builds a chain that, in theory, can go on growing indefinitely, as long as the supply of building blocks holds out. The process is simple but not easy to control.

One of the requisites of a polymerizable compound is the presence of an unsaturated group. Ethylene, the simplest monomer capable of polymerization, can be used for purposes of illustration:

$$
\begin{array}{cc}
\text{H} & \text{H} \\
| & | \\
\text{C} & \!\!=\!\! \text{C} \\
| & | \\
\text{H} & \text{R}
\end{array}
\qquad \text{where R=H}
$$

Theoretically, R can be almost any radical that one might choose. For example, it can be hydrogen, and the original ethylene gas can be polymerized under heat and pressure to polyethylene.

Activation of Addition Polymerization   The exact mechanism of polymerization reactions is still somewhat obscure, but for the purposes of the present discussion it can be assumed that the reactions are initiated by activated molecules. For example, the ethylene structure becomes activated, and the double bonds "open up":

$$
\begin{array}{cc}
\text{H} & \text{H} \\
| & | \\
-\text{C} & \!\!-\!\! \text{C}- \\
| & | \\
\text{H} & \text{R}
\end{array}
$$

This activated molecule then "collides" with another molecule, and the second molecule becomes activated:

$$
-\!\overset{\text{H}}{\underset{\text{H}}{\text{C}}}\!-\!\overset{\text{H}}{\underset{\text{R}}{\text{C}}}\!-\;+\;\overset{\text{H}}{\underset{\text{H}}{\text{C}}}\!=\!\overset{\text{H}}{\underset{\text{R}}{\text{C}}}\;\rightarrow\;-\!\overset{\text{H}}{\underset{\text{H}}{\text{C}}}\!-\!\overset{\text{H}}{\underset{\text{R}}{\text{C}}}\!-\!\overset{\text{H}}{\underset{\text{H}}{\text{C}}}\!-\!\overset{\text{H}}{\underset{\text{R}}{\text{C}}}\!-
$$

The process continues, and the polymer is finally formed:

$$
\cdots-\text{C}-\text{C}-\text{C}-\text{C}-\text{C}-\text{C}-\text{C}-\text{C}-\text{C}-\text{C}-\cdots
$$

The nature of the covalent bonding that is established between the two molecules has been previously discussed in Chapter 2.

The polymerization can be pictured as a series of chain reactions such as takes place during an explosion. The process occurs very rapidly, almost instantaneously. The reactions are exothermic, and considerable heat is evolved.

A further classification of polymers can be made on the basis of structural or spatial configurations. The polymerization procedure outlined demonstrates the formation of the simplest of all polymers, the *linear polymer*, in which the structural units are connected one to another in linear sequence. It might be represented simply by the type formula:

$$M'—[—M—]_{\overline{x-2}}-M''$$

in which the principal structural unit, or mer, is represented by M and x is the degree of polymerization. The *terminal* units are M' and M". All structural units except the terminal ones must be covalent.

In their simplest forms both addition and condensation types of polymerization should yield linear macromolecules. Such molecules are seldom realized in practice. In the case of addition polymers, branching side reactions may arise through chain transfer with the monomer or previously formed polymer molecules, to be explained later. Such structural units of the polymer may be connected together in a manner as to form a *nonlinear branched* or *cross-linked* polymer. In this type, some of the structural units must possess a valence greater than two. A typical branched polymer, in which the branching unit is represented by Y, might be indicated by:

$$
\begin{array}{c}
M' \\
| \\
M \\
| \\
M \\
| \\
M'—M—M—Y—M—M—Y—M—\cdots \\
| \\
M \\
| \\
M \\
| \\
\cdots—M—\cdots
\end{array}
$$

Highly ramified molecular structures may then be formed by further propagation of the branched structure.

The original activation of the monomer molecules can be effected by ultraviolet light and other active rays, by heat, or by an energy transfer from another activated compound. Since the last-named method is the one employed in dentistry, it will be discussed more fully.

The activation of the ethylene derivative by another activated compound $R_1 \cdot^*$ can be written as follows:

$$
R_1 \cdot + \ \begin{array}{c} H \quad H \\ | \quad | \\ C{=}C \\ | \quad | \\ H \quad R \end{array} \rightarrow R_1 - \begin{array}{c} H \quad H \\ | \quad | \\ C{-}C\cdot \\ | \quad | \\ H \quad R \end{array}
$$

or if M represents $\begin{array}{c} H \quad H \\ | \quad | \\ C{=}C \\ | \quad | \\ H \quad R \end{array}$, the reaction mechanism can be described as follows:

$$R_1 \cdot + M \rightarrow R_1 M \cdot \tag{1}$$

---

*Represents the activated condition.

The reaction then progresses:

$$R_1M\cdot \quad + M \rightarrow R_1MM\cdot$$
$$R_1MM\cdot \ + M \rightarrow R_1MMM\cdot$$
$$R_1M_{n-1}\cdot + M \rightarrow R_1M_n\cdot \qquad\qquad (2)$$

where n is any integral number.

It should be noted that the activating chemical R_1 is not a catalyst as the latter term is usually defined, since it enters into the chemical reaction and becomes part of the final chemical compound. It might better be termed an *initiator*.

This method of polymerization, then, is dependent upon the formation of *free radicals*. A free radical is a compound with an unpaired electron, usually a fragment of a larger molecule that has, for instance, been split by heating. This unpaired electron makes the radical very reactive. The conventional symbol $C=C$, of course, represents two pairs of electrons. When a free radical collides with a double bond, it may pair with one of the electrons in the extra bond, leaving the other member of the pair free. Thus the monomer itself then becomes a free radical.

A number of substances capable of generating free radicals are potent initiators for the polymerization of poly(methyl methacrylate) resins. The most commonly employed is benzoyl peroxide, which decomposes at relatively low temperatures to release free radicals.

The decomposition of benzoyl peroxide, which occurs quite rapidly between 50 and 100° C, may be represented as

$$(R—COO)_2 \rightarrow 2R—COO \cdot \rightarrow 2R \cdot + 2CO_2$$

Stages in Polymerization   The polymerization process can be described as occurring in four stages: induction, propagation, termination, and chain transfer.

Induction   The induction or initiation period is the time during which the molecules of the initiator become energized or activated and start to transfer their energy to the monomer molecules. This period is greatly influenced by the purity of the monomer. Any impurities present that can react with the activated groups can increase the length of this period. The higher the temperature, the shorter the length of the induction period.

The initiation energy for the activation of each monomer molecular unit is 16,000 to 29,000 calories per mol in the liquid phase.

Propagation   The propagation reactions are illustrated by reactions (1) and (2). Since only 5000 to 8000 calories per mol are required once the growth has started, the process continues with considerable velocity. Theoretically, the chain reactions should continue, with the evolution of heat, until all of the monomer has been changed to polymer. Actually the polymerization is never complete.

Termination   The chain reactions can be terminated either by direct coupling or by the exchange of a hydrogen atom from one growing chain to another.

The termination by direct coupling can be illustrated in terms of a diagrammatic reaction. Let R_1M_n represent a polymer of n monomer units, and R_1M_m signify a polymer of m monomer units. Then:

$$R_1 M_n \cdot + R_1 M_m \cdot \rightarrow R_1 M_{m+n}$$

or

$$R_1 M_n \cdot + R_1 M_m \cdot \rightarrow R_1 M_n + R_1 M_m$$

In other words, both molecules become deactivated by an exchange of energy.

Another means by which such an energy exchange can be effected is by the transfer of a hydrogen atom from one growing chain to another, for example:

$$
\begin{array}{c}
\quad\ \ \text{H} \ \ \text{H} \qquad\qquad\quad \text{H} \ \ \text{H} \qquad\qquad\quad \text{H} \ \ \text{H} \qquad\qquad\quad \text{H} \ \ \text{H} \\
\quad\ \ | \ \ | \qquad\qquad\quad\ | \ \ | \qquad\qquad\quad\ | \ \ | \qquad\qquad\quad\ | \ \ | \\
R_1 M_n\!-\!C\!-\!C\cdot + R_1 M_m\!-\!C\!-\!C\cdot \rightarrow R_1 M_n\!-\!C\!=\!C + R_1 M_m\!-\!C\!-\!C\!-\!H \\
\quad\ \ | \ \ | \qquad\qquad\quad\ | \ \ | \qquad\qquad\qquad\ | \qquad\qquad\quad\ | \ \ | \\
\quad\ \ \text{H} \ \ \text{R} \qquad\qquad\quad \text{H} \ \ \text{R} \qquad\qquad\qquad \text{R} \qquad\qquad\quad \text{H} \ \ \text{R}
\end{array}
$$

in which $R_1 M$ and R have the same significance as in the previous reaction. As before, m and n represent numbers of monomer molecules linked in the chain.

Chain Transfer Although chain termination can result from *chain transfer,* the process differs from the termination reactions described in that the active state is transferred from an activated radical to an inactive molecule, and a new nucleus for further growth is created.

For example, a monomer molecule may be activated by a growing macromolecule in such a manner that termination occurs in the latter:

$$
\begin{array}{c}
\quad\ \ \text{H} \ \ \text{H} \qquad \text{H} \ \ \text{H} \qquad\qquad \text{H} \ \ \text{H} \qquad\qquad \text{H} \ \ \text{H} \\
\quad\ \ | \ \ | \qquad\ | \ \ | \qquad\qquad\ | \ \ | \qquad\qquad\ | \ \ | \\
R_1 M_n\!-\!C\!-\!C\cdot + C\!=\!C \rightarrow R_1 M_n\!-\!C\!=\!C + H\!-\!C\!-\!C\cdot \\
\quad\ \ | \ \ | \qquad\ | \ \ | \qquad\qquad\ | \qquad\qquad\qquad | \ \ | \\
\quad\ \ \text{H} \ \ \text{R} \qquad \text{H} \ \ \text{R} \qquad\qquad \text{H} \qquad\qquad\quad\ \text{H} \ \ \text{R}
\end{array}
$$

Thus, a new nucleus for growth results.

In the same manner, an already terminated chain might be reactivated by chain transfer, and continue to grow:

$$
\begin{array}{c}
\quad\ \ \text{H} \ \ \text{H} \qquad\qquad \text{H} \ \ \text{H} \qquad\qquad \text{H} \ \ \text{H} \qquad\qquad \text{H} \ \ \text{H} \\
\quad\ \ | \ \ | \qquad\qquad\ | \ \ | \qquad\qquad\ | \ \ | \qquad\qquad\ | \ \ | \\
R_1 M_m\!-\!C\!-\!C\cdot + R_1 M_n\!-\!C\!=\!C \rightarrow R_1 M_m\!-\!C\!=\!C + R_1 M_n\!-\!C\!-\!C\cdot \\
\quad\ \ | \ \ | \qquad\qquad\qquad | \qquad\qquad\qquad | \qquad\qquad\quad | \ \ | \\
\quad\ \ \text{H} \ \ \text{R} \qquad\qquad\quad\ \text{R} \qquad\qquad\qquad \text{R} \qquad\qquad\quad \text{H} \ \ \text{R}
\end{array}
$$

Inhibition of Polymerization As noted in the previous section, the polymerization reactions are not likely to result in a complete exhaustion of the monomer, nor do they always form polymers of high molecular weight. Impurities in the monomer often inhibit such reactions.

Any impurity in the monomer that can react with free radicals will inhibit or retard the polymerization reaction. It can react either with the activated initiator or any activated nucleus, or with an activated growing chain to prevent further growth. The presence of such inhibitors markedly influences the length of the initiation period as well as the degree of polymerization.

For example, the addition of a small amount of hydroquinone to the monomer will inhibit polymerization if no initiator is present, and it will definitely retard the polymerization in the presence of an initiator.

The presence of oxygen often causes retardation of the polymerization, since the oxygen can react with the free radicals. It has been shown that the reaction velocity and the degree of the polymerization are less if the polymerization is conducted in the open air in comparison to the higher values obtained when the reaction is carried on in a sealed tube, for example.[4] The influence of oxygen on polymerization is governed by many factors, such as the concentration of oxygen, temperature, and light.

It is common commercial practice to add a small amount (approximately 0.006 per cent or less) of an inhibitor such as the methyl ether of hydroquinone to the monomer in order to aid in the prevention of polymerization during storage.

Copolymerization   In the addition polymerization reactions that have been described, the macromolecule was formed by the polymerization of a single type structural unit. In order to improve the physical properties, it is often advantageous to use two or more chemically different monomers as starting materials. The polymer thus formed may contain units of all of the monomers originally present. Such a polymer is called a *copolymer* and its process of formation is known as *copolymerization*. In a copolymer, the relative number and position of the different type units may vary among the individual macromolecules.

Copolymerization is best illustrated with two monomers, although it is possible to have more than two monomers involved. For example, two monomers consisting of ethylene derivatives might possess the following structural formulas:

$$
\begin{array}{cc}
\text{H} & \text{H} \\
| & | \\
\text{C} & = \text{C} \\
| & | \\
\text{H} & \text{R}_2
\end{array}
\qquad\qquad
\begin{array}{cc}
\text{H} & \text{H} \\
| & | \\
\text{C} & = \text{C} \\
| & | \\
\text{H} & \text{R}_3
\end{array}
$$

in which R_2 and R_3 are two different radicals. It is conceivable that after the polymerization occurs in the usual manner the following copolymer might result:

$$
\cdots-\underset{\underset{\text{H}}{|}}{\overset{\overset{\text{H}}{|}}{\text{C}}}-\underset{\underset{\text{R}_2}{|}}{\overset{\overset{\text{H}}{|}}{\text{C}}}-\underset{\underset{\text{H}}{|}}{\overset{\overset{\text{H}}{|}}{\text{C}}}-\underset{\underset{\text{R}_3}{|}}{\overset{\overset{\text{H}}{|}}{\text{C}}}-\underset{\underset{\text{H}}{|}}{\overset{\overset{\text{H}}{|}}{\text{C}}}-\underset{\underset{\text{R}_2}{|}}{\overset{\overset{\text{H}}{|}}{\text{C}}}-\underset{\underset{\text{H}}{|}}{\overset{\overset{\text{H}}{|}}{\text{C}}}-\underset{\underset{\text{R}_3}{|}}{\overset{\overset{\text{H}}{|}}{\text{C}}}-\cdots
$$

This copolymer structure is, however, highly idealized, since the occurrence of alternately placed radicals in the chain would seldom occur. It is more likely that their positions will be random — a matter of probability.

As a matter of fact, the composition of the copolymer seldom corresponds to the composition of the original monomer mixture. If the monomer given in the first formula is designated as *A*, and if the second monomer formula is called *B*, then the composition of the copolymer will depend upon the relative reactivities of the different molecules and the molecules of the same composition.

For example, if the tendency of monomer *A* to polymerize is so great that it polymerizes independently of *B*, no copolymerization will occur, and the resulting resin will be a mixture of two polymers. Such a condition seldom, if ever, occurs. On the other hand, *A* and *B* may exhibit a greater tendency to polymerize together than to polymerize separately. In such a case, all of the monomers present might enter into the copolymer with no independent polymerization taking place.

In the majority of cases, the final resin consists of a mixture of polymers and copolymers with varying degrees of polymerization or copolymerization.

Copolymers are of three different types–*random, graft,* and *block*. In the random type of copolymer the different mers are randomly distributed along the chain, such as

$$\cdots-M-M-M-Y-M-Y-M-M-Y-Y-M-M-\cdots$$

However, if identical monomer units occur in relatively long sequences along the main polymer chain, a block copolymer is formed:

$$\cdots-M-M-M-\cdots-M-M-Y-Y-Y-\cdots-Y-Y-Y-M-M-M-\cdots$$

In graft copolymers, sequences of one of the monomers are grafted onto a "backbone" of the second monomer species:

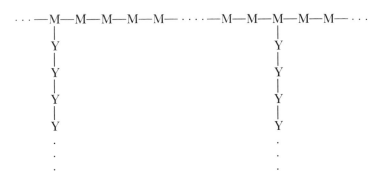

Copolymerization may alter the physical properties of the resulting resin considerably from those of the resins formed individually from the monomers involved. Many useful resins are manufactured by copolymerization. Methyl methacrylate and acrylic and methacrylic esters all copolymerize readily, with little inhibition between monomer pairs. For example, small amounts of ethyl acrylate may be copolymerized with methyl methacrylate to alter the flexibility of the denture.

Grafting of various polymer segments onto a linear chain provides an important mechanism for modifying or tailor-making macromolecules in order to obtain required properties for specific uses. For example, block and graft polymers often show improved impact strength. In small quantities they can modify the adhesive properties of resins as well as their surface characteristics. Although information is not available regarding the molecular configuration of commercial dental resins, it is likely that an increasing number of these copolymers or polymer blends fall within the realm of block and graft polymers.

Cross-Linking As described in the formation of calcium alginate from sodium alginate (Chapter 9) and in the curing of polysulfide rubber impression materials (Chapter 10), linear polymers may be joined, or bridged, through certain reactive side chains to form molecular networks. The cross-linked structure may be envisioned as:

$$
\begin{array}{c}
\cdots -M-M-M-Y-M-M-M-Y- \cdots \\
| \\
Y \\
| \\
Y \\
| \\
\cdots -M-Y-M-M-M-Y-M-Y- \cdots \\
| \qquad\qquad\qquad | \\
Y \qquad\qquad\qquad Y \\
| \qquad\qquad\qquad | \\
Y \qquad\qquad\qquad Y \\
| \qquad\qquad\qquad | \\
\cdots -M-Y-M-M-M-M-M-Y- \cdots
\end{array}
$$

Cross-linkage provides a sufficient number of bridges between the linear macromolecules to form a three-dimensional network that alters the strength, solubility, and water sorption of the resin. For example, cross-linkage has been used widely in the manufacture of acrylic teeth in order to increase their resistance to solvents and surface stresses.

The exact effect of cross-linking upon the physical properties varies with the composition and concentration of the cross-linking agent and the polymer system. In certain cases, cross-linking of a low molecular weight polymer may increase the glass transition temperature to the equivalent of a high molecular weight polymer. Other studies have shown that cross-linking has little influence on tensile strength, transverse strength, or hardness.[7]

Plasticizers Plasticizers are often added to resins to reduce their softening or fusion temperatures. For example, it is possible to plasticize a resin that is normally hard and stiff at room temperature to a condition in which it is flexible and soft. Plastic handbags, raincoats, etc., are often made from resins of this type. Often the plasticizer is added in relatively smaller amounts than would affect appreciably the flexibility of the resin at normal room temperatures. Although the softening temperature of the resin is somewhat reduced, in the case of dental resins, the function of the plasticizer is to increase the solubility of the polymer in the monomer and to decrease the brittleness of the polymer.

The action of the plasticizer is the partial neutralization of the secondary bonds or intermolecular forces that normally prevent the resin molecules from slipping past one another when the material is stressed. Its action may be considered analogous to that of a solvent, since it penetrates between the macromolecules. This type of plasticizer is referred to as an external plasticizer. It is an insoluble high-boiling compound. Its molecular attraction to the polymer should be extremely great so that it will not volatilize or otherwise leach out during the fabrication or the subsequent use of the resin. Such a condition is seldom realized in practice, so this type of plasticizer is used sparingly in dental resins.

Plasticizing of a resin can also be accomplished by copolymerization with a suitable comonomer. In this case the plasticizing agent is a part of the polymer and thus acts as an internal plasticizer. For example, when butyl acrylate is added to methyl methacrylate prior to polymerization, the polymerized resin is plasticized internally by the poly(butyl acrylate).

As might be expected from the theory, plasticizers usually reduce the strength and hardness of the resin, as well as the softening point.

Polymer Structure   As previously noted, the individual organic macromolecules are intramolecularly bonded by covalent bonds. These bonds are so well satisfied that only van der Waals forces bond the aggregate molecules. Since these bonds are easily disrupted, any increase in temperature will cause the polymers to soften their glass transition temperatures (T_g) at which they virtually liquefy. However, if the polymer has been stabilized, the macromolecule may degrade or depolymerize before its T_g is reached.

Characteristically, the dental linear polymers are disordered or noncrystalline in structure. The polymer chains form in a tangled mass as diagrammed in Figure 11–1. Their collective structure can be compared to that of cooked spaghetti, with each piece approximately a mile in length. Under such conditions, it is evident that the mers have little chance to diffuse or become mobile in the solid state. As in the case of glass, any ordering will be short range.

However, many polymers have some degree of crytallization depending upon the secondary valence bonds that can be formed, the structure of the polymer chain, the degree of ordering, and the molecular weight. The conditions for "crystallization" can be illustrated using ethylene derivatives or vinyl resins, of which the following generalized formula is characteristic:

$$\begin{array}{cc} H & H \\ | & | \\ C & = & C \\ | & | \\ H & R \end{array}$$

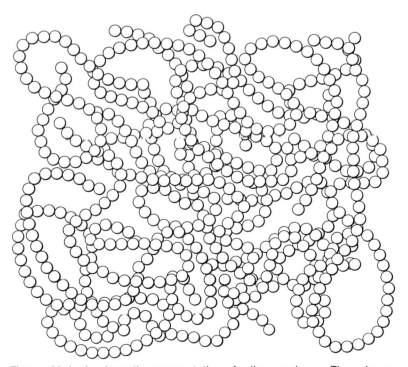

Figure 11–1   A schematic representation of a linear polymer. The spheres represent the mers in the polymer chain, not specific atoms. (From Moffat, Pearsall, and Wulff: The Structure and Properties of Materials, New York, John Wiley and Sons, Inc., 1964, Vol. 1.)

If R is a simple side group such as where R is OH, which forms polyvinyl alcohol, after polymerization the polymer chains may tend to form a short range ordered lattice. On the other hand, if the side chain is more complex, a noncrystalline structure results unless the mers in the polymer chains themselves are arranged symmetrically to each other. In such a case, a crystalline polymer may result, even with a complex side chain.

Usually, a dental resin is noncrystalline. Although polymer crystallinity may increase the tensile strength, it also may reduce the ductility of the resin as well as increase its molding temperature. Its solubility is also decreased and, as a result, its dental use, as outlined in the next chapter, may be rendered difficult.

The factors that favor noncrystallinity are:

1. Long, branched polymers
2. Random arrangement of side groups — particularly large side groups — which tend to separate the molecules
3. Copolymerization, which decreases the regularity of the polymer chains
4. Plasticizers, which tend to separate the chains (see previous section)[8]

Elastomers   Elastomers are polymers that may be stretched in a manner similar to rubber, and that will relax to their original dimensions when unstressed, as noted in Chapter 10. All of these polymers are noncrystalline at room temperature, but they may crystallize under tensile stress.

One of the requisites for the elastomers is that their T_g be below room temperature so that the chain segments are thermally agitated. In this manner the chains are rendered more flexible. In fact, almost any means can be used to impart elastomeric qualities, by which the polymer molecules are rendered more mobile. Another requisite is that the chains be long and bent, or coiled.

A third requisite is that the chains be cross-linked. Such cross-linking must occur only occasionally between the chains. If the cross-linking is complete, a network configuration prevails and the resin becomes rigid. The situation is completely analogous to that described in the formation of calcium alginate in alginate gels. Such cross-linked bonds cause the polymer to return to its original shape after the load is released, as in the case of the gels.

TYPES OF RESINS

As previously mentioned, in order for a synthetic resin to be useful in dentistry it must exhibit exceptional qualities regarding its chemical and dimensional stability, and yet it must possess properties that render it relatively easy to process; it must be strong, hard, and not brittle. A few resins of possible interest to the dentist will be discussed.

Vinyl Resins   Like most polymerization resins, the vinyl resins are derivatives of ethylene. Ethylene ($CH_2=CH_2$) is the simplest molecule capable of addition polymerization, yet a great number of commercial resins are derived from this monomer.

Two of the derivatives of ethylene of special interest are vinyl chloride

$$
\begin{array}{cc}
\text{H} & \text{H} \\
| & | \\
\text{C} & = \text{C} \\
| & | \\
\text{H} & \text{Cl}
\end{array}
$$

and vinyl acetate:

$$
\begin{array}{cc}
\text{H} & \text{H} \\
| & | \\
\text{C} & = \text{C} \\
| & | \\
\text{H} & \text{O} \\
 & | \\
 & \text{C} = \text{O} \\
 & | \\
\text{H} & -\text{C} - \text{H} \\
 & | \\
 & \text{H}
\end{array}
$$

Vinyl chloride polymerizes in the usual manner to form poly(vinyl chloride):

$$
\cdots - \overset{\displaystyle \text{H}}{\underset{\displaystyle \text{H}}{\text{C}}} - \overset{\displaystyle \text{H}}{\underset{\displaystyle \text{Cl}}{\text{C}}} - \overset{\displaystyle \text{H}}{\underset{\displaystyle \text{H}}{\text{C}}} - \overset{\displaystyle \text{H}}{\underset{\displaystyle \text{Cl}}{\text{C}}} - \overset{\displaystyle \text{H}}{\underset{\displaystyle \text{H}}{\text{C}}} - \overset{\displaystyle \text{H}}{\underset{\displaystyle \text{Cl}}{\text{C}}} - \cdots
$$

Vinyl acetate forms poly(vinyl acetate) on polymerization:

$$
\cdots - \text{C} - \text{C} - \text{C} - \text{C} - \text{C} - \text{C} - \cdots
$$

(with H above each carbon; O, H, O, H, O below alternating carbons, and $\text{C}=\text{O}$ groups bearing CH_3 substituents)

Poly(vinyl chloride) is a clear, hard resin that is tasteless and odorless. It darkens when exposed to ultraviolet light and, unless it is plasticized, it discolors when it is heated near its softening point for molding purposes.

On the other hand, the poly(vinyl acetate) is stable to light and heat, but it exhibits an abnormally low softening point (35 to 40° C). When monomers of vinyl chloride and vinyl acetate are copolymerized in varying proportions, many useful copolymer resins result.

A copolymer of approximate composition vinyl chloride 80 per cent and vinyl acetate 20 per cent was once used for the construction of denture bases. The resin was excellent for the purpose in every respect, except that the molecular weight distribution could not be controlled. The average molecular weight was so high that the molding temperature employed was not sufficient to soften the resin thoroughly during molding. As a result, many permanent stresses and strains were induced. Instead of being released by relaxation, the stresses reduced the endurance limit of the resin, and the dentures fractured along the midline of the anterior ridge and palate region after they had been in service for a limited time.

Polystyrene   When a benzene radical is attached to the vinyl grouping, styrene, or vinylbenzene, results:

$$
\begin{array}{cc}
H & H \\
| & | \\
C & = C \\
| & | \\
H & C_6H_5
\end{array}
$$

Such a monomer polymerizes to polystyrene [poly(vinylbenzene)] by addition in the regular manner:

$$
\cdots\cdots\;-\!\!\underset{\underset{H}{|}}{\overset{\overset{H}{|}}{C}}\!-\!\underset{\underset{C_6H_5}{|}}{\overset{\overset{H}{|}}{C}}\!-\!\!-\!\underset{\underset{H}{|}}{\overset{\overset{H}{|}}{C}}\!-\!\underset{\underset{C_6H_5}{|}}{\overset{\overset{H}{|}}{C}}\!-\!\!-\!\underset{\underset{H}{|}}{\overset{\overset{H}{|}}{C}}\!-\!\underset{\underset{C_6H_5}{|}}{\overset{\overset{H}{|}}{C}}\!-\!\cdots\cdots
$$

Polystyrene is a clear resin of the thermoplastic type. It is stable to light and many chemical reagents, although it is soluble in certain organic solvents. It is being used to a limited extent for the construction of denture bases.

Polystyrene can be copolymerized with a number of resins. Its copolymer with divinylbenzene is of interest in that a cross-linked polymer is formed. For example, as little as one mol of p-divinylbenzene copolymerized with 40,000 mols of styrene results in a cross-linked polymer that is insoluble and infusible.

Acrylic Resins   The acrylic resins are derivatives of ethylene, and contain a vinyl group in their structural formula. There are at least two acrylic resin series which are of dental interest. One series is derived from acrylic acid, $CH_2{=}CHCOOH$, and the other from methacrylic acid, $CH_2{=}C(CH_3)COOH$. Both of these compounds polymerize by addition in the usual manner.

Although the polyacids are hard and transparent, their polarity, related to the carboxyl group, causes them to imbibe water. The water tends to separate the chains and to cause a general softening and loss of strength. Consequently, they are not used in the mouth.

The esters of these polyacids are, however, of considerable dental interest. For example, if R represents any ester radical, the formula for a polymethacrylate would be:

$$
\cdots-\underset{\underset{H}{|}}{\overset{\overset{H}{|}}{C}}\!\!-\!\!\underset{\underset{\underset{\underset{\underset{R}{|}}{O}}{|}}{\overset{\overset{\overset{\overset{H-C-H}{|}}{H}}{|}}{C}}\!\!-\!\!\underset{\underset{H}{|}}{\overset{\overset{H}{|}}{C}}\!\!-\!\!\underset{\underset{\underset{\underset{\underset{R}{|}}{O}}{|}}{\overset{\overset{\overset{\overset{H-C-H}{|}}{H}}{|}}{C}}\!\!-\!\!\underset{\underset{H}{|}}{\overset{\overset{H}{|}}{C}}\!\!-\!\!\underset{\underset{\underset{\underset{\underset{R}{|}}{O}}{|}}{\overset{\overset{\overset{\overset{H-C-H}{|}}{H}}{|}}{C}}\!\!-\cdots
$$

When it is realized that theoretically R can be almost any organic or inorganic radical, it is evident that thousands of different acrylic resins are capable of formation. Such a consideration does not include the possibilities of copolymerization, which are even greater.

The effect of esterification on the softening point of a few of the polymethacrylate compounds[9] is shown in Table 11–1. This temperature is always definite for the noncrystalline polymers, such as the polymethacrylates.

Until the side chain becomes quite long, the longer the side chain, the lower the softening or glass transition temperature. For example, poly(methyl methacrylate) is the hardest resin of the series with the highest softening temperature. Ethyl methacrylate possesses a lower softening point and surface hardness; n-propyl methacrylate is still softer, and so on. If an isomer of a straight chain esterifying agent is used, it is interesting to note that the softening temperature is increased above that of the normal straight chain compound. For example, the softening temperature of poly(isopropyl methacrylate) is greater than that of poly(ethyl methacrylate), yet the softening temperature of poly(n-propyl methacrylate) is only 38° C. As the molecular weight of the straight chain alkyl groups increases further, the softening point continues to decrease until the liquid state is attained at room temperature. For example, poly(dodecyl methacrylate) [monomer, $CH_2{=}C(CH_3)COOC_{12}H_{25}$] is a viscous liquid at room temperature. Some resins, such as addition polymers of isobutylene, may be liquid at temperatures as low as $-70°$ C.

Esterification with an aromatic alcohol increases the softening point, even though the molecular weights of the aromatic and aliphatic esterifying compounds may be nearly the same; this is illustrated by the relatively high softening point of poly(phenyl methacrylate) as given in Table 11–1.

Methyl Methacrylate   Poly(methyl methacrylate) by itself is not used in dentistry to a great extent in molding procedures. Rather, the liquid monomer, methyl methacrylate, is mixed with the polymer, which is in the powdered form. The monomer partially dissolves the polymer to form a plastic dough. This dough is packed into the mold, and the monomer is polymerized by one of the methods previously discussed. Consequently, the monomer, methyl methacrylate, is of considerable importance in dentistry.

Methyl methacrylate is a clear, transparent liquid at room temperature with the following physical properties: melting point of $-48°$ C, boiling point of 100.8° C, density of 0.945 gm/ml at 20° C, and heat of polymerization of 12.9 kcal/mol. It exhibits a high vapor pressure, and is an excellent organic solvent. Although the polymerization of methyl methacrylate can be initiated by ultraviolet or visible light or heat, it is commonly polymerized in dentistry by the use of a chemical initiator, as previously described.

Table 11–1.   *Softening Temperatures of Polymethacrylate Esters*

POLYMETHACRYLATE	T_g (°C)
Methyl	125
Ethyl	65
n-Propyl	38
Isopropyl	95
n-Butyl	33
Isobutyl	70
sec-Butyl	62
tert-Amyl	76
Phenyl	120

The conditions for the polymerization of methyl methacrylate are not critical, provided that the reaction is not carried out at a too rapid rate. The degree of polymerization varies with the conditions of polymerization, such as the temperature, method of activation, type of initiator used and its concentration, purity of chemicals, and similar factors. Because they will polymerize readily under the conditions of usage, the methacrylate monomers have found particular usefulness in dentistry. Many other resin systems will not polymerize at room temperature in the presence of air.

A volume shrinkage of 21 per cent occurs during the polymerization of the pure methyl methacrylate monomer.

*Poly(Methyl Methacrylate)** Poly(methyl methacrylate) is a transparent resin of remarkable clarity; it transmits light into the ultraviolet range to a wave length of $0.25 \mu m$. It is a hard resin with a Knoop hardness number of 18 to 20. Its tensile strength is approximately 59 MPa (8500 psi) and its specific gravity is 1.19. Its modulus of elasticity is approximately 2400 MPa (350,000 psi).

The resin is extremely stable; it will not discolor in ultraviolet light, and it exhibits remarkable aging properties. It is chemically stable to heat; it will soften at 125° C, and it can be molded as a thermoplastic material. Between this temperature and 200° C, depolymerization takes place. At approximately 450° C, 90 per cent of the polymer will depolymerize to the monomer. Poly(methyl methacrylate) of high molecular weight will degrade to a lower polymer at the same time that it evolves to the monomer.

Like all acrylic resins, poly(methyl methacrylate) exhibits a tendency to take up water by a process of imbibition. Its noncrystalline structure possesses a high internal energy; thus, molecular diffusion can occur into the resin, since less activation energy is required. Furthermore, the polar carboxyl group, even though esterified, can form a hydrogen bridge with the water, if only to a limited extent.

Since both absorption and adsorption are involved, the term *sorption* is usually used to include the total phenomenon. It has been reported that typical dental methacrylate resins show an increase of approximately 0.5 per cent by weight after one week in water.[10] Higher values have been reported for a series of methyl methacrylate polymers.[11] The sorption of water is nearly independent of temperature from 0 to 60° C, but is markedly affected by the molecular weight of the polymer. The greater the molecular weight, the smaller the weight increase. Sorption is reversible if the resin is dried.

Since poly(methyl methacrylate) is a chain polymer, it can be expected that it will be soluble in a number of organic solvents, such as chloroform and acetone.

Epoxy Resins Another resin family of interest to dentistry is the epoxy resin. These thermosetting resins possess unique characteristics in terms of adhesion to various metals, wood, and glass.

---

*The nomenclature of *poly(methyl methacrylate)* has been retained throughout this edition. Frequently it is referred to as *polymethyl methacrylate* or *methyl methacrylate polymer*. However, the present rules of the International Union of Pure and Applied Chemistry state: "A polymer of unspecified chain length is named with the prefix 'poly' followed by, in parentheses or brackets, as appropriate, the name of the smallest repeating unit. The generic name for a single-stranded linear polymer is thus poly(bivalent radical)." (Macromolecules, *1*:19, 1968.)

The epoxy resin molecule is characterized by the reactive epoxy or oxirane groups

$$
\begin{array}{c}
\overset{\displaystyle O}{\diagup \diagdown} \\
-\underset{|}{C}\!-\!-\!-\!\underset{|}{C}-
\end{array}
$$

which serve as terminal polymerization points. In this group, the ring is in a somewhat unstable condition and prone to open and combine with compounds having an available hydrogen. Cross-linkage is easily accomplished.

A typical epoxy molecule is represented by the diglycidyl ether of bisphenol-A:

$$
\underset{CH_2}{\diagup}\!\!-\!\!-\!\!CH\!-\!CH_2\!-\!O\!-\!\!\left\langle\bigcirc\right\rangle\!-\!\underset{\underset{CH_3}{|}}{\overset{\overset{CH_3}{|}}{C}}\!-\!\!\left\langle\bigcirc\right\rangle\!-\!O\!-\!CH_2\!-\!CH\!-\!\underset{O}{\diagdown}\!CH_2
$$

Such epoxy resins, which are often viscous liquids at room temperature, may be cured by use of a reactive intermediate to join the resin chains. The primary cross-linking agents are polyfunctional primary and secondary amines, such as diethylenetriamine,

$$NH_2\!-\!CH_2\!-\!CH_2\!-\!NH\!-\!CH_2\!-\!CH_2\!-\!NH_2$$

Other agents such as polybasic acids, boron trifluoride, and certain anhydrides may also be employed, although the amines are the most common.

Several modified epoxy resins have been suggested as denture base materials. The mixed resin is poured into the flask and a low curing temperature is used. Although certain advantages were claimed for this type of resin, problems, such as color stability, water sorption, and patient sensitivity, were not completely eliminated in the dental products introduced.

A resin based upon an epoxy starting material is being used as the matrix for the commonly used composite restorative materials.[12] This resin formulation is actually a reaction product of methacrylic acid and diglycidal ether of bisphenol-A.[13] The backbone of the molecule is similar to that of an epoxy resin, but the functional reactive groups in the molecule are acrylic. This resin is often referred to as the BIS-GMA system. It is believed that the backbone of the molecule, as part of composite formulations, provides superior toughness and other desirable properties. The chemistry and characteristics of this and other restorative resins will be discussed further in Chapter 14.

Other Resin Systems   There are several other polymers of dental interest. Among these are the polycarbonates, polyurethanes, and cyanoacrylates.

The polycarbonates are polyesters of carbonic acid in which the carbonate is repeated in the linear chain. Polycarbonate resins have been employed as denture bases and as a direct filling resin. Their physical properties fall into the general range of poly(methyl methacrylate) resin denture base materials. The principal advantage of the polycarbonate resin as a denture base material is that it has greater resistance to fracture by impact than does poly(methyl methacrylate). However, it has the disadvantage of a high softening temperature and complicated apparatus. Temperatures in the range of 140 to 160° C are required to mold the material. The softened material is then injected into the mold.

Because of the more complicated procedure, these resins have not been widely used either for denture bases or for the restoration of teeth. There is no evidence that dentures or restorations fabricated from polycarbonate resins are superior to those made from acrylic resins.

When used in small amounts, the alkyl (methyl, butyl) cyanoacrylate resins may be polymerized by weak bases, such as water. Since they polymerize in the presence of moisture and are biodegradable, they have been employed experimentally as surgical sutures and for periodontal dressings.

Polyurethane resins have been investigated as adhesive lining agents. Some experimental compositions appear to have some adhesion to tooth structure, and they also have been tested as pit and fissure sealants. They will be discussed in Chapter 14, particularly as related to their use in composite restorative resins.

References

1. Brauer GM: The present and future of macromolecules for dental applications. Polym Plast Tech Eng 9:87, 1977.
2. Caul HJ and Schoonover ID: A method for determining the extent of polymerization of acrylic resins and its application for dentures. J Am Dent Assoc 39:1, 1949.
3. Gowman DJ, Cornell J, and Powers CM: Effect of composition on dimensional stability of denture bases. J Am Dent Assoc 70:1200, 1965.
4. Odian G: Principles of Polymerization. New York, McGraw-Hill Book Co., 1970.
5. Lenz RW: Organic Chemistry of Synthetic High Polymers. New York, Interscience Publishers (Division of John Wiley and Sons, Inc.), 1967.
6. Stille JK: Introduction to Polymer Chemistry. New York, John Wiley and Sons, Inc., 1962.
7. Wolff EM: The effect of cross-linking agents on acrylic resins. Aust Dent J 7:439, 1962.
8. Moffat WG, Pearsall GW, and Wulff J: The Structure and Properties of Materials. New York, John Wiley and Sons, Inc., 1964, Vol. 1.
9. Powers PO: Synthetic Resins and Rubbers. New York, John Wiley and Sons, Inc., 1943.
10. Peyton FA, and Mann WR: Acrylic and acrylic-styrene resins: Their properties in relation to their uses as restorative materials. J Am Dent Assoc 29:1852, 1942.
11. Brauer GM, and Sweeney WT: Sorption of water by polymethyl methacrylate. Mod Plast 32:138, 1955.
12. Bowen RL: Compatibility of various materials with oral tissues. I. The components of composite restorations. J Dent Res 58:1493, 1979.
13. Bowen RL: Properties of a silica-reinforced polymer for dental restoration. J Am Dent Assoc 66:57, 1963.

12 DENTURE BASE RESINS: TECHNICAL CONSIDERATIONS

A complete acrylic resin denture is shown in Figure 12–1. The artificial teeth are seated on the *denture base,* the part of the denture that retains the artificial teeth and rests on the soft tissues of the mouth. The denture base resin is tinted to imitate the natural gum tissues as closely as possible.

The better the fit of the denture base, the better will be the retention of the denture in the mouth, and the greater will be the comfort to the patient. Consequently, considerable attention will be given to the discussion of methods for improving the fit and the dimensional stability of the denture. There are, of course, many factors other than the fit of the denture base which determine its efficiency in function, but the fit is basically very important. The maximal biting force of a patient wearing an artificial denture may be only one-sixth of the force exerted by a person with natural dentition.[1] Thus, close adaptation of the denture base to the oral structures is imperative to prevent even further loss of chewing efficiency.

The artificial teeth are constructed either of porcelain or of resin, tinted to simulate the human teeth. Acrylic resin dentures can often be constructed so lifelike in appearance as to defy detection.

General Technique   Considerable discussion of the processing technique will be given in subsequent sections. Briefly, the process consists first of the construction of the base plate on the stone cast. A swaging method is frequently used to form the base plates from sheets of polystyrene. The base plate material may also be another type of resin or shellac. The artificial teeth are then placed in position with wax.

The cast, with the base plate and positioned teeth, is seated in freshly mixed dental stone or plaster in the appropriate denture flask. The type of flask used is determined by the technique employed in fabricating the denture. Typical flasks for three generally accepted techniques are shown in Figure 12–2.

When the flasks are separated, the wax and base plate are removed. The mold space that remains is filled with the resin denture base material. After it has been formed and cured, the denture is removed from the flask and finished, resulting in a final appliance, such as that seen in Figure 12–1.

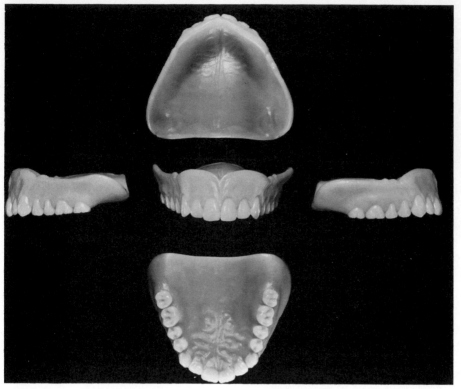

Figure 12–1 Various views of an upper acrylic resin denture. (Courtesy of L. Merritt and E. Lipawsky, Dentsply International, Inc.)

Acrylic Resin   Although denture base resins are available using polystyrene or vinyl copolymer resins as discussed later, the principal base resin employed at the present time is poly(methyl methacrylate):

$$\cdots-\overset{\overset{\displaystyle H}{|}}{\underset{\underset{\displaystyle H}{|}}{C}}-\overset{\overset{\displaystyle CH_3}{|}}{\underset{\underset{\displaystyle \underset{\displaystyle CH_3}{|}}{\underset{\displaystyle O}{|}}}{\underset{\displaystyle C=O}{C}}}-\overset{\overset{\displaystyle H}{|}}{\underset{\underset{\displaystyle H}{|}}{C}}-\overset{\overset{\displaystyle CH_3}{|}}{\underset{\underset{\displaystyle \underset{\displaystyle CH_3}{|}}{\underset{\displaystyle O}{|}}}{\underset{\displaystyle C=O}{C}}}-\overset{\overset{\displaystyle H}{|}}{\underset{\underset{\displaystyle H}{|}}{C}}-\overset{\overset{\displaystyle CH_3}{|}}{\underset{\underset{\displaystyle \underset{\displaystyle CH_3}{|}}{\underset{\displaystyle O}{|}}}{\underset{\displaystyle C=O}{C}}}-\overset{\overset{\displaystyle H}{|}}{\underset{\underset{\displaystyle H}{|}}{C}}-\overset{\overset{\displaystyle CH_3}{|}}{\underset{\underset{\displaystyle \underset{\displaystyle CH_3}{|}}{\underset{\displaystyle O}{|}}}{\underset{\displaystyle C=O}{C}}}-\cdots$$

The resin is transparent. It can be colored or tinted to almost any shade and degree of translucence. Its color and optical properties are stable under all normal conditions, and its strength and other physical properties are adequate. The properties of acrylic resins are not ideal, of course, any more than the properties of any other dental material are ideal. However, it is the combination of desirable characteristics which have made them so acceptable.

One decided advantage of poly(methyl methacrylate) as a denture base material is the comparative ease with which it can be processed. Although it is a thermoplastic resin, in dentistry it is not usually molded by thermoplastic means. Rather, the liquid (monomer) methyl methacrylate is mixed with the polymer, which is dispensed in the form of a powder. As will be discussed in detail in a subsequent section, the monomer plasticizes the polymer to a

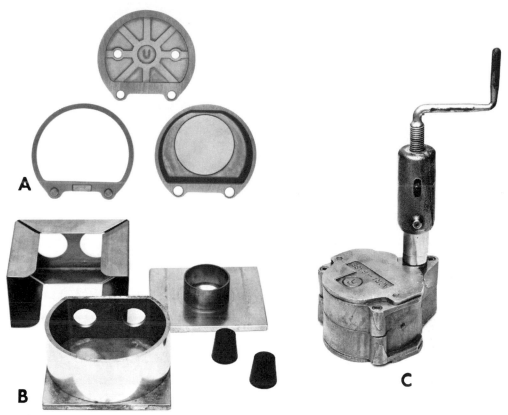

Figure 12–2 Typical denture flasks: *A*, for conventional compression molding; *B*, for fluid resin technique; and *C*, for injection molding.

doughlike consistency which can be easily molded initially in the mold space. The monomer is subsequently polymerized and the resulting denture base is composed of a solid, homogeneous resin. The polymerization can be effected either by heating the polymer-monomer mixture, usually in a water bath, or by chemical activation at room temperature.

HEAT-CURING DENTURE BASE RESINS

Probably more than 95 per cent of the complete dentures made today use one of the acrylic resins.[2] A number of other materials find occasional use as denture bases. These include other types of resins and metals. Because the use of acrylic resins is so prevalent in the construction of artificial dentures, emphasis will be placed on that system.

Composition-Acrylic Resin   The monomer is generally pure methyl methacrylate with a slight amount of hydroquinone (0.006 per cent or less), which aids in the inhibition of polymerization during storage.

The polymer usually consists of a powder composed of small spherical particles, as shown in Figure 12–3. The spheres (*pearls* or *beads*) can be polymerized from monomer which has been heated in some nonpolymerizing liquid under agitation.

Since the more desirable high molecular weight poly(methyl methacrylate) dissolves in the monomer very slowly, an additive is usually included

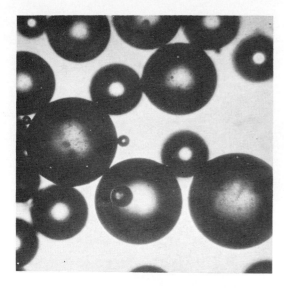

Figure 12–3 Polymer pearls are highlighted to show detail. The pearls are actually transparent.

to increase the solubility. For example, a copolymer of methyl methacrylate and ethyl acrylate ($CH_2{=}CHCOOC_2H_5$) may be employed, with the quantity of the ethyl acrylate limited to 5 per cent or less.

A second method for increasing the solubility is to add a plasticizer such as dibutyl phthalate [$C_6H_4(COOC_4H_9)_2$], either by ball milling it with the pearls or by adding it to the monomer. The quantity of plasticizer should be limited to 8 to 10 per cent in order to prevent a subsequent deterioration of the resin in the oral fluids. A third method is to blend the high molecular weight beads with poly(methyl methacrylate) of lower molecular weight which is more soluble in the monomer. Such a method, of course, lowers the average molecular weight of the resin.

An initiator (benzoyl peroxide) is always included in the polymer in a small amount, as previously discussed. Usually there is sufficient benzoyl peroxide left in the polymer pearls from their initial polymerization.

The pigment can be incorporated in the pearl during the initial polymerization, or it can be added after the polymerization by an impregnation into the pearls by means of a ball mill, for example. When the latter method is employed, the pigment is ground into the surface of the pearl.

Many acrylic resin denture base materials contain a cross-linking agent such as glycol dimethacrylate:

$$
\begin{array}{c}
\left[\begin{array}{cc}
\mathrm{H} & \mathrm{CH_3} \\
| & | \\
\mathrm{C}\!=\!\mathrm{C} \\
| & | \\
\mathrm{M} \quad \mathrm{H} & \mathrm{C}\!=\!\mathrm{O} \\
& | \\
& \mathrm{O} \\
& | \\
& \mathrm{CH_2}
\end{array}\right] \\
\hline
\left[\begin{array}{cc}
& \mathrm{CH_2} \\
& | \\
& \mathrm{O} \\
& | \\
\mathrm{M} \quad \mathrm{H} & \mathrm{C}\!=\!\mathrm{O} \\
| & | \\
\mathrm{C}\!=\!\mathrm{C} \\
| & | \\
\mathrm{H} & \mathrm{CH_3}
\end{array}\right]
\end{array}
$$

Glycol dimethacrylate

Note that the formulas above and below the dotted line are essentially methyl methacrylate. Thus there are two mers (M), one above and one below as indicated. Polymerization is through the double bonds. The polymer, poly(glycol dimethacrylate), is cross-linked through the $CH_2 — CH_2$ groups in at least two directions to form a bridged network, as was depicted in the previous chapter. The cross-linking agent is incorporated in the monomer, at a concentration of 1 to 2 per cent. These resins are generally labeled by the manufacturer as *cross-linked resins*.

Usually the monomer and polymer are combined immediately before the mixture is placed in the denture mold. However, the polymer and monomer can be pre-mixed by the manufacturer and supplied in the form of a flexible sheet or gel, ready to be packed into the mold. Unfortunately, in spite of the added inhibitor, the pre-mixed material may harden in its container during storage. Therefore, it possesses a short shelf life.

At least one denture resin is dispensed exclusively in the gel form. This particular material contains a vinyl resin in addition to poly(methyl methacrylate). Instead of employing poly(methyl methacrylate) for the solid component of the monomer-polymer mixture, a copolymer of vinyl chloride and vinyl acetate is used. The vinyl copolymer is processed to a plastic gel by saturation with methyl methacrylate monomer. The resulting gel is packed into the mold space and the resin is polymerized by heat in the usual manner. The resulting resin is a mixture of poly(methyl methacrylate) and, predominantly, vinyl copolymer resin.

Polystyrene is sometimes used to fabricate denture bases. A cylinder of polystyrene of the proper molecular weight distribution is softened under heat and forced into the mold space under pressure by a process known as *injection molding*. In other words, advantage is taken of the thermoplastic property of the resin.

It was previously noted that thin polystyrene sheets that can be heat softened and swaged directly against the cast are available for fabricating a tissue fitting base plate. The base plate can then be integrated into the denture base via the procedure just described.

Storage   A word of caution should be given in regard to storage of these materials. Responsible manufacturers of gel-type resins and of those products with monomer components that are subject to deterioration during storage usually recommend specific temperatures and time limits. Strict observance of these recommendations is essential. Most of the heat-curing liquid-powder resins and some of the self-curing materials are formulated to endure high temperatures over extended periods of time without harmful effects. However, there are other storage related problems that can affect the materials adversely if certain precautions are not observed.

The finer sized particles of the powdered polymer and pigment tend to migrate to the bottom of the container as a result of vibration that occurs during storage. The greater the disparity in particle sizes, the faster and the more thorough will be the separation of the particle sizes. Therefore, in order to obtain optimal results with polymer powders, it is necessary to tumble the powder about in the container, or in a larger one, to restore uniform distribution of the different particle sizes. Failure to redistribute the particle sizes uniformly will result in mixes that actually have different monomer-polymer ratios than those recommended by the manufacturers.

The container of the liquid monomer must be kept tightly sealed at all times to guard against evaporation of the most volatile ingredients and an imbalance in the chemistry of the liquid.

Compression Molding Technique

Because most of the denture resins are acrylic resins and are supplied in the form of a powder (polymer) and a liquid (monomer), the technique employed with this type of resin will be discussed in detail.

Preparation of the Mold   As previously noted, the stone cast, with the base plate and positioned teeth, is embedded in an investing medium in the lower half of the flask (Fig. 12–2A). After the investing material hardens it is coated with an agent, such as a sodium alginate, to prevent the stone or plaster mixture that is poured into the upper half of the flask from adhering to that in the lower half. A variation to the all-gypsum investment for the upper half of the flask is a layer of silicone placed over the teeth and external surface of the wax denture.

Although the top half of the flask may be filled with a single pour of the investing material, there may be some advantage to a two-pour or "capping" technique.[3] The advantage of the capping technique is appreciated during deflasking procedures. A one-piece pour requires that the technician locate the teeth and remove the investment without damage to the tooth surfaces. The two-piece investment permits easy removal of the cap, exposing the teeth. The investment may then be removed without danger of marring the teeth by the deflasking equipment.

The investment material is poured into the upper half of the flask, leaving the occlusal and incisal surfaces of the teeth exposed, as shown in Figure 12–4. When this initial pour has set, the surface is saturated with water to prevent moisture from being drawn from it by the second pour. A second mix of the investment material is used to complete the fill of the upper half of the flask.

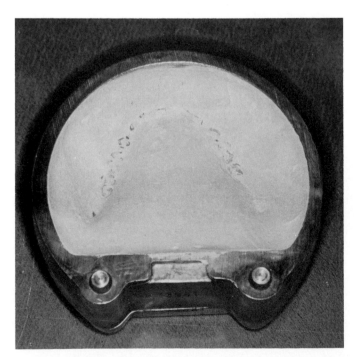

Figure 12–4   Occlusal and incisal edges of denture teeth exposed in top half of flask, ready to receive stone cap. (From Rudd, K. D., Dent Clin North Am, Nov., 1964.)

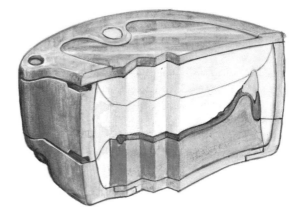

Figure 12–5 A cross section through a flask, showing the wax denture on the stone cast surrounded by investment with cap.

The result of the two-pour technique is diagrammed in Figure 12–5, in which the cap is shown immediately under the cover plate.

After the investing material has set in the top half, the flask is heated sufficiently to soften the wax, and then the halves are separated. The teeth remain in the upper half, since they are retained in the stone or plaster (Fig. 12–6). The wax is completely removed from the mold. Any residual wax is flushed out with boiling water containing an ordinary household detergent in proportions of one tablespoon to one pint of water.

Separating Media During its processing, the resin must be carefully protected from the gypsum surfaces surrounding the mold space for two reasons: (1) Any water incorporated into the resin from the gypsum during processing will definitely affect the polymerization rate and the color of the resin. The denture produced will craze readily because of the stresses formed by the evaporation of water after the processing, particularly if the resin is not cross-linked. (2) Dissolved polymer and free monomer must be prevented from soaking into the mold surface. If any liquid resin penetrates into the investing medium, portions of the gypsum material will be joined to the denture after polymerization, with the result that it will be virtually impossible to separate the investing material from the resin.

One of the first widely accepted means of protecting the denture base material was to line the mold with thin sheets of tin foil. A scarcity of tin foil during the early 1940's made it necessary to employ other *separating media.*

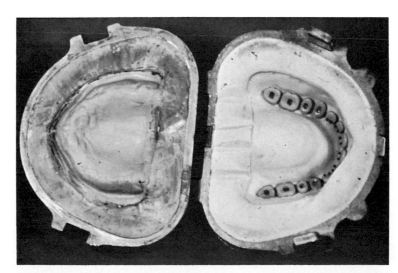

Figure 12–6 The appearance of the flask halves after the first opening. The artificial teeth are held by the plaster in the upper half. The holes and pins in the teeth provide anchorage in the finally cured resin. (Courtesy of A. H. Grunewald.)

Cellulose lacquers and solutions of alginate compounds, evaporated milk, soap, sodium silicate, and starches have all been used as paint-on tin foil substitutes.

The most popular separating agents are water-soluble alginates which produce a very thin water– and organic solvent–insoluble calcium alginate film on the gypsum surface.

The physical properties of most denture resins cured in molds lined with an alginate film are not significantly different from those of resins obtained with tin foil liners, provided the film is uniform and continuous throughout the mold.

The following factors should be taken into account in the use of such agents: (1) Waxes or oils remaining on the mold surface will not permit the solution to contact and react with the investment in order to form a satisfactory film over the contaminated areas. (2) Continuity of the film can be disrupted if the solution is applied while the mold is steaming. It is safe to apply the solution only when the flask can be held comfortably in the bare hand. (3) Puddling of the solution around and on the teeth, or on the cast surface, during application results in the formation of excessively thick films that prevent satisfactory adaptation of the denture base material in the critical areas. Coatings left on resin teeth obstruct bonding to the denture base material. Any such film existing between the necks of the teeth and the denture base will permit penetration of stains into the affected areas when the cured dentures are in use. Likewise, excessively thick layers of the separator covering the tissue copying surfaces of the cast will constitute discrepancies that prevent the reproduction of detail in the denture as an accurate negative copy of the oral tissue.

Monomer–Polymer Ratio   The proper monomer to polymer ratio is of considerable importance to the final structure of the resin. In general, the more polymer used, the shorter will be the reaction time. Furthermore, the shrinkage of the resin will be lower. However, sufficient monomer must be employed to thoroughly wet each polymer pearl.

The approximate proportions of polymer to monomer are generally 3 to 1 by volume. This is assuming that there is a uniform distribution of the different sized polymer and pigment particles throughout the powder increment. It is also assuming that the powder and liquid components will be thoroughly mixed so that the resultant dough will have a proper polymer-monomer balance. Failure to properly blend the powder and liquid can result in low strength, porosities, and poor color in the cured denture.

Monomer-Polymer Reaction   The function of the monomer in the polymer is to produce a plastic mass that can be packed into the mold. Such a plasticization is accomplished by a partial solution of the polymer in the monomer.

At least four stages can be identified during the physical reaction of the powder and liquid:

STAGE 1   The polymer gradually settles into the monomer and a somewhat fluid, incoherent mass is formed.

STAGE 2   The monomer attacks the polymer. This is accomplished by the penetration of the monomer into the polymer; the layer of polymer so penetrated sloughs off and either goes into solution or is dispersed in the monomer. This stage is characterized by a stringiness and adhesiveness if the mixture is touched or pulled apart.

STAGE 3   As the monomer diffuses into the polymer, and the mass becomes more saturated with polymer in solution, it becomes smooth and doughlike. It is no longer tacky, and it does not adhere to the walls of the mixing jar. It consists of undissolved polymer particles suspended in a plastic matrix of monomer and dissolved polymer. This stage is often called the *dough* or *gel stage*. While the mixture is in this stage, it is packed into the mold.

STAGE 4   The monomer seemingly disappears, by evaporation and by further penetration into the polymer. The mass becomes more cohesive and rubber-like. It is no longer completely plastic, and it cannot be molded by the methods used in dentistry. A word of caution should be added that any contamination of the liquid monomer storage container by particles of the polymer must be avoided. Even a minute amount of powder in the liquid will cause it to thicken and eventually solidify.

Dough-forming Time   The time required to reach stage 3 depends upon the solubility of the polymer pearls in this monomer. In addition to the factors already mentioned in this connection, the solution rate may be increased by increasing the temperature. The mixing jar may be heated in warm water (never over an open flame, as the monomer liquid or vapor is inflammable), but care must be taken that the water does not contact the resin. Under no circumstances should the jar be heated above 55° C (130° F), since polymerization begins at a rapid rate above this temperature and the resin becomes too difficult to mold by dental procedures.

Another factor that influences the dough-forming time is the size of the polymer particles. Since more area is presented for solution, the smaller the particle size of the polymer, the more rapid is the solution of the polymer in the monomer, and the shorter is the dough-forming period. However, this factor is apt to be of minor importance in comparison with some of the other factors mentioned.

Working Time   The *working time* is the time elapsing between stage 2 and the beginning of stage 4, or, in other words, the time that the material remains in the dough form. According to the American Dental Association Specification no. 12, the dough should be moldable for at least 5 minutes.

As already indicated, the working time is affected by the temperature; the lower the temperature, the longer is the working time. Some commercial denture resins can be preserved in a moldable condition in a refrigerator for many hours. An objection to this method is that moisture may condense on the resin when it is removed from the refrigerator. Such contamination can be avoided by storing the material in an airtight container. Following removal from the refrigerator, the container is not opened until the resin reaches room temperature.

There are a number of methods for increasing the time of the dough stage at room temperature. For example, it can be reasoned that a blend of molecular weights might prolong such a stage; the lower molecular weight fraction might conceivably result in an early dough stage, and as the monomer diffuses more slowly into the pearls of higher molecular weight, the dough stage might be prolonged.

Trial Closure   It is very important that the mold be filled properly at the time the resin is polymerized; consequently, the mold is packed with dough in several steps. A mold at room temperature is preferable, since the working time will be longer. Also, there will be less likelihood of stiffening by premature polymerization.

The resin is rolled into a ropelike form, bent into a horseshoe shape, and placed in the upper half of the flask. A polyethylene sheet is placed over the resin and the mold space. The purpose of such a sheet is to prevent the adhesion of the resin to the lower mold surface when the 2 halves of the flask are pressed together.

When the lower half is pressed against the upper half, it is very important that the pressure be applied slowly so that the dough will flow evenly throughout the mold space. When further application of pressure meets with considerable resistance, the 2 halves are separated. If too much material has been placed in the mold, it will be found to have overflowed onto the *land* surrounding the mold space, as shown in Figure 12–7. The excess material is called the *flash*. If a flash does not occur, it is possible that there was insufficient dough in the mold at the start; consequently, more resin is added, and the process is repeated.

The flash is carefully removed, and another trial closure is made; usually, the flask can be closed entirely during the second trial closure, although care should be taken not to force the closure unduly. The trial closures are repeated until no flash is observed. Heavy pressures are not needed. Only sufficient pressure for complete closure of the flask is required.

After all trial closures are completed, a mold-protecting medium is applied to the surfaces of the investment and cast in the lower half of the flask. The separating plastic sheet is then removed and the 2 halves are closed under pressure, which is maintained until the denture has been processed. A diagram of a cross section through the flask and associated materials at this stage is shown in Figure 12–8. The finished cured denture is also depicted in this sketch.

Injection Molding Technique

The mold space may be filled by injecting the resin under pressure before it hardens, using a flask such as is shown in Figure 12–2C. A vent in the flask permits the attachment of an outside injector, as seen in that figure. The soft

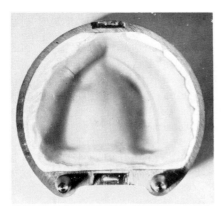

Figure 12–7   After the first trial closure, a flash of resin appears, spread over the land surrounding the mold space.

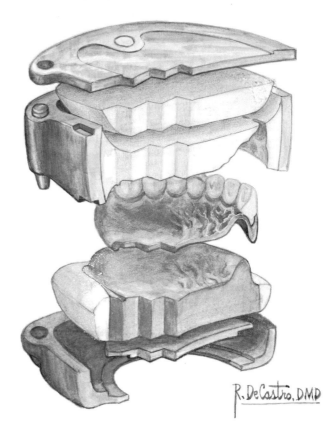

Figure 12–8 A diagram of a cross section through a flask showing the finished denture and the various auxiliary materials.

R. DeCastro, DMD

resin is contained in the injector and is forced into the mold space as needed.

In the case of the polystyrene resin previously described, the polymer is first softened under heat and injected while hot. The thermoplastic resin then solidifies in the mold upon cooling. If the usual monomer-polymer mixture is employed, the dough is injected in a similar manner at room temperature. In either case, the resin and flask are kept under pressure until the resin has hardened.

One advantage of the injection molding technique over the usual compression molding method already described is that no trial closure is necessary and that the mold is properly filled automatically, provided the proper pressure is employed. However, there appears to be no difference between the two methods in accuracy or the physical properties obtained.[4]

CURING PROCEDURE

Polymerization As previously noted, the dental resins usually contain benzoyl peroxide. When the temperature of the dough increases above 60° C (140° F), the molecules of benzoyl peroxide decompose to form free radicals. A free radical reacts with a monomer molecule, and a new free radical is formed, which in turn becomes attached to another monomer molecule; the chain reaction is thus propagated until a termination occurs, as described in the previous chapter.

The principal factor that governs the rate of polymerization is the rate at which the free radicals of the benzoyl peroxide are released, and, in the reaction under discussion, this factor is determined largely by the temperature.

Generally, the lower the temperature of the polymerization, the greater will be the molecular weight of the polymer, although the time required to complete the reaction may be greatly lengthened. Although this rule holds in the processing of dental resins, the other factors enumerated may also affect the polymerization to an appreciable extent, and higher temperatures with shorter curing times are often equally effective.

Temperature Rise   The polymerization reaction is exothermic, and the amount of heat evolved may be a factor in the proper processing of the denture. The temperature changes that may occur with time in water, in the investing plaster or stone, and in the resin itself are plotted in Figure 12–9. In this case, a 25.4 mm (1 inch) cube mold cavity was formed according to the procedure used for making dentures. Thermocouples were imbedded in the various media and the changes in temperature with time were noted.[5]

As can be noted from Figure 12–9, the temperature of the water and the plaster increased from room temperature to 100° C (212° F) in 60 minutes. The temperature of the acrylic resin increased at the same rate as the other two materials until a temperature slightly above 70° C (160° F) was reached, at which time the temperature of the resin began to increase rapidly. At this temperature, a sufficient number of molecules of benzoyl peroxide were activated to produce the chain reaction, and to cause the temperature of the interior of the resin to rise considerably above the temperature of the boiling water at which the resin was polymerized.

Internal Porosity   The general effect of the temperature rise above 100° C is to produce a porosity in the interior of a thick piece of the resin. The boiling point of the monomer (100.8° C or 213.4° F) is very slightly higher than that of the water. Although the rate of polymerization is extremely rapid, it is not instantaneous, and if the temperature rises above the boiling point of the residual monomer or some of the very low molecular weight polymers, these

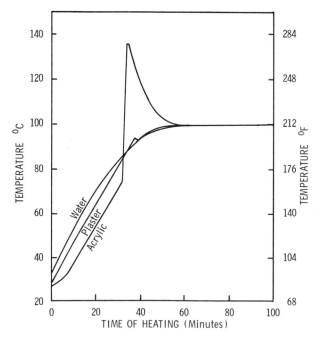

Figure 12–9 Temperature-time heating curves for the water bath, investing plaster, and acrylic resin during the polymerization of a 25.4 mm cube of denture resin. (Modified from Tuckfield, Worner, and Guerin, Aust Dent J, March, 1943.)

components may boil with the production of bubbles, as shown in Figure 13–3C in the next chapter.

This type of porosity will usually not be present on the surface of a denture. The reason is that the exothermic heat can be conducted away from the surface of the resin into the investing medium, and the temperature in this region is not likely to rise above the boiling point of the monomer. In the center of a thick portion, however, the heat cannot be conducted away with sufficient rapidity; therefore, the temperature in the center portion may rise considerably above the boiling point of the monomer.

Porosity of this type may occur in the thick ridge portions of an acrylic resin denture, but never in the thin palate portions of an upper denture, for example. If the resin section is thin, the exothermic heat can be conducted away with sufficient rapidity to prevent the formation of bubbles.

Curing Cycle   The *curing cycle* is the technical name for the heating process employed to control the initial propagation of polymerization in the denture mold. The curing cycle presented in Figure 12–9 is unsatisfactory because of the considerable temperature rise during the initial polymerization.

As previously noted, it is only in the thicker sections of the denture that the temperature during polymerization is apt to rise above the boiling point of the monomer. Furthermore, the temperature reached during polymerization obviously depends upon the bulk of the resin and the rate at which the exothermic heat is evolved, or, in other words, the curing rate. It follows, therefore, that a slower curing rate, effected by heating the denture more slowly above approximately 60° C (140° F), will result in a smaller temperature rise* during polymerization.

This effect of rate of heating on the temperature rise of the resin is illustrated in Figure 12–10. Certainly, the curing cycle indicated by the curve C in the figure (also, in the heating curve in Figure 12–9) would likely result in internal porosity of the thick ridge portions of the denture, since the temperature of the interior of the resin exceeds 100° C. On the other hand, the curing cycle indicated by curve A (Fig. 12–10) would not complete the curing in the thin portions of the denture, since the mold failed to reach 100° C.

---

*It should be remembered that the temperature rise is a function of the rate of polymer formation, or curing rate, rather than the rate of polymerization of a single polymer. Furthermore, the temperature rise is dependent on the rate of heat (calories) evolution and not necessarily upon the total heat evolved. For a given degree of polymerization, the amount (calories) of heat evolved will theoretically be the same regardless of the curing rate, but the temperature rise may be less with a slow curing rate because the heat of polymerization can dissipate to the surrounding investing media as it evolves.

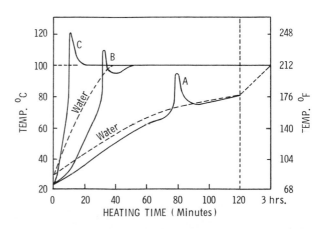

Figure 12–10 Temperature changes in acrylic resin during polymerization when cured at different rates. (Modified from Tuckfield, Worner and Guerin, Aust Dent J, March, 1943.)

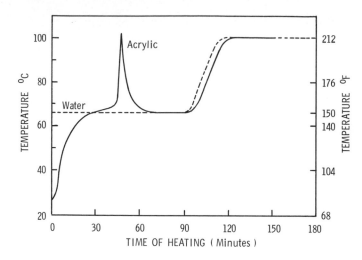

Figure 12–11 A recommended curing cycle to avoid internal porosity. (Modified from Tuckfield, Worner, and Guerin, Aust Dent J, March, 1943.)

The optimal curing cycle would, of course, depend upon the dimensions of the denture. However, it is estimated that the curing cycle shown in Figure 12–11 would result in a satisfactory cure. In this curing cycle, the denture flask is placed immediately in water at 65° C (150° F) and allowed to remain for 90 minutes to polymerize the thick areas of the dentures without causing porosity. The case is then boiled for 60 minutes to cure the thin palate areas. A more recent study, making use of smaller test specimens that are more realistic in terms of the thickness of dentures, corroborates the importance of processing initially at a maximum temperature of 70° C (160° F).[6] After most of the monomer has polymerized, the temperature can be raised to insure that the cure is complete. That investigation also stressed the temperature lag that occurs before the center of the curing denture base actually reaches the water bath temperature.

There are many variations of such a curing cycle, but the basic theory is the same. Theoretically, one should be able to polymerize the denture by curing it at 65 to 70° C (150 to 160° F) for a sufficient length of time. It has been shown that the curing time would be 48 hours to reach the same degree of polymerization throughout the denture as obtained by the 3-hour curing cycle shown in Figure 12–11.[7]

A generally accepted, long, low temperature curing cycle is one in which the denture is processed for 9 hours at 74° C (165° F), with no terminal boil.[8]

The flask should be cooled slowly from the final water bath temperature. If the flask is placed directly into tap water, warpage of the denture due to the differential thermal contraction of the resin and gypsum mold may result. Cooling overnight is ideal. However, removing the flask from the water bath, bench cooling it for 30 minutes, and then placing it in cold tap water for 15 minutes is generally satisfactory.

After deflasking and polishing, the denture is stored in water until it is delivered to the patient.

CHEMICALLY ACTIVATED DENTURE BASE ACRYLIC RESINS

Chemistry   Instead of using heat to activate the benzoyl peroxide, a chemical activator can be employed, so that the polymerization can be completed at room temperature. For example, a small amount of tertiary amine such as dimethyl-p-toluidine [$CH_3C_6H_4N(CH_3)_2$] can be added to the monomer before the monomer and polymer are mixed, as described for the heat-curing resins. After mixing, free radicals are formed from the benzoyl peroxide by a reaction with the dimethyl-p-toluidine, and the polymerization reaction proceeds as previously described.

These resins, first used for dental purposes in Germany during World War II, are known variously as "self-curing," "cold cure," or "autopolymer" resins, to distinguish them from the resins polymerized when heat is employed for activation. It should be noted that the fundamental difference between the two types of resins is the method of the activation of the benzoyl peroxide. As a general rule, not as great a degree of polymerization can be attained with a chemical activator as when the activation is effected by heat.

There are many systems other than the use of dimethyl-p-toluidine by which the room temperature polymerization can be effected, but the use of an amine of some nature is probably most common.

The type and concentration of both the activator and initiator influence the rate and degree of polymerization. There appears to be a maximal useful concentration of the amine at approximately 0.75 per cent; the maximal concentration for the peroxide is 2.0 per cent.[9] As with the heat-curing resins, the rate of polymerization is influenced by the particle size of the polymer. The smaller the particle size, the more rapid is the polymerization.

The color stability of the self-curing resins is apt to be inferior to that of the heat-curing type because of the subsequent oxidation of the tertiary amine. The condition can be minimized by the addition of certain stabilizing agents to prevent such oxidation, or the polymerization may be consummated by the use of a more stable activator, as will be discussed in Chapter 14.

Technical Considerations   The technique employed for the processing of the self-curing denture resins by compression molding is essentially the same as that previously described for the heat-curing resins. The same procedure is used in the mixing of the monomer and polymer. The same precautions should be observed in the preparation of the mold.

The monomer-polymer reactions, in the case of the self-curing resins, are likely to be complicated by a polymerization reaction that may begin before the dough stage is reached. The working time for the self-curing resins is invariably shorter than for the heat-curing materials. A lengthy initiation period before the polymerization begins is desirable so that there will be plenty of time for the trial closures. The production of a flash during the processing of this type of resin is apt to cause an increase of the vertical dimension of the denture, as described for the heat-curing resins. It should be noted that insofar as the importance of the proper filling of the mold is concerned, the technical considerations for the 2 types of resins are identical.

One method to prolong the initiation period is to decrease the temperature of the mixing jar. Such a procedure would delay the solution of the polymer in the monomer, and would prolong the dough-forming time. The material will, in most instances, remain in the dough form longer, and the working time will be increased. There are many methods by which the initiation period can be prolonged by chemical means. Unfortunately, the resin is likely to exhibit inferior strength properties if its initiation period is too prolonged by such methods. At best, the transverse strength will be approximately 80 per cent of that for the heat-cured resins. In any event, if the resin meets the requirements of the American Dental Association Specification no. 12, the dough will be workable for at least 5 minutes.

In the case of the self-curing resins with the minimal working time, it is doubtful that more than two trial closures can be made. Considerable care must be taken to insure that the proper amount of resin is employed, so that only the minimal number of trial closures will be necessary. The injection technique could be used to considerable advantage in the processing of self-curing denture bases, since no trial closure is needed in this instance, and the operation can be completed well within the 5-minute period.

Time and Temperature of Processing   It is very likely that the curing of these denture resins at room temperature aids in eliminating many of the processing stresses introduced during heat-curing, with the result that the denture may fit better and be more stable dimensionally.

The time to be allowed for the curing before the denture is removed from the flask will vary with different materials. Undoubtedly, the initial hardening of the material will occur within 20 to 30 minutes after the final closure of the flask, but it is doubtful that the polymerization will be complete.

Polymerization may actually continue for several hours.[6] A better dimensional stability of the denture base will be insured if the flask is held under pressure for 2 to 3 hours, or overnight. As previously mentioned, the polymerization of the self-curing resins is never as complete as that of the heat-curing type; 3 to 5 per cent of the self-curing resin is composed of free monomer, in comparison to approximately 0.2 to 0.5 per cent free monomer that may be found in a resin processed in boiling water. Consequently, it is most important that the polymerization reaction of the self-curing resins be as complete as possible before the pressure on the flasked denture is released. Otherwise, a subsequent warpage of the denture may occur in service.

The exothermic temperature change of a sphere of self-curing resin approximately 5 cm (2 inches) in diameter is shown in Figure 12–12. The curve is very similar to that shown in Figure 12–9, except that the temperature at the time of activation is that of the room. As in the case of the

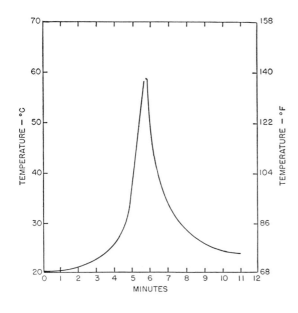

Figure 12–12 Temperature change of a self-curing denture resin during polymerization.

heat-curing resins, the temperature of the bulky portions will be higher at their centers than at their surfaces because of the poor thermal conductivity of the resin. It is to be expected, therefore, that the thinner portions of the denture will be less polymerized and, therefore, will be weaker than the thick portions. Only in a bulk not likely to occur in denture bases will the exothermic heat be sufficient to cause the monomer to boil; consequently, no porosity due to boiling monomer is to be expected in the processing of a denture with the self-curing resins.

Fluid Resin Technique

Innovative among the chemically activated systems are those known commercially as *pour-type* or *fluid* resins. The polymer powders formulated for this technique usually have a very fine particle size. They also have a high percentage of high molecular weight polymer as an aid to prevent an undue increase in viscosity during the mixing and pouring stages.

The fluid resin technique has now been in use for over 20 years. In the original technique the denture wax-up, sealed to the case, was positioned in a specially designed flask, such as the one shown in Figure 12–2B. The flask was then filled with a reversible hydrocolloid investment medium rather than conventional gypsum products. After gelation of the hydrocolloid, the cast with the attached wax-up was removed. Vents and sprues were cut from the outside of the flask into the mold space. After the wax and base plate were eliminated, the teeth and the cast (coated with a mold protecting medium) were replaced in the vented flask.

The fluid resin was mixed and then poured into the mold via the sprue openings. The filled flask was held in a pressurized chamber at room temperature until the resin hardened.

Advantages claimed for the fluid resin technique include better tissue fit, fewer open bites, less fracture of porcelain teeth during deflasking operations, reduced material costs, and simplification of the laboratory procedure for flasking, deflasking, and finishing of the denture.[10, 11]

However, there were some disadvantages reported:[2, 12] (1) air inclusions (bubbles), (2) shifting of the teeth during processing, (3) infraocclusion (closed bites), (4) occlusal imbalances not attributable to shifting of the teeth, (5) incomplete flow of the denture base material over the necks of anterior teeth, (6) formation of films of denture base material over cervical portions of plastic teeth that had not been previously covered with wax, (7) poor bonding to plastic teeth, and (8) technique sensitivity.

Subsequent approaches directed toward avoiding these problems have made use of improved spruing, centrifuging of the resin into the mold, more rigid hydrocolloid mold materials, modified gypsum molds to provide for improved retention of the teeth in their mold sockets, grinding of ridgelap surfaces on the teeth, more careful manufacturing practices in formulating the liquid, and greater time devoted to the supervision and training of technical personnel.[13, 14]

In general, these types of resins have somewhat lower mechanical properties than the conventional heat-cured resins.[15] This particular study also noted the sensitivity of the technique to laboratory variables. For example, the rheological properties of six commercial fluid denture resins were determined.[16] All showed initial non-newtonian flow behavior and increased viscosity with time. Thus early introduction of the resin into the mold is necessary to help in minimizing voids and loss of fine detail in the denture.

The current state of the art appears to indicate that clinically acceptable dentures can be obtained when using any of the fluid resin techniques, provided that proper precautions are exercised to avoid problems known to be inherent with the use of all of the materials and equipment involved.

References

1. Kapur KK and Somarn SD: Masticatory performance and efficiency in denture wearers. J Prosthet Dent 14:687, 1964.
2. Woelfel JB: Newer materials and techniques in prosthetic resin materials. Dent Clin North Am 15:67, 1971.
3. Rudd KD: Processing complete dentures without tooth movement. Dent Clin North Am Nov., 1964, p. 675.
4. Peyton FA and Anthony DH: Evaluation of dentures processed by different technics. J Prosthet Dent 13:269, 1963.
5. Tuckfield WJ, Worner HK, and Guerin BD: Acrylic resins in dentistry, Part II. Aust Dent J 47:172, 1943.
6. Faraj SAA and Ellis B: The effect of processing temperatures on the exotherm, porosity and properties of acrylic denture base. Br Dent J 147:209, 1979.
7. Smith DC: The acrylic denture base. Br Dent J 105:86, 1958.
8. Weaver RG and Ryge G: Advancements in processing techniques. J Ala Dent Assoc 53:22, 1969.
9. Rose EE, Lal J, and Green R: Effects of peroxide, amine and hydroquinone in varying concentrations on the polymerization rate of polymethyl methacrylate slurries. J Am Dent Assoc 56:375, 1958.
10. Winkler S: Pour technique for denture base processing. Dent Dig 73:200, 1967.
11. Shepard WL: Denture bases processed from a fluid resin. J Prosthet Dent 19:561, 1968.
12. Council on Dental Materials and Devices: Guide to Dental Materials and Devices. 8th ed., American Dental Association, Chicago, 1976, pp. 150–151.
13. Winkler S: Construction of denture bases from pour resins. Dent Clin North Am 19:243, 1975.
14. Civjan S, Huget EF, and deSimon LB: Modification of the fluid resin technique. J Am Dent Assoc 85:109, 1972.
15. Bates JF, Stanford GD, Huggett R, and Handley RW: Current status of pour type denture base resins. J Dent 5:177, 1977.
16. Vermilyea SG, Powers JM, and Koran A: The rheological properties of fluid denture-base resins. J Dent Res 57:227, 1978.

13 DENTURE BASE RESINS: TECHNICAL CONSIDERATIONS (CONTINUED). MISCELLANEOUS RESINS AND TECHNIQUES

When a resin is employed in a situation requiring dimensional precision, one of the properties given first consideration is its stability. As noted in the previous chapter, the fit of the denture in the mouth of the patient is of prime consideration. Consequently, any change in the dimension of the denture base, either during its processing or during its function in the mouth, is of considerable importance. Since the acrylic resins exhibit certain unavoidable dimensional changes, the dentist should appreciate these limitations so that he will not expect the impossible. Also, he should understand the variables that can minimize inaccuracy of fit and subsequent distortion.

Curing Shrinkage   When methyl methacrylate monomer is polymerized, the density changes from 0.94 gm/cm³ to 1.19 gm/cm³. This change in density results in a volumetric shrinkage of 21 per cent, usually called the *polymerization shrinkage*. When a conventional heat curing powder–liquid acrylic resin, as described in Chapter 12, is mixed at a P/L weight ratio of 2 to 1, there is an approximate true ratio of 1 part liquid to 1.6 parts of powder by volume. More than one third of the dough will be liquid. Consequently, the calculated volumetric shrinkage should be about 8 per cent.

There may be several reasons why materials having such a high volumetric shrinkage can be used to produce clinically satisfactory dentures. Behavior of these denture base resins over the years seems to indicate that the shrinkage will be distributed uniformly over all surfaces of the denture so that fit of the denture to the tissues is not seriously affected, provided the materials are handled properly.

The volumetric shrinkage, due to polymerization contraction, probably contributes very little to the linear shrinkage that has been observed with all of the resins used for denture bases. Linear shrinkage values are obtained by measuring the distance between reference points marked on the occlusal surface of the two second molar teeth in a denture waxup, or the distance between similar points marked on ridge crests of the cast. Then after removal of the cast, a comparable measurement is made on the cured denture. The negative difference between the pre- and post-cure measurements is recorded as the linear shrinkage. The greater the linear shrinkage, the greater is the discrepancy usually observed in the initial fit of the denture.

On the basis of probable volumetric shrinkage noted above, it can be calculated that an acrylic resin denture base should shrink linearly more than 2 per cent. However, such a shrinkage does not actually occur. All factors considered, it appears that thermal shrinkage of the resin is the chief contributor to the linear shrinkage phenomenon. As the denture base begins to cool after the cure, the resin remains soft while it is near the curing temperature, and the pressure inside the mold causes it to contract at approximately the same rate as the cast.

Then, as the soft resin approaches the glass transition temperature during cooling, its rigidity increases. Below the transition temperature it can be assumed that the denture will contract independently of the cast. Since the polymerizing shrinkage is likely to be complete at this stage, the shrinkage occurring below the transition temperature can be assumed to be thermal and will vary according to the composition of the resin.

As a specific example, let it be assumed that the transition temperature of a denture resin is 75° C (167° F). If the resin denture is cooled in the flask to a room temperature of 20° C (68° F), the thermal contraction can be calculated.[1] The generally accepted value for the linear coefficient of expansion of poly(methyl methacrylate) is $81 \times 10^{-6}/°C$. Consequently,

$$(75-20)\ 81 \times 10^{-6} = 0.0044 \text{ mm/mm} = 0.44 \text{ per cent}$$

This value is in general agreement with the linear shrinkages of from 0.2 to 0.5 per cent reported for various commercial denture base materials.

A curing shrinkage in a maxillary denture is often evidenced by a discrepancy in the palate region as shown in Figure 13–1. Presumably, during cooling, the resin shrinks toward the areas of the greatest bulk, which in this case are the ridge portions of the denture base. Such a shrinkage causes a tensile stress to occur in the thinner palate region. When this stress is relieved in upper dentures, the resin is pulled away from the palate, and with both upper and lower dentures the posterior teeth on opposite sides of the arch are pulled closer together. This accounts for the linear shrinkage phenomenon.

It is interesting to note that when the denture was constructed with a self-curing denture resin, in which during processing the thermal or "curing shrinkage" was negligible, the fit was superior (Fig. 13–1A) to that of the heat-cured resin (Fig. 13–1B). The processing shrinkage has been measured as 0.53 per cent for a heat-cured resin as compared to only 0.26 per cent for a self-cured resin.[2]

The greater shrinkage observed for the denture constructed from the injection resin (Fig. 13–1C) has been attributed either to the high curing temperature or the characteristic of the special resin system used. Fluid or pour resin denture bases processed in a hydrocolloid mold tend to have greater shrinkage than the self-curing resin bases processed by compression molding.[3]

A loss of vertical dimension of occlusion is generally associated with the processing of denture bases by fluid resin techniques when a hydrocolloid mold or flask is used. Generally, the opposite occurs in dentures processed from heat-cured, compression-molded resins and in fluid resin dentures when a gypsum rather than a hydrocolloid mold is used. However, the increase in vertical dimension is greater in the compression molding than in the fluid resin/gypsum mold technique.[4]

Compensation for the loss of vertical dimension could likely be made by means of adjustments in the pre-processing procedure. However, the increase in

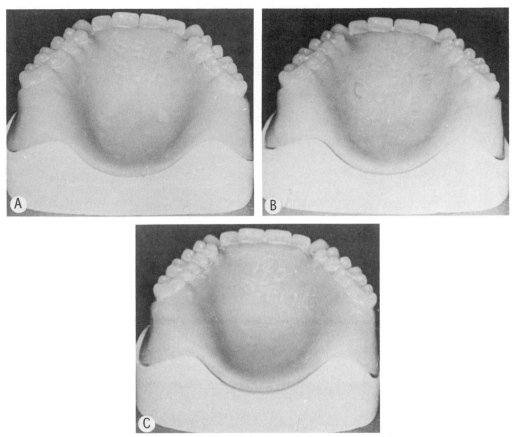

Figure 13–1 The fit of maxillary dentures constructed with *A*, a self-cured acrylic resin; *B*, a heat-cured resin; and *C*, an injection processed polystyrene resin. (From Anthony and Peyton, J Prosthet Dent, *12*:74, 1962.)

vertical dimension found with the heat-cured dentures seems to be more predictable and easier to correct following the cure.

The dimensional change occurring in dentures, fabricated from different resins, at various stages in processing is shown in Figure 13–2. All three of the heat-cured denture base materials were comparable in respect to the dimensional change that occurred during fabrication, all being somewhat inferior to the compression molded self-cured resin denture. It is important to note that the distortion occurring upon removal of the denture from the cast is much greater than any that will take place in subsequent clinical service.

Porosity   There are a number of causes of porosity that may occur during the processing of the denture base. If the porosity appears on the surface of the denture, proper cleansing will be difficult if not impossible. Also, the appearance of the denture base will be unsightly. Even though the porosity may be entirely internal, the denture base will be weakened. Furthermore, since each internal pore or bleb is an area of stress concentration, the denture may warp as the stresses relax.

It was previously noted that internal porosity may develop in the thick portion of a denture base as a result of the vaporization of the monomer or of the low molecular weight polymers, when the temperature of the resin increases above the boiling point of these phases.

This type of porosity may not occur equally throughout the section

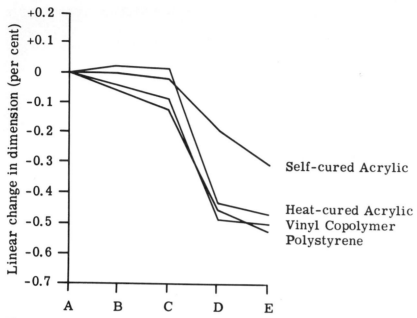

Figure 13–2 Dimensional change occurring in dentures fabricated from different resins at various stages in processing. *A*, Wax denture on gypsum cast; *B*, wax denture flasked to occlusal surfaces; *C*, cured denture unflasked down to occlusal surfaces; *D*, cured denture removed from cast; *E*, cured denture after polishing plus one day's storage in water. (From Woelfel, Paffenbarger, and Sweeney, J Am Dent Assoc, *61*:413, 1960.)

involved. For example, specimen *B* shown in Figure 13–3 exhibits a porosity only near one edge. The specimen was flasked so that the edge which is clear was nearer the metal wall of the flask. It is apparent that the metal in the flask conducted the exothermic heat away from this area with sufficient rapidity to prevent the occurrence of porosity. For this reason, the thick lingual posterior area of the lower denture base, for example, is more likely to exhibit porosity than is the buccal portion, because the latter is generally nearer the metal flask.

A second cause of porosity in an acrylic denture base is a lack of

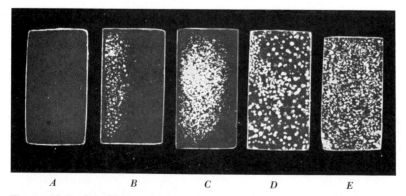

Figure 13–3 Specimens of heat-cured denture base resins showing different types and degrees of porosity. *A*, Properly cured, no porosity. *B* and *C*, Too rapid rate of heating. No porosity at the surface since heat of polymerization was conducted to investing medium in this area. *D*, Insufficient mixing of monomer and polymer. *E*, Insufficient pressure during curing. (From Tuckfield, Worner, and Guerin, Aust Dent J, March, 1943.)

homogeneity in the dough or gel at the time of the polymerization. It may be difficult, or even impossible, to obtain complete homogeneity in powder-liquid dough masses making use of the procedures usually available in a dental laboratory. It is probable then that some regions will contain more monomer than others. These regions will shrink more during polymerization than the adjacent regions, and such a localized shrinkage will tend to produce voids (Figure 13–3*D*).

The occurrence of such a type of porosity can be minimized by insuring that the greatest possible homogeneity of the resin is attained. Use of proper P/L ratios and the most favorable mixing procedures will aid in this connection. Furthermore, since the material is more homogeneous when in the dough stage as compared to the tacky stage, it is generally safer to delay packing the resin until the dough stage is reached.

In summary, the gel homogeneity is, therefore, primarily related to the dough-forming time. This factor can be controlled by the composition and molecular weight of the polymer beads. As previously explained, some of the newer resins can be mixed with monomer to such fluidity that they can be poured into the denture mold and the processing begun immediately after test packing. In such a case, a minimal dough-forming time probably is provided so that sufficient homogeneity is insured before the processing begins.

In evaluating the information and photographs in Figure 13–3 it should be understood that porosities of all the types shown can occur on the surfaces of dentures as well as in the internal parts. Furthermore, porosities resulting from heating the mold too rapidly (Fig. 13–3*B,C*) can be much larger than those shown in the photograph.

A third type of porosity, exemplified by specimen *E*, is caused by a lack of adequate pressure during the polymerization, or by a definite lack of dough or gel in the mold at the time of the final closure. The bubbles are not spherical. This type of porosity as well as the preceding type may be in such abundance as to cause the resin to appear white. A pigmented resin may appear lighter in color for this reason.

The surface and subsurface porosities occurring with the fluid and other self-curing resins appear to be caused by failure to expel air inclusions incorporated during mixing or pouring of the resin. Careful mixing, improved spruing and venting, centrifuging, and curing pressure increases seem to help reduce the incidence of such air inclusions. It has been shown that adequate density can be obtained for the self-curing relining resins when they are processed at room temperature under an air pressure of .07 MPa (10 psi). However, instructions for most of the fluid resins now recommend the use of higher temperatures and, therefore, higher pressures in order to obtain dentures having increased hardness and better reproduction of fine details of cast surfaces.[5]

Water Absorption   Poly(methyl methacrylate) absorbs water slowly over a period of time. The absorption is undoubtedly due primarily to the polar properties of the resin molecules. However, it has been shown that the mechanism is by diffusion of the water molecules according to the laws of diffusion. The diffusion coefficient *(D)* of a typical heat-cured denture acrylic resin is 1.08×10^{-12} m²/sec at 37° C (99° F). When the temperature drops to 23° C (73° F), *D* is reduced by one-half. For a self-curing acrylic resin, *D* is 2.34×10^{-12} m²/sec.[6]

The diffusion presumably occurs between the macromolecules, which are forced slightly apart. In this respect, the action of the water is not unlike that of a plasticizer. As can be deduced from the low values for D, the amount of water involved is very small even at saturation, which probably is determined in part by the number of polar groups. In spite of this fact, it has been estimated that for each 1 per cent increase in the weight of the water absorbed, the acrylic resin expands linearly 0.23 per cent.[7]

As might be concluded from the low values for the diffusion coefficient, the time required to reach saturation may be considerable. It depends, of course, on the thickness of the dental appliance. It has been calculated that a typical acrylic resin denture may require a period of almost 17 days to become fully saturated with water when immersed in water at room temperature.[6]

Because the macromolecules are forced apart by the diffusion of the water, they are rendered more mobile, with the result that inherent stresses can be relieved with a consequent relaxation and possible change in the shape of the denture. It has been shown that the increase in dimension by water absorption of stress-free acrylic resin strips is, for all practical purposes, equal to the curing shrinkage.[1] Similar measurements of acrylic resin dentures indicate that such a swelling may be less than the curing shrinkage because of the stress relaxation. When the acrylic resin is allowed to dry or desorb, the entire process is reversed quantitatively, provided the resin is stress free.

One method for the measurement of the water *sorption* is to determine the increase in weight of the resin per unit of surface area exposed to the water. Such a method is specified in the American Dental Association Specification no. 12. A disk of material with specified dimensions is prepared. The disk is first dried to constant weight, and then it is stored in water for seven days. According to the specification, the gain in weight by the resin during this treatment must not be greater than 0.8 mg/cm². There is no apparent difference between the heat-cured or the self-curing resins in this regard. The net result of the processing contraction, and the subsequent expansion due to water sorption, is that after several months in the patient's mouth the compression molded heat-cured acrylic resin denture will be very slightly undersize, molar to molar, whereas the compression molded self-curing acrylic resin denture will be very slightly oversize, molar to molar.[8]

Solubility   Although the denture base resins are soluble in many solvents, they are virtually insoluble in most fluids with which they will come in contact in the oral cavity.

When the disk employed for the determination of the water sorption, as described in the preceding section, is dried out the second time, any loss of weight observed would presumably be a measure of its solubility in the water during the test. According to the American Dental Association Specification no. 12, such a loss in weight must not be greater than 0.04 mg/cm² of surface. Such a loss is negligible from a clinical standpoint.

Processing Stresses   It is axiomatic that whenever a natural dimensional change is inhibited, the structure involved will be stressed, with the result that a distortion or warpage may subsequently occur if such stresses are relaxed. The dental acrylic resins are no exception to this rule, since stresses are invariably induced during processing.

For example, during the polymerization shrinkage, it is possible that the friction between the mold walls and the soft resin may inhibit the normal shrinkage of the resin. Since the resin is actually stretched by this inhibition, the resulting stresses are tensile in character.

Although the majority of these stresses can be relieved above the glass transition temperature while the resin is soft, it can be assumed that some of them will persist below the transition temperature. As a result, the thermal contraction, or curing shrinkage, seemingly will be reduced.

Other factors that enter into processing stresses are differences in the thickness of the denture in various areas, localized polymerization shrinkage such as around porcelain teeth, and water sorption, as just described.

Many processing techniques and denture resin formulas have been invented in an attempt to eliminate, or at least to minimize, such processing stresses and the resulting distortions, but the beneficial results claimed seldom materialize to an extent worthy of consideration. As a matter of fact, the distortions are quite small.[9] The total dimensional change that occurs in a typical resin denture during processing and in service is in the range of only 0.1 to 0.2 mm. It is doubtful that dimensional changes of that magnitude would be noted by the patient. It is not likely that dimensional stability of the denture base itself accounts for ill-fitting dentures. However, a gradual deterioration both in fit and efficacy of function is common. Probably this is the result of changes in the supporting tissues, not the resin. Such may not be the case, however, when the hard tissues of teeth are involved, as described in the next chapter.

Crazing   Although the warpage that may occur during the relaxation of processing stresses in dentures may not be of clinical importance, relaxation of surface stresses may result in the formation of cracks, or *crazing*, which may deleteriously affect the denture.

Crazing of the resin consists of the formation of small cracks, which may vary in size from microscopic dimensions to a size that is readily visible to the unaided eye. In some instances, the crazing in a clear resin is evidenced by a hazy or foggy appearance rather than by individual cracks. In any event, whenever such a crazing occurs, it has a weakening effect on the resin and reduces the esthetic qualities of the denture. Cracks formed on crazing may indicate the beginning of a fracture.

Crazing may occur under mechanical stress, or as the result of an attack by a solvent. The crazing appears to occur in poly(methyl methacrylate) only when a tensile stress is present. The cracks appear at right angles to the direction of the tensile stress. The modern concept is that crazing is an actual mechanical separation of the polymer chains or groups of chains under tensile stress.

Crazing usually starts on the surface in a region in which the polymer molecules are oriented at right angles to the direction of the applied tensile stress. It then gradually penetrates inward. Such a type of crazing is visible around the porcelain teeth in the denture shown in Figure 13–4. The tensile stress was probably induced by the contraction of the resin around the tooth during the cooling of the denture, after it had been processed under heat. The cracks became evident only after limited water immersion and may be the result of stress relaxation brought about by the water absorption.

Although crazing by solvent action also indicates the presence of surface stresses, the cracks are more randomly oriented than those shown in Figure 13–4. The crazing can appear in the presence of even weak solvents, such as alcohol. Cross-linking of the resin reduces that fault considerably.

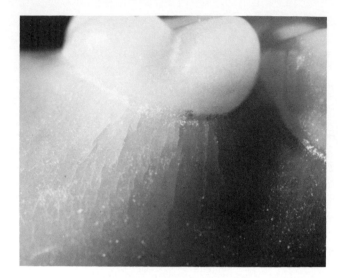

Figure 13–4 Crazing around porcelain teeth.

PHYSICAL PROPERTIES OF DENTURE RESINS

Strength   The strength of the acrylic resin denture base materials may fluctuate considerably, depending on the composition of the resin, the technique of processing, and the subsequent environment of the denture. The stress properties of the resin are generally measured by means of a transverse test, as described in the American Dental Association Specification no. 12. The specimen is subjected to a transverse loading at a specified rate. A typical load-deflection curve is shown in Figure 13–5. The requirement in Specification no. 12 stipulates certain maximal deflections in the center of the specimens between various load ranges. Thus, in actuality, the test evaluates a combina-

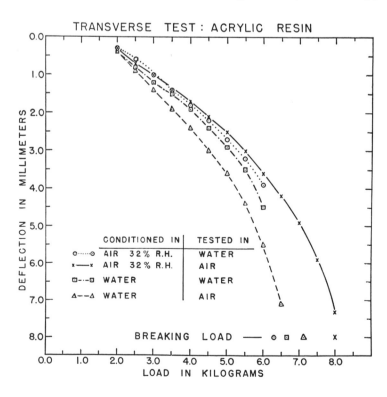

TRANSVERSE TEST : ACRYLIC RESIN

CONDITIONED IN	TESTED IN
o·····o AIR 32% R.H.	WATER
x——x AIR 32% R.H.	AIR
□–·–□ WATER	WATER
△——△ WATER	AIR

BREAKING LOAD —— o □ △   x

Figure 13–5 Transverse load-deflection curve for a typical denture base acrylic resin, showing the influence of different conditioning procedures and testing environments. All specimens were conditioned for three days as indicated before testing. (From Swaney, Paffenbarger, and Caul, J Am Dent Assoc, Jan., 1953.)

tion of properties, such as tensile and compressive strength and modulus of elasticity.

The interpretation of the lack of a straight-line portion in the curve is that a plastic flow of the resin is produced during the loading in addition to an elastic deformation. When the load is released, the stresses are relaxed slowly, and the structure may never recover completely from the original deformation.

It has been repeatedly stated that the lower the degree of polymerization of a given solid polymer, the less will be its strength. In this respect, the curing cycle employed with a heat-cured resin is most important. The transverse load-deflection curves shown in Figure 13–6 indicate the progressive weakening and decrease in stiffness of the resin as the curing time is reduced, the curing temperature being held constant at 71° C (160° F).

Owing to the lower degree of polymerization attained and to the residual monomer retained, the maximal strength and stiffness of the self-curing resins are lower than that of the heat-cured type. However, the difference in elastic modulus between heat-cured and self-cured denture resins is not great, with overlapping values between the two groups. Mean flexural modulus at 37° C for a water saturated conventional heat-cured resin would be 2500 MPa (360,000 psi). For a representative group of self-cured resins this value would be nearer to 2200 MPa (320,000 psi), with considerably greater variation as influenced by the cross-linking agent used.[10]

Those resins that are formulated to provide higher impact strength (polyvinyl acrylics and rubber reinforced acrylics) do have approximately a 20 per cent lower flexural modulus than the conventional heat-cured resins.[11]

The flexural modulus will decrease as the water saturation of the resin

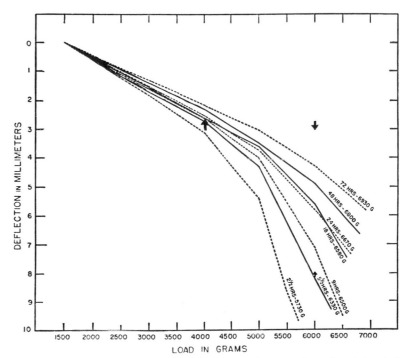

Figure 13–6 Transverse stress-strain curves for samples of poly(methyl methacrylate) cured for different periods at 71° C (160° F). Curing time and fracture load are noted on each curve. (From Harman, J Am Dent Assoc, Feb., 1949.)

and the temperature increase, the rate of decreasing modulus being especially great as the glass transition temperature is approached. The T_g of the matrix of a heat-cured resin is close to 100° C. For self-curing resins the T_g is 25 to 30 per cent less.[12] One group of four heat-cured resins had a flexural modulus change of -44 per cent between 23 and 70° C. In a group of self-curing resins, the loss in modulus was 76 per cent.[10]

However, all of the denture base materials, including the self-curing products, that appear on the American Dental Association List of Certified Dental Materials must comply with the same physical property requirements, including those for strength and stiffness. The self-cured resins used primarily for repairing denture bases are covered by American Dental Association Specification no. 13.

The strength and stiffness of the resin are reduced after the sorption of water, as can be noted from Figure 13–5. It is of further interest that its strength and stiffness are less if the resin is stressed under water than if it is stressed in air.

The properties of the resin may also be reduced by the finishing of the denture with abrasives and polishing agents. The heat from the polishing wheel, for example, may cause a warpage of the denture by a release of processing stresses. Excessive heat, incurred during polishing or abrading, may cause a partial depolymerization, with a resulting decrease in the degree of polymerization, and a decrease in strength and rigidity.

As discussed in the previous chapter, the exothermic heat evolved during the polymerization varies according to the bulk of the denture. On this basis, it can be expected that the bulkier portions of the denture may exhibit greater strength than the thinner portions. In other words, the ridge portions of an upper denture may be stronger than the palatal portions.

The stress-strain curve of an acrylic resin under tensile stress is similar to that obtained under a transverse test in that no portion of the curve is a straight line. However, if certain assumptions are made for the calculations, the approximate values for the tensile properties of the dry, heat-cured resin tested in air are: modulus of elasticity, 2350 MPa (340,000 psi); proportional limit, 27 MPa (3900 psi); and tensile strength, 52 MPa (7500 psi).[13] The self-curing resins generally exhibit tensile properties lower than those for the heat-cured resins.

The tensile strength of resin is much lower than that of alloys used for denture castings, but it seems adequate, judging by the relatively small number of dentures that fracture in service.

Creep   Denture resins are viscoelastic. When subjected to a constant load so that strain can be observed as a function of time, they show primary and secondary creep following the initial instantaneous elastic strain. The secondary creep rate increases with increase in temperature, stress, residual monomer, plasticizers, and cross-linking agents. Although the creep rates of heat-cured and self-cured acrylic resins are very similar at low stress (9.0 MPa, 1300 psi), the creep rate for the self-curing resins increases with stress more rapidly than for the heat-cured resins.[14]

Miscellaneous Properties   The Charpy impact strength of a heat-cured acrylic resin is approximately 0.98 to 1.27 joules, whereas that for a self-curing resin is approximately 0.78 J. The impact strength for a poly-vinyl acrylic or a rubber reinforced acrylic resin can be twice that of poly(methyl methacrylate).

These energy figures are useful for comparison only, since the energy absorbed by the test specimen during rupture will depend upon such factors as specimen size and geometry, distance between specimen supports, and the presence or absence of notching of the specimen, as well as certain mechanical properties.

The Knoop hardness number of self-curing resin is approximately 16 to 18, whereas that for a resin cured under heat may be as high as 20. Such differences are of academic interest only.

The color stability of the resin is usually tested by exposure to ultraviolet light. The heat-cured resins generally exhibit good color stability. The resins cured by chemical activation are sometimes not as color stable as the former type, but this deficiency can be minimized as previously described. The whole matter of the clinical significance of in vitro color stability tests will be discussed in further detail in the next chapter.

MISCELLANEOUS RESINS AND TECHNIQUES

Repair Resins If an acrylic denture is fractured in service, it can be repaired. Essentially, the technique involves fastening the fractured parts together with wax or by other means. A stone cast is then constructed in the denture base. The denture is removed from the cast, the wax is eliminated, and the edges of the fracture are trimmed, beveled, and smoothed. A rounded joint is superior in strength to a butt joint due to lower stress concentrations.

The area of the cast underlying the fracture is coated with a mold-protecting medium to facilitate the subsequent removal of the repaired denture. The repaired sections of the denture are then reassembled on the cast and held in position with wax or modeling compound.

Although the repair with a self-cured resin invariably has a lower transverse strength than that of the original heat-cured denture base resin,[15] the autopolymerizing resins are usually preferred. The use of a heat-cured resin will tend to warp the denture during processing.

Increments of monomer and polymer are alternately added to the repair area using a small sable-hair brush. Care must be taken to avoid flooding the denture surfaces that are not directly involved in the repair. Many old dentures are subject to crazing and subsequent weakening upon contact with monomer. The fresh repair is then allowed to cure in a pressure chamber, as described for fluid resins in the previous chapter. The processed repair is finished by conventional procedures.

Since the repair can be made at room temperature, no significant warpage of the denture is to be expected. If the denture is properly constructed so that there is no undue trauma in localized areas, the strength of the self-curing repair resin is not likely to be a clinical problem.

Rebasing of Dentures Because of soft tissue changes that occur during the wearing of the denture, it is often necessary to change the tissue surface of the denture to conform to the new tissue contours and occlusal relationships. Such a readaptation of the denture can be accomplished by either *rebasing* or *relining* the denture. When a denture reliner is used, new resin of some type is added to the existing denture base as described in the next section.

In rebasing the denture, an impression of the soft tissues is obtained, using the existing denture as an impression tray. A stone cast is then constructed in the corrected denture. The denture and cast are mounted in a specially designed device which will maintain the correct vertical and horizontal relationship between the cast and the denture teeth. After the teeth are thus indexed for position, the denture is removed and the teeth are separated from the old denture base. The teeth are then reassembled in the index of the mounting device and held in their original relationship to the cast while they are waxed to the new base plate.

From this point conventional procedures are followed and a new denture base processed. In other words, a new denture is constructed using the same teeth as before.

Denture Reliners   As in the previous procedure, an impression of the soft tissues is again obtained, using the existing denture as an impression tray. A stone cast is constructed in the corrected denture, after which the cast with the attached denture is invested in a flask. When the flask halves are separated, the impression material is removed from the denture, and new acrylic resin is cured against the old by the usual compression molding technique.

A low curing temperature for the relining process is necessary in order not to distort the denture. The use of a self-curing resin is preferred in this case as well. When a self-curing resin is used for relining the denture, a special mounting, which maintains the correct vertical and horizontal relationship between the cast and the denture, may be used instead of completely flasking the denture.

However, even though the denture is flasked during the relining procedure, there is a tendency for it to warp toward the relined side because of the diffusion of the monomer from the reliner before curing, and also because of the subsequent processing shrinkage of the liner. From the standpoint of denture stability, the rebasing process is preferred to the relining technique.

Self-curing materials are available for relining resin dentures directly in the mouth. Unfortunately, some of these materials generate enough heat to injure the oral tissues. Naturally the greater the bulk of the relining material, the greater is the heat generated. All such materials which appear on the American Dental Association List of Certified Dental Materials must comply with Specification no. 17, which places limits on the rate of temperature rise and the maximum temperature generated.

Some of these materials that are made for repair as well as for relining purposes will comply with Specification no. 13 for repairs; however, they may not comply with the temperature requirements of Specification no. 17. Others that may comply with Specification no. 17 are suitable only as temporary expedients because they tend to discolor, become foul, or may even loosen from the denture base. They often contain plasticizers or solvents to increase their fluidity during seating of the denture. Low molecular weight polymers may also be used for the same reason.

Similar types of relining materials are often advertised in newspapers and sold directly for home use. Such materials are generally inferior. Their use often results in damage to the oral tissues because the users do not possess the knowledge needed to establish the occlusal and jaw relationships required for effective denture function.

Soft or Resilient Liners   The purpose of the "permanent" soft liner is to absorb some of the energy, produced by masticatory impact, that would otherwise be transmitted through the denture to the soft basal tissue. As the liner returns to its predeformed shape the absorbed energy is more slowly released. Just how rapidly the resilient liner should recover is not known, but the delay in recovery will be greater for a soft acrylic material than for a silicone rubber.[16]

The types of liners are as follows.

1. The most common type is the plasticized acrylic resin, either self-curing or heat-curing. In the self-cured material, poly(ethyl methyacrylate), poly(methyl methacrylate) or an acrylate copolymer is mixed with an aromatic ester–ethanol liquid containing 60 to 80 per cent plasticizer, such as dibutyl phthalate. The liquid does not contain an acrylic monomer and the liner that is formed is essentially a tissue conditioner and not a so-called "permanent" type of soft liner.[17]

Although the heat-cured resin may be supplied in a sheet form, usually a powder and liquid are mixed to form a dough that is cured by the conventional flasking and pressure molding technique. The liner material may be cured along with the rigid acrylic base material or used in a reline procedure.

The powder is composed of acrylic resin polymers and copolymers selected so that when mixed with the appropriate acrylic monomer and plasticizer liquid the glass transition temperature of the cured resin will be below mouth temperature.[17]

Thus, as poly(methyl methacrylate) is replaced by higher methacrylates (ethyl, n-propyl, n-butyl) with lower T_g, less plasticizer is required in the liquid to produce a T_g of lower than 35° C.

If both the polymer and the monomer are higher methacrylates, the plasticizer content can be further reduced. This should be desirable in order to minimize the undesirable leaching of the plasticizer. A liner of this kind has been described as being made from a poly(ethyl methacrylate) polymer and an n-butyl ester monomer with up to 30 per cent phthalate plasticizer in the cured material.[16]

Also, acrylic polymers with hydrophilic groups, such as poly(hydroxyethyl methacrylate), may be supplied as a gel or as a powder and monomer of hydroxyethyl methacrylate. The cured dry polymer is hard and brittle but becomes soft upon exposure to water.

2. *Vinyl resins.* The plasticized poly(vinyl chloride) and poly(vinyl acetate) resins, like the plasticized acrylic resins, lose plasticizer and harden during use.

3. *Silicone rubbers.* These materials retain their elastic properties but may lose adhesion to the denture base.

Room temperature curing chairside silicones are intended as a temporary soft liner. The composition and curing reactions for this two component material are essentially the same as those of a condensation polymerizing silicone elastomeric impression material (Chapter 10). A primer or adhesive is required for bonding to the hard acrylic or vinyl denture base, which must be relieved and cleaned before application of the primer and the mixed silicone.

Heat-cured silicones are also available. These are generally one-component systems supplied as a paste or gel containing an oxygen catalyst, which is heat polymerized against an acrylic resin dough in the compression molding technique. The silicone gel can also be injected against the acrylic resin prior to heating of the flask.

For adhesion between silicone and denture base a rubber–poly(methyl methacrylate) graft polymer solution cement may be used. One of these heat-cured gels does not require an additional adhesive when cured in conjunction with the acrylic denture base. It is a copolymer of silicone and a second polymer that achieves adhesion to the acrylic resin.[18] A silicone polymer in a volatile solvent is also used as an adhesive, the solvent providing bonding to the acrylic or vinyl resin, and the silicone polymer to the silicone liner.[16]

When an adhesive coupling agent is used on clean cured acrylic, the heat-cured silicone gel can be processed against the adhesive-covered acrylic polymer as well as against the uncured acrylic dough.

There are a number of problems associated with all of these liners; for example, inadequate bonding to the denture base, especially for the silicone liners. The high rate of water diffusion through the silicone as compared to the diffusion rate through acrylic may be partially responsible for loss of adhesion.

Some, but not all, silicone liners also undergo a high volume change (up to ± 40 per cent) with gain and loss of water. The hydrophilic acrylics behave similarly.

The heat-cured soft acrylics bond well to the hard denture base but lose their softness as plasticizer is leached from the liner. The considerable difference in hardening rate for these acrylic liners may be associated with the manner in which a low T_g is achieved. A polymer that in itself has a lower T_g would require less plasticizer and should therefore retain softness for a longer period of time.

The apparent softness of the liner depends upon its thickness as well as its hardness and elastic modulus. A liner thickness of 2 to 3 mm is generally recommended. A further increase in thickness would have less effect in increasing apparent softness. For many dentures this is physically impossible.

The soft liner decreases the denture base strength of a heat-cured resin, not only because of reduction in base thickness but also by solvent action of the silicone adhesive and the soft acrylic monomer. Loss in the base strength can result in fracture in clinical service.

Trimming, cutting, adjusting, and polishing of a soft liner are difficult. The silicone surface, in comparison to that of a hard acrylic resin, is abrasive and irritating to the oral mucosa.[19]

The "permanent" soft liner, as well as the tissue conditioner, often has a characteristic and disagreeable taste and odor. Perhaps the greatest disadvantage of the soft liner is that it fouls more readily than the hard denture base resin, and it cannot be cleaned as effectively.[20] Both the oxygenating and hypochlorite type of denture cleaners will damage soft liners, especially the silicone type.

Although the silicone liner itself does not support mycotic growth, debris that accumulates in pores in the liner does. The most common fungal growth is *Candida albicans*. Immersion in a fungicidal solution for 20 minutes each day can help control the growth, which in one report was occurring on 81 per cent of the silicone liners.[20]

One of the room temperature curing silicone liners is supplied as a three-component system, one of the components being a dibutyltin dilaurate catalyst which will inhibit the growth of *C. albicans*. This growth-inhibiting activity undergoes exponential decay as the tin compound is washed from the liner. However, it has not been determined whether the growth inhibiting effect will persist throughout the life of the liner as testing was done in vitro.[21]

Mechanical cleaning of the soft liner can easily lead to damage but is often necessary. A soft brush and detergent should be used.

Thus, it can be seen that none of the soft denture reliners can be considered entirely satisfactory. Few of the materials will remain soft indefinitely, although some of them harden more slowly than others. Also, all of them stain with use and are difficult to clean. It must be concluded that at the present time these materials should be used only as a temporary expedient and not for an extended period.

Tissue Conditioners Tissue conditioners or temporary soft reliners are materials whose useful function is very short, generally a matter of a few days. Under certain conditions of health debilitation or ill-fitting dentures, oral tissues may become inflamed and distorted. Relining the ill-fitting denture with a tissue conditioner allows the tissue to return to "normal," at which time a new denture can be made.

These tissue conditioners are primarily highly plasticized acrylic resins. They are supplied as a powder and a liquid. The composition of the powdered polymer is generally a poly(ethyl methacrylate) or one of its copolymers, while the liquid is an aromatic ester (butyl phthalate butyl glycolate) in ethanol or an alcohol of high molecular weight.

These are mixed together to form a gel. As with other relining procedures, the denture base is relieved on the tissue surface and the dough or gel inserted. When the denture is placed in the mouth, the gel flows readily to fill the space between the denture base and the oral tissue.

The tissue conditioners, like the "permanent" resilient liners, can absorb energy elastically; however, unlike permanent resilient materials, the tissue conditioners also undergo viscous flow under load. Thus, they change their form with the changing contour of the supporting tissue so that good adaptation of the denture to the tissue is maintained. It also has been stated that the conditioner can massage the underlying tissue and stimulate blood circulation.

As tissue conditioners age they lose their plastic properties, and the elastic characteristic becomes dominant. When this occurs, if the problem has not been corrected, it may be necessary to replace the old tissue conditioner with new material. Some individuals may use the denture with the tissue conditioner as an impression from which a gypsum model is obtained for construction of the new denture.

Since the most important characteristics of the tissue conditioners are their rheological properties, research has been done to characterize their behavior in the oral cavity. The initial mix is a free-flowing liquid which requires 15 or 20 minutes to develop plastic properties (form a strain rate sensitive gel). The formation of elastic characteristics varies with different products, ranging from several hours to several days. In the end, the elastic properties are lost when the alcohol and plasticizer are leached from the resin.[22]

Resin Impression Trays Resin impression trays are constructed on stone casts prepared from mouth impressions. Base plate wax, or another suitable spacer material, approximately 2 mm thick, is spread over the surface of the cast and trimmed to the area to be covered by the impression.

A self-curing resin dough is formed by mixing the inorganically filled polymer and the monomer. The dough is flattened to a sheet approximately 2 mm in thickness. The sheet is then laid over the spacer and trimmed to the same dimensions. When the resin is cured and separated from the spacer, the tray will contain sufficient space for the impression material.

Such a tray offers a decided advantage for some impression materials, e.g., rubber or ZOE, in that a uniform thickness of the material over the entire tissue surface is ensured.

It should be noted that such custom-made acrylic trays may not be dimensionally stable until 20 to 24 hours after fabrication.[23] Thus it may not be prudent to use the tray before that time.

Denture Cleansers   A wide variety of agents are used by patients for cleaning artificial dentures. In approximate order of preference, they include dentifrices, proprietary denture cleansers, soap and water, salt and soda, household cleansers, bleaches, and vinegar. Either immersion in the agent or, more generally, brushing of the denture with the cleanser is employed.

The most common commercial denture cleansers are the immersion type and are usually marketed as a powder or tablet. Their composition includes alkaline compounds, detergents, flavoring agents, and sodium perborate. When the powder is dissolved in water, the perborate decomposes to form an alkaline peroxide solution, which in turn decomposes to liberate oxygen. The oxygen bubbles supposedly then act mechanically to loosen the debris.

The household bleaches (hypochlorites) also effectively remove certain types of stains. They do not influence the color of the denture. However, because of their effect on the metal, hypochlorites should not be employed with any base metal appliance. Also, certain of the soft relining materials, particularly the silicone variety, may be bleached by such chemicals.

The influence of abrasive agents on acrylic resin has been investigated. The toothbrush itself has little effect on the surface of the resin. Salt, soda, soap, and most commercial dentifrices are not harmful. However, household cleansers are definitely contraindicated. Prolonged use of such agents may affect the fit of the denture and the rough surface produced makes the maintenance of a clean surface most difficult. The patient should be warned accordingly.

Allergic Reactions   Possible toxic or allergic reactions to poly(methyl methacrylate) have long been postulated. Theoretically, chemical irritation could occur from either the polymer, the residual monomer, the benzoyl peroxide, the hydroquinone, the pigment or a reaction product between some component of the denture base and its environment. One such product is formaldehyde, which can form in several ways. Self-cured dough and pour-type resins release more formaldehyde than do heat-cured acrylics.[24] Also, increasing the polymer/monomer ratio will reduce formaldehyde release from self-curing resin. All of these ingredients have been subjected to biological evaluation.

It is probable that true allergic reactions to acrylic resins are seldom seen in the oral cavity. The residual monomer, approximately 0.5 per cent in a well processed denture, is the usual component singled out as an irritant. If the monomer content in the denture is measured after storage in water, it is found that the free monomer at the surface of the denture is leached out within 17 hours.[25] The remainder of the monomer is not readily extracted. Even if some of it were made available under continued stressing of the denture, the evidence suggests that it would wash away rapidly.

Thus, if residual monomer were a cause of a denture-sore mouth, its effect might be expected to appear comparatively rapidly, but the majority of clinical cases reporting irritation under the denture occur months, or even years, after insertion. Careful clinical evaluation of large numbers of so-called allergies to acrylic resins shows that the causative factor is either unhygienic conditions under the denture or an ill-fitting denture that is traumatizing the tissue.[26] A true allergy to acrylic resin can be recognized by a patch test.

A somewhat different biological effect from the monomer may occasionally be observed in dentistry. Direct contact of the monomer over a continuing period of time may provoke a dermatitis. Such a situation may occur in certain laboratory procedures, for example. Because of this possibility, the dentist or dental technician should refrain from handling the acrylic resin dough with the hands. The high concentration of monomer in the dough may produce a local irritation and even a serious sensitization of the fingers. Use of the monomer should be restricted to well ventilated areas to avoid possible toxic reaction due to inhalation of monomer vapor.

Toxicology   There is no indication that these dental resins could produce any systemic effect upon the patient. The quantity of methyl methacrylate monomer that might enter the circulation by passing through the oral mucosa would be extremely low. The half-life of methyl methacrylate in blood at 37° C is said to range between 20 and 40 minutes, clearance being by hydrolysis to methacrylic acid.[27]

Resin Teeth   It is estimated that at least 60 per cent of the preformed artificial teeth sold in the United States are made of acrylic or vinyl–acrylic resins. Tooth colored powder–liquid acrylic resins are also available for constructing custom tooth replacements.

The composition of resin teeth is essentially poly(methyl methacrylate) copolymerized with a cross-linking agent as described for denture resins. Usually a greater amount of the cross-linking agent is employed in resin teeth in order to reduce the tendency of the teeth to craze upon contact with the monomer-polymer dough during construction of the denture. The gingival ridge-lap area may not be as highly cross-linked as the incisal in order to facilitate chemical bonding to the denture base. Various pigments are utilized to produce a natural esthetic appearance. Recently, a microfilled urethane dimethacrylate resin tooth has been developed which is stated to have an improved resistance to abrasion.[28]

Chemical union between the acrylic resin teeth and heat-cured denture base resins can be easily obtained.[29] Also, an increased bond strength may be produced by removing the glossy surface of the ridge-lap through judicious grinding.[30] It should be noted that bond failures may occur if the ridge-lap area is contaminated with residual wax or by careless application of tin-foil substitutes. It is extremely important that the mold be flushed thoroughly with a detergent solution in order to obtain complete wax elimination.

The use of mechanical retention has been the primary means of securing resin teeth in cold-curing denture base acrylic resins. However, bond strengths similar to those obtained with heat-curing resins have resulted when a solution of equal parts by volume of methylene chloride and self-curing methyl methacrylate monomer is applied to the necks of the teeth for 4 to 5 minutes. This solution combines a solvent attack on the teeth with polymerization bonding.[31] The excess material must be removed from the teeth prior to packing in order to prevent porosity in the denture base material. Coating the teeth only with cold-curing monomer fails to produce the minimal bond strength required by the American Dental Association specification.

A discussion of resin teeth is not complete without a comparison with porcelain teeth, a summary of which is presented in Table 13–1. The resin teeth possess certain advantages over porcelain teeth in esthetic qualities, higher impact strength, and greater resistance to thermal shock. Acrylic anterior teeth can be ground and reshaped to look more natural. On the other hand, resin teeth possess a lower modulus of elasticity, lower resistance to cold flow, and a tendency for dimensional change through water sorption. Also, their low abrasion resistance is particularly evident when they are placed in occlusion against enamel or porcelain.

During the setting of the teeth in wax on the base plate, it is customary to smooth the wax with a flame. This should be done cautiously in the presence of resin teeth, since the surfaces may be melted or burned. The resultant surface stresses induced during cooling may contribute to crazing in service.

The selection between resin or porcelain teeth is dependent on the clinical situation. Resin teeth should be chosen to oppose gold occlusal surfaces or natural teeth, where there is diminished interocclusal distance, or when poor ridge support exists.[32] Porcelain teeth may be used when both maxillary and mandibular dentures are constructed for patients with good ridge conditions and interarch space.

Materials in Maxillofacial Prosthetics   The use of prosthetics for maxillofacial defects can be traced to ancient civilization. Egyptian mummies show artificial eyes, ears, and noses. The Chinese, too, used waxes and resins to reconstruct parts of the head and face. By the 16th century when the French surgeon Ambroise Paré wrote about the simple prostheses then in use, the art had been well established. Casualties in World Wars I and II established a great need for maxillofacial prosthetics. Today dentistry plays a major role in the construction of prostheses and in the rehabilitation process.[33]

Despite the fabrication skills of the surgeon, the success of prostheses is limited by the properties of the reconstruction materials. Although modern elastomers and polymers have greatly improved facial prostheses, there is still no ideal material that resembles or duplicates human skin.

Ideally, the materials used in extraoral prostheses need a varied complement of characteristics. They must be easy and inexpensive to fabricate, and be biocompatible, strong, and sufficiently stable to endure. The prosthesis must be skinlike in appearance, and soft to the touch, with such desirable qualities

Table 13–1.   *Comparison of Resin and Porcelain Denture Teeth*

RESIN	PORCELAIN
High fracture toughness	Brittle, may chip
Crazing if not cross-linked	Susceptible to crazing by thermal shock
Clinically significant wear	Insignificant wear
Easily ground and polished	Grinding difficult and danger of removing glaze
Silent on contact	Sharp impact (clicking) sound
Dimensional change with water sorption	Dimensionally stable
Cold flow under stress	No permanent deformation
Loss of vertical dimension	Stable
Self-adjusting	Difficult to fit in diminished interarch space
Chemical bond to denture	Mechanical retention necessary
Minimal abrasion of opposing dentition	Abrades opposing natural teeth and gold surfaces

as translucence, skin color and texture. As the finished prosthesis is subject to sunlight (including ultraviolet light), heat, and cold, it must be color stable, resistant to temperature cycling and chemicals, and resilient enough to prevent tearing. Additionally, it must be easy to cleanse and manage by the patient.

Obviously, no material has all of these characteristics.[34, 35] A brief description of the materials that have been successfully used follows.

The first modern material chosen because it was easy to work with, hygienic, and durable was poly(methyl methacrylate) resin. Its major drawback was its rigidity. Even when combined with plasticizers, the material soon became hard, severely limiting its usefulness in extra-oral prostheses.

Latexes   Latexes are soft, inexpensive, and easy to manipulate, and they form lifelike prostheses. However, because the finished product is weak, degenerates rapidly with age, and changes color, latex is no longer a major facial prosthetic material.

A synthetic latex developed recently is a tripolymer of butyl acrylate, methyl methacrylate, and methyl methacrylamide. Superior to natural latex, latex skin is almost transparent and the color is sprayed on the reverse or tissue side of the prosthesis, thus appearing more natural and blending well into the prosthesis. However, the technical process of combining the latex skin with foam rubber scaffolding is lengthy and the prosthesis will last only a few months. Hence latex has very limited use for this purpose.

Vinyl Plastisol   Vinyl resins, made more flexible by adding a plasticizer, are used in some prostheses. As a plastisol, the material is a thick liquid consisting of small vinyl particles dispersed in the plasticizer. Color pigments can be incorporated to match individual skin tones. Flexibility is achieved by heating the plastisol dispersion to partially dissolve the solid particles. However, the prosthesis becomes hard with age because the plasticizers migrate from the surface of the prosthesis. Ultraviolet light also has an adverse effect on this material.

Silicone Rubber   Although silicones (Chapter 10) were introduced around 1946, only in the past few years have they been used in the fabrication of maxillofacial prostheses. Both heat-vulcanizing and room temperature-vulcanizing silicones are in use today and both have advantages and disadvantages.

The room temperature-vulcanizing silicones are either transparent or opaque white, and, before the catalyst is introduced, dry earth pigments are added to match the color of the individual skin. The prosthesis can be cured in an artificial stone mold, but a more durable mold can be made from epoxy resin or metal. The prosthesis can be easily fabricated in the dental laboratory with little special equipment. However, such silicones are not as strong as the heat-vulcanized silicones and the intrinsic color is monochromatic.

Heat-vulcanizing silicone is a semi-solid or putty-like material that requires milling, packing under pressure, and 30-minute curing at 180° C (356° F). Pigments are milled into the material, which is then packed in discrete locations of the mold. In this manner a lifelike and intrinsic color texture may be achieved which may not require further extrinsic coloration. This is the material of choice, particularly in terms of strength and color stability.[36, 37] A major advantage of this material over RTV silicone and polyurethane is a faster coloring procedure that is generally entirely intrinsic and polychromatic.

Its major disadvantage is the requirement for a milling machine and a press. In addition, a metal mold is normally used, and fabrication of the mold is a lengthy procedure. A stone mold reinforced in a denture flask may be used; however, the tensile strength of such a silicone is such that there is a high risk of damaging the mold on withdrawal. A modification in formulation that permits repeated use of a stone mold has been reported.[37]

Polyurethane Polymers   Polyurethane is the most recent addition to the materials used in maxillofacial prostheses. Fabrication of a polyurethane prosthesis involves three components, which require accurate proportioning and mixing. One of the components is acrylate, which needs careful handling to prevent a toxic reaction to the operator. Although the material is cured at room temperature, it requires accurate temperature control because a slight change in temperature can alter the chemical reaction. Since moisture in the air can also affect the processing, a metal mold may be necessary. Although a polyurethane prosthesis has lifelike feel and appearance, it is susceptible to deterioration. However, the color stability of this material is better than that of polyvinyl chloride.

The reader is referred to texts in this discipline for details on coloring the prostheses and adhesives used to hold the appliances in place.[33, 35]

References

1. Skinner EW and Cooper EN: Physical properties of denture resins. Part I. Curing shrinkage and water sorption. J Am Dent Assoc 30:1845, 1943.
2. Faraj SAA and Ellis B: The effect of processing temperatures on the exotherm, porosity, and properties of acrylic denture base. Br Dent J 147:209, 1979.
3. Goodkind RJ and Schulte RC: Dimensional accuracy of pour acrylic resin and conventional processing of cold-curing acrylic resin bases. J Prosthet Dent 24:662, 1970.
4. Hardy F: Comparison of fluid resin and compression molding methods in processing dimensional changes. J Prosthet Dent 39:375, 1978.
5. Civjan S, Huget EF, and deSimon LB: Modifications of the fluid resin technique. J. Am Dent Assoc 85:109, 1972.
6. Braden M: The absorption of water by acrylic resins and other materials. J Prosthet Dent 14:307, 1964.
7. Vernonite Work Bench: Vol. 6, No. 3, 1947.
8. Woelfel JB: Processing complete dentures. Dent Clin North Am 21:329, 1977.
9. Paffenbarger GC, Woelfel JB, and Sweeney WT: Resins and technics used in constructing dentures. Dent Clin North Am, March, 1965, p. 251.
10. Ruyter IE and Svendsen SA: Flexural properties of denture base polymers. J Prosthet Dent 43:95, 1980.
11. Stafford GO and Handley RW: Transverse bend testing of denture base polymers. J Dent 3:251, 1975.
12. McCabe JF and Wilson HJ: The use of differential scanning calorimetry for the evaluation of dental materials. Part II. Denture base materials. J Oral Rehabil 7:235, 1980.
13. Sweeney WT and Schoonover IC: A progress report on denture base material. J Am Dent Assoc 23:1498, 1936.
14. Ruyter IE and Espevik S: Compressive creep of denture base polymers. Acta Odontol Scand 38:169, 1980.
15. Leong A and Grant AA: The transverse strength of repairs in polymethyl methacrylate. Aust Dent J 16:232, 1971.
16. Wright PS: Soft lining materials: Their status and prospects. J Dent 4:247, 1976.

17. McCabe, JF: Soft lining materials: Composition and structure. J Oral Rehabil 3:273, 1976.
18. Braden M and Clarke RL: Viscoelastic properties of soft lining materials. J Dent Res 51:1525, 1972.
19. Bell DH Jr, Finnegan FJ, and Ward JE: Pros and cons of hard and resilient denture base materials. J Am Dent Assoc 94:511, 1977.
20. Makila E and Honka O: Clinical study of a heat-cured silicone soft lining material. J Oral Rehabil 6:199, 1979.
21. Wright PS: The effect of soft lining materials on the growth of *Candida albicans*. J Dent 8:144, 1980.
22. McCarthy JA and Moser JB: Mechanical properties of tissue conditioners. Part I: Theoretical considerations, behavioral characteristics, and tensile properties. J Prosthet Dent 40:89, 1978.
23. Sieweke JC, Rogers LB, and Eames WB: Dimensional stability of custom tray acrylics: Effect on impression accuracy. IADR Program and Abstracts, No. 35, 1978.
24. Ruyter IE: Release of formaldehyde from denture base polymers. Acta Odontol Scand 38:17, 1980.
25. Smith DC and Baines MED: Residual methyl methacrylate in the denture base and its relation to denture sore mouth. Br Dent J 98:55, 1955.
26. Nyquist G: Study of denture sore mouth. An investigation of traumatic, allergic and toxic lesions of the oral mucosa arising from the use of full dentures. Acta Odontol Scand 10:154, 1952.
27. Corkill JA, Lloyd EJ, Hoyle P, Crout DHG, Ling RSM, James ML, and Piper, RJ: Toxicology of methyl methacrylate: The rate of disappearance of methyl methacrylate in human blood in vitro. Clin Chim Acta 68:141, 1976.
28. Michl RJ: Isosit — a new dental material. Quint Int 3:29, 1978.
29. Morrow RM, Matvias FM, Windeler AS, and Fuchs RJ: Bonding of plastic teeth to two heat-curing denture base resins. J Prosthet Dent 39:565, 1978.
30. Shepard WL: Denture bases processed from a fluid resin. J Prosthet Dent 19:561, 1968.
31. Rupp NW, Bowen RL, and Paffenbarger GC: Bonding cold-curing denture base acrylic resin to acrylic resin teeth. J Am Dent Assoc 83:601, 1971.
32. Ortman HR: Complete denture occlusion. Dent Clin North Am 21:308, 1977.
33. Chalian VA, Drane JB, and Standish SM: Maxillofacial Prosthetics: Multidisciplinary Practice. Baltimore, Williams & Wilkins Co., 1972.
34. Chalian VA and Phillips RW: Materials in maxillofacial prosthetics. J Biomed Mater Res 2:349, 1974.
35. Laney WR: Maxillofacial Prosthetics. Littleton, Massachusetts, PSG Publishing Co., 1979.
36. Chalian VA: Evaluation and comparison of physical properties of materials used in maxillofacial prosthetics. Thesis, Indiana University School of Dentistry, Indianapolis, 1976.
37. Lontz JF, Schweiger JW, and Burger, AW: Development and standardization of polysiloxane maxillofacial prostheses. Presented at 22nd Annual Meeting of the American Academy of Maxillofacial Prosthetics, Williamsburg, November 3–6, 1974.

14 RESTORATIVE RESINS

The chemistry of the resin systems pertinent to dentistry was discussed in Chapter 11. That discussion will be developed further in this chapter with particular attention to their use in operative procedures.

Synthetic resins have been developed as restorative materials principally because of their esthetic properties. The early resin restorations were made by cementing heat-cured acrylic inlays or crowns into the prepared cavity. However, the low modulus of elasticity and lack of dimensional stability of the resin invariably resulted in a fracture of the cement, with subsequent leakage and failure of the restoration.

The development of the self-curing acrylic materials in the late 1940's made feasible the direct restoration of teeth with resin. The monomer and polymer could be combined and the resultant dough or gel inserted into the prepared cavity, where it polymerized in situ.

The use of acrylic resin for tooth restorations has been the subject of much controversy. Certain properties, such as esthetic qualities and insolubility, made it superior to silicate cement (Chapter 30). On the other hand, inherent weaknesses that will be discussed have cast doubt as to its suitability as a restorative material.

With the advancements in polymer science, research has focused on the evolution of an improved resin system for use as a restorative material and preferably one that would adhesively bond to tooth structure. Although the latter goal has not as yet been achieved, new resins (i.e., the BIS-GMA systems referred to in Chapter 11) reinforced by means of fillers have been developed. In general the properties of these "composite" resins are superior to those of the conventional unfilled acrylic resin.

Thus two kinds of direct-filling resins are currently in use, although there is a strong preference for the composite resins. Requirements for these two classes of resins are set forth in American Dental Association Specification no. 27 for direct-filling resins.[1] The unfilled resins are classified as Type I and the composite resins as Type II. Actually there are two classifications of composite resins, the so-called "conventional" composites and the newer microfilled resins. Commercial products that are representative of each of these resin systems appear in Figure 14–1. Also discussed in this chapter are resins

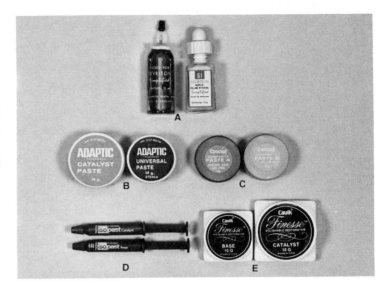

Figure 14–1 Commercial products representative of currently available resin systems. *A*, Unfilled resin. *B, C, D,* and *E*, Composite resins. *B* and *C* are conventional composites and *D* and *E* are microfilled resins.

employed for other purposes, such as pit and fissure sealants, as coatings for eroded areas, and for use in crown and bridge work.

ACRYLIC RESIN (TYPE I)

As indicated previously, the unfilled direct filling resins are no longer the materials of choice. However, their chemistry and inherent properties form the background for the now popular composite restoratives. Such information will continue to be of interest in the ever unfolding composite technology. Therefore, a discussion of these older materials is necessary and should be beneficial in understanding the newer resin systems.

In all fairness it should be recognized that improved compositions and techniques have eliminated some of the problems originally encountered in the use of the first acrylic restorative materials. However, even with these improvements, the inherent properties of acrylic resins restrict their use to selected situations. It is only by a knowledge of the basic chemical and physical properties of that system that one can intelligently evaluate its proper role in the restoration of the carious tooth. For that matter, any resin is a difficult material to master. The dentist must be prepared to acknowledge this fact and to assume a certain responsibility for acquiring the experience needed to familiarize himself with its characteristics and behavior.

Composition and Chemistry   The unfilled acrylic resins are supplied as a powder and liquid, as shown in Figure 14–1. The main ingredient of the powder is a polymer, in the form of beads or grindings, while the liquid is primarily a monomer.

In contrast to the curing of the denture base self-curing resins, it is highly desirable that the polymerization of a direct filling resin be completed in a comparatively short time. As the resin is polymerized directly in the prepared cavity, the chair time should be as short as possible. Also, the more rapid the polymerization, the less likely it is that the adaptation of the resin to the cavity walls will be disturbed during the finishing of the restoration. Consequently, a short induction period is desirable. Thus, the direct filling resins are compounded in such a manner that the induction period (gel time) is short.

Although there are various means by which active radicals can be supplied to initiate polymerization of resins at oral temperatures, two mechanisms are employed in the currently available unfilled direct filling resins. The older of the two mechanisms is the benzoyl peroxide–tertiary amine redox system and the other is the sulfinate system.

In addition to the polymer beads or grindings, the powder component of the acrylic resins contains the initiator, benzoyl peroxide (0.3 to 3 per cent). With the sulfinate system the powder usually contains the accelerator or cocatalyst. Proper shade is obtained in the same manner as for denture resins. Either polymer beads of the desired shade or color are mixed with clear beads or pigments are blended with the powder. A few manufacturers add a small percentage of inorganic filler, such as glass, to the powder. However, these additions do not appreciably improve the properties, so such formulations are still within the category of Type I resins. The amount of filler is much less than in the Type II resin (composite) and the resin matrix of the latter is also different, as will be discussed.

The liquid is methyl methacrylate (monomer) together with a cross-linking agent such as ethylene dimethacrylate, in an amount of 5 per cent or more. The monomer also contains a minute amount of inhibitor (e.g., monomethylether of hydroquinone), in concentrations of approximately 0.006 per cent.

If the peroxide-amine induction system is employed to accomplish polymerization of the resin, the amine (N–N dimethyl-p-toluidine or similar compound) is contained in the liquid. When the powder and liquid are mixed together, the peroxide reacts with the amine to form free radicals and thereby initiate polymerization of the monomer, as was discussed in Chapter 11.

The peroxide-amine polymerization system may be inhibited by phenolic compounds such as eugenol. Thus the resin would not polymerize properly in the presence of eugenol-containing materials such as zinc oxide–eugenol cements. Also the system is sensitive to oxygen. Excessive air incorporated into the resin mix will inhibit polymerization and can cause spongy spots to be present in the restoration.

A major problem encountered with early amine-containing resins was a lack of color stability of the restorations. The cured resin was sensitive to ultraviolet light and in time turned yellow or brown upon exposure to sunlight. The inclusion of ultraviolet absorbers in the material has remedied this problem to a large degree, although some color shift may occur in peroxide-amine cured resins during long exposure to water.

With the sulfinate curing system, p-toluene sulfinic acid ($CH_3 \cdot C_6H_4 \cdot SO_2H$) or its derivatives can be dissolved in the monomer. Actually, under certain conditions p-toluene sulfinic acid dissolved in monomer can initiate polymerization without the addition of benzoyl peroxide. However, usually salts of sulfinic acid are dispersed in the powder along with benzoyl peroxide. The system is quite complicated in its mechanism of polymerization and requires a variety of additives. In essence, these additives convert the sulfinate salts to sulfinic acid (RSO_2H) to produce free radicals.

The reaction products of the sulfinate system are colorless so that resins polymerized by this mechanism are relatively color stable. The system is less sensitive to inhibition by oxygen and phenolic compounds than is the amine-peroxide system. However, sulfinic acid and its salts are very unstable in the presence of water, or even moisture, which creates packaging and storage problems. In fact, polymerization can be completely inhibited by water. Thus, the powder that contains the sulfinate must be carefully stored and the operative technique exceedingly meticulous in order to avoid any moisture contamination of the resin.

Physical, Mechanical, and Chemical Properties A number of properties of unfilled acrylic direct filling resins, along with certain requisites set forth for Type I resins in American Dental Association Specification no. 27, are shown in Table 14–1.

Working time indicates the time from the start of the mix during which the material retains sufficient plasticity that it can be adapted to the walls and margins of the cavity preparation. As can be seen in Table 14–1, the specification requires a minimum working time of 1.5 minutes for such direct filling resins.

Setting or hardening time indicates the time at which the matrix can be removed. This can be evaluated in several ways. The specification test employs a penotrometer type of hardness tester (the Barcol instrument). Hardening time is stated as that time from the start of the mix when a specific hardness reading is obtained. The maximum time allotted is 8 minutes.

As has been discussed, polymerization is an exothermic reaction. Since most of the polymerization of the resin occurs before and at the peak temperature, determination of the time at which peak temperature is reached can also be used as an indicator of hardening time.[2] Obviously, as polymerization proceeds the amount of monomer present in the mass becomes less. Thus the rate at which the residual monomer decreases may be used to evaluate hardening time.[3]

The polymerization shrinkage, by volume, of unfilled acrylic restorative resins is from 5 to 8 per cent,[4, 5] which is in the same range as that of the denture resins, discussed previously. Variations in monomer–polymer ratio

Table 14–1. Direct Filling Resins*

| | | Type I (Unfilled) | | Type II (Composites) | | |
		ADA Specification	Acrylic	ADA Specification	Conventional	Microfilled
Working time — min		Minimum 1.5	1.5	Minimum 1.5	4	3
Compressive strength (24 hr)	— MPa		69		235	276
	— psi		10,000		34,000	40,000
Diametral tensile strength (24 hr)	— MPa	Minimum 24	24	Minimum 34	45	32
	— psi	3480	3500	4930	6500	4700
Modulus of elasticity	— GPa		2.4		13.7	4.5
	— psi		$.34 \times 10^6$		2.2×10^6	$.65 \times 10^6$
H₂O sorption (1 wk)	— mg/cm²	Maximum 1.7	1.7	Maximum 0.7	0.6	1.4
Polymerization shrinkage (by volume)	— %		7		1.4	1.7

*Comparison of the properties of representative unfilled acrylic, conventional composite and microfilled composite resins.

may influence the polymerization shrinkage to a certain extent, but the effects of such manipulative variables are relatively insignificant when compared to the magnitude of the shrinkage that is inherent in the material.

As will be stressed, a major goal of techniques used for insertion of the unfilled resins is to control the direction of the polymerization so that it does not occur in a critical area such as the cavo-surface margin. Shrinkage of the material away from the cavity margin would create a gap resulting in marginal leakage and all of the problems associated with microleakage.

The linear coefficient of thermal expansion across the crown of a tooth is 11.4×10^{-6} mm/mm/° C (Table 3–2). The coefficient of thermal expansion of an unfilled acrylic direct filling resin is 92×10^{-6} mm/mm/° C. Therefore, when an unfilled resin restoration is heated or cooled, it will change dimension approximately 8 times as much as does the tooth for each degree of temperature change. As can be seen in Table 14–2, the differential in thermal expansion between the tooth and the unfilled resin is greater than that of any other restorative material.

These values suggest that when cold food is consumed, the contraction of an unfilled resin restoration, as compared with that of the tooth, is considerably greater than that which would occur in restorations of other types of materials. Hence, the potential for marginal leakage from this source would appear to be enhanced with direct filling acrylic resin restorations.

However, the unfilled resin does have one characteristic that probably offsets to some degree the undesirable effects of the relatively high coefficient of thermal expansion. Unfilled acrylic resins have low thermal conductivity and diffusivity. Thus the restoration changes temperature quite slowly. Therefore, it takes considerably longer for the resin restoration to become hot or cold, as compared to metallic restorations, which have high thermal conductivity and diffusivity.[6]

Poly(methyl methacrylate) is virtually insoluble in water. Thus solubility is not a problem with unfilled acrylic restorations. However, the material does tend to sorb water, approximately 1.7 mg/cm². It has been suggested that the linear expansion of the material that occurs as the result of water sorption (in the range of 0.3 to 0.5 per cent) may aid in sealing the cavity.[7] Whether the marginal seal is actually improved by this phenomenon remains somewhat controversial.

As seen in Table 14–1, the compressive strength of the unfilled acrylic

Table 14–2. *Differential Thermal Dimensional Change Between Tooth Structure on Various Restorative Materials*

		FACTOR $\dfrac{\alpha^* \text{ for Material}}{\alpha \text{ for Tooth}}$
(Type I)	Unfilled acrylic resin	8.1
	Microfilled composite resin	5.3
(Type II)	Conventional composite resin	3.1
	Amalgam	2.2
	Gold inlay	1.9
	Gold foil	1.3
	Silicate cement	0.7

*α = linear coefficient of expansion.

resin is low, about 62 MPa (9000 psi). Yield strength and tensile strengths are even lower. For a Type I resin the American Dental Association specification requires a minimum diametral tensile strength of only 24 MPa (3480 psi). When compared with the occlusal stress that can be generated during mastication, the material is inordinately weak. In addition, the modulus of elasticity is 2.4 GPa (0.34×10^6 psi) as compared to a value of 46.2 GPa (6.7×10^6 psi) reported for cusp enamel (Table 3-3). Thus, masticatory stresses would likely produce more deformation in the resin than in the tooth and cause distortion of the resin at the margins.

The acrylic resin is the softest of all the restorative materials. A comparison of the Knoop hardness numbers of tooth structure and various restorative materials appears in Table 14–3. Although it has previously been noted that hardness does not always provide an exact index of abrasion resistance for any material, it would be expected that such a soft resin would be susceptible to abrasion. (The problem of wear and abrasion will be discussed later in this chapter.)

Because of these relatively low mechanical properties, use of unfilled acrylic resins has been limited to restoration of Class III and V cavities. They have also been employed with certain effectiveness as a temporary measure in Class IV cavities.

Esthetics is a primary concern of materials employed for the restoration of anterior teeth. A color change in the material that produces an obvious mismatch between the restoration and tooth may require replacement of the restoration. Thus it is appropriate that a test for color stability is included in the American Dental Association specification for direct filling resins. Since ultraviolet light produces a marked color change in many chemically activated resins, the test specified consists of exposing resin samples to ultraviolet light for 24 hours. The exposed specimen is then compared visually with an identical unexposed (control) specimen. If the difference in the color of the control and exposed specimens is greater than that which can be "perceived with difficulty," the resin is unacceptable.

Other tests for color stability include storage of the specimens in water at elevated temperature and also subjecting the resin to the combined effects of water, heat, and ultraviolet light in a weathering chamber. There are no direct data to indicate that a resin which shows color change by any one or all of these tests invariably will undergo the same degree of color shift in the oral cavity. However, these tests do indicate the propensity of the material for color change.

Table 14–3. *Comparative Knoop Hardness of Tooth Structure and Restorative Materials*

	KHN
Enamel	300
Dentin	65
Amalgam	90
Direct filling gold	70
Silicate cement	65
Conventional composite resin	55
Soft inlay gold	50
Microfilled composite resin	25
Unfilled acrylic resin	15

Biological Properties   All materials used for restoring carious teeth produce some degree of pulpal reaction, and generally an undesirable one. The acrylic resin is no exception. When the material was first introduced, pulpal injury and pathology were frequently observed and attributed to the toxic effects of components in the resin. However, the frequency of pulpal injury has been reduced as a result of improvement in the material itself and of refinement of the insertion techniques designed to reduce marginal leakage. Now it is generally agreed that, with a properly placed resin restoration, the reaction is a reversible one. However, since the acrylic resins initially induce pulpal irritation, protection of the pulp by means of a liner or base of calcium hydroxide on the pulpal wall is recommended, particularly in the deep cavity preparation. A zinc oxide–eugenol cement is not used, since the eugenol may prevent proper polymerization of the resin, as noted.

Manipulative Technique   A number of different techniques have been used for the insertion of direct acrylic resin restoration. They are the bulk pack or pressure technique, the non-pressure or bead technique, and the flow technique. Other procedures are basically variations of these three.

When the *bulk* technique is employed, the liquid is roughly measured and the powder is added to the liquid, just as with denture resins. The powder and liquid can be mixed on a glass slab or in a dappen dish. The mixture is stirred gently to minimize entrapment of air in the material, which could produce voids in the restoration and inhibit polymerization of a peroxide-amine cured resin. When the material reaches a doughy stage, the mass is quickly inserted into the cavity and held under pressure by means of a matrix strip. The matrix strip must be of a substance such as Mylar that will not be attacked by the monomer. It is clamped tightly in position and held immobile until polymerization is virtually completed. Any movement of the strip while the material is soft can pull the material away from the wall of the cavity, leaving the margins open and permitting gross leakage to occur along the tooth-restoration interface. A second purpose of maintaining pressure on the matrix strip is to prevent the resin from pulling away from the cavity margins when it contracts during polymerization.

A restoration placed by a properly executed bulk technique is shown in Figure 14–2. Note that polymerization shrinkage has been directed so that it

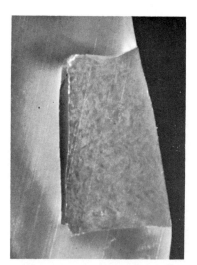

Figure 14–2   Cross section through an unfilled acrylic restoration inserted by a properly executed pressure technique. Polymerization shrinkage has resulted in a contraction of the material away from the cavity floor; however, the resin appears to be well adapted at the cavo-surface margins.

occurs along the pulpal wall while the material is closely adapted to tooth at the cavo-surface margins.

The *non-pressure,* or *bead,* technique is accomplished by applying the monomer-polymer mixture in increments, rather than by filling the cavity with the bulk mix. In this technique, the polymer is placed in one dappen dish and the monomer in another. The prepared cavity is first moistened with monomer. The tip of a small sable-hair brush is then dipped into the monomer and touched to the polymer so that a few particles cling to it to form a small bead or agglomerate of powder particles and monomer. The bead formed on the tip of the brush is immediately placed in contact with the cavity floor. The fluid mix flows readily over the cavity floor already wetted by the monomer. The process is repeated until the cavity is properly filled.

The surface of the restoration is then covered by some type of inert material, such as silicone grease, cocoa butter, wax, or oil. Such protective coatings are supplied by some manufacturers. The coating prevents evaporation of monomer and inhibition of polymerization by oxygen. In the case of resins polymerized by the sulfinate system, the coating reduces the danger of inhibition by moisture.

In the *flow* technique, a thin mix of resin is made and the fluid resin is then carried into the prepared cavity by means of a small instrument. After the cavity is filled, a matrix band is applied but is not held under pressure. The fluidity of the resin assists in securing intimate adaptation to the tooth surface. The matrix aids in containing the resin, ensuring proper contact and contour.

Another aid to improving adaptation of acrylic resins is use of the cavity lining agents that are often supplied by the manufacturer, particularly for those resins that employ the sulfinate curing system. These liners, often referred to by the manufacturer as "primers" or "cavity seals," should not be confused with the cavity varnishes described in Chapter 30. Conventional cavity varnishes are not used with acrylic resin restorative materials. Such varnishes contain solvents, such as chloroform and ether, which inhibit the polymerization of the resin, just as for eugenol. The cavity lining agents formulated for use with acrylic resins are solutions of methacrylic acid or the phosphoric acid ester of glycerin dissolved in methyl methacrylate monomer.

The liner is applied to the surface of the prepared cavity prior to insertion of the resin. The intended purpose is to wet-out the hydrophilic surface of the dentin and enamel in order to make it more attractive to the hydrophobic resin.

Likewise the advent of the acid etching techniques has markedly improved the mechanical bond of the resin to the enamel. That technique will be discussed later in the chapter.

COMPOSITE RESINS (TYPE II)

It is apparent from the foregoing discussion of the unfilled acrylic resins that certain inherent characteristics in poly(methyl methacrylate) limit its use and its effectiveness as a restorative material. The low hardness and strength, high coefficient of thermal expansion, and lack of adhesion to tooth structure place restrictions as to where it may be effectively employed. Considerable research has centered upon the formulation of resin systems with improved physical properties, and thus superior clinical performance.

Other resins that have been studied include the cyanoacrylates, polystyrene, polyamide, an aziridino polyester, and polycarbonate. Certain of the shortcomings of the acrylic resins have also been inherent in these systems. In addition, some pose technical problems. For example, as was noted in Chapter 11, the polycarbonates must be injected into the prepared cavity well above the glass transition temperature of the resin.

The properties of epoxy resins (e.g., their potential adhesive characteristics and the fact that they harden at moderate temperatures with low polymerization shrinkage) stimulated research on their applicability as restorative materials, particularly as binders for inorganic fillers. The end result was the composite restorative resin.[8]

Conventional Composite (Type II)   Technically the term "composite" refers to a material system composed of a mixture of two or more macro constituents which differ in form, in that they are essentially insoluble in each other. However, in dentistry the term "composite" initially referred to a restorative material, usually in paste form, consisting of an organic binder containing at least 60 per cent inorganic filler by weight incorporated into a system that would induce polymerization. (As will be discussed later in this chapter the microfilled resins do not contain as much inorganic filler as do the conventional composite resins.) Likewise, the filler particles are coated with a "coupling" agent to bond them to the resin matrix. Thus, the essentials of a composite are a resin binder, a filler, and a coupling agent. Incidentally, another example of a composite structure is tooth enamel, in which a high concentration of filler particles of inorganic apatite is bound into an organic matrix.

The foregoing statement implies a discreteness in the formulation of the composite. A number of parameters have a marked influence upon the properties that can be obtained by the addition of fillers to a resin matrix. The characterization of the dispersed phase in terms of its shape, size, hardness, concentration, and distribution is very important, as will be discussed. The composition of the continuous phase, i.e., the resin, is equally significant. Thus the term composite distinguishes this class of materials from the previously discussed unreinforced direct acrylic filling resins, including those materials to which small amounts of a filler have been added.

Let us first turn our attention to the continuous phase in the dental composite restorative materials.

Resin Matrix   The search for a suitable matrix for dental composite filling resins encountered numerous difficulties, among which were unsuitable curing agents and lack of the necessary color stability. These problems led to a compromise between epoxy and methacrylate resins. The research of Bowen is classic, and most of the currently popular composites are based on his concept.[9, 10]

The reaction sites (oxirane groups) of the epoxy molecule were replaced by methacrylate groups. In this way a hybrid molecule was produced that could be polymerized through the methacrylate groups. Thus it was possible to bring about polymerization by means of the convenient benzoyl peroxide–tertiary amine curing systems commonly employed for the self-cured acrylic resins.

The structural formula of the dimethacrylate monomer (BIS-GMA) is compared with that of methyl methacrylate (next page).[11]

$$H_2C = \underset{\underset{CH_3}{|}}{CCOCH_2} - \underset{\underset{H}{|}}{\overset{\overset{H}{|}}{C}} - CH_2O - \bigcirc - \underset{\underset{CH_3}{|}}{\overset{\overset{CH_3}{|}}{C}} - \bigcirc - OCH_2 - \underset{\underset{H}{|}}{\overset{\overset{H}{|}}{C}} - CH_2O\underset{\underset{CH_3}{|}}{CC} = CH_2$$

BIS - GMA

$$H_2C = \underset{\underset{CH_3}{|}}{\overset{\overset{O}{\|}}{CCOCH_3}}$$

Methyl methacrylate

As discussed in Chapter 11, the dimethacrylate monomer (BIS-GMA) can be synthesized by the reaction between bisphenol-A and glycidyl methacrylate. It also can be obtained by the reaction of the glycidyl ether of bisphenol-A and methacrylic acid. This hybrid molecule is classified as a thermo-setting methacrylate resin. It has proved to be suitable for use as a binder for reinforcing fillers. It has a somewhat lower polymerization shrinkage than does methyl methacrylate and hardens rapidly under oral conditions.

The resin for the matrix of commercial composite resins must be modified even further in order to improve certain properties. The dimethacrylate resin is too viscous for convenient use at ambient temperatures, so it is diluted by the addition of other methacrylate monomers of low viscosity. These monomers may be difunctional so as to form a cross-linked polymer. Stabilizers are added to improve shelf life. Since polymerization is generally accomplished by means of the peroxide-amine system, ultraviolet light absorbing compounds must be added to minimize color change in the material when exposed to sunlight.

The resins are supplied as two components, a powder and a liquid, a paste and a liquid, or two pastes. Just as with the unfilled acrylic resins, the amine is incorporated in one component and the peroxide in the other. When the two are combined, polymerization occurs. As noted, most of the present composite restorative materials make at least partial use of the BIS-GMA molecule.

Although Bowen's BIS-GMA resin does have advantages as a binder for a composite restorative, it also has several disadvantages. These include a high viscosity that requires use of diluent monomers, difficulty in synthesizing a pure composition, strong air inhibition to polymerization, and high water sorption because of the diluents used and the hydroxyl groups in the BIS-GMA molecule. These problems have long been recognized and have led to extensive research on new binders. Present composites are formulated with or without BIS-GMA and usually contain adducts of BIS-GMA with diisocyanates, urethane methacrylates, BIS-GMA-type structures without hydroxyl groups, and even more exotic combinations of methacrylates of alkane epoxides and resorcinol ethers. For the next generation of products, polyfluorinated polymethacrylates, stabilizing phenolic methacrylates, and monomers polymerizing by a ring opening mechanism have been suggested.

Light Cured Resins   As noted, most of the conventional commercial composites are chemically activated via the peroxide-amine induction system. The two pastes are identical except that one contains the benzoyl peroxide initiator and the other the tertiary amine activator or accelerator. When the two pastes are mixed together the material polymerizes.

Conventional composite resins are also now being marketed whose cure is based upon light activation. While photocuring has had extensive use in industry, it has only recently been applied to dental restoratives. The first system used in dentistry employed *ultraviolet light*. In the ultraviolet curing system, benzoin methyl ether $(C_6H_5 \cdot C:O \cdot C \cdot (OCH_3) \cdot C_6H_5)$ or higher alkyl benzoin ethers are employed as the activator for the peroxide curing system. Upon exposure to light waves in the ultraviolet range, the ether decomposes to form free radicals that trigger the polymerization.

Some products make use of *visible light* activation, using radiation greater than 400 nanometers. The activating compounds for visible light are usually diketones and aromatic ketones such as camphoroquinone and biacetyl, used in conjunction with reducing agents, i.e., tertiary amines.

An advantage of visible light curing systems, as compared to ultraviolet light systems, is that a greater depth of resin can be cured by visible light. Also the resin can be polymerized through enamel, which is particularly advantageous in Class III restorations. In addition, the intensity of ultraviolet light tends to decrease with time. Thus the light must be tested continually to assure that the resin is being properly polymerized. The intensity of the visible lights remain relatively constant until the bulb fails completely.

An advantage of light-curing systems is that the dentist has complete control over the working time and is not confined to the built-in curing cycle of the self-cure. This is particularly beneficial when large restorations are placed, e.g., Class IV. There are still some attendant difficulties with light curing. With certain light-curing systems there is a lower percentage of conversion of the monomer, a lower degree of polymerization, and a limited depth of cure. However, when properly cured, the properties of light-cured composite resins are in the same general range of chemically cured materials.

Fillers   The filler in a composite must be in high concentration if the dispersed particles are to inhibit deformation of the matrix. Also, another function of the filler is to reduce the coefficient of thermal expansion of the resin matrix. The higher the ratio between the dimensionally stable filler and the dimensionally unstable resin, the lower will be the coefficient of thermal expansion of the composite. Although the filler concentration varies from one commercial product to another, it is generally present in the amount of 70 to 80 per cent.

Current products most often contain crystalline quartz and/or lithium glass ceramics. However, other fillers, such as calcium silicate, glass beads, glass fibers, and beta-eucryptite, have been used. Very recently calcium fluoride has been introduced as a filler. The hardness of the fillers varies from big, hard particles of quartz to small, soft particles of glass. As some radiopacity is desirable in a restoration, this is achieved by filler blends containing barium and strontium glasses and most recently lanthanum glass. The latter two glasses are characterized by low solubility and toxicity.

Particle size distribution is an important consideration for the filler. In most conventional composites, the distribution ranges from 1 to 100 microme-

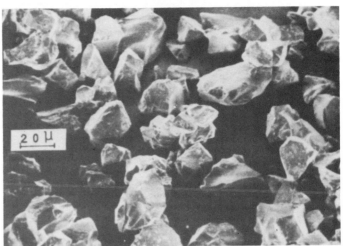

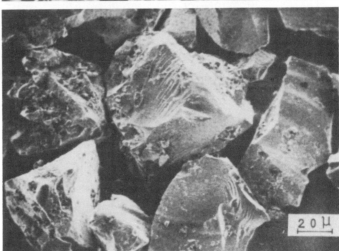

Figure 14–3 Scanning electron microscope picture of inorganic fillers employed in two commerical composite restorative materials. (Courtesy of L. N. Johnson.)

ters. Generally, blends of fine particles (1–20 μm) and coarse particles (<100 μm) are employed. Examples of fillers used in a popular conventional composite resin are shown in Figure 14–3.

Coupling Agents A stable, adhesive bonding of the filler to the resin is essential for strength and durability in the composite. Lack of an adequate bond will permit dislodgment of the filler from the surface or ready penetration of water along the filler–matrix interface. Thus, the manufacturer coats the surface of the filler with a suitable *coupling* or *keying agent*. Such agents may also act as a stress absorber at the filler–resin interface.

Vinyl silane coupling agents were first used. These have now been replaced by more reactive compounds, such as gamma-methacryloxy propyl silane.

Physical, Mechanical, and Chemical Properties Naturally, the properties of commercial composite resins vary to some degree from one product to another.[12, 13] These variations are due principally to the differences in the monomers and the concentration and nature of the fillers employed.

Typical values for certain of the mechanical and physical properties of conventional composites, as compared with those of unreinforced resins, are shown in Table 14–1. This table includes data from several reports and for a variety of materials. For ease in comparing the types of resins, the numbers represent values in the middle range.

As can be seen, the American Dental Association Specification for Type II Direct Filling Resins stipulates a working time of at least 1.5 minutes and a maximum hardening time of 8 minutes, just as it does for Type I resins. However, the requirements for other properties, such as diametral tensile strength and water sorption, are more stringent for the Type II resins.

It is obvious that the composite resins are superior to the unreinforced acrylic resins in respect to most mechanical and physical properties. This would be anticipated because of the strengthening effect of the filler and the difference in the properties of the resin matrix. For example, the molecular weight of the BIS-GMA molecule is approximately 512, while that of the methyl methacrylate monomer is only 100.

Because of the higher molecular weight of the monomer and the high concentration of inorganic filler, the polymerization shrinkage of approximately 1.4 per cent for the conventional composites is much less than that of the unfilled acrylic resins, which is in the range of 7 per cent (Table 14–1). Thus it would be expected that the conventional composite resins should have less tendency to pull away from the walls of the cavity as the material hardens.

For these same reasons the coefficient of thermal expansion is appreciably lower than that of an unfilled acrylic resin. The linear coefficient of thermal expansion of the conventional composite resin is approximately 37×10^{-6} as compared to 92×10^{-6} for unfilled acrylic resins. As shown in Table 14–2, for each degree of temperature change, the average conventional composite resin restoration changes dimension only three times as much as does the tooth when subjected to temperature change, as compared to a dimensional change differential of approximately eight for an unfilled acrylic resin.

Just as with the unfilled acrylic direct filling resins, solubility of composite resins in oral fluids is not of consequence. As shown in Table 14–1, the water sorption of the conventional composites is less than that of an unfilled acrylic resin. The American Dental Association specification specifies a maximum water sorption of 1.7 mg/cm^2 at one week for a Type I resin as compared with only 0.7 mg/cm^2 permissible for a Type II resin.

The conventional composite resins are appreciably stronger than unfilled resins when loaded in compression (235 MPa [34,000 psi] as compared with 69 MPa [10,000 psi]). The composites also have a higher tensile strength. The fatigue limit is approximately 65 per cent of the compressive strength.[14] The American Dental Association specification requires a diametral tensile strength of at least 24 MPa (3480 psi) for unfilled acrylic (Type I), while the minimum acceptable strength for a composite resin (Type II) is 34 MPa (4930 psi). The conventional composite resins also have a much higher modulus of elasticity than do the unfilled acrylic resins. This would suggest that the stiffer material would be less susceptible to elastic deformation when subjected to masticatory forces.

The composites are also much harder than the unfilled acrylic resins (Table 14–3), approximately 55 KHN as compared to 15 KHN. The composite resins appear to withstand abrasion by a tooth brush and a dentifrice somewhat better than the unfilled resins.[15] However, wear problems have been encountered when composites were used to restore occlusal surfaces of teeth, as will be discussed later.

Biological Properties The irritational characteristics of composite resins are comparable to those of the unfilled acrylic resins. Thus, the same protective measures should be used as was described for those materials. As for many other restorative materials, whenever the cavity preparation is deep, the pulp must be protected from possible injury from irritants in the resin. A calcium hydroxide cement base is the preferred material for placement on the cavity floor before insertion of the resin. As a general rule, cavity varnish or a zinc oxide–eugenol cement is contraindicated because of the potential softening of the resin at the interface by the eugenol or solvent in the varnish, as for acrylic resins.

Manipulative Techniques As stated, self-curing composite direct filling resins can be supplied commercially in a variety of forms, including powder and liquid, two paste systems, and paste-liquid combinations. Because of the convenience, the powder-liquid system does have the advantage of longer shelf life without the need to store the material under refrigeration.[16] The two-paste system, examples of which are shown in Figure 14–1, is by far the most popular. One of the reasons for the success of composites is the relatively non-critical proportions of the components used. However, as with all dental materials, they should be handled according to the manufacturer's directions.

There are some general rules that are common to all products. The jars of paste must not be cross contaminated, since one contains the activator and the other the initiator. If the material of one jar is contaminated by material from the other jar, partial polymerization of the contaminated material will occur. The resin will become crumbly and unusable. The paste should never be removed from the two jars with the same instrument.

The fillers used in composite resins are relatively hard and will abrade metal mixing instruments. Any metal particles abraded from the instruments become incorporated into the resin mix and discolor the material. Therefore, plastic or wooden spatulas should be used.

The self-curing resins polymerize rapidly; thus, the working time is very short. For this reason they must be mixed quickly, the mix being completed within 30 seconds. It is important that the material be thoroughly mixed in order to insure a homogeneous distribution of the curing agent (activator) throughout the mass, yet not so vigorously that air is incorporated.

The method of insertion is similar to that of the bulk or pressure technique described for the unfilled acrylic resins. Immediately following mixing, the material is carried to the mouth by means of plastic-tipped instruments and wiped or "teased" into the cavity. Some products are suitable for injection into the cavity by means of a plastic tipped syringe.

The mixing and insertion procedure must be completed within 60 to 75 seconds to insure that the working time of the material has not been exceeded.

The presence of voids is a greater problem in composite resin restorations than in unfilled acrylic resin restorations. The material is relatively viscous and does not flow readily; therefore, it tends to trap air. Voids within the body of the restoration reduce the strength and impair the esthetics. A void at the margin is particularly serious, since such an area would be exceedingly vulnerable to secondary caries. The technique of inserting the material should be one that will minimize trapping of air. If a void is apparent, it may be necessary to remove the material and insert a new restoration.

Contour of the restoration is achieved by use of a properly prepared matrix, which is held in place until the material hardens.

The light-cured composites do give the clinician more latitude in technique and ease of manipulation. The mix of the components is made and inserted into the preparation. In the case of the preactivated products, the paste is merely wiped into the prepared cavity. When placement is completed, a matrix, if required, is adjusted and the light source is applied for the prescribed time. Ultraviolet light and visible light sources designed for intraoral use in curing a light-activated resin restoration are shown in Figure 14–4. The light intensity incident on the surface of the restoration is dependent on the source and the distance of that source from the restoration. Intensity varies inversely as the square of the distance. Therefore, the light must be held close to but not touching the restoration.[17]

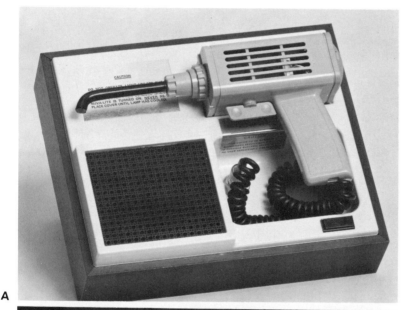

A

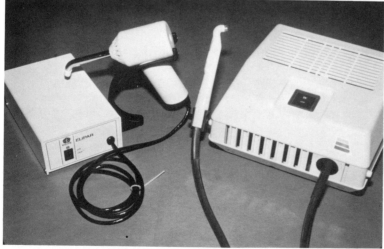

B

Figure 14–4   *A*, An ultraviolet light for polymerization of restorative resins. *B*, Two devices for polymerizing resin with visible light.

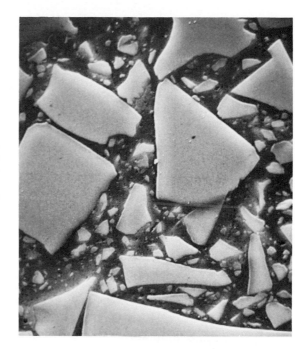

Figure 14–5 Scanning electron microscope picture of the surface of a composite resin after finish. The resin matrix has been abraded away but the hard filler particles have not been worn. The result is a rough surface. (Original magnification 1800 ×.)

Finishing   There is not complete agreement as to the time that should elapse following insertion of the resin and final finishing. Most manufacturers state that finishing can be initiated upon removal of the matrix, 5 minutes or so from the start of the mix or 1 minute after removal of the light in the case of a light activated system. However, some have suggested that when finishing is delayed for 24 hours better marginal adaptation is achieved. Despite these observations, finishing is usually done at the same seating that the restoration is placed.

The traditional composites are very difficult to finish. The fillers are exceedingly hard and resistant to abrasion, while the resin matrix is soft and abrades readily. Thus, during finishing, the resin matrix wears away rapidly, leaving the hard filler virtually untouched so that the particles project above the resin, as can be seen in Figure 14–5. The end result is a rough surface that is susceptible to the accumulation of debris and plaque.[18] The ease of finishing varies with the different products, depending upon the size, hardness, and fracture resistance of the filler particles. The smoothest finish that can be achieved on the surface of composite restorations is that left by the matrix band.

Optimal instruments and agents for providing a truly acceptable finished surface have not as yet been developed. However, 12-fluted burs are commonly used. Final finishing can be done with white rubber abrasive points lightly coated with silicone grease, a rubber cup and pumice paste, or aluminum oxide and zirconium silicate strips or discs.

Glazing agents consisting of dilute solutions of BIS-GMA, or whatever the resin matrix might be of the composite itself, are marketed for the purpose of alleviating roughness in the finished composite restoration surface. The glazing agent is painted on the surface of the restoration after final finishing to provide a smooth coating. For a period of time the glazes will accomplish that goal. However, since the glazing agents are resins, their resistance to abrasion, i.e., that produced by a tooth brush and dentifrice, is no greater than that of the composite resin matrix itself. Although disagreement[19, 20] still exists as to the length of time that glazed restorations will retain their initial smoothness, the application of a glaze agent is not contraindicated.

Clinical Behavior   One of the advantages of the conventional composites is their ease of manipulation. The paste form of the resin and the lower polymerization shrinkage facilitate the use of the convenient pressure or bulk technique for insertion of the resin, rather than the somewhat complicated bead-brush technique that is usually recommended for use with the unfilled acrylic resins. The esthetics of the materials is acceptable.

When color stability is tested in the usual manner by exposing specimens to UV light, the composites show little color shift. However, with time, slight yellowing is often observed in clinical restorations. (Recall that the clinical significance of in vitro color stability tests was discussed earlier in this chapter.) In addition to such color change within the material, discoloration may also be due in part to surface stain that results from the rough surface that remains after finishing. On occasion, discoloration is seen at the margins of the restoration which would suggest some loss of adaptation of the material to the tooth with time. However, the use of the acid etching techniques, to be described, provides a better resin-enamel bond and could reduce the incidence of marginal stain.

Although the strength properties are in general inferior to those of dental amalgam, gross fracture seldom occurs, even if the resin is used in Class II restorations which are subjected to masticatory stress. Neither does marginal breakdown appear to be a problem with composites, even when used for posterior restorations.

However, in time such resins often show definite evidence of wear.[21, 22] The wear is manifested by a change in the anatomical contour of the restoration. In Class IV restorations, wear is seen by loss of resin at the incisal. This observation may seem somewhat surprising, since abrasion resistance tests employing brushing of the resin by a tooth brush and abrasive slurry show superior wear resistance for the composite as compared with amalgam. However, as was discussed in Chapter 3, wear is a complex mechanism, involving an interaction of properties of both the abrading substance and the substrate that is being abraded, in this case the composite. Therefore, tooth brushing tests predict only the ability of the material to withstand that particular type of attrition and not necessarily that induced by opposing dentition and/or food stuffs.

The exact causative factor involved in this loss of material in stress-bearing restorations has not been identified but it probably involves a number of mechanisms. Unquestionably some of it may be attributed to a loss or "plucking" out of the filler particles under masticatory attrition. Research progresses on better coupling agents to retain the filler in the resin binder. Since the wear pattern is usually typified as a general erosion of the entire occlusal surface, it is possible that a chemical corrosion of some type also occurs in the resin binder. This leads to a loss of the resin itself.

There is a great deal of research now focused upon the development of a wear resistant composite for use in posterior teeth. One 3-year clinical study, making use of a strontium glass filled BIS-GMA resin, showed minimal wear in Class II restorations.[23] However, until there is additional documentation as to the performance of that system, the dentist is well advised to use restraint in substituting composite resins for amalgam in those situations. If esthetics is a predominant consideration and if the preparation is small, as in a bicuspid, then in such selected cases such a resin might be employed. However, the restoration should be checked periodically and replaced if a change in contour is noted. It should be emphasized that a Class II resin restoration is a difficult one in terms of the design and placement of a matrix to insure proper contour, and control of the insertion technique in order to attain good mechanical bonding of the resin to the cavity preparation.

MICROFILLED COMPOSITES

The newest series of composite resins is based upon the use of extremely small inorganic filler particles, and they are referred to as *microfilled, microfine,* or occasionally as *polishable* composites. The rationale for their development is that the small filler particles permit the resin to be finished to a much smoother surface than is possible with the coarse fillers found in the traditional composites. Thus, they are sometimes referred to as polishable composites. Representative commercial microfilled resins are shown in Figure 14–1.

Resin Matrix   The resins that serve as a matrix for these materials are the same as those in use for the conventional composites, BIS-GMA and/or adducts thereof. Several of the commercial products employ urethane dimethacrylate as the principal resin constituent. The resins are polymerized by the traditional peroxide-amine induction system.

Fillers   The microfilled resins differ from conventional composites primarily with respect to filler size and, in most instances, the manner in which the filler is incorporated into the resin paste.

The filler is pyrolytic or precipitated silica particles in the range of 0.04 to 0.06 μm, which is below the wavelength of visible light. If one assumes an average size of 20 μm for the fillers of conventional composites, such filler particles would have a diameter 500 times greater than the silica particles in the microfilled resins.

The silica particles may be dispersed directly into the resin paste as is done with the fillers of conventional composites. However, in order to increase the filler load, the filler particles, surface treated with a coupling agent, are predispersed in monomer in conjunction with chloroform. The chloroform is evaporated and the monomer polymerized to leave an agglomeration of silica filler (approximately 60 per cent by weight) in a polymerized binder. This is then pulverized by the manufacturer into particles that are approximately the size of particles of the quartz in a typical composite, for example. These particles of polymerized resin, which contain the inorganic colloidal silica filler, are then incorporated into a resin binder that may or may not also include a certain amount of colloidal silica.

The structure of the microfilled composite resin is diagrammed in Figure 14–6. Since the polymerized resin particles are dispersed in the pastes, this type of dispersion is sometimes referred to as an "organic filler." Obviously this is not strictly so since the inorganic colloidal silica is present in the "organic" resin fragments.

The ultrafine particle size markedly increases the surface area. Therefore, not as much filler can be incorporated and still maintain proper rheological characteristics. The filler concentration ranges from approximately 34 per cent

Filler (<50μ)
[60% SiO₂ (<.10μ) + BIS - GMA]

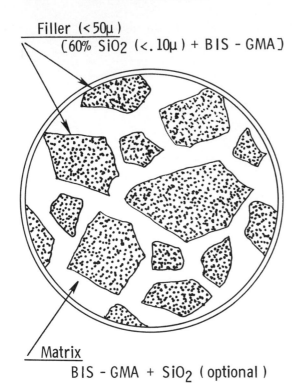

Figure 14–6 Diagram illustrating the structure of a microfilled resin.

Matrix
BIS - GMA + SiO₂ (optional)

by weight up to 50 per cent, as compared with 70 or 80 per cent for conventional composite resins.

Another type of resin system being marketed makes use of a very small particle size inorganic filler (1–5 μm), and generally it contains a small percentage of microfine filler as well. These are often referred to as "small particle" filled resins. Obviously this combination is used in an effort to capture the physical properties of the conventional composite and yet attain a relatively smooth surface. After finishing, the surface of such resins is considerably smoother than that of the traditional composite but not quite as smooth as that of a true microfilled material.

Physical and Mechanical Properties The outstanding characteristic of the microfine resins is, of course, the extremely smooth finished surface on the restoration. As has been discussed previously, surface roughness and the resultant problems of stain and plaque collection have constituted a major problem with conventional composite resins. During finishing, the cutting tool or abrasive instrument continually encounters the relatively large filler particles, which are harder and have greater abrasion resistance than does the surrounding resin matrix. As a consequence, the resin material is abraded away and the filler is either left standing above the matrix or plucked out, producing the rough surface as is diagrammed in Figure 14–7.

In the microfilled resins the filler particles are smaller than the abrasive particles used for finishing the restorations. Thus the silica filler is removed along with the resin in which it is embedded, possibly as shown in Figure 14–8. Even if the particles should be dislodged they are so small that the irregularities could not be detected by the eye or with a tactile instrument such as an explorer.

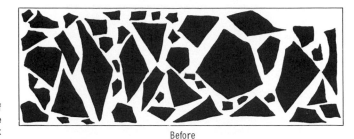

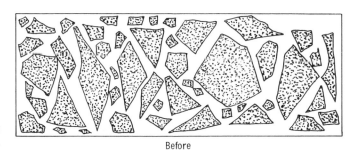

Figure 14–7 Diagram of the surface of a conventional composite resin before and after finishing. Note that the matrix has been worn away by the finishing procedure, leaving some filler particles projecting above the surface while others have fallen out.

The superior smoothness of the finished surface of the microfilled resin (Fig. 14–9) as compared with that of a conventional composite resin (Fig. 14–5) is obvious. Certainly this superior surface following finishing has appealed to the profession and resulted in a rapid growth in the popularity of the microfilled materials.

Generally, when changes are made in the formulation of a material in order to enhance one characteristic, other properties are altered. In the case of the microfilled composites, the improvement in surface finish is accompanied by a certain degree of trade-off in other traits. The differences that are to be cited in properties between the conventional composite and the microfilled system are principally related to the lower inorganic filler concentration, or higher resin content, of the microfilled materials. In certain properties the microfilled resins do not meet requirements set forth for Type II resins in the American Dental Association specification.

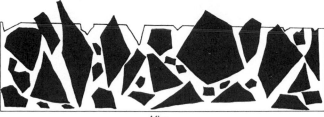

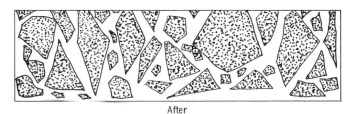

Figure 14–8 Diagram of the surface of a microfilled resin before and after finishing. Note that the finishing procedure produces a smoother surface, since the matrix and filler are cut at the same rate.

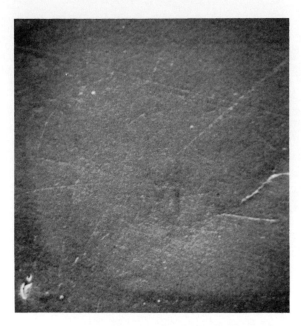

Figure 14–9 Scanning electron microscope picture of the surface of a microfilled resin after finishing. The surface is quite smooth. (Original magnification 1800 ×.)

The polymerization shrinkage may not be greatly different from that of conventional composite resins (Table 14–1). However, because of the higher resin content, the coefficient of thermal expansion is higher. Therefore, the thermal differential between the tooth and material is greater than that of the conventional composites but it is less than that of unfilled materials (Table 14–2).

The compressive strength of the microfilled resins is not adversely affected since it is as high as or higher than that of conventional composite (Table 14–1). However, the remaining properties generally tend to fall into a range between that of the conventional composite and unfilled resin.[24, 25] The tensile strength and modulus of elasticity are greater than that of the unfilled acrylic but less than that of the conventional composite. The average hardness is approximately 25 KHN as compared with an average value of 55 for conventional composites (Table 14–3). Although water sorption values vary to some degree from one product to another, the increased resin content as compared with conventional composites results in appreciably higher water sorption. It is comparable to that of unfilled resins.

When specimens of microfilled resins are exposed to UV light, as well as when stored in water at elevated temperatures, they have a greater tendency to change color (yellow) than do conventional composites or the unfilled acrylic resins polymerized by the sulfinic acid induction system. Also, tooth brush wear tests indicate that the microfilled resins might be somewhat more vulnerable to that type of abrasion than are conventional composite resins.[24]

Biological Properties   The degree of pulpal response irritation produced by microfilled resins is comparable to that of conventional composite resins. Therefore, the same protective measures should be exercised as was recommended with the other restorative resins; i.e., a calcium hydroxide base should be used in a deep cavity.

Manipulation   The microfilled resins usually are supplied as two pastes, just as are most chemically activated conventional composite resins. As shown in

Figure 14–1, the pastes are packaged in jars or syringes to facilitate dispensing two pastes in equal amounts. Also, the technique of mixing and insertion into the cavity is the same as described for those materials, and the same precautions should be observed with respect to porosity and voids in the restoration. Actually, microscopic subsurface porosity is more obvious in the microfilled resins than in the conventional composites but this may well be due to the greater translucence of the material.

Clinical Behavior There is no doubt that the dentist and often the patient appreciate the smooth finished surface that can be achieved in microfilled resin restorations. However, whether factors such as increased water sorption, a greater tendency for color change, and lower hardness and modulus of elasticity as compared with conventional composite resins will compromise clinical performance warrants further investigation and experience with these materials.

ACID ETCH TECHNIQUE

It should be apparent to the reader that the problem of microleakage is more acute with restorative resins than it is with any other type of material. Most provide some type of mechanism to counteract marginal leakage. For example, amalgam forms corrosion products along the tooth-restoration interface to provide a mechanical seal (see Fig. 3–16). Fluorides are present in some materials, as will be discussed in later chapters, and act beneficially to inhibit secondary caries.

However, the present direct restorative resins are inert and have no built-in capability to resist the dangerous effects of marginal penetration of deleterious agents. This is not to intimate that such materials do not serve a useful function in many areas of restorative dentistry. Rather, it is meant to emphasize that they are "unforgiving." A high premium for success is the attainment of good mechanical bonding to tooth structure and to maintain it in the heroic oral environment. This is the challenge to the dentist and the auxiliary.

One of the most effective ways of improving the marginal seal and mechanical bonding of the resin to tooth structure is to condition or pretreat the enamel with an acid prior to insertion of the resin.[26] The procedure is referred to as the *acid etch technique*. It has provided an added dimension in extending the use of restorative resins, simplifying procedures, and improving clinical performance.

The following discussion touches only on the principal fundamentals associated with the procedure. In-depth treatment of the scientific basis of the technique and details of the total technology can be found in other publications.[27-29]

Mechanism The improved bonding achieved via acid etching can probably be related to a number of factors. As was seen in Chapter 3, for various reasons, enamel is a poor adherend for bonding. For example, it is covered with a microscopic layer of debris left after cavity preparation. The acid cleanses the surface of such debris, providing an opportunity for better wetting of the enamel by the resin.

Even more important, though, is that a selective dissolution of the enamel occurs during etching. While enamel is normally porous, the acid removes calcium salts, increasing both the size and number of the microspaces present. An etched surface of enamel can be seen in Figure 14–10. In this instance the centers of the enamel rods have been preferentially dissolved. Other etch patterns show an attack on the rod periphery, or on both the rod core and the periphery.

The resin can now penetrate into these surface irregularities to form resin "tags," as seen in Figure 14–11. These are polymerized taglike extrusions of resin that form *within* the enamel surface. This mechanical interlocking of the resin filaments markedly increases the resin–tooth bond strength. Varying tag lengths have been reported, depending upon factors such as methodology of measurement, etching time, and the resin used. A length probably somewhere in the range of 10 to 20 μm is reasonable.[29]

Likewise, the etching markedly increases the total surface area of the enamel, which is always desirable for maximum bonding.

The technique is particularly useful when a resin is used to restore a fractured incisor (Class IV restoration). The improved retention via the etching increases the stability of the restoration. It also simplifies the procedure, since less retention is required in the cavity preparation itself. In most situations the use of auxiliary metal pins, which were previously employed to increase retention of the resin, may also be eliminated.

The more intimate bonding of the resin to enamel should reduce the incidence of marginal stain of any resin restoration, as such discoloration is indicative of microleakage. An example of stain at the margins of a resin restoration, no doubt due to microleakage, is seen in Figure 14–12.

Etching   The dentin must be protected against the acid, particularly if the preparation is deep. Only the enamel is treated. Therefore, wherever possible a protective layer of a calcium hydroxide base is placed over the exposed dentin.

Phosphoric acid is used as the etchant. Most manufacturers supply "acid etch" kits that include solutions which vary in concentration between 30 and

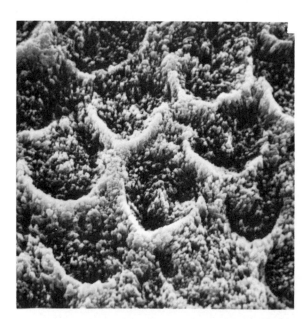

Figure 14–10 Scanning electron microscope picture of enamel surface that has been etched by phosphoric acid. (Original magnification 5000 ×.)

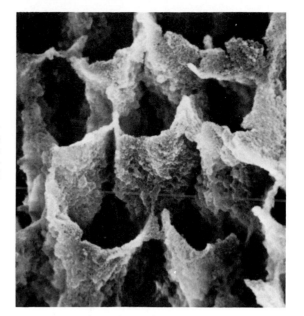

Figure 14–11 Scanning electron microscope picture of tags formed by penetration of resin into etched areas of enamel. The resin was applied to the etched enamel and the enamel was then dissolved by acid in order to reveal the tags. (Original magnification 5000 ×.)

50 per cent. Perhaps surprisingly, the depth of etch is greater at lower acid concentrations.[30] There is still some controversy as to the optimal concentration or the exact relationship between the length of resin tag and bond strength. Probably any concentration between 30 and 50 per cent is appropriate. Certainly concentrations above 50 per cent should not be used. A monocalcium phosphate monohydrate rapidly forms on the enamel which then protects the tooth from further dissolution.[31]

The acid is applied by a cotton pellet or mini-sponge, continually being dabbed gently onto the enamel. The surface should not be scrubbed or rubbed during the etchant application, as this may damage the fragile enamel latticework or simply push the decalcified material back into the pores that are being formed.

The application time varies somewhat with the particular history of the tooth. A more highly calcified mature enamel, as for an adult, or one that has a

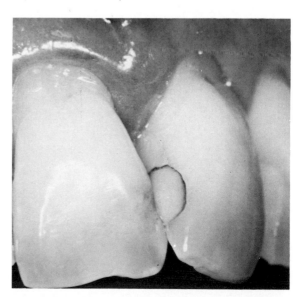

Figure 14–12 Clinical resin restoration with severe marginal discoloration, which resulted from poor adaptation and subsequent leakage. (Courtesy of J. Osborne.)

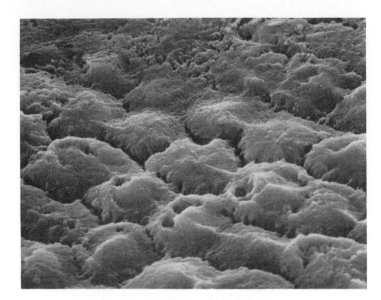

Figure 14–13 Enamel surface that has been "over-etched." Note the deposition of insoluble products on the surface. (Courtesy of J. Gwinnett.)

high fluoride content is more difficult to decalcify. Thus the optimum time to produce the topography such as seen in Figure 14–10 may differ for certain patients. Generally one minute is adequate. A properly acid-conditioned surface will have an opaque, matte appearance as compared with the glossy translucency of normal enamel. Once the enamel attains that appearance, the etching is stopped. Over-etching must be avoided since a layer of tenacious insoluble reaction product forms that prevents tag formation, as seen in Figure 14–13.

The next critical step in the technique is to remove the precipitants produced during etching by use of a stream of water. If this debris is not flushed off the enamel surface, the resin tags cannot form. The resin–enamel

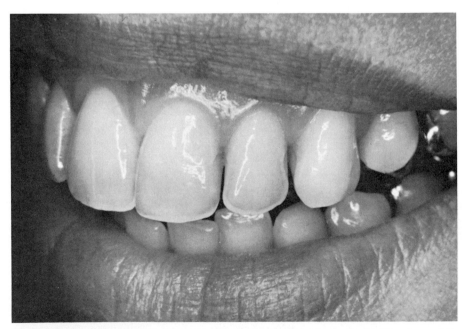

Figure 14–14 Anterior Class III resin restorations that are six years old. (Courtesy of H. Wm. Gilmore.)

bond strength is directly related to the wash time. For example, it has been shown that the mean tensile bond strength of one resin to enamel doubled when the wash time was extended from 15 seconds to 1 minute.[32] A minimum wash time of 45 seconds is recommended. The surface must then be dried for at least 15 seconds.

Any film of moisture on this cleaned surface will inhibit resin penetration into the etched area. If saliva contamination should occur, the saliva film cannot be completely removed by washing. Rather the surface should be dried, re-etched for 10 seconds, rewashed, and dried.[33]

In summary, the introduction of acid etching techniques has resulted in a simple, conservative, and more effective use of resin in many dental treatments, as will be noted in various places in this text. However, strict adherence to the basic principles of application, as described, is essential to its success.

The end result obtained by the use of a sound resin technology is a clinical restoration whose performance is most gratifying, as shown in Figure 14–14.

BONDING AGENTS

As compared with the unfilled acrylic resins, the composite resins are more viscous; hence they do not wet the tooth surface as readily. Because of the higher viscosity and the presence of the fillers, it has been theorized that they might not readily penetrate into the discrepancies produced in the enamel by acid etching. The accompanying reduction in the depth of penetration into the etched areas could reduce the resin tag length and the total surface area of the tooth in contact with the resin. In such a case the bond strength at the resin-tooth interface, mechanical retention, and marginal adaptation of the restoration could be impaired. On the basis of such reasoning, *bonding agents* were developed for use in conjunction with composite resins.

In most instances the composition of the commercial bonding agent is basically that of the matrix of its companion composite resin. Therefore, it has no true adhesion to the tooth structure. However, the resin in the bonding agent has been diluted by other monomers to a degree that it has low viscosity and readily wets the tooth surface. When painted on the cavity walls it freely penetrates into the tiny porosities produced by the acid etching where it polymerizes. It is rationalized that when the composite restorative resin is then inserted into the cavity, it will polymerize to the bonding agent present on the cavity surface. In this way, it is hoped, better adaptation to the enamel walls of the cavity is achieved with improved mechanical retention of the restoration.

Bonding agents generally are supplied as two liquids. As with the composites, the components are the same except that one contains the benzoyl peroxide initiator and the other the amine activator. A drop of each component is mixed together and a thin coat is painted onto the walls of the prepared cavity. Under no circumstance should the cavity be flooded with the bonding agent to an extent that it adds any bulk to the restoration. Because of the large amount of diluent and the lack of any filler, the properties are inferior to those of the composite resin. Naturally, a calcium hydroxide base should be placed in the deep cavity in order to prevent irritation of the pulp by the resin.

Since such bonding agents have no potential for adhesion, any benefit must occur by improvement in mechanical bonding via acid etching. The efficacy of bonding agents in improving retention and marginal seal of restorations beyond that achieved by acid etching alone is still controversial.[34-36] Some investigators have reported an additive effect in improving marginal seal and retention of composite restorations by the use of a bond agent in conjunction with acid etching. On the other hand, other studies have obtained comparable results with the acid etch technique with and without the use of a bonding agent.

The differences in these data may well be related to the degree of plasticity of the composite resin at the time it is inserted into the cavity and the matrix strip applied. If the material can be placed while the composite resin still has maximum plasticity, then the composite itself probably will penetrate readily into the etched areas and little measurable advantage will be achieved by use of a bonding agent. Conversely, if the resin has started to gel and the plasticity is reduced, the bonding agent could offer a distinct advantage in ensuring marginal seal and retention. It has been suggested that if more than one minute is required to place the composite, then a bonding agent should be used. Since clinical restorations often take at least this long to insert, routine use of a bonding agent undoubtedly provides a safety factor.

RESINS FOR RESTORING ERODED AREAS

Cervical lesions with exposed areas of cementum and dentin are not particularly common. However, when present they are of real concern to the patient. They are often unsightly and sensitive to thermal shock and/or tooth brush abrasion. The traditional method of treatment has been by the insertion of a Class V restoration, e.g., foil, resin or amalgam. Recently two more conservative procedures have become popular. One makes use of a glass ionomer cement for adhesive bonding to the underlying tooth structure, again without the use of a cavity preparation. That cement, and its use for that purpose, will be discussed in Chapter 30. The other procedure involves the use of an acid etching technique for mechanically bonding a restorative resin to tooth structure, as was just described, without the aid of retention via a cavity preparation.

At least two resins have been introduced, in conjunction with acid etching, specifically for the restoration of the so-called eroded area. Both are BIS-GMA based, while one product also advocates the use of an "adhesion promoter," which is claimed to provide a bond to the dentin and cementum. That agent is *n*-phenyl glycine-methacrylate.

If enamel is present at all the margins of the eroded area, one can anticipate a high success rate. Properly done, acid-etching will produce a sufficiently satisfactory enamel bond with any resin system to ensure a certain longevity of the restoration. Unfortunately, one seldom finds enamel surrounding the entire lesion. At the gingival margin, cementum or dentin is usually present.

As yet no satisfactory agent has been developed whereby cementum or dentin can be routinely *safely* etched in order to secure the required mechanical bonding of the resin to that surface. Thus, even though the restoration may remain in place for a year or longer because of the bond of the resin to the enamel that is present at the incisal or occlusal, microleakage is unquestionably occurring at the gingival. One should not be lulled into a false sense of security. Even though the resin may still be intact, leakage may well be occurring at the gingival margin. In time, this leakage pattern could contribute to a degradation of the bond and loss of the restoration. Equally important, it will be remembered that gross microleakage is always a possible contributor to secondary caries, pulpal irritation, and postoperative sensitivity.

Nonetheless, it is to be admitted that such a technique does merit consideration because of the conservative nature of the procedure and the esthetics of restorative resins as compared with metallic materials. Recognizing the problem that exists in the lack of an adequate bond to cementum or dentin, several suggestions can be offered if an acid etch-resin restoration is to be used. Certainly the patient should be advised that this is not a truly permanent restoration and repair or replacement may in time be required.

Relative to the technique itself, pumice pastes are often used for the initial cleansing of the area of plaque and debris. A paste should not be employed, since the glycerine type of vehicle used to make the paste may leave a film on the tooth surface even if subsequently washed and cleansed by water. That oil film will prevent proper etching of the enamel and/or wetting of the resin to the tooth. A pumice wash, not a paste, should be used.

It is also advisable to do a modest amount of instrumentation to the area.[37] At the incisal, or occlusal, a slight bevel can be placed in the enamel by a 33½ inverted cone bur, for example. The removal of the glazed surface exposes fresh enamel that is readily etched. Likewise, beveling provides the proper orientation of the enamel rods to the etching solution. The etch pattern on beveled enamel is markedly superior to that produced when the enamel rods are lying somewhat at right angles to the action of the acid. Thus the bevel will enhance retention and reduce the likelihood of marginal stain caused from microleakage.[38]

Improving the retention at the gingival is even more important, as has been discussed. This can be accomplished by a slight scoring of the cementum or dentin by means of a chisel. Not only is retention enhanced but microleakage may also be reduced.

These modest alterations to the tooth structure are valuable aids in coping with the microleakage phenomenon in such a restorative procedure, of course, in conjunction with attention to the other factors previously discussed that control the nature of the etch pattern and the bond of the resin to the enamel.

PIT AND FISSURE SEALANTS

Various materials and techniques have been advocated for preventing caries in the susceptible pit and fissure areas of molar teeth in the child patient. The most recent and most popular technique makes use of resin systems that can be applied to the occlusal surfaces of the teeth. The objective is for the resin to penetrate into the pits and fissures, polymerize, and seal these areas against the oral flora and debris. A cross-section of a tooth to which a pit and fissure sealant has been applied is shown in Figure 14–15.

Several types of resin, filled and unfilled, have been employed as pit and fissure sealants.[39] These resin systems include cyanoacrylates, polyurethanes, and the bisphenol-A-glycidyl methacrylate (BIS-GMA) reaction product. The commercially available products have been based upon either the polyurethane resin or, generally, the BIS/GMA resin. The BIS-GMA material may be polymerized in the conventional manner by means of the amine-peroxide system. At least one type of sealant makes use of light activation to accomplish polymerization.

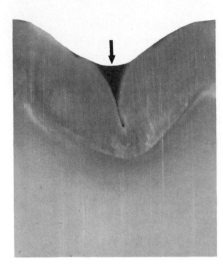

Figure 14–15 Cross section of a tooth showing penetration of a sealant into an occlusal fissure.

The success of the sealant technique is very dependent upon obtaining and maintaining an intimate adaptation of the sealant to the tooth surface and thereby hopefully sealing it. Therefore, the sealants must be of relatively low viscosity so that they will flow readily into the depths of the pits and fissures and wet the tooth. In order to enhance wetting and mechanical retention of the sealant, the tooth surface is first conditioned by etching with acid. The effects of acid etching were described earlier. The physical properties of the sealants have been investigated.[40] The properties of the sealants were closer to those of unfilled direct resins than to those of composite resins.

Reductions in occlusal caries resulting from the careful use of pit and fissure sealants have been impressive.[41, 42] Most of the studies reported involve careful case selection and meticulous application of the material to surfaces which appear to be free of caries. Apparently if the surface is noncarious and reasonably accessible it can be cleaned and etched with sufficient adequacy to provide intimate adaptation of the material and an effective seal, at least for a limited time. The in-place sealant should be examined every six months. If the sealant is entirely missing, reapplication by the recommended technique should be carried out.

If the pit or fissure is one that is not reasonably accessible, or if it is carious, it is unlikely that the surface can be cleansed sufficiently to obtain the necessary mechanical bonding of the resin to the tooth. It could be postulated that in such a situation the subsequent leakage might actually enhance the progression of caries.

Until further research resolves these and other questions, the sealant materials should be used under carefully controlled conditions, e.g., in offices where the emphasis is placed upon preventive dentistry.

CROWN AND BRIDGE RESINS

Jacket crowns and veneers for cast gold restorations are constructed from either dental porcelain (Chapter 31) or resin. The resin which has conventionally been used is poly(methyl methacrylate) or one of the acrylic resin copolymers and recently microfilled systems. In most cases, the resins are monomer-polymer mixtures, molded under heat and pressure.

The principal advantage of acrylic resin when employed for these purposes is low cost, ease of manipulation, and ability to match tooth structure. Acrylic resin is translucent in varying degrees. This translucency imparts a natural appearance in the mouth because the resin is capable of picking up the shades of the adjoining teeth. In addition, the resin restoration may be conveniently fabricated in the dental laboratory. On the other hand, the manipulation of procelain requires unusual artistic skill and considerable experience on the part of the technician.

Unfortunately, the many disadvantages of the restorative resins previously mentioned are generally enhanced in crown and bridge applications, as compared with their use in simple operative dentistry procedures. Because of low proportional limit and modulus of elasticity of the resin, it must be reinforced with a metallic framework in order to resist the stresses involved. Therefore it is used principally as a thin veneer, or facing, over a gold alloy casting. The lack of bulk and high surface area to volume ratio results in a high degree of dimensional change due to water sorption, as well as thermal dimensional change.

The acrylic resin facing does not adhere to the alloy and must be retained by mechanical means, either by cementation or by direct polymerization to metal retainers of some type. However, even though its adaptation may be adequate at first, its dimensional change during water sorption tends to reduce such adaptation. Furthermore, the considerable differential thermal expansion and contraction between the resin and the gold alloy allows considerable percolation to occur. The result is likely to be a notable leakage between the facing and the gold alloy backing, resulting in discoloration.

Of greater importance is the poor resistance of resin to abrasion. A resin veneer abrades rapidly under the retentive clasp arm of a partial denture, for example. Clinical experience has shown that acrylic resin veneers and crowns are often severely abraded during tooth brushing. For this reason, patients are advised to use a soft toothbrush, a non-abrasive tooth paste, and a proper brushing technique. Such patient education does not completely resolve the problem, however.

There are several types of resins employed for veneering cast gold restorations. The older conventional type of material is similar in composition to heat-cured denture resins. The dough is packed into a gypsum mold and then polymerized by heat. Some attempts to change the abrasion resistance have appeared in some products recently, containing other methacrylate monomers and small amounts of fine quartz particles or microfine silica in the polymer. Only marginal improvements have been noted.

As a conservative alternative to crown and bridge restorations for interim esthetic treatment, i.e., masking tooth discoloration, malformation, etc., a preformed laminate veneer system has been marketed. After contour adjustment of the prefab shell by grinding, the facing is cemented onto acid etched enamel by self-cure or ultraviolet cure sealant-type resins.

In summary, as compared with porcelain, the principal merits of current resins in crown and bridge prostheses are ease of fabrication and cost.

References

1. American Dental Association Specification No. 27 for direct filling resins. J Am Dent Assoc 94:1194, 1977.
2. Wolcott RG, Paffenbarger GC, and Schoonover IC: Direct resinous filling materials. Temperature rise during polymerization. J Am Dent Assoc 42:253, 1951.

3. Scheerer EW, Swartz ML, Norman RD, and Phillips RW: Residual monomer of restorative resins. J Dent Res 43:672, 1964.
4. Smith DL and Schoonover IC: Direct filling resins: Dimensional changes resulting from polymerization and water sorption. J Am Dent Assoc 46:540, 1953.
5. Stanford JW: The current status of restorative resins. Dent Clin North Am 15:57, 1971.
6. Harper R, Schnell RJ, Swartz ML, and Phillips RW: In vivo measurements of thermal diffusion through restoration of various materials. J Prosthet Dent 43:180, 1980.
7. Asmussen E, and Jorgensen KD: A microscopic investigation of the adaptation of some plastic filling materials to dental cavity walls. Acta Odontol Scand 30:3, 1972.
8. Bowen RL: Dental filling material comprising vinyl silane treated fused silica and a binder consisting of a reaction product of bisphenol and glycidyl acrylate. U.S. Patent No. 3066,112, Nov., 1962.
9. Bowen RL: Properties of silica reinforced polymer for dental restorations. J Am Dent Assoc 66:57, 1963.
10. Bowen RL: Compatibility of various materials with oral tissues. I: The components in composite restorations. J Dent Res 58:1493, 1979.
11. Bowen RL: Crystalline dimethacrylate monomers. J Dent Res 49:810, 1970.
12. Dennison JB and Craig RG: Physical properties and finished surface of composite restorative resins. J Am Dent Assoc 85:101, 1972.
13. Macchi RL and Craig RG: Physical and mechanical properties of composite restorative materials. J Am Dent Assoc 78:328, 1969.
14. Draughn RA: Compressive fatigue limits of composite restorative materials. J Dent Res 58:1093, 1979.
15. Heath JR and Wilson HY: Abrasion of restorative materials by toothpaste. J Oral Rehabil 4:165, 1977.
16. Leinfelder KF and Taylor DF: Current status of composite resins. North Carolina Dent J 61:17, 1978.
17. Kilian RJ: Visible light cured composite — dependence of cure on light intensity. IADR Program and Abstracts, No. 603, 1979.
18. Weitman RT and Eames WB: Plaque accumulation on composite surfaces after various finishing procedures. J Am Dent Assoc 91:101, 1975.
19. Garman TA, Fairhurst CW, Heuer GA, Williams HA, and Beglau DL: A comparison of glazing materials for composite restorations. J Am Dent Assoc 95:950, 1977.
20. Charbeneau GT, Bandau HE, and Bozell RR: A comparative clinical evaluation at two years of glaze materials with conventional finishing for composite resin. J Am Dent Assoc 60:357, 1978.
21. Phillips RW, Avery DR, Mehra R, Swartz ML, and McCune JR: Observations on a composite resin for Class II restorations: Two year report. J Prosthet Dent 28:164, 1972.
22. Leinfelder KF, Sluder TB, Sockwell CL, Strickland WD, and Wall JT: Clinical evaluation of composite resins as anterior and posterior restorative materials. J Prosthet Dent 33:407, 1975.
23. Moffa JP and Jenkins WA: Three year posterior clinical evaluation of three experimental composite resins. IADR Program and Abstracts, No. 206, 1978.
24. Swartz ML, Moore BK, Phillips RW, and Rhodes BF: Direct filling resins — a comparative study. IADR Program and Abstracts, No. 201, 1980.
25. Raptis CN, Fan PL, and Powers JM: Properties of microfilled and visible light cured composites. J Am Dent Assoc 99:631, 1979.
26. Buonocore MG: A simple method of increasing the adhesion of acrylic filling materials to enamel surfaces. J Dent Res 34:849, 1955.
27. Simonsen RJ: Clinical Application of the Acid Etch Technique. Chicago, Quintessence Publishing Co., 1978.
28. Buonocore MG: The Use of Adhesives in Dentistry. Springfield, Ill., Charles C Thomas, 1975.
29. Silverstone LM and Dogon IL (eds): The Acid Etch Technique: Proceedings of an International Symposium. St. Paul, Minn., North Central Publishing Company, 1975.
30. Silverstone LM: Fissure sealants: Laboratory studies. Caries Res 8:2, 1974.

31. Chow LC and Brown WE: Phosphoric acid conditioning of teeth for pit and fissure sealants. J Dent Res 52:1158, 1973.

32. Soetopo DR, Beech DR, and Hardwick JL: Mechanism of adhesion of polymers to acid-etched enamel. J Oral Rehabil 5:69, 1978.

33. Hormati AA, Fuller JL, and Denehy GE: Effects of contamination and mechanical disturbance on the quality of acid-etched enamel. J Am Dent Assoc 100:34, 1980.

34. Mitchum JC and Turner LR: The retentive strengths of acid-etched enamel. J Am Dent Assoc 89:1107, 1974.

35. Ortiz RF, Phillips RW, Swartz ML, and Osborne JW: Effect of composite resin bond agent on microleakage and bond strength. J Prosthet Dent 41:51, 1979.

36. Galan J, Mondelli J, and Coradazzi JL: Marginal leakage of two composite resin systems. J Dent Res 55:74, 1976.

37. Phillips RW: The restoration of eroded cervical areas. CDS Review 73:31, 1980.

38. Jordon RE, Suzuki M, Gwinnett AJ, and Hunter JK: Restoration of fractured and hypoplastic incisors by the acid etch technique: A three-year report. J Am Dent Assoc 95:795, 1977.

39. Council on Dental Materials and Devices and Council on Dental Therapeutics: Pit and fissure sealants. J Am Dent Assoc 82:1101, 1971.

40. Dennison JB and Powers JM: Physical properties of pit and fissure sealants. J Dent Res 58:1430, 1979.

41. Boudreau GE and Jerge CR: The efficacy of sealant treatment in the prevention of dental caries: A review and interpretation of the literature. J Am Dent Assoc 92:383, 1976.

42. Brooks, JD, Mertz-Fairhurst EJ, Della-Giustiana VE, Williams JE, and Fairhurst CW: A comparative study of two pit and fissure sealants: Three year results in Augusta, Ga. J Am Dent Assoc 99:42, 1979.

15 METALS: SOLIDIFICATION AND STRUCTURE

The next few chapters are devoted to an introduction to the theory of physical metallurgy. Only those principles of value to the dentist are discussed.

Metals Although metals are very common chemical elements, they are often more difficult to characterize than are other elements in the periodic table. Ordinarily, in a normal environment they are crystalline solids with the exceptions of mercury and possibly gallium (m p 30° C), which are liquids. Hydrogen, a very active metal, is, of course, a gas at normal room temperatures. If the normal room temperatures were about 982° C (1800° F), many of the ordinary metals would be liquids and some would be gases.

There are some properties of a metal that are characteristic in the solid state, however. A clean metallic surface exhibits a luster that is difficult to duplicate in other types of solid matter. A metal exhibits a certain metallic ring when it is struck, although certain silica compounds can be made to emit a similar sound. Generally, solid metals are harder, stronger, and denser than other chemical elements. They also are more ductile and malleable than the nonmetals. The unique characteristic of metals is that they are good thermal and electrical conductors.

Of the 103 elements currently listed in the periodic table of the elements, about 80 could be classed as metals. It is of scientific interest that these metallic elements group themselves into various types, e.g., light, very ductile, high melting point, noble, etc. The groupings can be seen in Table 15–1.

To the chemist and physicist all these metallic elements have one thing in common. The outermost electrons around the neutral atom are easily given up. For example, the chemist knows that sodium, zinc, and aluminum all tend to sacrifice their few valence electrons to become positive ions in solution. Also, if two different metals are the electrodes of a galvanic cell, the negative electrode, i.e., the one supplying the electrons to an outer circuit, is the more metallic. This ease of giving up the valence electrons is indeed responsible for the luster, or mirror-reflecting property, of metals and their malleability.

Most metals are "white," e.g., silver, nickel, tin, aluminum, and zinc. However, there is a slight difference in tint among the white metals and with a little practice they are distinguishable from one another. Two metals in the periodic table are nonwhite — gold and copper — and both happen to be rather important, in dentistry.

The properties of the pure elements do not change abruptly from metallic

Table 15–1. *Periodic Chart of the Elements*

Light Metals		Heavy Metals											Nonmetals					Inert Gases
1 H					High Melting												1 H	2 He
3 Li	4 Be			Brittle					Ductile				5 B	6 C	7 N	8 O	9 F	10 Ne
11 Na	12 Mg												13 Al	14 Si	15 P	16 S	17 Cl	18 A
19 K	20 Ca	21 Sc	22 Ti	23 V	24 Cr	25 Mn	26 Fe	27 Co	28 Ni	29 Cu	30 Zn	31 Ga	32 Ge	33 As	34 Se	35 Br	36 Kr
37 Rb	38 Sr	39 Y	40 Zr	41 Cb	42 Mo	43 Tc	44 Ru	45 Rh	46 Pd	47 Ag	48 Cd	49 In	50 Sn	51 Sb	52 Te	53 I	54 Xe
55 Cs	56 Ba	57-71 Rare Earths	72 Hf	73 Ta	74 W	75 Re	76 Os	77 Ir	78 Pt	79 Au	80 Hg	81 Tl	82 Pb	83 Bi	84 Po	85 At	86 Rn
87 Fa	88 Ra	89-96 Radio-Active					Noble				Low Melting						

Rare Earth Elements (Lanthanide Series)	57 La	58 Ce	59 Pr	60 Nd	61 Il	62 Sm	63 Eu	64 Gd	65 Tb	66 Dy	67 Ho	68 Er	69 Tm	70 Yb	71 Lu
Radioactive Elements (Actinide Series)	89 Ac	90 Th	91 Pa	92 U	93 Np	94 Pu	95 Am	96 Cm	97 Bk	98 Cf	99 Es	100 Fm	101 Md	102 No	103 Lw

Modified after Grosvenor AW (ed): Basic Metallurgy Principles. Cleveland, American Society for Metals, 1954, Vol. I. The preferred symbol for element 41 is now Nb.

to non-metallic as one moves to the right in the periodic chart (Table 15–1). Rather, the boundary between metals and non-metals is somewhat arbitrary, and the elements near the boundary exhibit characteristics of both metals and non-metals. The elements carbon, boron, and silicon are often alloyed with metals to form important combinations. Silicon and germanium are termed *semi-conductors* because their electrical conductivity is intermediate between that of a metal and that of a non-metal (insulator). These two elements form the basis for nearly all of the modern electronic devices.

Alloys The use of pure metals for dental purposes is quite limited. Pure metals are apt to be soft or, like iron, tend to corrode. Fortunately, metallic elements of the periodic table maintain their metallic behavior even when not pure and can tolerate a considerable addition of other elements in the liquid or solid state.

Thus, in order to optimize the properties, most of the "metals" commonly used are mixtures of two or more metallic elements. Although such mixtures can be produced in a number of ways, they are generally produced by a fusion of the metals above their melting points. Such a solid mixture of two or more metals is called an *alloy*. The early alloys evolved by trial and error, but today special purpose alloys are the result of technological skill. The metals most useful to civilization can be alloyed. A list of such metals with some of their physical constants is presented in Table 15–2.

The term "metal" is often used all-inclusively, to include alloys as well as pure metals. If the phenomenon discussed does not apply to both alloys and pure metals, a distinction should be made as to which is meant. In a later

Table 15–2.   *Physical Constants of the Alloy-forming Elements**

ELEMENT	SYMBOL	ATOMIC WEIGHT	MELTING POINT (°C)	BOILING POINT (°C)	DENSITY (gm/cc)	LINEAR COEFFICIENT OF THERMAL EXPANSION (PER °C $\times 10^{-4}$)
Aluminum	Al	26.98	660.2	2450	2.70	0.236
Antimony	Sb	121.75	630.5	1380	6.62	0.108
Bismuth	Bi	208.98	271.3	1560	9.80	0.133
Cadmium	Cd	112.40	320.9	765	8.37	0.298
Carbon	C	12.01	3700.0	4830	2.22	0.06
Chromium	Cr	52.00	1875.0	2665	7.19	0.062
Cobalt	Co	58.93	1495.0	2900	8.85	0.138
Copper	Cu	63.54	1083.0	2595	8.96	0.165
Gold	Au	196.97	1063.0	2970	19.32	0.142
Indium	In	114.82	156.2	2000	7.31	0.33
Iridium	Ir	192.2	2454.0	5300	22.5	0.068
Iron	Fe	55.85	1527.0	3000	7.87	0.123
Lead	Pb	207.19	327.4	1725	11.34	0.293
Magnesium	Mg	24.31	650.0	1107	1.74	0.252
Mercury	Hg	200.59	−38.87	357	13.55	0.40
Molybdenum	Mo	95.94	2610.0	5560	10.22	0.049
Nickel	Ni	58.71	1453.0	2730	8.90	0.133
Palladium	Pd	106.4	1552.0	3980	12.02	0.118
Platinum	Pt	195.09	1769.0	4530	21.45	0.089
Rhodium	Rh	102.91	1966.0	4500	12.44	0.083
Silicon	Si	28.09	1410.0	2480	2.33	0.073
Silver	Ag	107.87	960.8	2216	10.49	0.197
Tantalum	Ta	180.95	2996.0	5425	16.6	0.065
Tin	Sn	118.69	231.9	2270	7.298	0.23
Titanium	Ti	47.90	1668.0	3260	4.51	0.085
Tungsten	W	183.85	3410.0	5930	19.3	0.046
Zinc	Zn	65.37	420.0	906	7.133	0.397

*Compiled from Lyman T (ed): Metals Handbook, 8th ed., Cleveland, American Society for Metals, 1964, Vol. 1.

chapter, in order to understand alloying, the importance of constitutional diagrams will be discussed. However, before proceeding to alloys, the fundamentals of how a solid emerges from a melt will be described.

Metallic Bonds   As stated in Chapter 2, a third type of primary bonding exists, known as the *metallic bond*.

One of the chief characteristics of a metal, as previously noted, is its ability to conduct heat and electricity. Such energy conduction is due to the mobility of the so-called *free electrons* present in metals. The outer shell valence electrons can be removed easily from the metallic atom, leaving the balance of the electrons tied to the nucleus, thus forming a positive ion.

The free valence electrons are able to move about the metal space lattice to form what is sometimes described as an electron "cloud" or "gas." These electron "clouds" and the positive ions provide the forces of attraction that bond the metal atoms together.

The "free electrons" act as conductors of both thermal energy and electricity. They transfer energy by moving readily from areas of higher energy to those of lower energy, under the influence of either a thermal gradient or an electrical field (potential gradient).

Since both the bonding and transport properties of a metal depend on an interaction between the positive ion cores on the space lattice and the surrounding cloud of "free" electrons, one would expect the properties of a metal to be dependent on the form and dimensions of the space lattice. As an example, carbon can exist in two different crystal structures, either as graphite or as diamond. Graphite is a good electrical conductor and has metallic properties; diamond is an insulator and behaves like a non-metal. Similarly white tin, which is the familiar crystalline form, is a good metal. Gray tin, however, is a semi-conductor.

Solidification of Metals   Metals, in common with other chemical elements, can be identified by their melting points, boiling points, and similar basic physical and chemical properties. Some of these properties for most of the metals of dental interest are tabulated in Table 15–2.

The solidification phenomena that occur during the freezing of a pure metal will be considered first. The solidification of alloys will be discussed in a subsequent chapter.

If a metal is melted and then allowed to cool, and if its temperature during cooling is plotted as a function of the time, a graph similar to that in Figure 15–1 results. As can be noted, the temperature decreases regularly from A to B'. An increase in temperature then occurs to B at which time the temperature becomes constant until the time indicated by C. After C time has elapsed, the temperature decreases normally to room temperature.

The temperature T_f, as indicated by the straight or "plateau" portion of the curve at BC, is the freezing point, or solidification temperature. This is also the melting point, or *fusion temperature*. As can be noted, during melting or freezing the temperature remains constant. During freezing or solidification, heat is evolved as the metal changes from the liquid to the solid state. This

Figure 15–1 A time-temperature cooling curve for a pure metal showing supercooling.

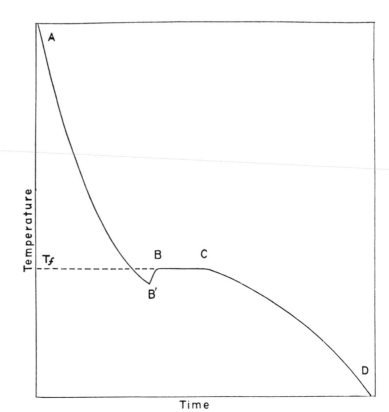

heat is the familiar *latent heat of solidification* and is equal to the *heat of fusion* studied in the course in physics. It is defined as the number of calories of heat liberated from 1 gram of a substance when it changes from the liquid to the solid state.

The interpretation of the curve in Figure 15–1 is that at all temperatures above T_f, as indicated by the plateau BC, the metal is molten, and at all temperatures below this temperature, it is a solid. The initial cooling to B′ is called *supercooling*. During the period of supercooling, the crystallization begins. Once the crystals begin to form, the latent heat of fusion causes the temperature to rise to the temperature T_f, where it remains until the crystallization is completed.

The fusion temperature of metals and alloys is of considerable interest to the dentist. Many metallic dental structures are *cast*. A *pattern* is prepared which is an exact duplication of the dental appliance or restoration to be cast. A mold is prepared from the pattern, into which a molten alloy can be forced under pressure. When the alloy solidifies, the original pattern is thus reproduced in a metallic form, known as a *casting*. The procedures and materials involved are discussed in subsequent chapters.

Nucleus Formation   Although the surface tension of liquid metals is approximately 10 times greater than that of water, molten or liquid metals are very little different in structure from any other liquids. Like other liquids, they can diffuse with a coefficient of diffusion of approximately 10^{-5} cm²/sec. Liquid metals do not differ in structure as much as do solid metals. The liquids all exhibit a tendency toward a short-range order arrangement.

As the molten metal approaches its melting temperature or "plateau" (Fig. 15–1), its energy relationships change. During supercooling below the freezing point (BC), the atoms begin to diffuse toward the regular space lattice arrangement and an interface tends to form between the liquid and the embryo solid phase.

As previously explained, the surface energy of a solid is greater than its internal energy because the unequal attraction of the surface atoms tends to draw them closer together (i.e., surface tension). It follows, therefore, that the solid space lattice arrangement cannot be permanent and a liquid-solid interface created until a proper relationship is established between the surface energy and the internal energy of the system. The internal energy can be related to what is known as the *volume free energy** which, at this stage of the solidification, is decreasing because of the change from the liquid to the solid state. On the other hand, the *surface free energy* increases as the supercooling increases (i.e., as the surrounding temperature decreases below the fusion temperature.)

The liquid state can be imagined as one of a multitude of random atoms or molecules surrounding numerous unstable atomic aggregates or clusters which are attempting to form crystal nuclei. These temporary nuclei are usually called embryos.

The embryos at high temperatures are few in number and generally very small in size. Thus, they dissolve readily back into the matrix of the random atoms. On approaching the solidification temperature these embryos increase in density and get larger, but they are still unstable and tend to dissolve into the matrix. However, once the supercooled region is penetrated, there is a

*For the benefit of the advanced chemistry student, the volume free energy is the Gibbs free energy in this case.

tendency for some of these embryos to survive and thus form a *solidification nucleus.*

To understand this in detail one needs to make use of the discipline of thermodynamics. Fortunately, there is a rather revealing device that makes the mechanism of nucleation relatively easy to understand. The phenomenon may be explained by a study of Figure 15–2.

Imagine an embryo to be a sphere of radius γ, as scaled on the horizontal axis in the figure. Envision about 50 atoms making up such an enbryo at the start. The vertical axis is the difference in the average useful energy per atom as compared with that which it possesses at precisely the melting temperature (the pressure is assumed to be constant). The word "useful" is somewhat important, as this energy must be used in order for the nucleus to form. This free energy is positive in the upper half of the graph and negative in the lower half. At the horizontal line it is zero, i.e., there is true equilibrium between liquid and solid.

Three curves are shown, all three representing a specific amount of supercooling. The volume free energy of the embryo is shown in curve F_v. The atoms in the interior of the embryo have a little negative free energy. Since the number of atoms in a sphere is proportional to the value of r^3, the negativity of this curve increases rapidly as the radius gets larger. Because it would take "work" to break up the embryo, it desires to be stable when the free energy is very negative.

Meanwhile, something else is going on. The surface of the embryo is also increasing. Every surface atom has a little positive surface free energy, because it takes "work" to hold an atom on the surface of the embryo away from the interior. (It has a compulsion to hide within the embryo, where less energy is needed to remain immersed among its neighbors.) The curve F_s represents the increase in the surface free energy as a function of the increase in the radius of the embryo.

Now, since the embryo is ambiguously increasing and decreasing in its free energy while it is growing, one would like to know what the net result will

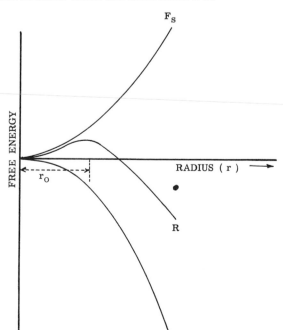

Figure 15–2 Free energy of formation of a nucleus as a function of its radius.

be. As the surface energy increases proportionately to only the square of the radius, the F_s curve goes up mildly with the increase in radius. This means that eventually the steeply descending F_v curve dominates the situation and the embryo becomes stable.

The curve R is drawn to represent the resultant free energy existing at any instant. The *critical radius,* indicated as r_0 in the figure, is the embryo radius obtained when the resultant free energy first begins to decrease with an increase in radius. It is also the minimal radius at which a *nucleus of crystallization,* or the first permanent solid space lattice, is formed.

The greater the supercooling, or the rate of temperature decrease, the smaller is this critical radius, r_0. Hence, more and more embryos are stable as supercooling is increased. If the melt is cooled rapidly so that solidification must occur at a low temperature, there will be a tendency for many solidification centers to form. If one wants a single crystal, very little supercooling is needed.

This general method of nucleus formation is called *homogeneous nucleation* since the formation of nuclei in the molten metal is a random process and has equal probability of occurring at any point in the melt.

Another method for reducing the surface energy of the embryo is for the atoms to contact some surface or particle or particles in the melt which it can wet; thus, the surface energy can be reduced and a nucleus formed. Such a process is known as *heterogeneous nucleation,* heterogeneous because a foreign body "seeded" the nucleus. For example, if the metal is gold, very fine particles of gold sifted into the molten metal can cause nucleation. Even the walls of the containing vessel or particles of dust and other impurities in the melt may produce heterogeneous nucleation.

It should be noted that supercooling is not necessary for heterogeneous nucleation. In fact, this type may account for most of the nucleation, with no supercooling being observed. The uniformity of distribution of heterogeneously formed nuclei is difficult to control because the distribution of the "seeds" is not likely to be uniform.

Mechanism of Crystallization   The crystallization is effected by atomic diffusion from the melt to the nuclei. The crystals do not form regularly, a plane at a time, but rather the atomic diffusion to lattice positions is pictured as being irregular, with lattice discontinuities and imperfections being constantly formed or repaired randomly.

Characteristically, a pure metal may crystallize treelike from a nucleus. Such crystal formations are called *dendrites.* In three dimensions, they are not unlike that of the two-dimensional frost crystals that form on a window pane in the winter. Figure 15–3 shows the dendritic structure that can be seen in alloys.

A schematic representation of such a crystallization in two dimensions is shown in Figure 15–4. As can be observed, the growth starts from the nuclei of crystallization, and the crystals grow toward each other. When two or more crystals collide in their growth, the growth is stopped. Finally, the entire space is filled with crystals as diagrammed in Figure 15–4F. However, each crystal remains a unit in itself. It is oriented differently from its neighbors. The metal is, therefore, made up of thousands of tiny crystals. Such a metal is said to be *polycrystalline* in nature, and each crystal is known technically as a *grain.*

If any metal is highly polished, and if the polished surface is etched with an appropriate reagent, the grain structure can be made visible in a microscope. The *photomicrograph* of the grain structure of a gold ingot prepared in

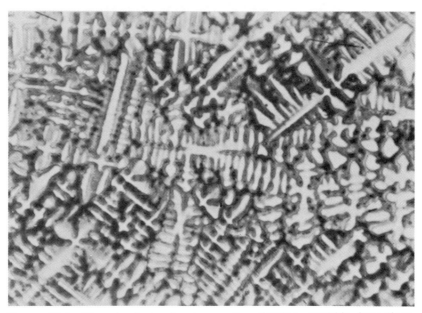

Figure 15–3 Microstructure of a brass alloy showing dendritic formations. (From Eisenstadt MM: Introduction to Mechanical Properties of Materials, New York, Macmillan Co. 1971.)

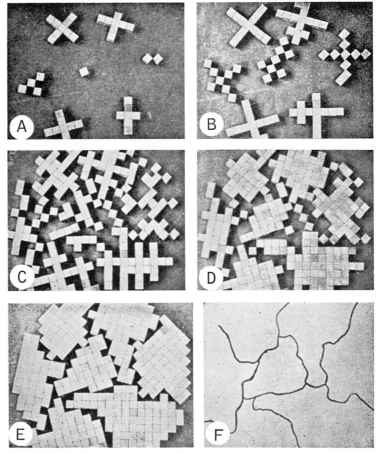

Figure 15–4 Stages in the formation of metallic grains during the solidification of a molten metal. (From Rosenhain: Introduction to Physical Metallurgy, 3rd ed., Constable and Co., Ltd., 1935.)

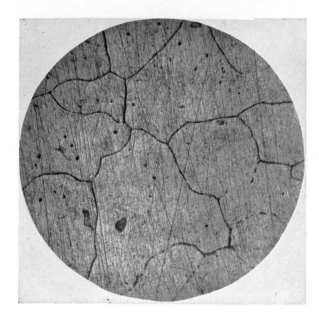

Figure 15–5 Microstructure of an ingot of gold. × 100. (Courtesy of S. D. Tylman.)

this manner is shown in Figure 15–5. The resemblance between the grain structure in Figure 15–5 and that of the diagram in Figure 15–4*F* is evident. The lines in Figure 15–5, somewhat indistinct in certain areas, represent the periphery of the grains, or the boundaries at which the grains met during their original growth.

Grain Size   The size of the grains depends upon the number and location of the nuclei at the time of the solidification. If the nuclei are equally spaced with reference to each other, the grains will be approximately equal in size.

The solidification can be pictured as proceeding from the nuclei in all directions at the same time in the form of a sphere which is constantly increasing in diameter. When these spheres meet, they are flattened along various surfaces. The tendency for each grain to remain spherical still exists, however, and the grain tends, therefore, to be the same diameter in all dimensions. Such a grain is said to be *equiaxed*. Dental castings generally tend to exhibit an equiaxed grain structure, and such a structure is of considerable dental importance.

Control of Grain Size   In general, the smaller the grain size of the metal, the better are its physical properties. For example, the yield strength of many types of materials has been found to vary inversely with the square root of the grain size. Consequently, obtaining a small grain size during casting is an advantage.

Because the grains crystallize from nuclei of crystallization, it follows logically that the number of grains formed is directly related to the number of nuclei of crystallization present at the time of solidification. As pointed out, this factor can be controlled to a degree by the amount of supercooling and the rate of cooling. In other words, the more rapidly the liquid state can be changed to the solid state, the smaller or *finer* the grains will be.

Another factor of equal importance is the rate of crystallization. If the crystals form faster than do the nuclei of crystallization, the grains will be larger than if the reverse condition prevails. Consequently, if the nuclear formation occurs faster than the crystallization, a small grain size can be obtained. Conversely, a slow cooling results in large grains. For example, some

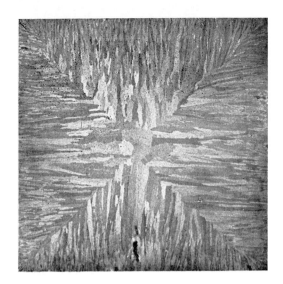

Figure 15–6   Metallic grains formed by the solidification of a metal in a square mold. (From Williams and Homerberg: Principles of Metallography, 5th ed., New York, McGraw-Hill Book Co., Inc., 1948.)

metals can be held at their fusion temperatures and caused to crystallize in contact with a crystal or "seed" of the metal. If the crystal is withdrawn at a constant speed as the crystallization proceeds, a rod or bar made up of a single grain can be formed. Such a metal is known as a *single crystal* in contrast to the polycrystalline form usually present.

In a polycrystalline metal, the shape of the grains may be influenced by the shape of the mold in which the metal solidifies. The latent heat of solidification of the metal must be absorbed by the surroundings. This heat transfer requires the existence of temperature gradients, which in turn greatly influence the size and shape of the solidifying grains. For example, if a metal solidifies in a square mold that is at a temperature considerably below the melting temperature of the metal, the crystal growth may proceed from the edges to the center, as shown in Figure 15–6. The grains are called *columnar grains* and are the result of heterogeneous nucleation. If the mold had been cylindrical, the grains would have grown perpendicular to the wall surface, thereby giving the radial grain structure appearance. Such grains are called *radial grains*.

Grain Boundaries   As previously noted, the orientation of the space lattice of the various grains is different, although each grain may possess the same space lattice as its neighbor. The probability is very small for two neighboring grains to grow from different nuclei and to meet so that the planes of their space lattices join in exact continuity. Consequently, there must be a discontinuity of lattice structure at the *grain boundaries,* as this area is designated.

It follows logically that the structure of the grain boundaries is different from that in the grain proper. The grain boundary is assumed to be a region of transition between the differently oriented crystal lattices of the two neighboring grains. The structure is more nearly noncrystalline, particularly toward the central region of the grain boundary. This region, therefore, must be considered to be of higher energy than the interior of the grain. Its tendency toward amorphism indicates a possible greater rate of diffusion. As a consequence, impurities in the metal may be found in greater concentration at the grain boundaries than in the grain proper. Also, the region is more readily attacked by chemicals, as indicated by the photomicrograph in Figure 15–5.

16 WROUGHT METAL: DEFORMATION. STRAIN HARDENING. RECRYSTALLIZATION AND GRAIN GROWTH

In the preceding chapter, the discussion was limited to cast metal. Most of the dental structures placed in the mouth are castings. However, wires are used by the orthodontist and are sometimes used for clasps in connection with partial dentures. Wires are not castings. Rather, wires are made from castings by drawing a cast metal through a die. Many of the accessory dental materials and tools have been rolled to form plate metal, or forged or ground to form knives, burs, and many other dental instruments.

Whenever a casting is worked in any manner to form any type of structure of a different type or shape, it is no longer a cast metal, but rather it becomes a *wrought metal,* and it exhibits certain metallurgical phenomena not generally associated with a cast structure. The differences are so marked that the dentist should always analyze any situation presented in terms of whether he or she is concerned with cast metal or wrought metal before proceeding with any dental operation or procedure.

Although, as stated, most dental appliances are of cast metal, the proper treatment of the many wrought metal tools employed in the preparation of the oral structures for the reception of the cast dental appliance is of equal importance to the success of the operation as the fabrication of the appliance itself. Actually, if one considers the many useful metallic articles encountered in everyday life, most of them are wrought metal and are not castings, although all wrought metal structures originate from cast metal.

Deformation of Metals In Chapter 3, it was assumed that two types of deformation may exist according to the stress-strain curve. At stresses below the proportional limit, it was assumed that the atoms in the crystal lattice are displaced in amount only so that, when the stress is relieved, they can return to their original positions. However, once the proportional limit is exceeded, a permanent deformation takes place and the structure does not return to its original dimensions when the load is released. Eventually, this displacement becomes so great that the atoms are separated completely and a fracture results.

A simple model illustrating plastic deformation of a *perfect* lattice under an applied shear stress is illustrated in Figure 16–1. Notice that the deformation or "slip" process requires the simultaneous displacement of an entire plane of atoms A relative to the plane B below it. If the elastic modulus in shear for a given metal is known, this model can be used in a very simple

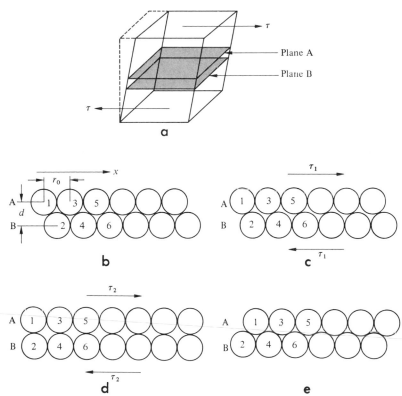

Figure 16–1 Slip between adjacent planes of atoms. *(a)* A solid subjected to a shear stress. Planes A and B are adjacent. *(b)* The configuration of planes A and B when the solid is not stressed. *(c)* Application of a shear stress, τ_1, causes plane A to move with respect to plane B. *(d)* Increasing the shear stress increases the relative displacement of the two planes. This configuration corresponds to the maximum storage of elastic energy. *(e)* The two planes have been displaced by a distance r_0 with respect to each other. This configuration will be maintained if the load is removed. If the load remains, the planes will continue to slip past each other. (From Eisenstadt MM: Introduction to Mechanical Properties of Materials. New York, Macmillan Co., 1971, p 175.)

calculation to determine the maximum theoretical shear strength of the metal.

Unfortunately, when this is done, the results are not even close to the strength values measured on bulk polycrystalline materials. As can be seen in Table 16-1, the discrepancies are on the order of 40 to 150 times larger for the calculated values. In fact, values approaching the theoretical shear strengths

Table 16–1. *Theoretical and Observed Shear Strength*

MATERIAL	SHEAR MODULUS (*psi*)	OBSERVED ULTIMATE SHEAR STRENGTH (POLYCRYSTALLINE) (*psi*)	CALCULATED ULTIMATE SHEAR STRENGTH (*psi*)	OBSERVED ULTIMATE SHEAR STRENGTH (WHISKER) (*psi*)*
Copper	7.0×10^6	32,000	1,120,000	302,000
Iron	11.6×10^6	42,000	1,805,000	1,380,000
Nickel	11.0×10^6	69,000	1,750,000	395,000
Al_2O_3	24.7×10^6		3,950,000	2,120,000
BeO	19.7×10^6	40,000 (tension)	3,150,000	1,340,000
SiC	29.3×10^6	25,000 (tension)	4,690,000	2,120,000

*The shape of the whiskers is not conducive to shear testing. The tabulated values were calculated from tensile strength data given by Broutman IJ and Krock RH: Modern Composite Materials, Reading, Mass., Addison Wesley, 1967. (Table from Eisenstadt MM: Introduction to Mechanical Properties of Materials. New York, Macmillan Co., 1971.)

are found only in measurements made on "whisker" specimens. These are tiny single-crystal filaments (approximately 2.5 μm in diameter) and are used as reinforcing agents in various commercial composite materials. They have been investigated for dental applications.[1]

The key to the difference in behavior of the "whiskers" and bulk polycrystalline specimens of the same material is the presence of *lattice imperfections* in the bulk material. Whiskers have nearly perfect lattice structures.

Lattice Imperfections   As described in the preceding chapter, crystallization from the nucleus does not occur in a regular fashion, lattice plane by lattice plane. Instead, the growth is likely to be more random, with some lattice positions left vacant and others overcrowded with atoms deposited interstitially between neighboring atoms and out of line with the principal lattice planes. These imperfections may be of many types, but they can be generally classified as *point defects* or *line defects.*

The defects already described are point defects; the simpler types are diagramed in Figure 16–2. Vacancies may occur in the space lattice singly, as shown in *a,* or two or more vacancies may condense as a di-vacancy or tri-vacancy, as shown in *b.* An interstitial point defect is illustrated in *c.*

It should be remembered that each defect results in a change in energy in the space lattice at its point of occurrence. The ultimate result is, of course, a weakening effect in regard to cleavage strength but a strengthening so far as further deformation is concerned.

Vacancies are sometimes referred to as equilibrium defects, since a crystal lattice that is in equilibrium will contain a certain number of these defects. The vacancy fraction depends on the temperature of the lattice and increases with increasing temperature. The presence of vacancies is necessary for the process of diffusion in a solid metal.

Dislocations   Probably the chief difference in physical properties between the single "perfect" crystal and the polycrystalline form is due to the formation of line defects or *dislocations* in the latter.

The simplest type of dislocation, known as an *edge dislocation,* is illustrated diagrammatically in Figure 16–3a. It can be noted that the lattice is regular except for the one plane of atoms that is discontinuous, forming a *dislocation line* at the edge of the half plane.

Dislocations are not equilibrium defects and the formation of a dislocation requires significant energy, which is stored in the strained crystal lattice surrounding the defect.

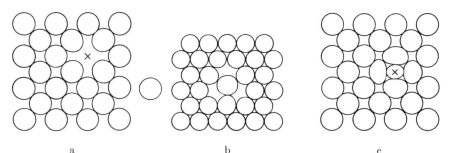

a   b   c

Figure 16–2   Point defects: *(a)* vacancies; *(b)* di-vacancy (two missing atoms); *(c)* interstitial. (From Van Vlack: Elements of Materials Science, 4th ed., Reading, Mass., Addison-Wesley Publishing Co., Inc., 1980.)

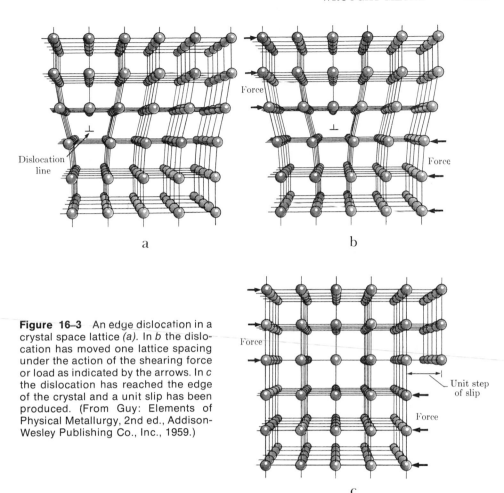

a

b

Figure 16–3 An edge dislocation in a crystal space lattice *(a).* In *b* the dislocation has moved one lattice spacing under the action of the shearing force or load as indicated by the arrows. In *c* the dislocation has reached the edge of the crystal and a unit slip has been produced. (From Guy: Elements of Physical Metallurgy, 2nd ed., Addison-Wesley Publishing Co., Inc., 1959.)

c

If a shearing force is applied to the crystal, the atoms in the plane above the dislocation easily break old bonds and establish new bonds with the lower atoms, and the dislocation shifts one lattice spacing, as indicated in Figure 16–3*b*. A continued application of the shear stress causes successive *slipping* of the atomic "edge" until finally the dislocation reaches the edge of the crystal and disappears, leaving one unit of slip at the edge of the crystal, as shown in Figure 16–3*c*. The plane along which a dislocation moves is known as a *slip plane*.

The final result is actually the establishment of equilibrium from a condition of energy concentration at the dislocation. Owing to the dislocation, the force necessary to cause the lattice deformation is very much less than it would be if a "perfect" crystal existed because only one line of atomic bonds has actually been disrupted. However, as has been shown previously, in a perfect crystal a whole plane of bonds must be ruptured to cause slipping. Thus, the difference between the tensile strength of a "whisker" and of a structure containing dislocations can be explained on the basis of lattice imperfections. Whiskers do not contain dislocations because their physical dimensions are too small to accommodate the strain field which surrounds a dislocation.

There are many other types of dislocations aside from the edge dislocation, but the mechanism of slip is essentially the same. When the slip planes occur in groups, the metal surface may become sufficiently irregular to cause a

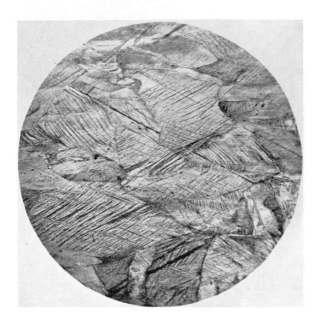

Figure 16–4 A photomicrograph of gold after cold working, showing slip bands. 100 ×. (Courtesy of S. D. Tylman.)

diffuse reflection of the light, when viewed through a metallurgical microscope, to reveal *slip bands* as shown in Figure 16–4.

Strain Hardening   So far, it has been assumed that any slip can occur in a given slip plane unimpeded so that the dislocation can be relieved. However, as might be deduced from Figure 16–3, if the dislocation during translation meets some other type of lattice discontinuity, its gliding movement under stress might be inhibited. Such discontinuities might be (1) point defects, (2) collision of one dislocation with another of a different type, (3) a foreign atom or groups of atoms of different lattice characteristics as in an alloy (see Chapter 17), or, possibly most important, (4) meeting grain boundaries in a polycrystalline metal. In addition, the process of slip consumes dislocations, as can be seen in Figure 16–3. If plastic deformation is to continue at relatively high strain rates, sources must be present within the metal in order to rapidly generate new dislocations.

In polycrystalline metal, the dislocations tend to build up at the grain boundaries. Also, the barrier action to slip at the grain boundaries causes the slip to occur on other intersecting slip planes. Point defects increase and the entire grain may eventually become distorted. Greater stress is required to produce further slip and the metal becomes stronger and harder. The process is known as *strain hardening* or *work hardening*. The latter term is derived from the fact that the process is a result of *cold work,* i.e., deformation at room temperature, in contrast to the effect of working at a higher temperature, such as in forging. In the latter case, the increase in rate of atomic diffusion occasioned by the increase in temperature may entirely prevent strain hardening. The ultimate result of strain hardening, with further increase in cold work, is fracture. This will be discussed in a later section.

The phenomenon of cold work and strain hardening is familiar to everyone. For example, one way to "cut" a wire is to bend it back and forth rapidly between the fingers. When all the slip possible has occurred, the wire fractures. When a nail is flattened with a hammer, the first few blows are quite effective. However, as the blows are continued, it is noted that they are not so effective, until finally no further deformation occurs. Instead, the metal cracks or fractures.

The surface hardness, strength, and proportional limit of the metal are increased with strain hardening, whereas the ductility and resistance to corrosion are decreased. However, the elastic modulus is not changed appreciably.

The change in physical properties of a metal effected by strain hardening is often a practical method in dentistry for the control of such properties. For example, it will be shown in another chapter that strain hardening of a gold foil restoration is necessary to provide proper strength and hardness.

An illustration of the effect on the grain structure of the flattening of a metal between rollers is shown in the first row of photomicrographs at the top of Figure 16–5. The rolling took place in a direction perpendicular to the plane of the photomicrographs, and it can be observed that the thinner the specimen, as designated above each photomicrograph, the flatter or thinner the grains appear to be. If the specimens were observed in a plane 90 degrees to that shown (i.e., parallel to the direction of rolling), the area of the grains would, of

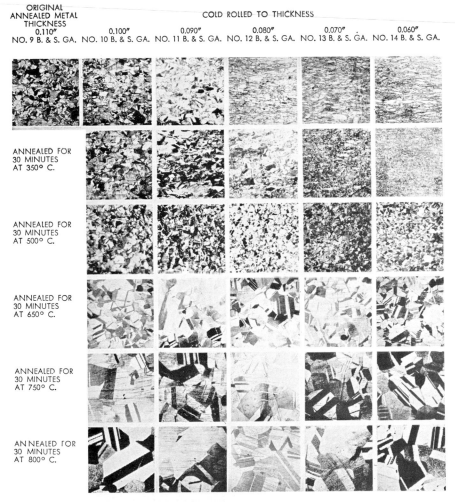

Figure 16–5 Grain size of brass (copper 66%, zinc 34%) after cold working and annealing. 40 ×. (Prepared by L. H. DeWald.)

course, be greater. Although brass was used, the same effect would be present with wrought gold alloys.

An interesting side effect of cold working or strain hardening is the tendency for preferred orientation in the distorted grain structure. The slip planes tend to line up in the shear planes of the deformation process. Thus, the strength of deformed metal, such as a rolled sheet, is usually greater in the transverse direction than in the direction of the rolling.

ANNEALING

The effects associated with cold working — e.g., strain hardening, lowered ductility, and distorted grains — can be eliminated by simply heating the metal. The process is called *annealing*. The more severe the cold working, the more readily does annealing occur.

Annealing in general comprises three stages: *recovery, recrystallization,* and *grain growth*. The effects of each of these three stages upon the tensile strength and ductility of a metal are shown in Figure 16–6. The microstructural changes that accompany such annealing were shown in Figure 16–5. Annealing is a relative process; the higher the melting point of the metal, the higher is the temperature needed for annealing. A rule of thumb is to use a temperature approximately one-half that necessary to melt the metal on the absolute temperature scale.

Recovery   Recovery might be considered the stage at which the cold work properties begin to disappear before any significant visible changes are observed in the microscope. As can be seen in Figure 16–6, during this period there is a very slight decrease in tensile strength and no change in ductility. However, there is a rather pronounced change in the recovery of the electrical conductivity. Also, a cold-worked metal is filled with stresses. Machining such material frequently results in warping. This tendency for warping on machining disappears in the recovery stage. If the deformation is mild — less than 3 per cent elongation — the anneal that takes place on heating is entirely recovery. Incidentally, this is approximately the deformation that occurs during a slight adjustment of a partial denture clasp. Orthodontic appliances fabricated by bending wrought wires are often subjected to a stress relief anneal prior to

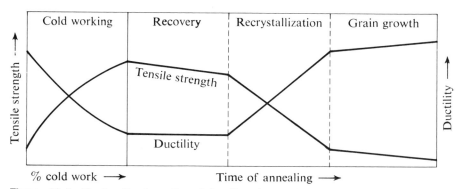

Figure 16–6   The tensile strength and ductility of a metal as a function of the per cent of cold work and annealing time. Tensile strength increases and ductility decreases during cold working. These properties change only slightly during recovery. During recrystallization the tensile strength decreases and the ductility increases rapidly. Only slight changes occur during grain growth. (From Richman MH: Introduction to the Science of Metals, Waltham, Mass., Blaisdell Pub. Co., 1967.)

their placement. Such a process stabilizes the configuration of the appliance and allows accurate determination of the force the appliance will deliver in the mouth.

Recrystallization   When a severely cold-worked metal is annealed, then recrystallization occurs after some recovery. This involves a rather radical change in the microstructure, as can be seen in Figure 16–5. It seems that recovery alone simply cannot remove the effects of excessive cold working. The old grains disappear completely and are replaced by a new set of strain-free grains. These recrystallization grains emerge from the most severely cold-worked regions in the metal, usually at grain boundaries, or where the lattice was most severely bent on deformation. The physical metallurgist interprets this as a process in which strain-free nuclei consume the severely distorted matrix faster than the matrix recovers.

On the completion of recrystallization, the material essentially attains its original soft and ductile condition (Fig.16–6).

Grain Growth   The recrystallized structure has a certain grain size, depending upon the number of nuclei. The more severe the cold working, the greater are the number of such nuclei. Thus, the grain size for the completely recrystallized material can range from rather fine to fairly coarse.

If now the fine grain form is further annealed, the grains begin to grow, as illustrated in Figure 16–5. It can be shown that this grain growth process is simply a boundary energy minimizing process. In effect, the big grains "eat up" the little grains. It does not progress indefinitely to a single crystal. Rather, an ultimate coarse grain structure seems to be reached, and then, for all practical purposes, the grain growth stops.

In any case, excessive annealing can lead to larger grains. It should be emphasized that this phenomenon occurs only in wrought materials. When a large grain structure does occur in a casting it is primarily the result of excessive casting and mold temperatures.

A large grain structure is generally detrimental to the strength properties of a metal. As previously noted, the grain boundary is a barrier to the movement of dislocations. With small or fine grains, the concentrations of inhibited dislocations per grain are greater. Consequently, with small grains a greater increase in strength, hardness, and proportional limit occurs during cold work than with large grains. However, under such a condition, it is to be expected that a lower ductility may result with smaller grains.

On the other hand, with a sufficiently large grain size, particularly in a dental appliance of small diameter or thickness, the space lattice of one large grain may be oriented in such a manner that a high ductility with a low proportional limit may result.

This effect is strikingly shown in Figure 16–7. A gold alloy rod 2.5 mm in diameter was cast. One of the grains occupied the entire cross section of the rod. A reduction in area occurred and the percentage elongation was approximately 64 per cent, whereas the average elongation was found to be 15 per cent when a typical polycrystalline structure was present. Consequently, from the standpoint of uniformity of stress distribution during cold work, the small grain size is preferred because grain orientation will be more equally distributed.

Cast Structure vs. Wrought Structure   Generally, all metals and alloys originate from castings. The composition of the alloy is determined during the

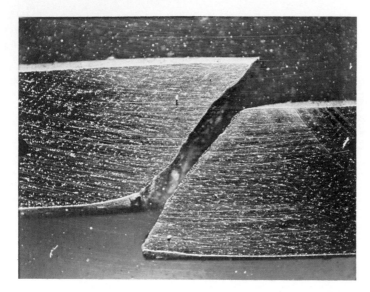

Figure 16–7 A cast rod showing a shear fracture through one large grain which occupied the entire cross-sectional area of the rod. Although ductility was high, fracture occurred because of high stress concentration. 24 ×.

casting procedure. The casting may then be machined, forged, drawn, extruded, or worked in some manner to provide the required article or appliance. It then becomes a wrought metal in contrast to a cast metal.

The influence of grain size on the physical properties of the metal is equally important in both cases. However, as described in the previous chapter, the grain size of the cast metal is normally established at the time of solidification. Apparently, the cast structure is so close to equilibrium conditions that heat treatments are virtually ineffective in changing the grain size.

Most dental appliances are cast and not wrought. Consequently, the factors that affect the grain size of the casting are very important. However, if the dentist bends a cast clasp during adjustment, for example, or burnishes the margin of a cast gold alloy inlay, the structure may be cold worked sufficiently to be changed to a wrought metal.

In the dental applications where wrought materials are used, e.g., orthodontic bands and wires, the strength values may depend on the wrought structure. An extended anneal into the recrystallization stage could seriously compromise the properties.* Prolonged heating of stainless steels to high temperatures can also markedly affect their corrosion resistance.

Such considerations become very important during soldering operations (Chapters 33 and 37) and similar procedures in which a high temperature is employed. Also, such theories should be applied during dental procedures at the chair and in the laboratory. Before heating any instrument, the dentist should consider the possibility that it might be ruined by grain growth or by other metallographic changes, to be described in a subsequent chapter.

Fracture   If the cold work is continued, the structure eventually fractures. However, as previously noted, the stress required for fracture (e.g., tensile strength) is much less in the polycrystalline metal, or in an ordinary imperfect single crystal, than would be expected theoretically.

The reason generally given for this difference is that submicroscopic

---

*It should be noted that wire should never be recrystallized, only recovery heat treated. If the fibrous grain structure is not preserved, the wire loses its identity as a wire structure.

cracks are present in the polycrystalline metal which cause stress concentrations. Such stresses, in turn, cause an elongation or propagation of the crack to rupture. Such microcracks may be the result of solidification faults or a concentration of dislocations, for example.

It is of interest that the observed tensile strength of a structure may increase with the rate of stress application because there is less time for plastic flow to occur near the microcrack, and thus to relieve the stress concentration. Such a fracture is known as a *brittle fracture* in contrast to a *ductile fracture,* in which plastic deformation of the grains can occur before fracture during a slower loading. A brittle fracture has the appearance of a more granular structure at the fracture surface than does a ductile fracture, with little necking or reduction in area at the site of the fracture.

As previously noted, the fracture is generally *transgranular* when it occurs at room temperature, rather than *intergranular,* such as occurs at elevated temperatures.

Reference

1. Grant AA and Greener EH: Whisker reinforcement of dental materials. IADR Program and Abstracts, No. 92, 1966.

17 CONSTITUTION OF ALLOYS

An alloy is defined for dental purposes as a combination of two or more metals which are generally mutually soluble in the molten condition. So far as the general principles of cast and wrought structure are concerned, the reactions of alloys are not essentially different from those of the pure metals already described. However, the addition of other metals to the pure metal complicates the picture in relation to certain fundamental aspects not yet considered.

For example, most alloys solidify over a range in temperature rather than at a single temperature as does a pure metal. Within this range a two phase (solid and liquid) system exists. The range of the solidification temperature is as typical for any one particular alloy composition as is the constant fusion temperature for the pure metal.

The presence of more than one metal may also bring about certain reactions in the solid state that cannot occur in the presence of a single metal, and that directly affect the properties of the alloy. These and other alloy phenomena will now be discussed.

Definitions A few terms that are used in metallurgy are also familiar in other branches of science. Some of these terms have been used in previous discussions. Before the technical discussion proceeds further, these terms will be explained to insure that a common ground of understanding is reached.

An alloy *system* is an aggregate of two or more metals in all possible combinations. For example, the "gold-silver system" means that all of the possible concentrations of gold with silver, and vice versa, are being considered.

From a metallurgical standpoint, a *phase* is any physically distinct, homogeneous, and mechanically separable portion of a system. Everyone is familiar with the fact that matter can exist in three different states or phases — liquid, solid, or gas. However, in metallurgy it is not uncommon to find that more than one phase is present in the solid state. For example, grains of two different compositions may be present which are mechanically separable.

Actually, the system must be in *equilibrium* before a true phase can exist.

Polycrystalline metals and alloys never reach true equilibrium conditions in the solid state. There are at least three reasons for this condition: (1) The rigidity of the metal prevents the ready diffusion of the atoms to attain equilibrium. (2) At temperatures of approximately one-half the melting temperature on the absolute scale the diffusion may be virtually arrested. If the alloy has been quenched in water from a high temperature at which the rate of atomic diffusion is considerable, an unstable structure at the high temperature may be made permanent and apparently stable at room temperature. (3) The energy at the grain boundaries described in Chapter 15 is not relieved as long as any grain boundaries persist; therefore, complete equilibrium is never attained in this area.

Nevertheless, equilibrium conditions are assumed in the subsequent discussions. The conditions to be described are approached as a limit only under conditions of slow cooling and prolonged annealing, with ample opportunity for atomic diffusion.

Classification of Alloys   Alloys can be classified according to the number of alloying elements. For example, if two elements are present, a *binary* alloy is formed; if three metals are present, a *ternary* alloy results, and so on. As the number of elements increases above two, the structure becomes increasingly complex. Consequently, only binary alloys will be studied in detail.

For dental purposes, the alloys can also be classified on the basis of the miscibility of the atoms in the solid state. The simplest alloy is one in which the atoms of the two metals intermingle randomly in a common space lattice. Under the microscope the grains of such alloys may resemble those of pure metals; the structure is entirely homogeneous. The metals are said to be *soluble* in each other in the solid state, and the alloys are called *solid solutions*. Most of the useful gold alloys used in dentistry are of the solid solution type.

Like the components of many liquid solutions, the metals that form solid solutions may not be completely soluble in each other in all proportions; they may be only partially soluble. In such a case, certain *intermediate phases* may appear which are not mutually soluble in the solid state.

Some of the intermediate phases that will be studied are the *eutectic alloys, peritectic alloys, valency* or *intermetallic compounds,* and combinations.

SOLID SOLUTIONS

By far the greatest number of alloys which are useful as dental restorations are solid solutions. Therefore special attention should be given to this type of alloy.

The term "solution" as applied to liquids is familiar to everyone. For example, a solution of sugar and water connotes a homogeneous system in which molecules of sugar diffuse through and intermingle with those of the water. The same is true of a molten solution of silver in palladium. However, if the sugar and water are frozen, each component crystallizes separately, but a palladium-silver alloy crystallizes in such a manner that the silver atoms are scattered randomly through the space lattice of the palladium, replacing the palladium atoms in a manner analogous to the molecular arrangement of the solute in the liquid solution. Such an alloy is called a solid solution. Because the atoms of silver enter directly into the space lattice of the palladium, the system is not mechanically separable and has only one phase. Furthermore, if the atoms of silver are segregated for any reason, and are not scattered randomly throughout the palladium space lattice, they may be made to diffuse in a manner quite analogous to that of undissolved sugar in water until equilibrium is reached.

Solute and Solvent   When sugar is dissolved in water, the water is known as the solvent and the sugar as the solute. When two metals are soluble in one another in the solid state, the solvent is that metal whose space lattice persists and the solute is the other metal. In palladium-silver alloys, the two metals are completely soluble in all proportions, and the same type of space lattice persists throughout the entire system. In such a case, the solvent may be defined as the metal whose atoms occupy more than one-half the total number of positions in the space lattice.

The configuration of the space lattice of solid solutions may be of several types: in the *substitutional* type, the atoms of the solute occupy the space lattice positions that normally are occupied by the solvent atoms in the pure metal. For example, in a palladium-silver alloy in which the palladium is the solvent, the silver atoms replace the palladium atoms randomly in lattice positions.

Another type of solid solution of considerable importance is the *interstitial solid solution*. In this case the solute atoms are present in positions between the solvent atoms (the interstices between regular lattice positions). This type of solid solution ordinarily requires that the solute atoms be much smaller in diameter than the solvent atoms. These solid solutions usually are limited to relatively small concentrations of solute. The interstitial solid solution of carbon in iron is one of the most important, since it forms the basis for the family of alloys called steels.

In some substitutional solid solutions the solvent and solute atoms have a slight affinity for each other. From an energy point of view, the random arrangement of atoms represents a higher energy than if the atoms are ordered in such a way as to have unlike nearest neighbors. For such an alloy, at a sufficiently low temperature, diffusion may bring about an ordering of a random solid solution. Since the order process implies a definite proportion of solute and solvent atoms, such ordered structures usually exist over very small compositional ranges.

For example, the gold-copper alloys exhibit a random or substitutional solid solution structure of the face-centered type at high temperatures (Fig. 17–1a), but if an alloy of the composition 50.2 per cent gold and 49.8 per cent copper by weight is allowed to cool slowly to below 400° C (752° F), the gold atoms are found at the corners of the cube of the unit lattice cell and the copper atoms on the faces (Fig. 17–1b).

When the unit cells are combined to form the space lattice, there are three times as many copper atoms as there are gold atoms, and as a result such a structure is represented as $AuCu_3$. The structure is called a *superlattice,* or an ordered structure.

Conditions for Solid Solubility   In any substitutional type of solid solution, the distance between the atoms changes according to the size of the solute atom. The entire lattice may be expanded or contracted, sometimes non-uniformly, according to the size of the solute atom in relation to the solvent atom.

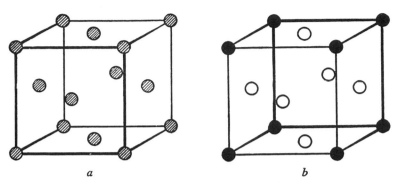

Figure 17-1 In a unit cell of a face-centered cubic space lattice of a copper-gold substitutional type, *a*, the positions of the copper atoms cannot be distinguished from the positions of the gold atoms. In the superlattice or ordered arrangement, *b*, the gold atoms are situated at the corners and the copper atoms are on the faces of the cube. (From Barrett: Metals and Alloys, Sept., 1937).

Generally, however, such changes in atomic distances are not great because one of the primary requisites for two or more metals to form solid solutions is that their sizes be approximately the same.

There are at least four factors which determine the extent of solid solubility of two or more metals.

1. Atom Size. If the sizes of two metallic atoms differ less than approximately 15 per cent, they are said to possess a *favorable* size factor for solid solubility. If the size factor is greater than 15 per cent, intermediate phases appear upon solidification. Probably none of the metals is completely lacking in solid solubility with another. Although the solid solubility may be only a fraction of a per cent, even such a limited solubility can be of importance in certain instances.

2. Valence. Metals of the same valence and size are more likely to form extensive solid solutions than are metals of different valences. If the valences differ, the metal with the higher valence may be more soluble in a metal of lower valence.

3. Chemical Affinity. When two metals exhibit a high degree of chemical affinity, they tend to form an intermetallic compound upon solidification rather than a solid solution.

4. Lattice Type. Only metals with the same type of lattice can form a complete series of solid solutions, particularly if the size factor is less than 8 per cent. Most of the metals used for dental restorations are face-centered cubic and can form a continuous series of solid solutions.

The size factor is possibly of first consideration in the estimation of whether two or more metals will be mutually soluble in the solid state. Once this requirement is met, the other factors are considered. Unfortunately, there are exceptions to these rules, but they are not likely to be of importance in dentistry.

Examples of Solid Solutions   Some of the atomic properties of metals used in dental alloys are given in Table 17-1. The first five metals are commonly used in dental gold alloys. All of these metals belong to the face-centered cubic system, and this factor, at least, is favorable for the formation of solid solutions. As might be expected from both the size and valence factors, silver and gold form a continuous series of solid solutions with each other, with very

Table 17–1. *Atomic Diameters of Metals of Dental Interest**

METAL	ATOMIC DIAMETER (ANGSTROMS)	CRYSTAL STRUCTURE
Gold	2.882	Face-centered cubic
Platinum	2.775	Face-centered cubic
Palladium	2.750	Face-centered cubic
Silver	2.888	Face-centered cubic
Copper	2.556	Face-centered cubic
Tin	3.016	Body-centered tetragonal
Zinc	2.665	Close-packed hexagonal
Silicon	2.351	Diamond cubic

*From Lyman T (ed): Metals Handbook, 8th ed., Cleveland, American Society for Metals, 1964, Vol. I.

little disturbance of the lattice dimensions. Silver and palladium also form a continuous series of solid solutions.

Although the diameter of the copper atom differs as much as 12 per cent from that of the other four metals under consideration, it is an important alloy component. As will be discussed later, it forms a limited series of solid solutions with silver. Solid solutions of copper in gold, platinum, and palladium are continuous at high temperatures, but upon cooling, superlattice changes take place, as already discussed in connection with the formation of the $AuCu_3$ superlattice.

According to Table 17–1, the difference between the silver and the tin atomic diameters is in the neighborhood of 4 per cent. However, the two metals are different in valence, and they are not closely associated in the electromotive series. It will be shown in a subsequent chapter that silver is a limited solvent for tin. As the tin content increases, an intermetallic compound forms, which is an important factor in the hardening of dental amalgams.

Physical Properties of Solid Solutions   It was previously noted that the lattice structure of a solvent metal is expanded or contracted by the introduction of solute atoms by substitution. Such a statement is true only if the situation is considered as an average condition over the entire space lattice. Actually, wherever a solute atom displaces or substitutes for a solvent atom, the difference in size of the solute atom results in a localized distortion or strained condition of the lattice, and slip becomes more difficult. As a consequence, the strength, proportional limit, and surface hardness are increased, whereas the ductility is decreased.

In other words, the alloying of metals may be a means of strengthening the metal. The general theory of slip interference in alloys is the same as in strain hardening, except that a different type of lattice distortion is present initially to inhibit slip before the structure is stressed or worked.

A number of useful alloys in dentistry are examples of this. Gold itself cannot be used as a restorative material unless it is strain hardened, as in the compaction of gold foil. Gold in the cast condition is too weak and ductile. However, if as little as 5 per cent by weight of copper is alloyed with the gold, the latter loses practically none of its ability to resist tarnish and corrosion, yet a strength and hardness is imparted to it so that it can be used for the casting of inlays.

In general, the hardness and strength of any metallic solvent are increased by the atoms of a solute. The nearer alike the atoms are in size, the less is the effect of the solute atoms, but some increase in strength can be expected nevertheless.

Generally, the more of the solute metal added to the solvent, the greater are the strength and hardness of the alloy. In two metals which form a continuous series of solid solutions with one another, the maximal hardness is reached at approximately 50 atomic per cent* of each metal. As might be expected from the theory, the ductility usually decreases progressively as the strength and hardness increase.

The density of a solid solution under conditions of complete solubility can be calculated from the composition. In the cases of limited solubility, however, the calculated density is likely to be lower than the density determined by experiment.

Constitution Diagrams — Equilibrium Phase Diagrams   The concept of a constitution or equilibrium phase diagram will be introduced, using as an example a system that should be familiar. The dissolution of ordinary table salt (NaCl) in water to form a true solution called brine is the starting point for the discussion. It is observed that at a particular temperature, a limit exists in how much salt can be dissolved before crystals begin to settle out. The chemist would refer to a solubility (or miscibility) limit. Notice that a pure single phase (brine) becomes a two-phase mixture (brine and salt) as the solubility limit is exceeded. If the temperature of the system is increased, the amount of salt that can be dissolved increases. If the temperature is decreased sufficiently, eventually another phase appears, called ice. Although pure water solidifies to form ice at 0° C, it is common knowledge that the addition of salt will depress the freezing point.

All of this information concerning the water-salt system can be assembled in an orderly fashion to form a "map" showing what phases are present at a particular temperature and composition (amount of salt). Such a diagram is presented in Figure 17–2. It should be emphasized that this diagram assumes that equilibrium conditions have been established.

In this figure can be seen one single phase region (brine); two liquid-solid two phase regions (ice plus brine and salt plus brine); and one solid-solid two phase regions (ice plus salt). The region labeled "ice plus brine" is likely not as familiar as the others. At salt concentrations below 23.3 per cent, as the temperature of a salt solution is lowered almost pure water settles out of solution as ice — to form the ice-brine mixture. This can be utilized to desalinate sea water (a 1.7 per cent salt solution) and is an economical alternative to distillation.

Atomic per cent is calculated on the basis of the atomic weight of each metal, rather than the gravity weight. When the latter is employed, the percentage is known as *weight per cent*.

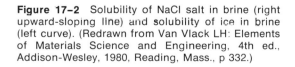

Figure 17–2 Solubility of NaCl salt in brine (right upward-sloping line) and solubility of ice in brine (left curve). (Redrawn from Van Vlack LH: Elements of Materials Science and Engineering, 4th ed., Addison-Wesley, 1980, Reading, Mass., p 332.)

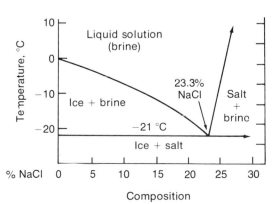

Now let us turn to the alloy system of pure metal A and pure metal B. As previously noted, such a system is composed of all possible combinations of A and B, ranging from 100 per cent A to 100 per cent B. Further assume that A and B are completely soluble at all compositions in both solid and liquid states.

Cooling curve experiments like the ones discussed in Chapter 15 will now be performed on a series of alloys from the A-B system as follows: (1) 100% A, (2) 80% A–20% B, (3) 60% A–40% B, (4) 40% A–60% B, (5) 20% A–80% B, (6) 100% B. These are shown in Figure 17–3a. Curves 1 and 6 for the pure metals A and B are familiar from Chapter 15. Curves 2 through 5 illustrate that solid solution alloys do not have a solidification temperature, but instead solidify over a temperature range. The region labeled L + S is a two-phase region composed of liquid and solid analogous to the brine and salt region in our first example.

These cooling curves can now be used to determine the equilibrium phase diagram for the A-B alloy system, as shown in Figure 17–3b. The temperature at which the *first* solid begins to form (called the *liquidus* temperature) for each composition is determined from the cooling curves in Figure 17–3a and then plotted in the temperature-composition diagram (Figure 17–3b). Similarly, the temperature at which the *last* liquid solidifies (called the *solidus*) is determined and plotted. When these points are connected with a smooth curve, the *equilibrium phase diagram* in 17–3b results.

The upper solid line in 17–3b is called the liquidus line, since the alloys are entirely liquid above this line. The lower line is called the solidus, since the alloys are entirely solid below this line. The region between is, of course, the two-phase liquid plus solid region.

Consider now an alloy system that has considerable dental interest and resembles the theoretical system just described. Figure 17–4 presents the phase diagram for palladium-silver. These metals exhibit complete solubility

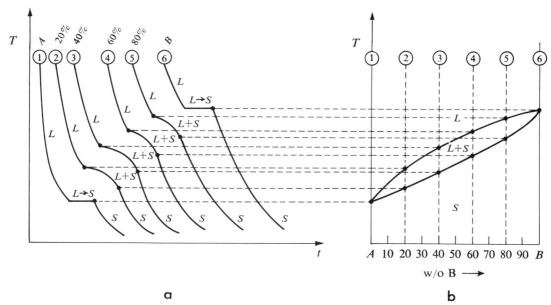

Figure 17–3 Determination of a phase diagram by thermal analysis. *(a)* The cooling curves of six alloys of various compositions are determined experimentally, and *(b)* the temperature of fusion and the liquidus and solidus temperatures are plotted as a function of composition to form the phase diagram. (From Richman, M.: An Introduction to the Science of Metals. Waltham, Mass., Blaisdell Pub. Co., 1967, p 213.)

in both liquid and solid states. Note the liquid, liquid-solid, and solid regions separated by the liquidus and solidus lines.

Interpretation of the Constitution Diagram As an illustration of how the constitution diagram can be used to advantage, consider an alloy of composition 65 per cent palladium and 35 per cent silver as indicated by the dotted line PO, erected perpendicularly to the base line through the chemical composition 65 per cent palladium (Fig. 17–4). If the point on the line PO corresponding to the temperature 1500° C (2732° F) is considered, it is evident that only a liquid is present with a composition of 65 per cent palladium and 35 per cent silver.

When the temperature decreases to approximately 1400° C (2552° F) at the point R which is situated on the liquidus, the first solid forms.* In order to determine the composition of the alloy first solidifying, the line RM, called the *tie line,* is drawn through R, parallel to the base line. If the point of intersection (M) with the solidus is projected to the base line, the composition of the first solid can be determined as 77 per cent palladium. Similarly, if the point R is so projected, the composition of the remaining liquid is found to be 65 per cent palladium.

Now assume that the temperature decreases to approximately 1370° C (2498° F) as denoted by the point S. At this temperature, the material is partially solid and partially liquid. As before, the composition of the solid and liquid at this stage may be determined by drawing the tie line YW, and locating its point of intersection with the liquidus and solidus respectively in terms of composition as before. Hence, the approximate composition of the liquid is 58 per cent palladium, as given by the projection of the point Y on the

---

*As a matter of convention, any point on the liquidus or solidus is considered to be in the two phase region between the liquidus and the solidus.

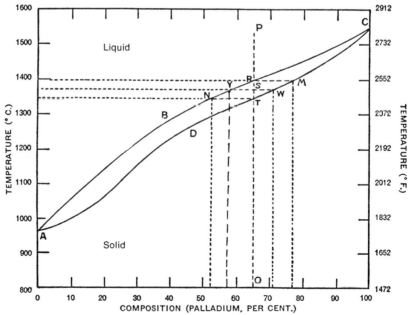

Figure 17–4 Constitution diagram for the palladium-silver system. Only the percentage composition for the palladium is given; the percentage composition for the silver is determined by subtracting the palladium composition from 100.

base line, whereas that of the solid is about 71 per cent palladium, determined by projecting the point W to the base line. At the temperature corresponding to the point T on the graph (approximately 1340° C, or 2444° F), the last portion of liquid solidifies. This liquid has the composition of 52 per cent palladium, and the solid phase is 65 per cent palladium. It should be re-emphasized that this is an equilibrium phase diagram and that the system would have to be held at each of these temperatures for a time sufficient that diffusion can produce equilibrium conditions. After equilibrium has been achieved, the compositions of liquid and solid and the amounts of each phase present are stable.

When the temperature decreases to below point T, the alloy is entirely solid, with a composition of 65 per cent palladium. Thus, the chemical composition of any phase of the palladium-silver system at any temperature can be obtained in a similar manner. The percentage of each phase that is present at a given temperature with a given base composition can also be calculated.

Coring   It can be noted from Table 17–2 that the composition of the dendrite or grain is not uniform. For example, the first embryo or nucleus that forms at the temperature R (or slightly below) in Figure 17–4 is rich in palladium, but as the temperature decreases, the palladium content decreases with an increase in the silver content as each succeeding "layer" solidifies. The liquid phase, of course, is "robbed" of palladium but its silver content increases as the solidification temperature is approached.

At the solidus temperature T (Fig. 17–4) the composition of the outermost "layer" of the dendrite is 65 per cent palladium and 35 per cent silver. The last liquid to solidify is rich in silver and solidifies between the dendrites. It can be recognized, therefore, that a cored structure results, with the core consisting of the dendrites composed of the higher melting alloy constituents and the matrix containing the lower melting components.

Excellent examples of cored structures can be observed in the photomicrograph in Figure 17–5a. The dark dendritic structure represents the core composed of the high melting alloys. The matrix which solidified last between the dendrites is lighter in shade. Note that this cored structure is *not* an equilibrium structure. The cooling rates involved in normal casting procedures do not allow time for sufficient diffusion to achieve equilibrium. Note also that the larger the temperature range between liquidus and solidus, the greater is the tendency toward coring.

Homogenization   In the previous discussion, rapid cooling was assumed. Actually, the atoms tend to diffuse to relieve the segregation as much as

Table 17–2.   *Chemical Compositions and Phase Amounts of the Alloy of 65 Per Cent Palladium and 35 Per Cent Silver*

TEMPERATURE			CHEMICAL COMPOSITION	
(°C)		(°F)	Liquid %Pd	Solid %Pd
1500		2732	65	*
1400		2552	65	77
1370		2498	58	71
1340		2444	52	65
900		1652	*	65

*Phase not present at this temperature.

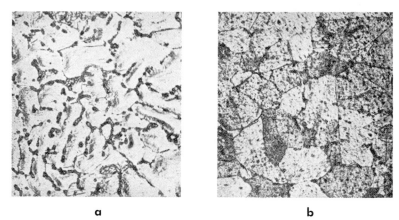

a   b

Figure 17–5   Copper-silver alloy (1 per cent) as cast, *a,* and same structure after homogenization, *b,* 100 ×. (From Avner SH: An Introduction to Physical Metallurgy, New York, McGraw-Hill Book Co., Inc., 1964.)

possible. Under conditions of equilibrium, the composition of the palladium-silver alloy should be 65 per cent palladium and 35 per cent silver throughout, and the atomic diffusion during cooling tends to produce such a situation. However, the faster the alloy is cooled from its liquidus temperature, the more nearly the compositions in Table 17–2 are approached; on the other hand, during a slow cooling, the greater is the amount of atomic diffusion toward equilibrium conditions.

If the alloy is cooled rapidly from its liquidus temperature, the coring can be relieved by a heat treating process similar to that described for wrought metal. The alloy is held at a temperature near its solidus so that the atomic diffusion can occur. Little or no grain growth occurs when a casting is heat treated, and higher temperatures are often employed than would be used with a wrought metal. The process of heating a cast alloy to eliminate composition differences (coring) is called *homogenization.*

A second difference is the time necessary for the homogenization. The rate of atomic diffusion in the cast structure is much less than that in a cold-worked structure. The former may require hours whereas, at the same high temperature, the latter may recrystallize in minutes. Consequently, if the cast structure can be cold worked, it can be homogenized much faster by recrystallization. However, often a casting cannot be cold worked and it must be homogenized, a process which requires 6 hours at a high temperature (Fig. 17–5*b*).

It will be shown in another chapter that an inhomogeneous dental gold alloy is more subject to tarnish and corrosion than the same alloy after it has been homogenized. This consideration is also important for silver-palladium alloys, since silver-rich phases tend to tarnish readily in the mouth.

As might be expected, the heterogeneous grain structure offers more resistance to slip than does the homogenized structure. Consequently, although the difference is not considerable, the ductility of the alloy is usually greater after homogenization.

EUTECTIC ALLOYS

Many binary alloy systems are not as simple as the one just considered in that they do not exhibit complete solubility in both the solid and liquid states.

As previously discussed, in such cases intermediate phases are formed. The *eutectic* system is an example in which the components exhibit complete liquid solubility but limited solid solubility.

The simplest illustration of a eutectic alloy is of two metals, A and B, which are completely insoluble in each other in the solid state. In such a case, some of the grains are composed solely of metal A, whereas the remainder of the grains are composed of metal B. The situation is analogous to a frozen sugar solution. Although in solution, the sugar and the water molecules intermingle randomly, upon freezing the result is a mixture of sugar crystals and ice crystals which form independently of each other.

However, all metals are probably soluble in one another, if only in a minute amount. Therefore, a binary eutectic system in which the two metals are partially soluble in each other will be used for purposes of illustration. One such system of interest to dentistry is the silver-copper system.

Silver-Copper System   The constitution diagram for the silver-copper system is presented in Figure 17–6. The solidus can be identified by the boundary line ABEGD and the liquidus as AED. The limited solid solubility of Cu in Ag and Ag in Cu is evident in that the major portion of the diagram below 780° C is composed of a two-phase region labeled $\alpha + \beta$. This region is a mechanical mixture of α, the silver-rich alloy, and β, the copper-rich alloy.

The first difference to be noted in comparison with Figure 17–4 is that the liquidus and solidus meet at E. This composition (71.9% silver, 28.1% copper) is known as the *eutectic composition* or, simply, the *eutectic*. It should be noted that (1) the temperature (779.4° C, or 1434.9° F) at which the eutectic occurs is lower than the fusion temperature of either silver or copper (eutectic literally means lowest melting), and is the lowest temperature at which any alloy composition of silver and copper is entirely liquid, and (2) there is no solidification range for this composition. In other words, it solidifies at a constant temperature, which is characteristic of the particular eutectic. In this respect only, it is similar to a pure metal. Eutectic alloys are often used when a lower fusion temperature is desired. In other respects they are generally inferior to solid solution alloys.

When a eutectic alloy solidifies, the atoms of the constituent metals must segregate to form regions of nearly pure parent metals. This results in a very distinctive structure, as can be seen in Figure 17–7A. The layered structure

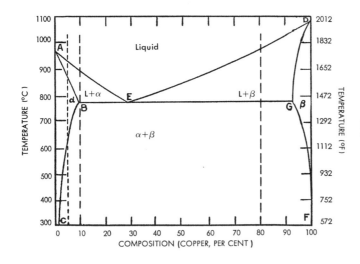

Figure 17–6 Constitution diagram for the silver-copper system.

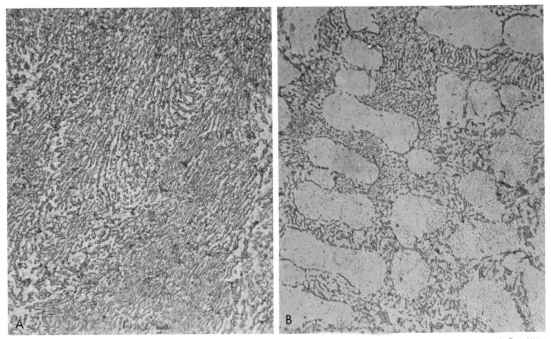

Figure 17–7   Microstructure of two lead-tin alloys. *A,* The alloy has the eutectic composition (62% Sn, 38% Pb). The structure is composed of alternating layers (lamellae) of α- solid solution (dark) which is Pb rich and β-solid solution (light) which is Sn rich (1280×). *B,* The alloy has a high tin content (75% Sn, 25% Pb). The light islands arc primary β, which solidified first. They are surrounded by the eutectic, which solidified when the eutectic temperature was reached (560 ×). (Courtesy of P. G. Winchell.)

forms because it requires the least amount of diffusion to produce the required segregation.

The eutectic reaction is sometimes written schematically as follows:

$$\text{Liquid} \rightarrow \alpha\text{-solid solution} + \beta\text{-solid solution}$$

It is referred to as an *invariant transformation,* since it occurs at one temperature and one composition only.

Another feature of the diagram is that the solidus at first gradually changes composition with a decrease in temperature until the eutectic temperature is attained. Its temperature then remains constant even though there is a phase change. For example, along the solidus from A to B, the silver becomes richer in copper as the temperature decreases. As a matter of fact, the copper content increases from 0 to 8.8 per cent at B with the reduction in temperature. At the copper end of the diagram, as the alloy cools from D to G, the number of silver atoms in the copper space lattice increases until 8 per cent silver has alloyed with the copper. It is evident that the silver lattice contains the copper atoms in solution in the first instance, and that the copper lattice contains the silver atoms in solution at the other end of the diagram. In other words, the copper is soluble in the silver to an extent of 8.8 per cent provided the system is held at the eutectic temperature E or, what is the same thing, the temperature indicated by the point B.

As with any solutions in which the solute solubility in the solvent is limited, the solubility decreases with the decrease in temperature. The *solvus lines* BC and GF indicate the change in solid solubility of the copper in silver and the silver in copper respectively as the temperature of the totally solid phase decreases. The solid solution of copper in silver is called the α-*solid solution,* and the solid solution of silver in copper is called the β-*solid solution.*

The compositions of the various alloys and the amount of each phase present can be determined in the same manner as for solid solutions of silver and palladium. For example, if a silver-copper alloy of 10 per cent copper is melted at a temperature above the liquidus and allowed to cool along the second dotted vertical line (Fig. 17–6), the first solid crystallizes at approximately 900° C (1652° F). If a tie line* is drawn from the liquidus at this point to the solidus, the first solid is the α-solid solution of the approximate composition 4 per cent copper and 96 per cent silver.

If the temperature is allowed to fall to 850° C (1562° F), the points of intersection of a tie line on the solidus and liquidus indicate an α-solid solution composition of 5 per cent copper; the remaining liquid is 15 per cent copper.

When the temperature decreases to the eutectic temperature, the tie line becomes BE. As the eutectic temperature is reached, the last liquid to solidify has the eutectic composition and solidifies forming α and β in the typical eutectic structure.

If the copper composition is greater than that of the eutectic, the composition change is similar except that the β-solid solution is the first solid solution to form instead of the α-solid solution as in the previous case. Such an effect is evident if the compositions of the alloy, 80 per cent copper, and 20 per cent silver, are calculated during cooling as indicated by the dotted vertical composition line to the extreme right in Figure 17–6.

In summary, the first solids to form above the eutectic temperature are always either of the solid solutions α or β. The first grains so formed are large, at least compared with the intimate mixture of small grains that form the eutectic. The larger grains are called *primary grains* because they form first. The α or β formed above the eutectic temperature is referred to as *primary* α or β. Figure 17–7B illustrates large grains of β surrounded by small amounts of eutectic structure.

To this point, the compositions below the eutectic temperature have not been considered. This is best illustrated by a cooling of the composition 5 per cent copper, as indicated by the first vertical dotted line in Figure 17–6. It begins to solidify at a temperature slightly above 900° C (1652° F), and it freezes completely as an α-solid solution at approximately 860° C (1580° F). As the temperature falls, the solid solution phase remains intact until a temperature of 630° C (1166° F) is reached; then the copper-rich β phase appears in a mixture with the α-solid solution as a precipitated phase. The reason for this change is related to the solid solubility of copper in silver. Just as the line AB (liquidus) represents the solubility limit of the copper in the silver at the respective solidus temperatures, so does the line BC (solvus) represent the solubility limit of the two metals in the solid state. Again it must be emphasized that this occurs only if very slow cooling has permitted equilibrium to be achieved. Rapid cooling of the 5 per cent copper alloy will result in almost pure α phase being retained at room temperature. As previously noted, if more than 8.8 per cent copper is added to the melt, the eutectic appears upon solidification. But the solubility of the copper in the silver becomes less as the temperature decreases below the eutectic solidification temperature, as indi-

---

*The student should draw the tie lines to verify the values quoted.

cated by the line BC. Consequently, when this alloy is slowly cooled below 630° C, the solid solution becomes *supersaturated* with copper, and the excess phase (copper) is *precipitated*. The process is analogous to similar phenomena in supersaturated liquid solutions.

At the other end of the diagram, it can be expected that silver precipitates from a supersaturated solution upon cooling in the same manner.

It should be emphasized that the eutectic structure does not appear in alloys of less than 8.8 per cent copper. Only the α-solid solution is present with varying amounts of β according to the temperature involved.

Physical Properties Unlike the palladium-silver system, the mechanical properties of the eutectic alloys do not vary linearly with the composition. For purposes of convenience, alloys with a composition less than that of the eutectic are called *hypoeutectic* alloys and those with a composition greater than the eutectic are known as *hypereutectic* alloys. The primary crystals of the hypoeutectic alloys in the copper-silver systems are composed of α-solid solution, and those of the hypereutectic alloys are β-solid solution; therefore, a linear relationship between composition and physical properties cannot be expected because the two phases differ in this respect.

The eutectic alloys are apt to be brittle because the presence of insoluble phases definitely inhibits slip. Consequently, the strength, and sometimes the hardness, of these alloys may surpass that of the constituent metals because of the composite structure of the alloy. On the other hand, if the recrystallization temperature of the matrix metals (*e.g.*, lead) is very low, a flow or creep may occur even at room temperature.

Except for the gold alloy solders (Chapter 33), the eutectic systems do not generally occur in dental precious metal alloys because of their low tarnish and corrosion resistance. However, α-solid solution alloys of silver and copper may be used to some extent in pedodontics as casting alloys. The tarnish resistance of these alloys is superior to that of the alloys containing the eutectic (see Chapter 19). The silver-copper eutectic is found as the admixed component in some types of high copper amalgam alloys (Chapters 20–21).

It has been found that the grain size of a cast gold alloy can be reduced under certain conditions by the addition of a trace of another metal of very low solubility and high fusion temperature.[1] It can be in the form of eutectic alloy with a eutectic composition very close to that of the pure gold side of the binary constitution diagram.

For example, iridium forms a eutectic alloy with gold that has a eutectic composition of approximately 0.005 per cent iridium. If approximately 0.005 per cent iridium is added to pure gold, nucleation occurs, with a resulting grain refinement. The iridium reduces the critical radius for nucleus formation. For example, the grain size of the unnucleated cast gold is 40 grains per square centimeter, whereas after nucleation with 0.005 per cent iridium, it is 84 grains per square centimeter. If greater amounts of iridium are added than its eutectic composition with gold, the iridium tends to segregate and a non-uniform grain size may result.

PERITECTIC SYSTEMS

In addition to the eutectic system just described, limited solid solubility of two metals can result in a transformation referred to as peritectic. *Peritectic*

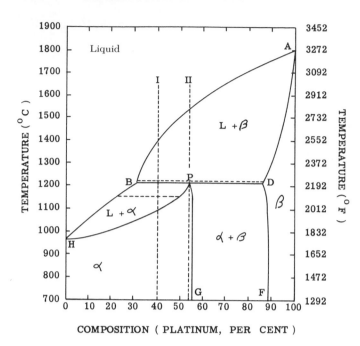

Figure 17–8 Constitution diagram of the platinum-silver system.

COMPOSITION (PLATINUM, PER CENT)

systems are not common in dentistry, the exception being the silver-tin system, which is the basis for traditional dental amalgam alloys. However, the platinum-silver phase diagram exhibits a very simple peritectic transformation; and since these metals are found in many of the gold casting alloys, the system is quite appropriate for study.

Like the eutectic transformation, the peritectic reaction is an invariant reaction, i.e., it occurs at a particular composition and temperature. The reaction can be written as:

$$\text{Liquid} + \beta \longrightarrow \alpha$$

Figure 17–8 is the phase diagram for the platinum-silver alloy system. The α phase is a silver-rich phase, the β phase is platinum-rich, and $\alpha + \beta$ is the two-phase region due to limited solid solubility. The peritectic transformation occurs at the point P where the liquid plus the platinum-rich phase β transforms into the silver-rich α phase. The substantial composition change involved can lead to large amounts of coring if rapid cooling occurs.

If the alloy has a hypoperitectic composition, as alloy I in Figure 17–8, cooling of the alloy through the peritectic temperature results in the transformation Liquid + $\beta \rightarrow$ Liquid + α. Rapid cooling results in precipitation of α phase around the β grains before diffusion can occur. The solid α phase inhibits diffusion, and substantial coring occurs. The cored structure is more brittle and has inferior corrosion resistance to the homogeneous α phase.

SOLID STATE REACTIONS

The alloy systems discussed so far have involved either total solid solubility or limited solid solubility. However, another possibility exists in which the elements are completely soluble in the liquid state and at high temperatures in the solid state. At lower temperatures the attraction of the solvent and solute

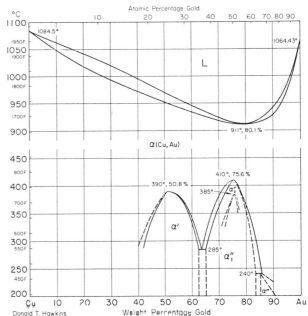

Figure 17-9 Constitution diagram for the gold-copper system. (From Metals Handbook, 8th ed., Metals Park, Ohio, American Society for Metals, 1973, Vol 8, p 267.)

atoms may be sufficient to convert the random solid solution into an ordered solid phase. The gold-copper alloy system exhibits this phenomenon at certain compositions.

Gold-Copper System   The phase diagram is shown in Figure 17-9. Note that the melting range is very narrow for all compositions, and that the liquidus and solidus actually touch at 80.1 per cent gold. Also addition of as little as 10 per cent copper to the gold lowers the liquidus temperature substantially. Both of these facts are advantageous in the use of the alloy system for dental casting procedures. At temperatures below the solidus but above 410° C, gold and copper exhibit complete solid solubility.

Below 410° C new solid phases appear. The phase α' is the ordered solid, previously described and illustrated in Figure 17-1. It has the composition $AuCu_3$. The large amount of copper in this phase would not be compatible with dental applications. The α'' phase is another ordered structure and is shown in

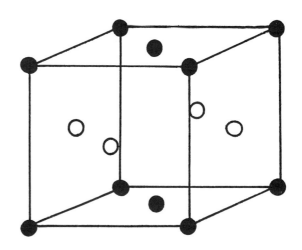

Figure 17-10 A unit cell of the face-centered tetragonal superlattice of AuCu. The open circles represent the gold atoms.

Figure 17–10. This phase is face centered tetragonal and has the composition AuCu.

The composition of most of the harder casting gold alloys is compatible with the compositional limits for this phase to form. The transformation from the cubic lattice type at high temperatures to the tetragonal low temperature phase produces localized strains that inhibit dislocation motion, effectively hardening the alloy. As is usually the case, if a gold-copper alloy is cooled rapidly (quenched) from the solidus temperature, the disordered solid solution is retained at room temperature, and the alloy is relatively soft. Slow cooling through the transition temperature, however, allows diffusion to occur. The alloy would partially transform to the ordered phase and would be harder than the quenched alloy.

OTHER SYSTEMS

The platinum-gold system exhibits a considerable spread in temperature between the liquidus and solidus, and an undesirable cored structure results. Platinum and gold exhibit total solid solubility only at temperatures very near the solidus. At lower temperatures a large two-phase region develops in a manner similar to a eutectic structure. At 400° C (752° F), this heterogeneous structure may be spread over compositions which range from 4 to 90 per cent gold.

The palladium-copper system is characterized by a relatively short melting range, particularly in comparison with that of the platinum-gold system. Although the liquidus is never less than the melting temperatures of the constituents, the copper effectively reduces the liquidus and solidus temperatures over a considerable range of composition. In some respects, this system resembles that of the gold-copper system. Transformations that correspond to the superlattice compositions PdCu (62.6 per cent palladium) and $PdCu_3$ (36 per cent palladium) occur. The range of the PdCu transformation is approximately from 48 to 63 per cent palladium, and it involves an atomic diffusion to an ordered body-centered cubic structure of essentially the same dimensions as the parent lattice.

The platinum-copper system resembles the palladium-copper system to some extent. The melting range is again fairly narrow. Alloys with less than 20 per cent platinum have liquidus temperatures only slightly above the melting point of copper. At least two intermediate phases appear upon slow cooling: PtCu (75.5 per cent platinum) and $PtCu_3$ (44 per cent platinum). The precipitation of the PtCu phase results in slip interference.

Reference

1. Nielsen JP and Tuccillo JJ: Grain size in dental gold alloys. J Dent Res 45:964, 1966.

18 SOLID STATE REACTION HEAT TREATMENT

Two methods for the control of the physical properties of metals have been discussed. The metal can be strengthened by strain hardening and then the strain-hardened metal can be rendered more ductile by recrystallization. The latter method is, of course, attained by a heat treatment or annealing process. In addition, the strength and toughness of a metal can be increased by making the grain structure fine.

It has been shown that the physical properties can also be controlled by alloying two or more metals. Each metal constituent contributes certain properties to the alloy. Such a method can be applied to any metal whether cast or wrought. A fourth and very practical method is to cause atomic diffusion by heat treatment in the solid state, as discussed briefly in the previous chapter. This method will now be discussed in more detail. It, too, can be employed in either the cast or wrought condition.

At this point, two terms need to be clarified. *Heat treatment* means that a metal is elevated to a temperature above room temperature and held there for a length of time. The effects of such a treatment depend entirely on the temperature, the metal, and its previous history. Heat treating may harden a metal, soften a metal, change its grain size or corrosion resistance, etc.

The second term is *quenching*. This term means that a metal is rapidly cooled from an elevated temperature to room temperature or below. This is usually done for one of two reasons: the first is to preserve at room temperature a phase ordinarily stable only at elevated temperatures, and the second is to rapidly terminate a process that only occurs at elevated temperatures.

Solid State Reaction In the preceding chapter, it was noted that in a number of cases certain atoms diffuse in the solid state to produce a new phase. Although in theory such precipitation solid-solid reactions may be similar to the liquid-solid precipitation, certain differences are to be expected.

For example, rates of diffusion to form the solid precipitate from the liquid are much greater than they are in the analogous solid state reaction. Consequently, the formation of the new phases or precipitates requires a longer time for completion. As might be expected, the higher the temperature, the more rapid is the diffusion rate.

Aside from composition, temperature is one of the most important considerations. A solution of sugar in water was used as an illustration of this effect. If the sugar solution is saturated at the boiling point of the solution, sugar precipitates or crystallizes upon cooling because the solution is supersaturated. If the solution is again heated to its boiling point, the precipitated sugar again goes into solution. However, there is no method by which the concentration of the sugar solution at the boiling point can be preserved at room temperature without sugar precipitation.

Such is not the case with a solid solution. A constituent that is soluble at a high temperature, but less so at a lower temperature, may be prevented from precipitating by plunging the alloy into water at this temperature (quenching). The atomic diffusion is effectively prevented so that the supersaturated condition is preserved at room temperature.

On the other hand, if the solid solution is cooled slowly from the high temperature, atoms of the partially soluble metal diffuse to form a new phase which is precipitated in the parent or solid solution phase. Typically, the reaction is reversible; the alloy can again be heated to the higher temperature and the precipitated phase again becomes soluble in the solvent metal. If the alloy is again quenched from this temperature, the solid solution structure persists.

The practical application of this theory is that the physical properties of the alloy can be controlled to a degree in this manner. For example, if the alloy is cooled slowly, the precipitated phase may require a volume change. The precipitation usually occurs at random either in various areas of the grains or, more likely, at the grain boundaries. As a result of the stress created by the volume change, localized lattice distortions of the remaining parent solid solution inhibit slip, and the ductility is reduced. At the same time, the strength, hardness, and proportional limit are increased. If the alloy is reheated so that the precipitated phase becomes soluble again, the original solid solution is restored and, after quenching, the ductility is increased to its original value, with a corresponding reduction in strength, etc. Such a procedure is a second example of heat treatment. Although such a quenched condition is not stable, the rate of atomic diffusion at room temperature is so low as to be negligible.

Heat Treatment   In summary, then, the dentist can control the physical properties of some of the dental alloys, whether cast or wrought, by heat treatment. It should be noted that a partial solubility of the constituents is a requisite for such heat treatments in dental gold alloys. For example, the physical properties are essentially the same for the palladium-silver system (Fig. 17–3) whether the alloys are quenched or cooled slowly because there is complete solid-solubility (assuming a homogenized structure).

A number of heat treatments have already been described. As noted previously, the recrystallization of a cold-worked structure is a type of heat treatment. After the structure is recrystallized, the ductility is increased and the hardness, strength, and proportional limit are reduced. In this type of annealing, the process is not reversible; the strain-hardened structure cannot be restored by heating or cooling.

A second heat treatment mentioned was homogenization, but, again, the process is not reversible by heating without a change in state. Nevertheless, these two heat treating processes can be used effectively by the dentist under certain conditions. A few typical examples of heat treatment by solid state reaction of dental importance will be described.

Table 18-1.   *Heat Treatment for Sterling Silver*

| HEAT TREATMENT | ULTIMATE TENSILE STRENGTH | | YIELD POINT | | ELONGATION |
	(MPa)	(psi)	(MPa)	(psi)	(%)
Solution	258	37,400	135	19,680	42
Age hardening	299	43,400	207	30,000	26

Silver-Copper System   The silver-copper alloys were possibly the first system investigated in which the changes in physical properties by precipitation hardening from a solid solution were demonstrated. For example, as already discussed in the previous chapter, when the alloy of 5 per cent copper in Figure 17–6 is allowed to cool slowly, copper is precipitated at 630° C (1166° F) at the point where the dotted line intersects the solvus line. Of course, additional copper precipitates as the alloy cools further, but to a limited extent because the diffusion rate decreases rapidly with the decrease in temperature.

Although, theoretically, a new phase should appear, it is not necessary for the precipitation to occur to the extent that it is evident metallographically. Any concentration of copper atoms in the space lattice of the silver-copper solid solution is sufficient to inhibit slip.

As previously noted, if the alloy is again heated above the temperature indicated by the solvus line for a sufficient time period to allow the copper atoms to rediffuse to random positions in the silver space lattice, a single phase solid solution structure again forms.

The heat treatment of "soaking" the alloy at the high temperature to produce the solid solution, followed by quenching, is known as the *solution heat treatment*. After a solution heat treatment, heating to produce precipitation of a second phase is known as an *age hardening heat treatment*.

One particularly famous silver-copper alloy, sometimes used for inlay purposes in deciduous teeth, is known as *sterling silver*. It is used extensively in fine silverware. It is 7.5 per cent copper and 92.5 per cent silver. As can be rationalized from the silver-copper phase diagram in Figure 17–6, on slow cooling from the melt the 7.5 per cent copper alloy first solidifies as an α-solid solution, which precipitates out a copper-rich β-phase on continued cooling. If a specimen of this alloy could be solution heat treated at 775° C (1427° F) for 30 minutes and then after quenching to room temperature be brought back up to 325° C (617° F) for two hours, it would give the age-hardening effect (see Table 18–1), and the microstructure should exhibit a fine dispersed phase.

Order-Disorder Heat Treatments   As noted in the gold-copper system, instead of a metal constituent precipitating, the atoms diffuse to form the superlattices $AuCu_3$ or $AuCu$ (Fig. 17–9). The superlattice $AuCu_3$ is of little aid in changing the physical properties of the alloy during age hardening because its lattice has essentially the same dimensions as that of the disordered lattice. Also, the comparatively high copper content alloys from which it precipitates are not suitable for oral use because of their low tarnish resistance.

On the other hand the formation of the $AuCu$ tetragonal crystal lattice contributes to the age-hardening process in an interesting manner. The ordered phase *per se* is not particularly strong or hard. However, the tetragonal structure precipitates out in the age-hardening temperature range in thin alternate layers. The alteration is necessary because the short C axis of the

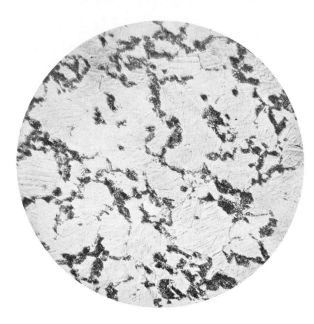

Figure 18–1 A photomicrograph of a dental alloy which was age hardened at 450° C for 100 hours. 250 ×. (Courtesy of E. M. Wise.)

tetragonal structure tends to produce elastic strain in the face-centered cubic parent structure. The strain is then relieved by a follow-up precipitated layer with the C axis perpendicular to the previous C axis. These alternations continue until the structure has precipitated the equilibrium quantity of the ordered structure.

These thin layers are seen as striations in the microstructure (Fig. 18–1), which represents the aged structure for a gold-copper-silver alloy for a type IV gold dental alloy. The dark gray constituent is a silver-rich phase, and the white matrix phase is the copper-rich phase. The gray precipitate hardens by dispersed phase hardening; the striations harden by obstructing slip due to lattice alternations.

It should be noted that the time for heat treatment is also important. Presumably, the longer the time of the age hardening treatment, the greater is the change in physical properties.

It should be emphasized that the precipitated phase is not necessarily harder than the parent lattice. The slip interference can be attributed to the lattice distortions caused by the precipitated phase. Theoretically, if the parent lattice could be entirely transformed to the precipitated phase, it is conceivable that the properties of strength would be less than those obtained during a proper age hardening treatment, but with an increase in ductility. That such a condition is not expected in the gold-copper system is evidenced by the photomicrograph shown in Figure 18–1. Even though the alloy was age hardened for 100 hours, the amount of precipitated phase was minimal and apparently occurred near the grain boundaries.

Usually, the time for age hardening is limited according to the desired properties of resulting structure. A low ductility in a dental alloy results in a brittleness that may prevent necessary adjustments of the dental appliance by the dentist. On the other hand, an increase in proportional limit is desirable in order to increase the modulus of resilience of the appliance. Practically, therefore, the time and temperature for age hardening should be specified for the particular alloy in order to provide a reasonable balance between the properties of strength and ductility.

In a solution heat treatment, the alloy should be held at the treatment temperature for sufficient time to allow the diffusion of the copper atoms to a random substitutional arrangement. Usually an arbitrarily selected time of 10 minutes at 700° C (1292° F) is employed, followed by quenching.

Miscellaneous Hardening Phases   As previously noted, dental casting gold alloys may contain as many as six metals, including gold, platinum, silver, palladium, copper, and zinc. As mentioned in the previous chapter, many of these metals in binary combinations can furnish precipitation phases during age hardening, with certain compositions.

The ordered lattice PtCu is known to produce age hardening. PdCu is not as effective unless silver is present when a ternary superlattice forms.

A particularly effective age-hardening constituent in gold alloys is a platinum-iron intermetallic compound. It is useful in strengthening the gold alloys used in the porcelain fused to gold restoration when platinum is used to increase the melting range and lower the coefficient of thermal expansion of the alloy. Such alloys are discussed in Chapters 24 and 31.

The Ternary Au-Ag-Cu System   Most dental gold alloys, as has been mentioned, are basically ternary alloys of gold, silver, and copper, containing minor additions of platinum, palladium, zinc, etc. A majority of these alloys can be hardened by heat treatment. They are usually homogeneous solid solutions when quenched immediately after solidification from the melt. In effect, this is the same as quenching for a solid solution heat treatment.

These alloys can be age-hardenable primarily because two phases precipitate out. One is a copper-rich phase and the other the typical AuCu ordered phase. In both precipitates no doubt silver is also present, thus adding to the solid solution hardening of each precipitated phase, as well as to the residual random solid solution phase.

There are other ternary combinations, and possibly quaternary, etc. Such systems are very complex and are not entirely understood.

19 TARNISH AND CORROSION

Metals undergo chemical reactions with nonmetallic elements in the environment to produce chemical compounds. Commonly known as corrosion products, these compounds may accelerate, retard, or have no influence on the subsequent deterioration of the metal surface. Unfortunately, many of the most commonly used metals derive little or no protection from the corrosion products that form under normal circumstances. The rusting of iron is a familiar example of the effects which may be produced by such a process.

One of the primary requisites of any metal or alloy that is to be used in the mouth is that it should not produce corrosion products that will be harmful to the structure. If not too marked, these products are often not recognized because they are not deleterious. However, when they are present in a more noticeable form, they not only lead to loss of aesthetic qualities but they may even alter the physical properties of an alloy to such an extent that the appliance may be weakened or may fail.

Unfortunately, the oral environment is very conducive to the formation of corrosion products. The mouth is moist and continually subjected to fluctuations in temperature. The foods and liquids ingested have wide ranges of pH. Acids are liberated during the breakdown of foodstuffs. This food debris often adheres tenaciously to the metallic restoration, thus providing a localized condition that is extremely conducive to an accelerated reaction between the corrosion products and the metal or alloy. All of these environmental factors contribute to the degrading process known as *corrosion*.

Gold resists chemical attack of this nature very well; therefore, it was natural that this "noblest of the metals" was employed early for the construction of dental appliances.

Causes of Tarnish and Corrosion A differentiation should be made between tarnish and corrosion. Even though there is a definite technical difference, it is difficult clinically to distinguish between the two phenomena, and the terms are often used interchangeably in the dental literature.

Tarnish is a surface discoloration on a metal or even a slight loss or alteration of the surface finish or luster. In the oral cavity, tarnish usually occurs from the formation of hard and soft deposits on the surface of the restoration. Calculus is the principal hard deposit and its color varies from light yellow to brown. The longer it remains on the surface, the darker it becomes. Its color varies also with the oral hygiene of the patient and is especially dark in the mouths of heavy smokers. The soft deposits are plaques and films composed mainly of microorganisms and mucin. Stain or discoloration arises from pigment-producing bacteria, drugs containing such chemicals as iron or mercury, and adsorbed food debris. These hard and soft deposits, and thus tarnish, may be found anywhere in the mouth but are more apt to be on surfaces that are protected from the abrasive action of foods and the toothbrush.

Although such deposits are the main cause of tarnish in the oral cavity, surface discoloration may also arise on a metal from the formation of thin films, such as oxides, sulfides, or chlorides. This phenomenon may then be only a simple deposition on the surface, and such a film may even be protective, as will be discussed subsequently. However, usually it is the first step leading to corrosion.

Corrosion in the specific sense is not merely a surface deposit but is an actual deterioration of a metal by reaction with its environment. In some perverse but frequent cases, especially with surfaces under stress or with intergranular impurities in the metal or with corrosion products that do not completely cover the substrate metal, the corrosion attack rate may actually increase with time. In due course it causes severe and catastrophic disintegration of the metal body. In addition, corrosion attack that is extremely localized may cause rapid mechanical failure of a structure even though the actual loss of material is quite small.

This disintegration of a metal may occur through the action of moisture, atmosphere, acid or alkaline solutions, and certain chemicals. Tarnish is often the forerunner of the more serious condition of corrosion. The film that is deposited and produces tarnish may in time form, or accumulate, elements or compounds that chemically attack the metallic surface. For example, eggs and certain other foods contain significant amounts of sulfur. Various sulfides, such as hydrogen or ammonium sulfide, corrode silver, copper, mercury, and similar metals present in dental alloys and amalgam.[1]

Also, water, oxygen, and chloride ions are present in saliva and contribute to corrosion attack. Various acids such as phosphoric, acetic, and lactic are present at times. At the proper concentration and pH these can lead to corrosion.

As will be seen in the following chapters, various ions play a major role in the corrosion of various alloys. For example, oxygen and chlorine are implicated in the corrosion of amalgam at the tooth interface and within the body of the alloy.[2] Sulfur is probably most significant in surface tarnish developed on casting alloys that contain silver, although chloride has also been identified as a contributor.

Classification of Corrosion The exact phenomenon of corrosion is often complex and not completely understood. The less homogeneous the metal or alloy and the more complex the environment, the more complicated is the corrosion process. The composition, physical state, and surface condition of the metallic material, as well as the chemical components of the surrounding medium — their phases and concentrations — determine the nature of the corrosion reactions. Other important variables affecting corrosion processes are the temperature, temperature fluctuation, movement or circulation of the medium in contact with the metal surface, and the nature and solubility of the corrosion products. In spite of all these complexities, if the general mechanism of corrosion is understood, it is usually possible to recognize the controlling variables in a given instance of corrosion.

There are two general classifications of corrosion reactions. One type is so-called *chemical corrosion* in which there is a direct combination of metallic and nonmetallic elements. This type is exemplified by oxidation, halogenation, or sulfurization reactions. A good example is the discoloration of silver by sulfur. The formation of Ag_2S in this reaction is chemical corrosion. Silver sulfide appears to be the principal corrosion product of dental gold alloys that contain silver. Such corrosion is also referred to as "dry" corrosion, since it occurs in the absence of water or other fluid electrolytes.

Chemical corrosion is seldom isolated and almost invariably is accompanied by a second type of corrosion known as *electrolytic* or *electrochemical corrosion*. This type is also referred to as "wet" corrosion, since it requires the presence of water or other fluid electrolytes. It also requires a pathway for the transport of electrons, an electrical current, if the process is to continue. Since the oral cavity is a wet environment, the remaining discussion will be principally concerned with wet corrosion.

The starting point for the discussion of electrolytic corrosion is the electrolytic cell illustrated in Figure 19–1. Such a cell is composed of four components.

The anode is the surface where positive ions are formed, that is, the metal surface which is corroding. The reaction may be described as:

$$M^0 \longrightarrow M^+ + e^- \qquad (1)$$

Notice that free electrons are produced; hence, this is sometimes referred to as the *oxidation reaction*.

At the cathode a reaction must occur which will consume the free electrons produced at the anode. Numerous possibilities exist and are dependent on the environment in the electrolyte. For example, metal ions may be removed from the solution to form metal atoms, hydrogen ions may be converted to hydrogen gas, or hydroxyl ions may be formed:

$$M^+ + e^- \longrightarrow M^0 \qquad (2)$$

$$2H^+ + 2e^- \longrightarrow H_2\uparrow \qquad (3)$$

$$2\,H_2O + O_2 + 4e^- \longrightarrow 4(OH)^- \qquad (4)$$

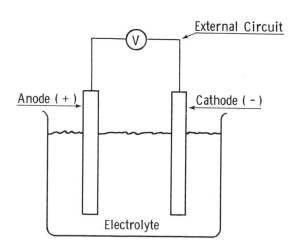

Figure 19–1 Diagram of an electrolytic cell.

All of these processes are referred to as *reduction reactions*. The electrolyte serves to supply the ions needed at the cathode and to carry away the corrosion products at the anode.

The external circuit serves as a conduction path to carry electrons (the electric current) from the anode to the cathode. If a voltmeter is placed into this circuit, an electrical potential difference, a voltage V, can be measured. This voltage has considerable theoretical importance, as will be discussed next. It should also be pointed out that this simple electrolytic cell is in principle a battery, since the flow of electrons in the external circuit is capable of lighting a light bulb in a flashlight or producing a physiological sensation, i.e., pain.

In order for electrolytic corrosion to be an ongoing process, the production of electrons by the oxidation reaction at the anode must be exactly balanced by the consumption of electrons in the reduction reaction at the cathode. This is a very important consideration in determining the rate of a corrosion process and can be used to advantage in order to reduce or eliminate corrosion.

The basis for any discussion of electrolytic corrosion is, of necessity, the *electromotive force series* (EMF). This classification is an arrangement of the elements in the order of their dissolution tendencies. The values for potential are calculated for the elements in solutions containing in effect one atomic weight, in grams, of ions in 1000 gm of water at 25° C. These standard potentials may be considered as the voltage of electrolytic cells in which one pole is the hydrogen electrode (equation 3), designated arbitrarily as zero, and the other is the electrode of the element designated. The sign of the electrode potential indicates the polarity in such a cell. The series for the elements that might be useful to the dentist is seen in Table 19–1.

The same series may be called an electrode potential or an oxidation potential series. In such a case the signs would be reversed. Potassium would be +2.92 and gold −1.50, for example. Such a sign designation is consistent with thermodynamics and indicates the propensity of the element to give up electrons (oxidize) and go into solution as positive ions. In a complete cell, the

Table 19–1. *Electromotive Series of the Metals*

Metal	Ion	Electrode Potential (Volts)
Gold	Au^+	+1.50
Gold	Au^{+++}	+1.36
Platinum	Pt^{++}	+0.86
Palladium	Pd^{++}	+0.82
Mercury	Hg^{++}	+0.80
Silver	Ag^+	+0.80
Copper	Cu^+	+0.47
Bismuth	Bi^{+++}	+0.23
Antimony	Sb^{+++}	+0.10
Hydrogen	H^+	0.00
Lead	Pb^{++}	−0.12
Tin	Sn^{++}	−0.14
Nickel	Ni^{++}	−0.23
Cadmium	Cd^{++}	−0.40
Iron	Fe^{++}	−0.44
Chromium	Cr^{++}	−0.56
Zinc	Zn^{++}	−0.76
Aluminum	Al^{+++}	−1.70
Sodium	Na^+	−2.71
Calcium	Ca^{++}	−2.87
Potassium	K^+	−2.92

metal that gives up its electrons and ionizes is called the anode. The metal that accepts electrons from the external circuit is called the cathode. Regardless of sign designation, the more active metal is the anode and the more noble metal is the cathode when a standard electrolyte is present.

Thus, according to this theory, if two metals are immersed in an electrolyte and are connected by an electrical conductor, an electric couple is formed. With the sign designation used in Table 19–1, the metal with the lowest electrode potential goes into solution. (Only when the signs are reversed do solution and electrode potential correspond.) The strength and direction of the current thus depend primarily upon the electrode potential of the individual metals.

A familiar example of this phenomenon is the dissolving of the zinc electrode in a voltaic cell when it is in electric contact with copper or some metal with a greater electrode potential than itself. Thus, the solution of the zinc and the corresponding disintegration of the surface are an example of the process of corrosion.

It should be emphasized that the relative position of any of the elements in the series is dependent not only on the inherent solution tendencies but also upon the effective concentration of ions of that element that are present in the environment. As the ionic concentration of the element increases in the environment, the tendency for that element to dissolve decreases. The significance of the concentration factor in determining the position of a metal in the electromotive series is well illustrated again by zinc and copper. In a zinc cyanide solution, under certain circumstances the copper actually dissolves and corrodes more readily than the zinc and it displaces zinc from the solution. It should also be pointed out that although theoretically the EMF or the galvanic series provides information about whether a corrosion reaction can occur, in an actual case neither will predict the occurrence or rate of corrosion.

This increase in metal content in the environment may finally prevent further corrosion. Metals usually cease corroding merely because their immediate environments have become saturated with ions of the metals. Such a situation does not usually occur in dental restorations because the dissolving ions are removed by food, fluids, and the toothbrush. Thus, the corrosion continues.

Electrolytic Corrosion   Electrolytic corrosion is of greater significance and is usually associated also with chemical corrosion; therefore, it will be discussed in greater detail and with special reference to the oral cavity.

Provided an electrolyte is present, four general types of electrolytic corrosion are possible and all may occur to some extent in the oral cavity because saliva, with the salts it contains, is a weak electrolyte. The electrochemical properties of saliva depend upon its composition, concentration of its components, pH, surface tension, and buffering capacity. All these factors may influence the strength of any electrolyte and thus the magnitude of the resulting corrosion.

In a wet corrosion environment in which the corroding metal replaces hydrogen or another metal from a compound, two reactions take place simultaneously on the surface of the metal. Metal ions pass into solution, and hydrogen ions pass out of solution. However, because ions have dimensions, it is obvious that both reactions cannot take place at the same point. There must be two independent areas, those at which the metal dissolves (anodic) and those at which hydrogen ions are discharged (cathodic). In such a postulation, it must be assumed that the interface between a metal and its environment is not entirely homogeneous. In other words, there are two types of interfaces between the metal and the environment at which different corrosion tendencies exist. In actual practice, it is safe to assume that perfectly homogeneous metals or surfaces are not possible and even if they were, the chances of their environment being equally homogeneous are remote.

The types of electrolytic corrosion are, therefore, based upon the mechanisms that produce these inhomogeneous areas and, thus, the electric couple action.

Dissimilar Metals   The first type of electrolytic corrosion is that found with combinations of *dissimilar metals*. Here the dental reference is to two separate restorations in which the metal surfaces are chemically dissimilar. The metallic combinations that may produce *electrogalvanism* or "galvanic currents" may or may not be in intermittent contact.

The effect of "galvanic shock" is well known in dentistry. For example, assume that an amalgam restoration, as discussed in the following chapters, is placed on the occlusal surface of a lower tooth directly opposing a gold inlay in an upper tooth. Because both restorations are wet with saliva, an electric couple exists, with a difference in potential between the dissimilar restorations. Such a situation is diagrammed in Figure 19–2. When the two fillings are brought into contact, the potential is suddenly short-circuited through the two alloys. The result is sharp pain. A similar effect may be observed by touching the tine of a silver fork to a gold foil or inlay restoration, and at the same time allowing some other portion of the fork to come in contact with the tongue.

When the teeth are not in contact, the difference in electrical potential or electromotive force between the two fillings still exists. A circuit also exists. The saliva forms the electrolyte, and the hard and soft tissues can constitute the external circuit. The resistance of the external circuit is considerable in comparison with that which exists when the two fillings are brought into contact. The electric currents measured under these conditions between a gold and an amalgam restoration in the same mouth, but not in contact, appear to be approximately 0.5 to 1 microampere or a corresponding electromotive force of approximately 500 millivolts.[3] These currents are somewhat greater when dissimilar metals are present, but they also occur between restorations of similar metals, which are never exactly comparable in surface composition or

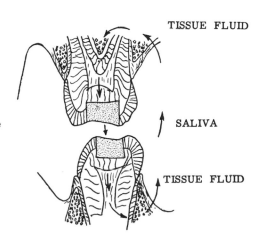

Figure 19–2 Possible path of an electric current in the mouth.

TISSUE FLUID

SALIVA

TISSUE FLUID

structure. A current of less intensity is present even in a single isolated metallic restoration. In the single restoration the cell is created between the two electrolytes, saliva and the tissue fluid. The term "tissue fluid" has been used to denote the dentin, soft tissue, and blood which provide the means for completing the external circuit.

Although the magnitude of these currents usually diminishes somewhat as the restoration ages, it remains indefinitely at the approximate value cited. The clinical significance of these currents, other than their influence on corrosion, will be discussed later in this chapter.

Heterogeneous Composition   A second type of electrolytic corrosion is that due to the *heterogeneous composition* of the metal surface. Examples of this type may be the eutectic and peritectic alloys. It was previously stated that the corrosion resistance of such alloys is generally less than that of solid solution. The reason should now be evident. When an alloy containing a eutectic is immersed in an electrolyte, the metallic grains with the lower electrode potential are attacked and corrosion results. Likewise, in a solid solution, any cored structure is less resistant to corrosion than the homogenized structure because of differences in electrode potential caused by segregation and variation in composition between the individual dendrites. Even a homogenized solid solution is somewhat susceptible to corrosion because of the difference in structure between the grains and their boundaries. The grain boundaries may act as the anodes and the interior of the grains as the cathodes. This results in the corrosion of the material in the anodic region at the grain boundaries.

Solder joints may also corrode because of the inhomogeneous composition of the alloy-solder combination. In this case, corrosion is more likely to occur because of the combined effects of dissimilar metals and the difference in composition of the alloy and the solder.

Impurities in any alloy enhance corrosion. They usually collect in the grain boundary, which in itself is more easily attacked by virtue of being in an inherently stressed condition. The impurities, such as mercury contamination of gold, have potentials different from the grains themselves. Pure metals corrode at much slower rates than alloys, since there is less chance of impurities or second phases, which act as microsize dissimilar electrode cells.

Inhomogeneous Surface   A third condition that produces electrolytic corrosion is the presence of an *inhomogeneous surface* structure. A common situation for this type of corrosion would be an amalgam restoration with polished and unpolished areas. The polished area could be anodic to the unpolished area.

This type is primarily associated with a stress condition in the alloy or metal. For example, even in a pure metal not previously subjected to external forces, a certain amount of stress is always present. The grain boundaries of the pure metal are chemically attacked in preference to the grain itself because of the lattice distortion in the boundary which produces a stressed condition.

Of course, any cold working of an alloy by bending, burnishing, or malleting localizes stress in some parts of the structure such as areas of stress dislocations. A couple composed of the stressed metal, saliva, and the unstressed metal is thus formed. The stressed area is then more readily dissolved by the electrolyte. This is one of the reasons why unnecessary burnishing of the margins of metallic restorations is contraindicated.

Stress Corrosion On most dental appliances, the deleterious effects of stress and corrosion are most apt to occur because of fatigue of the metal when associated with a corrosive environment. Repeated removal and insertion of a partial denture, for example, may build up a severe stress pattern in certain types of alloys, especially at the grain boundaries. Combined with an oral condition that promotes corrosion, the stressed appliance develops *stress corrosion*. Slight surface irregularities at that point, such as a notch or pit, can accelerate the process so that ordinary fatigue starts below the normal limit and failure results. Stress corrosion is characterized by the fact that the eventual fracture occurs intergranularly.

Concentration Cell Corrosion The fourth type of electrolytic corrosion is called *concentration cell corrosion*. This situation exists whenever there are variations in the electrolytes or in the composition of the given electrolyte within the system. For example, there are often accumulations of food debris in the interproximal areas of the mouth, particularly if oral hygiene is poor. This debris then produces one type of electrolyte in that area and the normal saliva provides another electrolyte at the occlusal surface. Therefore, electrolytic corrosion occurs.

A similar type of attack may be produced from differences in oxygen tension between parts of the same restoration. A cell is produced with the greatest activity occurring around the areas containing the least oxygen. Irregularities, such as pits, contribute to this phenomenon. The areas at the bottom of the surface concavities do not have oxygen because they are covered with food debris and mucin. The material at the bottom of the pit then becomes the anode and the material at the periphery the cathode, as diagramed in Figure 19–3. In this manner, metal atoms at the base of the pit ionize and go into solution, causing the pit to deepen. The rate of such corrosion may be very rapid, and failure may occur much before what would be anticipated if only a uniform surface attack were expected.

For this reason all metallic dental restorative materials should be polished. For example, a polished amalgam restoration will corrode less than one left unpolished.

Seldom are any of these four types of electrolytic corrosion found alone. Generally two or more act simultaneously and thus compound the problem. This situation can be illustrated by dissimilar metal corrosion between an inlay and an amalgam restoration. Owing to the surface changes that can occur during this type of electrolytic corrosion, differences in oxygen tension arise. At the same time, if the tarnished layer is incomplete or porous, as is usually the case with dental alloys, an inhomogeneous surface results which produces new corrosion cells.

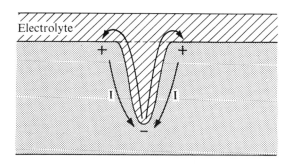

Figure 19–3 A pit is actually a small corrosion cell. The material at the bottom acts as the anode and that around the rim of the pit acts as the cathode. The ionic current flows through the electrolyte and the electronic current through the metal. (From Richman MH: An Introduction to the Science of Metals. Waltham, Mass., Blaisdell Pub. Co., 1967.)

Likewise, if the tarnished layer is not resistant to oral fluids, a direct chemical attack may occur. Depending on the location of the phenomena, a concentration cell corrosion may then be initiated. As a matter of fact, even in the very early stages of tarnish, apparently the principle of concentration cells, and thus localized galvanic action, operate. Careful microscopic examination of the progress of tarnish on dental gold alloys reveals that initially the deposited tarnish film is not actually continuous.[4] Rather, it is a discrete or discontinuous deposit. The apparent continuity is an overlapping of these numerous microdiscrete tarnish regions.

Such a situation exists even when the conditions remain constant. Unfortunately the oral environment is not stable because of pH fluctuations, oral hygiene habits, characteristics of the saliva, and continual stress exerted on the restoration. All of these variables, then, accelerate the multiple corrosion processes.

Protection Against Corrosion   A coating of a noble metal applied to the surface of a second metal may be used to prevent corrosion. The coating material must be less active than the base metal; that is, the coating material must be cathodic to the base metal. Although coatings of gold or silver have been used, any metal may be employed as long as it is less active than the metal which it is to protect.

If a noble metal casting is applied to a base metal surface and becomes scratched or pitted to such a depth that the base metal is exposed to the environment, the base metal will be corroded at a rapid rate. This occurs, of course, because of the dissimilar electrode cell formed between the exposed base metal and the noble metal of the coating.

Paints or other types of inorganic or organic coatings behave as noble coatings. Again, any pit or scratch in the protective layer may lead to rapid corrosion of the base metal. In the case of dissimilar metal corrosion, a paint or other non-conductive film can be used to advantage if it is applied to the more *noble* of the two metals. The corrosion rate of the more active metal will be reduced because the surface area available for the reduction reaction will have been decreased. A scratch in this type of coating will *not* lead to rapid attack on the active metal.

Such metallic and other coatings have been attempted on low carat dental gold alloys. Generally, they were ineffective because they were too thin, were incomplete, did not adhere to the underlying metal or alloy, or were readily scratched or attacked by oral fluids.

Certain metals develop a protective coating by oxidation, or some other chemical reaction, which protects them from further corrosion; such a metal is said to be *passive*. Practically, it is a form of tarnish in which the adhering coating protects the metal underneath from further tarnish and corrosion.

Chromium is the best example of passivity. This important metal does not readily corrode because it has already corroded so rapidly and so uniformly that the film of corrosion product formed does not mar its reflectivity. It is probable that this film consists of either a continuous layer of adsorbed oxygen or a closely packed chromic oxide with each molecule being oriented so that the oxygen is on the outside. Iron, steel, and certain other metals which are subject to corrosion may be electroplated with chromium so that they are rendered noncorrosive. The so-called "stainless steels" are alloys of steel with chromium in amounts sufficient to passivate the alloy.

Aluminum and titanium are other metals which passivate that have found application in dentistry.

Noble metals resist corrosion because their EMF is positive in respect to any of the common reduction reactions found in the oral environment. In order to corrode a noble metal under such conditions, an external current (overpotential) would have to be imposed.

The Dental Restoration It is apparent from this discussion that the oral environment and dental structures present complex conditions that can promote corrosion and discoloration. The variables of diet, bacterial activity, drugs, smoking, and oral hygiene habits unquestionably account for a great portion of the differences in corrosion often noted in different patients in whom the same dental alloy, handled in the same manner, was employed.

Corrosion resistance is, of course, an important consideration in the composition of the alloy itself. Unfortunately, there is no laboratory test that duplicates oral conditions exactly and thus accurately predicts the susceptibility of the material to corrosion. Various accelerated tests involving hydrogen peroxide, egg yolk, and ammonium sulfide have been advocated. The most common test has been the use of a warm sulfurized oil bath. Using these various test methods, it has been shown that the noble metal content, particularly gold, influences the resistance to corrosion. Alloys with a noble metal content below 65 per cent usually tarnish.[5] For this reason, it is estimated that at least half the atoms in a dental alloy should be gold, with platinum and palladium, to insure against corrosion.[6] However, it is possible to increase the tarnish resistance by adding palladium to the alloy.[7] As mentioned previously, silver sulfide appears to be the common corrosion product of gold alloys that contain silver. Palladium tends to retard the formation of silver sulfide and thus has become a common addition to silver containing dental gold alloys. With certain formulations, in this manner it may be possible to decrease the noble metal content down to perhaps 50 to 55 per cent. If noble metals are used to avoid corrosion, it is important that the more active constituents of the alloy be uniformly dispersed (random solid solution). The formation of a second phase which is rich in active metal obviously will produce a galvanic corrosion cell.

Certain base metal alloys, such as the chromium base alloys to be discussed later, are also especially resistant because of the passivity of the chromium.

In addition to proper compounding of the alloy itself, the surface condition of the restoration must be considered. Before the patient is finally dismissed, the surface of the restoration should be smooth and lustrous. This type of surface is not only desirable esthetically but also it minimizes subsequent corrosion. A polished, smooth surface provides easier cleansing and minimizes accumulation of debris.

As seen earlier, notches, pits, and porosity are to be avoided because they provide sources of stress and the risk of stress corrosion.

Clinical Significance of Galvanic Currents It has been proven that small galvanic currents associated with electrogalvanism are continually present in the oral cavity.[8] Their influence on corrosion was discussed earlier. As long as metallic dental restorative materials are employed, there seems to be little possibility that these galvanic currents can be eliminated. The cement base itself, although it is a good thermal insulator, has little effect in minimizing the current that is carried into the tooth and through the pulp. Although many of these base materials are good electrical insulators when dry, they lose this property when they become wet through marginal seepage or from moisture in the dentin.

Until materials or techniques are developed that will provide perfect adaptation to the cavity walls, the possibility of blocking such currents is highly unlikely. For all practical purposes, the metallic restoration cannot be isolated electrically from the tooth. While the cement base does not appreciably reduce the total quantity of current, it may alter its path through the tooth. In situations in which the metallic restoration is extremely close to the pulp, the current concentration and pulpal stimulation may be reduced somewhat by replacing the deepest portion of the metal restoration with a lower conduction base material.

Although the postoperative pain due to galvanic shock is not a common occurrence in the dental office, it can be a real source of discomfort to an occasional patient. However, such postoperative pain usually occurs immediately after insertion of a new restoration and generally it gradually subsides and disappears in a few days. It has often been suggested that the reason the pain does not last indefinitely is because of the formation of a layer of tarnish on the restoration or that the cement base, such as zinc oxide–eugenol cement, becomes a better insulator as setting progresses. However, it has been clearly shown that these currents continue in old as well as new restorations, and that the cement base itself is not an effective insulator to electrical energy. Therefore, it is more likely that the physiologic condition of the tooth is the primary factor responsible for the pain resulting from this current flow. Once the tooth has responded from the injury of preparing the cavity and returned to a more normal physiologic condition, the same magnitude of current flow then produces no response.

Practically, the best method for reducing or eliminating galvanic shock seems to be to paint an external varnish on the surface of the restoration. As long as the varnish remains, the restoration is insulated from saliva and no cell is established. By the time the varnish has worn away, the pulp has usually healed sufficiently so that no pain is evidenced. In the amalgam restoration, polishing of any corroded surface has also been recommended as a possible expedient. It is possible that the more homogeneous surface created by polishing might reduce the magnitude of the current.

It has been suggested that these currents, or the metallic ions that are liberated from the restoration because of the galvanic current, could account for many types of dyscrasias, such as lesions, ulcers, leukoplakia, cancer, and kidney disorders.[9] Other research, particularly a statistical analysis of 1000 patients, has failed to correlate any relationship between dissimilar metals and tissue irritation.[10] One study is of particular interest.[11] A high galvanic current flow of approximately 5 microamperes was induced through the tongue and lips of rats each time they drank water through a stainless steel tube. After a period of one year, there was no gross or microscopic evidence of tissue changes induced by a current of this magnitude.

The effects of these currents in pathologic changes in oral, or other, tissues have possibly been exaggerated. The problem will remain controversial as long as dissimilar metals are used in the mouth, but the efforts that would be necessary to resolve this issue seem not to be worthy of the time and energy required. It is the opinion of the majority of research workers in pathology and dental materials that these currents exist, but that they are probably deleterious only from the standpoint of possible discomfort to an occasional patient. Until it can be clearly substantiated that there is a correlation between these currents and the many dyscrasias attributed to them, it seems logical to assume that such undiagnosed instances are related to more logical, fundamental, and established factors.

On the other hand, until the situation is more definitely clarified, it seems that the conservative procedure would be to avoid situations that might obviously produce an exaggerated condition. For example, the insertion of an amalgam restoration directly in contact with a gold crown seems to be contraindicated. Mercury released from the corroding amalgam (the anode) certainly alloys with the gold alloy (the cathode) and weakens it. A discoloration of both restorations will probably occur. Furthermore, whether it is harmful or not, a metallic taste is always present subsequent to the dental operation, and, as previously stated, it may persist indefinitely.

The previous discussion has referred primarily to electrogalvanism associated with amalgam and noble metal restorations. When contacting dissimilar base metal alloys are present in the oral cavity, spectacular examples of corrosion and soft and hard tissue destruction have been reported.[12, 13] In dental prostheses involving the use of dissimilar base metals, the biological effects of these phenomena appear to warrant further investigation.

References

1. Swartz ML, Phillips RW, and El Tannir MD: Tarnish of certain dental alloys. J Dent Res 37:837, 1958.
2. Marshall GW Jr, Jackson BL, and Marshall SJ: Copper-rich and conventional amalgam restorations after clinical use. J Am Dent Assoc 100:43, 1980.
3. Reed GJ and Willman W: Galvanism in the oral cavity. J Am Dent Assoc 27:1471, 1940.
4. Tuccillo JT and Nielsen JP: Observations of onset of sulfide tarnish on gold-base alloys. J Prosthet Dent 25:629, 1971.
5. Souder W and Paffenbarger GC: Physical properties of dental materials. National Bureau of Standards Circular C433. Washington, DC, US Government Printing Office, 1942, pp. 24–25.
6. Lane JR: Survey of dental alloys. J Am Dent Assoc 39:414, 1949.
7. Burse AB, Swartz ML, Phillips RW, and Dykema RW: Comparison of the in vitro and in vivo tarnish of three gold alloys. J Biomed Mater Res 6:267, 1972.
8. Schriever W and Diamond LE: Electromotive force and electric currents caused by metallic dental fillings. J Dent Res 31:205, 1952.
9. Lain ES, Schriever W, and Gaughnon GS: Problems of electrogalvanism in the oral cavity caused by dissimilar dental materials. J Am Dent Assoc 27:1765, 1940.
10. Mills RB: Study of incidence of irritation in mouths having teeth filled with dissimilar metals. Northwest Univ Bull 39:18, 1939.
11. Phillips RW, Schnell RJ, and Shafer WG: Failure of galvanic current to produce leukoplakia in rats. J Dent Res 47:666, 1968.
12. Bradley P: Electrolyte action around bone pins in the "halo" frame. Br Dent J Oral Surg 7:69, 1969.
13. Oehlers FAC: Electrolytic action related to metal bridge restorations in the treatment of jaw fractures. Br Dent J 102:494, 1957.

20 DENTAL AMALGAM ALLOYS AND AMALGAM STRUCTURES

An *amalgam* is a special type of alloy in that one of its constituents is mercury. Inasmuch as mercury is liquid at room temperature, it can be alloyed with other metals that are in the solid state. This type of alloying is known as *amalgamation*.

Before these alloys combine with mercury they are known as *dental amalgam alloys*. Historically, amalgam alloys were required by American Dental Association Specification no. 1 to contain at least 65 weight per cent silver and 29 weight per cent tin. This composition is close to that which was first recommended by G. V. Black in 1896.[1] Copper, if present at all in alloys, was limited to less than 6 weight per cent. During the 1970's, many amalgam alloys containing between 6 weight per cent and 30 weight per cent copper were developed. Many of these high copper *alloys* produce amalgams (*high copper amalgams*) that are superior in many respects to the traditional *low copper amalgams*. In 1977, the composition limitations of American Dental Association Specification no. 1 were modified to permit the compositions that included much more copper.

Probably few materials have the intrigue of dental amalgam. Its history,[2] the complexity of its reactions and structure, and its importance to dental health care have occupied, and still occupy, the attention of scientists and practitioners.

To make amalgam, mercury is mixed with a powder of the amalgam alloy. The powder may be produced by milling or lathe cutting a cast ingot of the amalgam alloy. The particles of this *lathe-cut* powder are irregularly shaped, as seen in Figure 20–1. Alternately, the powder may be produced by atomizing the liquid alloy. The particles of this *atomized powder* are essentially spherical. As can be seen in Figure 20–2, they may not be true spheres and can even take an oblong shape, depending on the atomizing and solidification technique employed. As will be seen later, the alloy may also be supplied as a mixture of lathe-cut and spherical particles.

The powder may also be supplied in the form of pellets or pills. In this case, the fine particles are subjected to sufficient pressure to cause them to form a "skin" over the outside of the pellet and to cohere slightly on the inside. Yet the

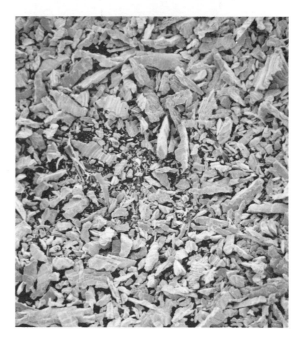

Figure 20–1 Particles of a conventional lathe cut (filing) type amalgam alloy (100 ×).

cohesion is not so great that the particles cannot be readily separated when they are properly amalgamated.

Amalgam alloy is mixed with mercury by the dentist or by the assistant. The mixing procedure is technically known as *trituration*. The product of trituration is a plastic mass similar to that which occurs in the melt of alloys at temperatures between the liquidus and solidus. Special instruments are used to force the plastic mass into the prepared cavity by a process known as *condensation*. The complete technique will be discussed in detail in a subsequent chapter.

During trituration of an alloy powder with mercury, the mercury dissolves

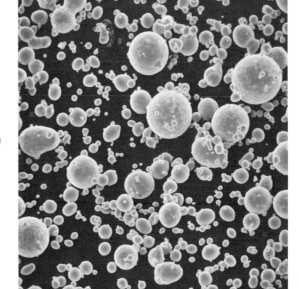

Figure 20–2 Particles of a spherical amalgam alloy (500 ×).

the surface of alloy particles (*dissolution*) and the new phases form (*precipitation*). These new phases have melting points well above any temperature that might normally occur in the mouth. The transformation of the mercury-powder mixture to a precipitate-powder mixture (a *composite*) brings about the setting and *hardening* of the amalgam.

Clinical Performance of Amalgam Restorations   Dental amalgams are used more than any other material for the restoration of lost tooth structure. More than 160 million amalgam restorations are placed each year.[3] These restorations make up approximately 80 per cent of all single tooth restorations.

One of the reasons for dental amalgam's exceptionally fine record of clinical performance may be the tendency of the amalgam restoration to minimize marginal leakage. It has been frequently pointed out in other chapters that one of the greatest hazards associated with restoring teeth is the microleakage that may occur between the cavity walls and the restoration. As repeatedly stated, no restorative material truly adheres to the tooth structure; consequently, penetration of fluids and debris around the margins may be the greatest cause for recurrence of caries. At best, amalgam affords only a reasonably close adaptation to the walls of the prepared cavity. For this reason, cavity varnishes (Chapter 30) are used to reduce the gross leakage that occurs around a new restoration.

The small amount of leakage under amalgam restorations is unique. Apparently, if the restoration is properly inserted, leakage decreases as the restoration ages in the mouth. It is believed that this is caused by corrosion products which form in the interface between the tooth and the restoration.[4] The nature of these products will be discussed later in connection with the structure of the amalgam. The corrosion products apparently seal the interface, thereby preventing leakage. The presence of calcium and phosphorus and the demineralization of tooth structures adjacent to the amalgam restoration also strongly suggest a possible biological interaction in this corrosion process.[5]

The ability to seal against microleakage is shared by both the older low copper amalgams and the newer high copper amalgams.[6-7] However, the accumulation of corrosion products is somewhat slower with the high copper alloys, so the use of a cavity varnish (Chapter 30) is even more essential with these newer systems.

At any rate, the reduced microleakage may be the significant characteristic which accounts for the optimal clinical results experienced through the years with this material.

Nevertheless, daily observations in the dental office reveal many amalgams that exhibit less than optimal performance. Problems that are encountered include secondary caries, gross fracture, "ditched" or fractured margins, and excessive tarnish and corrosion. The ultimate lifetime of an amalgam restoration is determined by a number of factors: (1) the material, (2) the dentist and the assistant, and (3) the patient.[8] The dominant factors that control the performance during the early life of the restoration are the first two. As time proceeds, differences in the dynamics of the oral environment between patients contribute significantly to the variability of deterioration, particularly marginal ditching.[9]

It has been said that the clinical success of the amalgam restoration is based upon meticulous attention to detail. Each manipulative step from the time the cavity is prepared until the restoration has been polished can have an effect upon the physical and chemical properties of the amalgam and the success or failure of the restoration. Certainly, violation of the fundamental principles of cavity preparation have contributed substantially to failure. These matters are treated in texts in operative dentistry. The following discussions will be concerned with failures associated with the alloy itself and the manipulation of it.

In a sense, the dentist and the assistant manufacture the amalgam. The two components, the alloy and mercury, are purchased. However, in the process of combining the two and fashioning the restoration, the amalgam is formed. The precise manner in which this is accomplished will then control the properties and performance of the amalgam.

Therefore, it is convenient to divide the factors governing the quality of a dental amalgam restoration into two groups: those that can be controlled by the dentist and those that are under the control of the manufacturer. The factors governed by the dentist are: (1) mercury-alloy ratios, (2) trituration procedures, (3) condensation technique, (4) marginal integrity and anatomic characteristics, and (5) final finish.

The manufacturer controls (1) the composition of the alloy; (2) the heat treatment of the alloy; (3) the size, shape, and method of production of the alloy particles; (4) the surface treatment of the particles; and (5) the form in which the alloy is supplied. Generally, the factors that are the responsibility of the dentist, or the assistant, will be discussed in the following two chapters. Those factors that are controlled by the manufacturer require some discussion of the metallurgical characteristics of amalgam alloy.

LOW COPPER ALLOYS

American Dental Association Specification no. 1 requires that amalgam alloys be predominantly silver and tin. However, unspecified amounts of other elements (such as copper, zinc, gold, and mercury) are allowed as long as they are present in concentrations less than the silver or tin content. Alloys containing zinc in excess of 0.01 per cent are required to be designated "zinc-containing." Those alloys containing zinc equal to or less than 0.01 per cent are designated as "non-zinc." There is no specification for a low or high copper alloy per se.

It has now become less common to use the G. V. Black[1] silver-tin alloys (the low copper alloys) in preparing amalgam restorations. Nevertheless, the silver-tin alloy is still an important alloy for amalgam, since a silver-tin alloy powder makes up the largest part of some high copper alloy powders. Therefore, it is important to understand the characteristics of both low copper and high copper alloys.

The Silver-Tin System An examination of Figure 20–3 will be necessary to fully understand parts of the following discussion. This is an equilibrium phase diagram of the silver-tin alloy system. Since silver and tin make up the major portion of low copper amalgam alloys, the phase relations shown in this diagram are very close to those found in low copper amalgam alloys.

The low copper alloys have a narrow range of compositions which falls within the $\beta+\gamma$ and γ areas of the diagram shown in Figure 20–3. These areas are enclosed by the lines ABCDE. At point C is the intermetallic compound Ag_3Sn, γ phase, which forms by peritectic reaction (Chapter 17) from the liquid

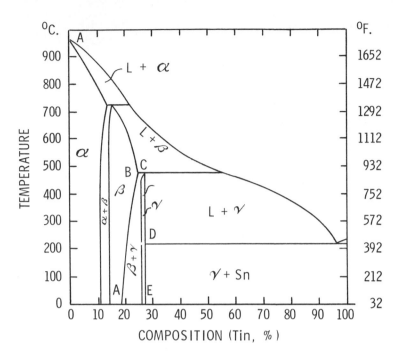

Figure 20–3 Equilibrium phase diagram of the silver-tin system.

plus β area above it. The more silver-rich β phase is a solid solution of tin in silver that crystallographically is similar to the γ phase.

The Influence of Ag-Sn Phases on Amalgam Properties   In the range of compositions around the γ phase, increases or decreases of silver will influence the properties. Increased silver produces more β phase. Decreased silver produces more γ phase. Most commercial alloys fall within the limited composition range of B to C and are not exactly at the peritectic composition. Since the effect of these phases is relatively pronounced, their control is essential if an alloy of uniform quality is to be produced.

If the tin concentration exceeds 26.8 weight per cent, a mixture of γ phase and tin is formed. Presence of the tin phase increases the amount of the tin-mercury phase that is formed when the alloy is amalgamated. The tin-mercury phase lacks corrosion resistance and is the weakest component of dental amalgam. Amalgams of tin-rich alloys display less expansion than silver-rich alloys.

The Influence of Other Elements on Ag-Sn Alloys and Amalgams Silver-tin alloys are quite brittle and are difficult to comminute uniformly unless a small amount of copper is included to "replace" silver atoms. The degree of this atomic replacement is limited to about 4 or 5 weight per cent. Thereafter, the excess copper is seen in metallographic sections as a separate phase, probably as Cu_3Sn. Within the limited range of copper solubility, increased copper content hardens and strengthens the silver-tin alloy.

The use of zinc in an amalgam alloy is a subject of controversy. Zinc is seldom present in an alloy to an extent greater than 1 weight per cent. Alloys without zinc are more brittle than alloys with zinc and their amalgams tend to be less plastic. The chief function of zinc in amalgam alloy is that of a deoxidizer. It acts as a scavenger during melting, uniting with oxygen to minimize the formation of oxides. Unfortunately, the zinc, even in small amounts, causes an abnormal expansion of the amalgam if the amalgam is condensed in the presence of moisture. This effect will be explained in the next chapter.

The American Dental Association specification for amalgam alloys allows mercury in the alloy powder. Some pre-amalgamated alloys are sold in Europe, but these alloys have not been marketed extensively in the United States. These alloys amalgamate very rapidly, but otherwise are similar to alloys that have not been preamalgamated. Elements other than silver, tin, copper, zinc, and/or mercury may be included in amalgam alloy if the manufacturer furnishes adequate clinical and biological data to show that the alloy is safe to use in the mouth.

HIGH COPPER ALLOYS

The popularity of the low copper alloys just described has decreased markedly in recent years. For reasons to be discussed, the high copper alloys are becoming the materials of choice. Actually, a suggestion of the potential of this system appeared in the literature as early as 1941.[10] However, it was not until the early 1960's that the subject surfaced again, leading in time to commercial products.

Two different types of high copper alloy powders are available. The first is an *admixed alloy* powder and the second is a *single-composition alloy powder*. Both types contain more than 6 weight per cent copper.

Admixed Alloys   In 1963, Innes and Yondelis added spherical silver-copper eutectic alloy (71.9 weight per cent Ag and 28.1 weight per cent Cu) particles to lathe-cut low copper particles.[11] This was the first major change in the composition of alloy for dental amalgam since Black's work. The spherical silver-copper particles were intended to dispersion harden amalgams made from the admixed powder; consequently, amalgams of this type are often called *dispersion* or *dispersant* amalgams. However, such alloys are better termed *admixed alloys* because the final powder is a mixture of at least two kinds of particles. An admixed powder, showing lathe-cut low copper alloy particles and spherical silver-copper alloy particles, is seen in Figure 20–4.

It was found that amalgam made from the admixed powders was stronger than amalgam made from lathe-cut low copper powder. The investigators hypothesized that the silver-copper particles "dispersion hardened" the amalgam. Dispersion hardening is a strengthening that is observed in metals when a large volume fraction of ultrafine particles (typically less than 1 μm) is dispersed throughout the metal.[12] It seems unlikely that the silver-copper particles in admixed amalgams (Fig. 20–4) are either small enough or closely enough spaced to produce dispersion hardening. It is more likely that hardening of admixed amalgams is due to the strength of the silver-copper particles. It is known that composite materials (materials that consist of a matrix and a filler) can be strengthened by the addition of strong fillers, as was discussed in Chapter 14. It is probable that the silver-copper particles act as strong fillers, strengthening the amalgam matrix.

It was almost 10 years after this prototype admixed amalgam was developed that its clinical performance became known. Two independent studies[13, 14] showed that restorations made with this prototype admixed amalgam were clinically superior to low copper amalgam restorations when the

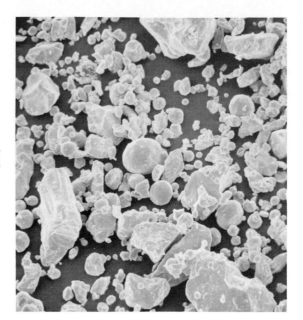

Figure 20–4 Typical admix high copper alloy powder showing the lathe-cut silver-tin particles and the silver-copper spheres (500 ×).

restorations were evaluated for resistance to marginal breakdown. The suggested characteristics of the alloy that bring about this improved clinical performance will be discussed later. It is sufficient to say that these studies[11, 13, 14] are classic, since they triggered the era of the high copper alloy.

Admixed alloy powders usually contain 30 to 55 weight per cent spherical high copper powder. The total copper content in admixed alloys ranges from approximately 9 to 20 weight per cent.

The phases present in the copper-containing particles will depend on their composition. The silver-copper alloy consists of mixtures of two phases, a silver phase and a copper phase. These phases have the crystal structures of pure silver and pure copper, respectively. A small amount of copper is dissolved in the silver phase. In the atomized powder (which is fast cooled), the eutectic two-phase mixture forms very fine lamellae. Compositions on either side of the eutectic will form relatively large grains of copper phase or silver phase amid a eutectic mixture (see Chapter 17).

Single Composition Alloys   Success of the admixed amalgams has led to the development of another type of high copper alloy. Unlike admixed alloy powders, each alloy particle of these alloy powders has the same chemical composition. Therefore, they are called *single composition alloys*. The major components of the particles are usually silver, copper, and tin. (Thus, they are frequently referred to as ternary alloys.) For example, the first alloy of this type contained 60 weight per cent silver, 27 weight per cent tin, and 13 weight per cent copper.[15] The copper content in these alloy particles ranges from 13 to 30 weight per cent, depending on the brand. In addition, small amounts of indium or palladium are also found in some of the currently marketed single composition alloys.

The phases found in the single composition alloys include β Ag-Sn, γ Ag-Sn, and ϵ Cu-Sn (Cu_3Sn). Some of the alloys may also contain some Cu_6Sn_5, the η phase of the copper-tin system, as will be discussed.[16] Atomized particles have dendritic microstructures. Within the dendrites are single phase lamellae less than 50 μm thick.[17]

MANUFACTURE OF ALLOY POWDER

Lathe-Cut Powder   To make lathe-cut powder, an annealed ingot of alloy (either low or high alloy) is placed in a milling machine or in a lathe and is fed into a cutting tool or bit. Since the chips removed are often needle-like, some manufacturers reduce the chip size by ball-milling.

Homogenizing Anneal   Due to the rapid "as cast" cooling conditions the ingot of a silver-tin alloy has a cored structure and contains nonhomogeneous grains of varying composition. In order to re-establish the equilibrium phase relationship, a homogenizing heat treatment is performed (Chapters 17 and 18). The ingot is placed in an oven and heated at a temperature below the solidus for sufficient time to allow diffusion of the atoms to occur and the phases to reach equilibrium. Although the solidus is 480° C (900° F), the danger of incipient melting within the ingot exists at temperatures above 450° C (840° F). Therefore, homogenizing heat treatments usually take place at temperatures below 450° C (840° F). The time of heat treatment may vary, depending on the temperature used and the size of the ingot, but 24 hours at the selected temperature is not unusual.

At the conclusion of the heating cycle, the ingot is brought to room temperature for the succeeding steps in manufacture. The proportion of β and γ phases present in the ingot after cooling will be affected by the manner in which the ingot is cooled. If the ingot is withdrawn from the heat treatment oven rapidly and then quickly quenched, the phase distribution will remain essentially unchanged. On the other hand, if the ingot is permitted to cool very slowly, the proportions of β and γ phases will continue to adjust toward the room temperature equilibrium ratio.

In general, then, rapid quenching of the alloy ingot results in the maximum amount of β phase retained, while slow cooling results in the formation of the maximum amount of the γ phase.

Aging   Once the alloy ingot has been reduced to cuttings, many manufacturers perform some type of surface treatment to the particles. Although specific details of the treatment of the particles are considered proprietary, it is generally accepted that treatment of the alloy particles with acid has been a manufacturing practice for many years. The exact function of this treatment is still not entirely understood, but it is probably related to the preferential dissolution of specific components from the alloy. Amalgams made from acid-washed powders tend to be more reactive than those made from unwashed powders.

The microstresses induced into the particle during the cutting and ball-milling must be relieved. If they are not removed by the manufacturer, they will slowly release over a period of time, causing a change in the alloy; particularly in the rate at which amalgamation will occur and the dimensional change that will occur during hardening. The process is called *aging* and involves an annealing cycle at a moderate temperature (Chapter 16). Usually "aging" is done for several hours at approximately 100° C. A properly "aged" alloy will generally then be stable in its reactivity and properties when stored for an indefinite time.

Atomized Powder   Atomized powder is made by melting together the desired elements, to produce either a low or high copper composition. The liquid metal is then atomized into fine spherical droplets of metal. If the droplets solidify before hitting a surface, the spherical shape is preserved. Whether or not they are truly spherical, atomized powders are frequently called *spherical powders*.

Like the lathe-cut powders, spherical powders are given a heat treatment. The heat treatment coarsens the grains and slows the reaction of these particles with mercury. The reasons necessitating this heat treatment are not fully understood at this time. As with the lathe-cut alloys, spherical powders are usually washed with an acid.

Particle Size   Maximum particle size, and the distribution of sizes within an alloy powder, are controlled by the manufacturer. The average particle sizes of modern powders range between 25 and 35 μm.

The most significant influence on amalgam properties is not the average particle size but rather the distribution of sizes around the average. For example, very small particles (less than 3 μm) greatly increase the surface area per unit volume of the powder. A powder containing tiny particles requires a greater amount of mercury to form acceptable amalgam.

In producing lathe-cut alloys, the cutting rate is precisely controlled to maintain the desired average particle size and size distribution. Similarly, parameters of the atomizing process are controlled to produce the desired particle sizes of spherical alloys. In addition, the particles may be graded according to size and the graded particles remixed to produce a powder with an optimum size distribution.

The present trend in amalgam technique favors the use of a small average particle size. Other factors being equal, a smaller average particle size tends to produce a more rapid hardening of the amalgam with a greater early strength than does the use of larger alloy particles.

As will be seen, the bulk of the finished restoration is composed of particles of the original alloy surrounded by reaction products. The particle size distribution can affect the character of the finished surface. When the amalgam has partially hardened, the tooth anatomy is carved in the amalgam with a sharp instrument. During this carving, the larger particles may be pulled out of the matrix, producing a rough surface. Such a surface is probably more susceptible to corrosion than a smooth surface.

Lathe-Cut Compared to Atomized Alloys   Amalgams made from lathe-cut powders, or admixed powders of a blend of lathe-cut and spherical powders, tend to resist condensation better than amalgams made entirely from spherical powders. Since amalgams of spherical powders are very plastic, one cannot rely upon the pressure of condensation to establish proximal contour. A contoured and wedged matrix band is essential in order to prevent flat proximal contours, improper contacts, and overhanging cervical margins. Of course, good technique requires a matrix band, regardless of the amalgam's resistance to condensation.

Spherical alloys require less mercury than typical lathe-cut alloys because spherical alloys have a smaller surface area per volume than do the lathe-cut alloys. As will become apparent in the next chapter, amalgams with a low mercury content have better properties.

When using lathe-cut powder, higher condensation pressures are necessary than with spherical alloys. One study compared the tensile strength of amalgams prepared from lathe-cut and spherical low copper powders.[18] Low pressure condensation of spherical powder amalgams produced satisfactory tensile strengths. To obtain the same strength level in amalgams of lathe-cut powder required condensation pressures 10 times higher.

AMALGAMATION AND RESULTING STRUCTURE

Low Copper Alloys Amalgamation occurs when mercury comes into contact with the surface of the silver-tin alloy particles. When a powder is triturated, the silver and tin in the outer portion of the particles dissolve into mercury. At the same time, mercury diffuses into alloy particles. The mercury has a limited solubility for silver (0.035 weight per cent)[19] and tin (0.6 weight per cent).[20]

When that solubility is exceeded, crystals of two binary metallic compounds precipitate into mercury. These are the body-centered cubic silver-mercury compound, Ag_2Hg_3,[20] and the hexagonal tin-mercury compound (approximately Sn_8Hg).[21] These phases are called the γ_1 (gamma-one) phase and the γ_2 (gamma-two), respectively. Since the solubility of silver in mercury is much lower than that of tin, the γ_1 phase precipitates first and the γ_2 phase precipitates later.

Immediately after trituration, the alloy powder coexists with the liquid mercury, giving the mix a plastic consistency. γ_1 and γ_2 crystals grow as the remaining mercury dissolves the alloy particles. As the mercury disappears, the amalgam hardens. As the particles become covered with newly formed crystals, mostly γ_1, the reaction rate decreases. The alloy is usually mixed with mercury in about a 1:1 ratio. This is insufficient mercury to completely consume the β and γ alloy particles; consequently, unconsumed particles are present in the set amalgam. Alloy particles (smaller now, because their surface has dissolved in mercury) are surrounded by and bound together by solid γ_1 and γ_2 crystals.

Thus, a typical low copper amalgam is a *composite* in which the unconsumed particles are embedded in γ_1 and γ_2 phases. The sequence of amalgamation of the silver-tin alloy is shown schematically in Figure 20–5.

The micrograph shown in Figure 20–6 illustrates the features found in a typical amalgam made from a lathe-cut low copper alloy. The features include: β and γ Ag-Sn phases labeled (P), ϵ Cu-Sn particle (E), γ_1 Ag-Hg areas (G1), γ_2 Sn-Hg grains (G2), and voids (V). These voids are always formed during γ_1 and γ_2 crystal growth when amalgam is condensed by the usual methods.

The final equilibrium condition is demonstrated in the following equation in which all of the Ag-Sn is considered as Ag_3Sn.[22]

$$16.78\ Ag_3Sn + 37\ Hg \leftrightarrow 12\ Ag_2Hg_3 + Sn_8Hg + 8.78\ Ag_3Sn$$

The 8.78 Ag_3Sn is the amount of unconsumed original alloy, which is 0.31 volume fraction of the hardened amalgam. The reaction can also be conveniently expressed in terms of the phases that form during amalgamation:

$$\beta + \gamma + Hg \rightarrow \gamma_1 + \gamma_2 + \beta + \gamma$$

The physical properties of the hardened amalgam depend upon the relative percentages of each of the microstructural features. The unconsumed Ag-Sn particles have a very strong effect. The more of this phase that is retained in

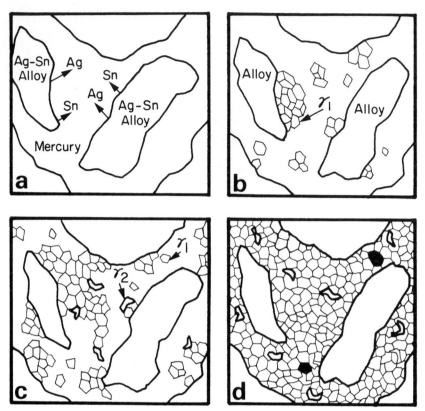

Figure 20–5 These schematic drawings illustrate the sequence of development of amalgam microstructure when lathe-cut low copper alloy particles are mixed with mercury. In order these show: *a*, dissolution of silver and tin into mercury; *b*, precipitation of γ_1 crystals in the mercury; *c*, consumption of the remaining mercury by growth of γ_1 and γ_2 grains; and *d*, the final set amalgam. (Courtesy of T. Okabe, R. Mitchell and C. W. Fairhurst.)

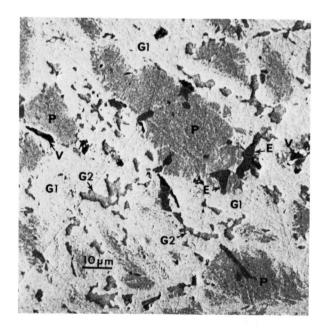

Figure 20–6 A scanning electron micrograph of a low copper silver-tin amalgam (1000 ×). (Courtesy of T. Okabe and M. B. Butts.)

the final structure, the stronger will be the amalgam. Physically and mechanically, the weakest component is the γ_2 phase.[21, 23] The hardness of γ_2 is approximately 10 per cent of the hardness of γ_1, while the γ phase hardness is somewhat higher than that of γ_1.[21]

The γ_2 phase is also the least stable in a corrosion environment, consequently, the γ_2 phase may suffer corrosion attack, especially in "crevices" of the restorations.[24] In general, γ Ag_3Sn is stable in an oral environment. Also the pure Ag_2Hg_3 γ_1 phase is relatively stable. However, γ_1 in amalgam does contain small amounts of tin which can be lost in a corrosion environment.[24]

The interface between the γ phase and the matrix is important.[25] The high proportion of the unconsumed γ phase will not strengthen the amalgam unless the particles are bound to the matrix.

Admixed High Copper Alloys   When mercury is reacted with an admixed powder, silver enters the mercury from the silver-copper alloy particles and both silver and tin enter the mercury from the silver-tin alloy particles. The tin in solution diffuses to the surfaces of the silver-copper alloy particles and reacts with the copper phase to form η Cu-Sn (Cu_6Sn_5). A layer of η crystals forms around unconsumed silver-copper alloy particles. The η Cu-Sn layer on Ag-Cu alloy particles is believed to also contain some γ_1 Ag-Hg crystals.[26, 27] The γ_1 phase forms simultaneously with the η phase and surrounds both the η covered silver-copper alloy particles and the silver-tin alloy particles. As in the low copper amalgams, γ_1 is the matrix phase, i.e., the phase that binds the unconsumed alloy particles together.

Figure 20–7 illustrates the microstructure of an admixed amalgam. Included in the structures are Ag-Sn γ phases, Ag-Cu particles, ϵ Cu-Sn particles, γ_1 matrix areas and η reaction layers. In some admixed amalgams, a small number of η Cu-Sn crystals are also found amid the γ_1 matrix.[28]

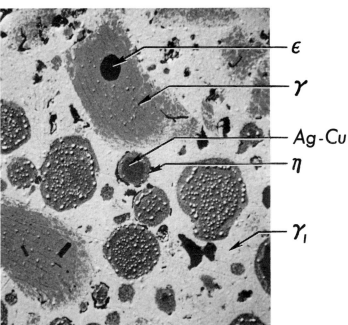

Figure 20–7 Scanning electron micrograph of an admix high copper amalgam. The various phases and reaction layer are labeled. The small, very light, drop-shaped areas are high in mercury due to the freshly polished specimen (1000 ×).

Thus the reaction of the admixed alloy powder with mercury can be summarized as follows:

$$\beta + \gamma + \text{Ag-Cu eutectic} + \text{Hg} \rightarrow \gamma_1 + \eta + \text{unconsumed alloy}$$
$$\text{of both types of particles}$$

Note that γ_2 has been eliminated in this reaction. Incidentally, as yet there is not a precise definition of the characteristics required in an amalgam alloy for it to qualify as a "high copper" system. However, it is generally accepted that it is a formulation whereby the γ_2 is virtually eliminated during amalgamation and the hardening reactions. In order to accomplish this, it is probably necessary to have a net copper concentration of at least 12 per cent in the alloy powder.

Some admixed amalgams do contain γ_2, although the percentage of γ_2 is typically less than is found in low copper amalgams. The effectiveness of the copper-containing particles in preventing γ_2 formation depends on the percentage of copper-containing particles in the mix. The η Cu-Sn phase apparently forms in preference to the γ_2 Sn-Hg phase. If there is insufficient copper to react with the tin dissolved in mercury, the excess tin reacts with mercury to form γ_2.

Single Composition Alloys   Single composition alloy particles may contain both β and γ phases and the ϵ Cu-Sn phase (Cu_3Sn). Very little or no copper dissolves in mercury; as a result, ϵ may not dissolve.

Silver and tin from the Ag-Sn phases dissolve in mercury. The Ag-Hg phase γ_1 crystals grow, forming a matrix that binds together the partially dissolved alloy particles. The η Cu-Sn crystals are found as meshes of rod crystals at the surfaces of alloy particles.[29] These are much larger than the η crystals found in the reaction layers surrounding Ag-Cu particles in admixed amalgams.

Figure 20–8 shows the microstructure of a typical single composition amalgam. The structure includes unconsumed alloy particles labeled P, γ_1 grains (G1), and η Cu-Sn crystals (H).

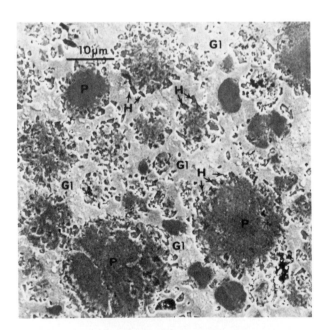

Figure 20–8 A scanning electron micrograph of a high copper single composition amalgam. A relief polish technique was used to reveal the structure[30] (560 ×). (Courtesy of M. B. Butts, T. Okabe, and C. W. Fairhurst.)

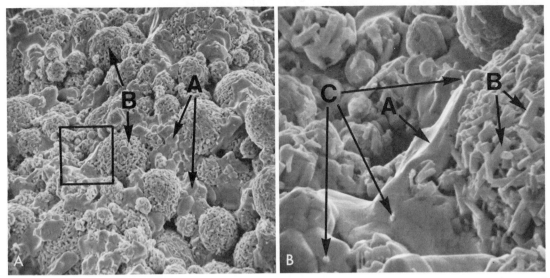

Figure 20–9 A, Scanning electron micrograph of a high copper single composition amalgam fractured shortly after condensation, showing reaction products being formed-γ, (A) and η (B). (1000×). B, Higher magnification of marked area. η rods embedded in γ, crystals can be identified (C). (5000×) (Courtesy of T. Okabe, R. Mitchell, M. B. Butts, and C. W. Fairhurst.)

Figure 20–9A shows a scanning electron micrograph of a high copper single composition amalgam fractured a few minutes after condensation when the amalgamation reaction was still taking place.[29] Two kinds of crystals are seen on the surface: γ_1 polyhedral crystals, shown by arrow A, between the unconsumed alloy particles, and meshes of η Cu-Sn rod crystals, shown by arrow B, which cover the unconsumed alloy particles.

Figure 20–9B shows details of the marked area in Figure 20–9A. In addition to a mesh of η Cu-Sn crystals (B) which formed on an unconsumed particle, η Cu-Sn rods (C) are seen to have embedded in a γ_1 crystal (A). Meshed η crystals on unconsumed alloy particles may strengthen bonding between the alloy particles and γ_1 grains, and η crystals dispersed between γ_1 grains may interlock γ_1 grains. These interlockings are believed to improve the amalgam's resistance to deformation, as will be discussed in Chapter 21.

To summarize, the reaction of the single composition alloy powder with mercury is as follows:

$$\text{(Ag-Sn-Cu alloy particles)} + \text{Hg} \rightarrow \gamma_1 + \eta + \text{unconsumed alloy particles}$$

The undesirable γ_2 phase can also form in single composition amalgams. This is particularly true if the atomized powder has not been heat treated or if the powder has been treated for too long at too high a temperature.[17] Nevertheless, in most single composition amalgams little or no γ_2 forms.

References

1. Black GV: The physical properties of the silver-tin amalgams. Dent Cosmos 38:965, 1896.
2. Greener EH: Amalgam — yesterday, today, and tomorrow. Oper Dent 4:24, 1979.
3. Moen BD and Poetsch WE: More preventive care, less tooth repair. J Am Dent Assoc 81:25, 1970.

4. Swartz ML and Phillips RW: In vitro studies on the marginal leakage of restorative materials. J Am Dent Assoc 62:141, 1961.
5. Sarkar NK, Brice C, and McTique D: Corrosion of Dispersalloy amalgam restorations. IADR Program and Abstracts, No. 1028, 1980.
6. Andrews JT and Hembree JH: In vitro evaluation of marginal leakage of corrosion-resistant amalgam alloy. J Dent Child 42:367, 1975.
7. Boyer DB and Torney DL: Microleakage of amalgam restorations with high-copper content. J Am Dent Assoc 99:199, 1979.
8. Vrijhoef MMA, Vermeersch AG, and Spanauf AJ: Dental Amalgam. Chicago, Quintessence Publ. Co., 1980.
9. Goldberg J, Munster E, Rydinge E, Sanchez L, and Lambert K: Experimental design in the clinical evaluation of amalgam restorations. J Biomed Mater Res 14:777, 1980.
10. Schoonover IC and Souder W: Corrosion of dental alloys. J Am Dent Assoc 28:1278, 1941.
11. Innes DBK and Youdelis WV: Dispersion strengthened amalgams. Can Dent Assoc J 29:587, 1963.
12. Dieter GE: Mechanical Metallurgy. 2nd ed, New York, McGraw-Hill Book Co., Inc., 1976.
13. Duperon DF, Nevile MD, and Kasloff Z: Clinical evaluation of corrosion resistance of conventional alloy, spherical-particle alloy, and dispersion-phase alloy. J Prosthet Dent 25:650, 1971.
14. Mahler DB, Terkla LG, Van Eysden J, and Reisbick MH: Marginal fracture versus mechanical properties of amalgam. J Dent Res 49:1452, 1970.
15. Asgar K: Amalgam alloy with a single composition behavior similar to Dispersalloy. IADR Program and Abstracts, No. 23, 1974.
16. Mahler DB: Dental Amalgam. Dental Materials Review (R.G. Craig, Ed.), Ann Arbor, University of Michigan Press, 1977.
17. Okabe T, Butts MB, Heffernan JJ, Kepler EE, Mitchell RJ, and Asgar K: Effects of annealing alloy powder on high copper amalgam properties. IADR Program and Abstracts, No. 329, 1980.
18. Eden GT and Waterstrat RM: Effects of packing pressures on the properties of spherical alloy amalgams. J Am Dent Assoc 74:1024, 1967.
19. Hansen M and Anderko K: Constitution of Binary Alloys. New York, McGraw-Hill Book Co., Inc., 1958.
20. Fairhurst CW and Cohen JB: The crystal structures of two compounds found in dental amalgam: Ag_2Hg_3 and Ag_3Sn. Acta Cryst B28:371, 1972.
21. Fairhurst CW and Ryge G: X-ray diffraction investigation of the Sn-Hg phase in dental amalgam. Advances in X-ray Analysis (W.M. Mueller, Ed.) Vol. 5, New York, Plenum Press, 1962.
22. Fairhurst CW: PhD Dissertation, Northwestern University, Illinois, 1966.
23. Young FA and Wilsdorf, HGF: The tensile failure of dental amalgam. Proceedings of a symposium on research in dental and medical materials. (E. Korostoff, Ed.), New York, Plenum Press, 1969.
24. Marek M, Hockman RF, and Okabe T: In vitro corrosion of dental amalgam phases. J Biomed Mater Res 10:789, 1976.
25. Wing G: Modern concepts for the amalgam restoration. Dent Clin North Am 15:43, 1971.
26. Mahler DB, Adey JD, and Van Eysden, J.: Quantitative microprobe analysis of amalgam. J Dent Res 54:218, 1975.
27. Okabe T, Mitchell R, Butts MB, Bosley JR, and Fairhurst CW: Analysis of Asgar-Mahler zone in Dispersalloy amalgam of electron diffraction. J Dent Res 56:1037, 1977.
28. Okabe T, Mitchell RJ, and Fairhurst CW: A study of high copper amalgams. IV. Formation of η Cu-Sn (Cu_6Sn_5) crystals in a high copper dispersant amalgam matrix. J Dent Res 58:1087, 1979.
29. Okabe T, Mitchell RJ, Butts MB, and Fairhurst CW: A study of high copper amalgams. III. SEM Observations of amalgamation of high copper powders. J Dent Res 57:975, 1978.
30. Butts MB, Okabe T, and Fairhurst CW: Metallographic polishing technique for high-copper amalgam. J Japan Soc Dent Apparatus Mater 22:5, 1981.

21 DENTAL AMALGAM: DIMENSIONAL CHANGE, STRENGTH, AND CREEP

The manipulation of an amalgam by the dentist can influence its physical and mechanical properties. This chapter focuses on how and why manipulation influences the dimensional change, strength, and creep of an amalgam.

DIMENSIONAL CHANGE

Amalgam can expand or contract, depending on its manipulation. Ideally, the dimensional change should be small. Severe contraction can lead to microleakage and to caries under a restoration. Excessive expansion can produce pressure on the pulp and postoperative pain. Protrusion of a restoration can also result from excessive expansion.

Measurement of Dimensional Change The dimensional change of amalgam depends on how much the amalgam is constrained during setting[1] and on when the measurement is initiated.[2] Constraining a specimen will decrease the expansion or increase the contraction. A delay in the beginning of measurement will decrease the measured contraction or, conversely, increase the measured expansion.

American Dental Association Specification no. 1 requires that amalgam neither contract nor expand more than 20 μm/cm. This expansion is measured between 5 minutes and 24 hours after the beginning of trituration with a device that is accurate to at least 0.5 μm. The test is conducted at 37° C using specimens that are 8 mm long and 4 mm in diameter, a bulk of amalgam essentially equivalent to that used in large amalgam restorations.

Theory of Dimensional Change Most modern amalgams exhibit a net contraction when triturated with a mechanical amalgamator and evaluated by this procedure.[2, 3] The classic picture of dimensional change is one in which the specimen undergoes an initial contraction for about 20 minutes after the

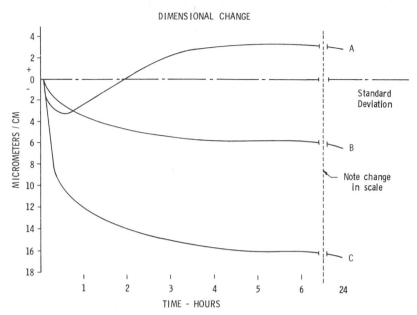

Figure 21–1 Dimensional change curves for three amalgam alloys. *A* is a high copper admixed amalgam, *B* is a high copper single composition, and *C* is a lathe-cut low copper amalgam.

beginning of trituration and then begins to expand. However, as Figure 21–1 illustrates, modern amalgams do not exhibit such simple behavior.[4]

When mercury is mixed with alloy particles, silver and tin dissolve into the mercury. Within the first 2 to 3 seconds, γ_1 Ag-Hg crystals precipitate from the silver saturated mercury, as was described in the previous chapter. Contraction results as the particles dissolve (and hence become smaller) and the γ_1 grows. Calculations show that the final volume of γ_1 is less than the sum of the initial volumes of dissolved silver and liquid mercury that go into making the γ_1.[5, 6] Therefore, contraction will continue as long as growth of γ_1 continues. As γ_1 crystals grow, they will impinge against one another. If conditions are right, this impingement of γ_1 can produce an outward pressure tending to oppose the contraction.

Expansion will occur when γ_1 crystals impinge, if there is sufficient liquid mercury present to provide a plastic matrix. After a rigid γ_1 matrix has formed, growth of γ_1 crystals cannot force the matrix to expand. Instead of growing so as to force other γ_1 crystals outward, γ_1 crystals will grow into interstices containing mercury. This growth will consume mercury, producing continued reaction.

According to the above model, if sufficient mercury is present in the mix when the measurement of dimensional change begins, expansion will be observed. Otherwise, contraction is seen. Therefore, manipulation that results in less mercury in the mix will favor contraction. Such manipulative factors include lower mercury-alloy ratios and higher condensation pressures. In addition, manipulative procedures that accelerate the setting of the amalgam, and accelerate consumption of mercury, also favor contraction. Such procedures include longer trituration times and use of alloys having smaller particles.

The influence of condensation pressure and particle size may require explanation. Higher condensation pressures will squeeze mercury out of the amalgam. Since this produces a lower mercury-alloy ratio, such condensation will favor contraction. Smaller particle size accelerates the consumption of mercury because small particles have a larger surface area per unit mass than larger particles. Since a larger surface area is dissolving, silver enters the solution faster, γ_1 grows from the solution faster, and the consumption of mercury is accelerated.

Measurements of the dimensional change of many modern amalgams reveal a net contraction, whereas in the past measurements invariably indicated that an expansion occurred. Two reasons for the difference is that older amalgams contained larger alloy particles and were mixed at higher mercury-alloy ratios than present-day amalgams. Likewise, hand trituration was used in preparing the specimens. Now high speed mechanical amalgamators are employed. The change to the modern method is equivalent to a large increase in trituration time. All these factors tend to favor expansion of specimens prepared some years ago and contraction of the specimens prepared by modern techniques.

The γ_2 crystals that usually form later in amalgamation are believed to be sufficiently plastic that they will flow into pores and voids instead of pushing γ_1 crystals apart during growth.[6] Therefore, growth of γ_2 does not seem to contribute to the dimensional change of amalgam.

Effect of Moisture Contamination   All of the observations thus far presented have been concerned with the dimensional change during the first 24 hours only. Some admixed amalgams continue to expand for at least 2 years.[1] It has been suggested that this expansion may be related to the disappearance of some or all of the γ_2 in these high copper amalgams. Nevertheless, if manipulated properly, most amalgams exhibit little further dimensional change after 24 hours.

If, however, a zinc-containing amalgam is contaminated by moisture during trituration or condensation, a large expansion, such as that shown in Figure 21–2, can take place. This expansion usually starts after 3 to 5 days and may continue for months, reaching values greater than 400 μm (4%). This type of expansion is known as *delayed expansion* or *secondary expansion*.

The delayed expansion is associated with the zinc in the amalgam. However, the zinc content per se is not directly responsible for the delayed expansion. The effect is due to some type of reaction of "zinc" with water. The effect is not present in non-zinc amalgams. It has been clearly demonstrated that the contaminating substance is water, regardless of whether it is pure or contains an inorganic salt.

One of the products of the reaction of water and zinc is hydrogen. It is produced by electrolytic action between the zinc, the electrolyte, and the anodic elements present. This hydrogen does not combine with the amalgam constituents but, rather, collects within the restoration. It has been shown that the internal pressure of the hydrogen may build up to levels high enough to cause the amalgam to creep, thus producing the observed expansion.[7]

The delayed expansion also occurs in zinc-containing high copper amalgams.[8] If the zinc is not present, the expansion does not occur. It should be noted that the contamination must occur during trituration or condensation; after the amalgam is condensed, the external surface may come in contact with saliva with no ill effect so far as its dimensional change is concerned.

The contamination of the amalgam can occur at almost any time during its manipulation and insertion into the cavity. If the zinc-containing amalgam

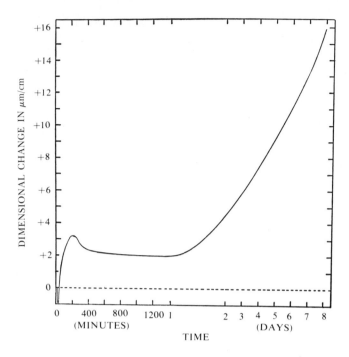

Figure 21–2 Delayed expansion of an amalgam.

is touched with the hands during trituration or condensation, skin secretions are likely to be introduced. If the operative area is not kept dry, the amalgam may become contaminated with saliva during condensation. In short, any contamination of the amalgam with moisture, whatever the source, before it has been inserted into the prepared cavity causes a delayed expansion if zinc is present. This matter will be discussed further in the next chapter.

STRENGTH

It is obvious that sufficient strength to resist fracture is a prime requisite for any restorative material. Fracturing of even a small area, especially at the margins, hastens corrosion, secondary caries, and subsequent clinical failure. A lack of truly adequate strength to resist masticatory forces has long been recognized as one of the inherent weaknesses of the amalgam restoration.

An example of gross fracture of an amalgam restoration is shown in Figure 21–3. If the restoration is properly designed, such failures are relatively rare. More common are defects at the margins of amalgams. Although there is division of opinion on this subject, it is possible that many such defects are the result of fracture of the amalgam. One 4-year study, which examined more than 1000 amalgam restorations in deciduous teeth, found that marginal defects were the most frequently occurring defects in the amalgams.[9] Moreover, a recent study has found that the incidence of secondary caries increases as the integrity of restoration margins decreases.[10]

Measurement of Strength   It is difficult to identify the principal property, or properties, responsible for the failure shown in the restoration in Figure 21–3. Traditionally, the strength of dental amalgam has been measured under compressive stress, using cylindrical specimens of dimensions comparable to the volume of typical amalgam restorations. When measured in this manner,

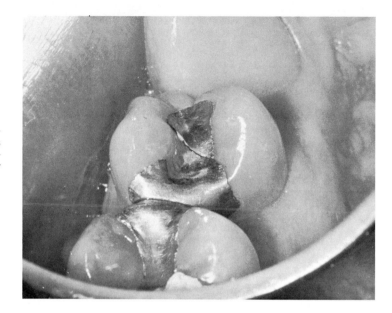

Figure 21–3 A fractured amalgam restoration. Such failures may occur from improper manipulation of the material. (Courtesy of J. T. Andrews.)

the compressive strength of a satisfactory amalgam probably should be at least 310 MPa (45,000 psi). When manipulated properly most amalgams will exhibit a compressive strength in excess of this value.

In Table 21–1, typical compressive strengths at 1 hour and 7 days after preparation are given for a low copper amalgam and two high copper amalgams. After 7 days the compressive strengths of high copper amalgams are generally higher than that of low copper amalgams. In addition, note that the 1-hour compressive strength of the single composition amalgam is almost double of that of the other two amalgams. This trend is generally true for other single composition amalgams.

The significance of the 7-day compressive strength to clinical performance has been questioned. The strength of amalgam is more than adequate to withstand potential compressive loads. Unfortunately, amalgam is much weaker in tension than in compression. Both low and high copper amalgams have tensile strengths that range between 48 and 70 MPa (7000 to 10,000 psi)[11] (Table 21–1).

Tensile stresses can easily occur in amalgam restorations. For example, on

Table 21–1. *Comparison of Compressive Strength and Creep of a Low Copper Silver-Tin Amalgam and High Copper Amalgams*

AMALGAM	COMPRESSIVE STRENGTH MPa (psi)		CREEP — %	TENSILE STRENGTH — 24 HR. MPa (psi)
	1 Hour	*7 Day*		
Low copper*	145 (21,100)	343 (49,800)	2.0	60 (8700)
Admix†	137 (19,800)	431 (62,600)	0.4	48 (7000)
Single composition‡	262 (38,000)	510 (73,900)	0.13	64 (9300)

*Fine Cut, L. D. Caulk Company.
†Dispersalloy, Johnson and Johnson Dental Products.
‡Tytin, S. S. White Dental Manufacturing Company.

the isthmus of a compound restoration, any compressive stress on the adjacent restored cusp induces a shear that in turn produces a tensile stress in the isthmus area. The tensile strength of the dentin that surrounds the restoration is approximately 280 MPa (40,000 psi). Therefore, if the cross-sectional area of the dentin in the isthmus is sufficient, the dentin will compensate for the relatively low tensile strength of the amalgam. On the other hand, dentin has a relatively low modulus of elasticity. Therefore, as much tooth structure as possible should be preserved to prevent the dentin from bending away from the restoration, or even fracturing under masticatory forces.

It is important to re-emphasize that amalgam cannot withstand high tensile stresses. The design of the restoration should include supporting structures whenever there is danger that it will be bent or pulled in tension. Use of a high copper amalgam will not help. The tensile strengths of high copper amalgams are not significantly different from those of the low copper amalgams (Table 21–1).

Effect of Trituration   The effect of trituration on strength depends on the type of amalgam alloy, on the trituration time, and on the speed of the triturator.[12] Either undertrituration or overtrituration will decrease the strength. Both traditional and high copper amalgams show the same effect.

Effect of Mercury Content   A very important factor in the control of the strength is the mercury content of the restoration. Sufficient mercury should be mixed with the alloy to coat the alloy particles and to allow a thorough amalgamation. Each particle of the alloy must be wetted by the mercury; otherwise, a dry, granular mix results. Such a mix results in a rough, pitted surface that invites corrosion. However, any excess of mercury left in the restoration can produce a marked reduction in strength.

The effect of the mercury content upon the compressive strength of an

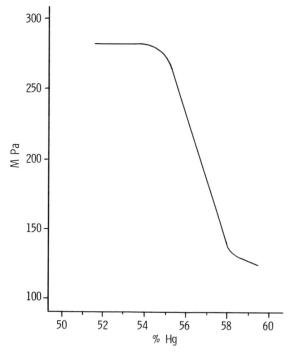

Figure 21–4 Compressive strength of an amalgam as related to the mercury content.

amalgam prepared from a lathe-cut low copper alloy is shown in Figure 21–4. There appears to be no important effect of the mercury content on the strength of the silver-tin amalgam within the limits of approximately 45 to 53 weight per cent. Above approximately 55 per cent mercury content, the strength decreases markedly with an increase in mercury content.[13] In amalgams containing 59 weight per cent mercury, the compressive strength is reduced to 125 MPa (18,000 psi) from a maximum strength of more than 280 MPa (40,000 psi) in amalgams with a mercury content of approximately 54 per cent. Similar decreases in strength with increased final mercury content have been observed for spherical low copper amalgams and for high copper amalgams.

The strength of an amalgam is a function of the relative volume fractions of unconsumed alloy particles and matrix phases (γ_1 and γ_2).[14] Low mercury content amalgams contain more of the alloy particles, which are stronger, and less of the matrix phases, which are weaker. Increasing the final mercury content increases the volume fraction of the matrix phases at the expense of alloy particles. As a result, amalgams containing higher amounts of final mercury are weaker.

The amount of γ_2 that forms affects the strength of high copper amalgams. The lowest mercury content at which the γ_2 phase appears ranges from 44 to as high as 60 per cent in some commercial high copper amalgams.[15] As noted in Chapter 20, the γ_2 is the weakest phase within dental amalgam. Consequently, a very small volume fraction of γ_2 within high copper amalgam will severely weaken it.[16] To avoid this problem, low mercury-alloy ratios should be used when triturating high copper amalgams.

Effect of Condensation   The condensation pressure, as well as technique, affects the strength. When typical condensation techniques and lathe-cut alloys are employed, the greater the condensation pressure, the higher is the compressive strength, particularly the early strength, e.g., at one hour. Good condensation techniques will express mercury, and thereby result in a smaller volume fraction of matrix phases. Because of their irregular shapes, lathe-cut amalgams resist condensation more than do spherical amalgams. Higher condensation pressures are required to minimize porosity and to express mercury from lathe-cut amalgams. On the other hand, spherical amalgams condensed with lighter pressures produce adequate strength.

Effect of Porosity   Voids and porosity have been advanced as possible factors influencing the compressive strength of hardened amalgam.[17] In the preceding chapter, voids were seen in micrographs of a low copper amalgam (Fig. 20–6), an admixed amalgam (Fig. 20–7), and a single composition amalgam (Fig. 20–8).

This porosity is considered to be related to a number of factors, including the *plasticity* of the mix.[18] Plasticity of amalgam mixes decreases with increased time from the end of trituration and condensation (delayed condensation) and with undertrituration. It could be anticipated that porosities would thereby be greater, and strength lower, under such conditions.

Increased condensation pressure improves adaptation of the amalgam to the cavity preparation. As illustrated in Figure 21–5, a 1-pound thrust on the condenser produced poor adaptation. A large number of voids are seen in the amalgam. Increasing the condensation pressure steadily improves the adaptation at the margins and decreases the number of voids.

The above comments are related to lathe-cut or admix amalgams, which

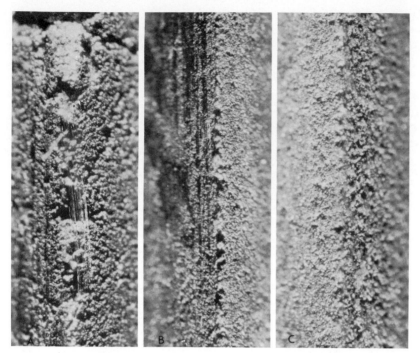

Figure 21–5 Photomicrographs of edges (cavosurface margins) of specimens of amalgam condensed by one-pound thrust on the condenser *(A)*, two-pound thrust *(B)*, and eight-pound thrust *(C)*. There is less porosity and superior adaptation to the mold as the condensation pressure is increased. (From Eames WB, J Amer Dent Assoc 75:629, 1967.)

offer resistance to condensation. With spherical alloys, the condenser will simply punch through the amalgam if heavy pressures are employed. Fortunately, voids are not such a problem with these amalgams. Thus, lighter pressure can be used without danger of sacrificing properties.

Effect of Rate of Hardening The rate of hardening of the amalgam is of considerable interest to the dentist. Since a patient may be dismissed from the dental chair within 20 minutes after trituration of the amalgam, a vital question is whether the amalgam has gained sufficient strength for its function. It is likely that a high percentage of amalgam restorations that fracture (Fig. 21–3) do so shortly after insertion. The clinical manifestation may not be evident for some months, but the initial crack within the restoration may occur within the first few hours.

Amalgam does not gain strength as rapidly as might be desired. For example, at the end of 20 minutes, its compressive strength may be only 6 per cent of its strength in one week. A good index of the rate of hardening is the 1 hour compressive strength test required in American Dental Association Specification no. 1. The test is conducted on specimens only 1 hour old. The specification stipulates a minimum strength of 80 MPa (11,600 pounds per square inch).

The 1 hour compressive strength of high copper single composition amalgams is exceptionally high (Table 21–1). This strength may have some advantages clinically. For example, fracture is less likely if the patient accidentally bites on the restoration soon after leaving the dental office. Also these amalgams may be strong enough shortly after placement to permit amalgam buildups to be prepared for crowns and to permit the taking of impressions for crowns.

Even if a fast hardening amalgam is used, ths strength of the amalgam restoration is likely to be low initially. Patients should be cautioned not to subject the restoration to high biting stresses for at least 8 hours after placement. By that time a typical amalgam has reached at least 70 per cent of its strength. Recommendation of liquids for the meal following placement is probably a sound safety precaution.

It is of interest to note that even at the end of a 6 month period, some amalgams may still be increasing in strength. Such observations suggest that the reactions between the matrix phases and the alloy particles may continue indefinitely. It is doubtful that equilibrium conditions between them are ever attained.

CREEP

The Significance of Creep to Amalgam Performance   During the 1970's, dental researchers discovered that data obtained from tests which measured the resistance of hardened dental amalgams to slow strain rate deformation seemed to correlate with long-term clinical performance. One such test measures the *static creep* of amalgam (Chapter 3). An amalgam specimen is placed under a constant load which is less than that needed to produce either instantaneous plastic deformation or fracture. When subjected to such a load, a specimen will slowly deform. The rate of deformation will depend on the magnitude of the stress in the specimen and on the temperature at which the test is conducted.

As mentioned earlier in this chapter, marginal breakdown is the most commonly observed defect in amalgam restorations. It is now well established that creep rate correlates well with marginal breakdown of the traditional low copper amalgams; i.e., the higher the creep, the greater is the degree of marginal deterioration.[19-21] This is illustrated in Figure 21–6, which shows marginal breakdown in amalgam restorations placed with high and low creep rate amalgams. The margins of the high creep amalgam are severely ditched.

Unfortunately, with the high copper amalgams creep is not a precise indicator of marginal fracture.[15, 22, 23] Many of these amalgams have creep rates of 0.4 (Table 21–1) or less. However, exceptions have been found in the clinical performance of different amalgams as would be predicted on the basis of their creep rates.

Nevertheless, creep is a useful tool to be included in the criteria employed in selecting a commercial alloy and it is prudent to select one that has a relatively low creep rate. The matter of the exact mechanism by which marginal deterioration occurs, as related to creep rate and other factors, will be explored in greater depth in the next chapter.

Incidentally, static creep is not the only measure of slow strain rate deformation that has been correlated with marginal breakdown. Both dynamic creep and compressive strength, as determined by slow strain rates, have been related to this phenomenon.[24, 25] However, the correlation between static creep and marginal breakdown has been better than that of the other two tests.

Measurement of Creep   American Dental Association Specification no. 1 contains a test for creep. This test subjects a 1-week-old amalgam cylinder, 8 mm long and 4 mm in diameter, to a compressive load of 36 MPa (5200 psi) in a

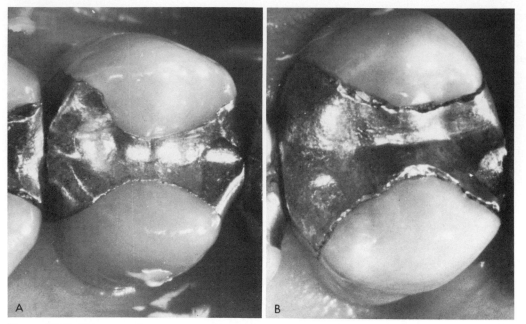

Figure 21–6 Four-year-old amalgam restorations. *A,* Amalgam placed with an alloy having minimal dynamic creep. *B,* Amalgam restoration of an alloy having a high creep value. (Courtesy of D. B. Mahler.)

37° C environment. The change in length of the cylinder that occurs between the first and fourth hour of testing is divided by the original length and multiplied by 100. This gives the per cent strain during this 3 hour period. This "per cent creep" is proportional to the creep rate.

American Dental Association creep values of low copper amalgams range between 0.80 and 8.00 per cent. As just noted, the high copper amalgams have much lower creep values, some even less than 0.1 per cent. Nevertheless, there are no data available which suggest that reducing the American Dental Association creep value below approximately 1.0 per cent will influence marginal breakdown.

The Influence of Microstructure on Creep The γ_1 Ag-Hg phase has been found to exert a primary influence on low copper amalgam creep rates.[26] Creep rates increase with larger γ_1 volume fractions[27] and decrease with larger γ_1 grain sizes.[28] Pure γ_2 has a higher creep rate than pure γ_1.[29] Although creep rate is not directly proportional to the volume fraction of γ_2,[28] it is clear that the presence (or absence) of γ_2 can dramatically affect the creep rate. For example, high copper amalgams that contain little or no γ_2 have low creep rates, as noted.

The dependence of creep rate on the inverse of the grain size is consistent with mechanisms of creep which involve grain boundary sliding (GBS).[27] At slow strain rates, plastic deformation and diffusion change grain shapes in a manner to permit GBS. Such GBS has been observed in the matrix of dental amalgams.[30, 31]

Figure 21–7 shows the microstructure of a low copper amalgam before the beginning of an American Dental Association creep test (Fig. 21–7*A*) and after 7 hours under creep load (Fig. 21–7*B*). (The stress axis in this micrograph is parallel to the bottom of the micrograph.) Gamma-one grains throughout Figure 21–7*B* have been delineated by grain boundary sliding (GBS). In this process of plastic deformation, the γ_2 phase increases the creep rate because it

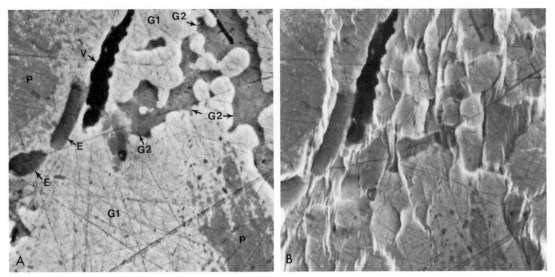

Figure 21–7 Grain boundary sliding during a creep test of a low copper amalgam (5700 ×). *A,* An area before creep test: Unconsumed particles (P), ϵ Cu$_3$Sn areas (E), γ_1 matrix areas which consist of a larger number of γ_1 grains (G1), γ_2 areas (G2), and a void (V). *B,* The same area after 7 hours under load. (Courtesy of T. Okabe, M. B. Butts, R. J. Mitchell, and C. W. Fairhurst.)

is extremely plastic, easily changing shape to make way for sliding γ_1 grains. If γ_2 is not present, the rate at which sliding occurs is reduced.

Likewise, the η crystals may play a role in contributing to the slowness of sliding in high copper amalgams. The suggested mechanism is diagrammed in Figure 21–8 for a single composition amalgam.[32] Numerous η Cu$_6$Sn$_5$ crystals are found embedded in and between γ_1 grains in such amalgams (see Fig. 20–9), and they interlock the γ_1 grains. Before the grain boundary sliding can occur, grains must flow plastically and by diffusion around these crystals. Thus, these η crystals inhibit GBS and thereby decrease the creep rate of single composition amalgams.

In addition, meshes of η crystals at the surfaces of unconsumed alloy particles in single composition amalgams (Fig. 20–9) seem to restrict the sliding of γ_1 grains adjacent to these particles.[32] It is clear that the mesh of η crystals improves the bonding between the alloy particles and the γ_1 matrix in single composition amalgams. The reaction layer around the Ag-Cu particles in admixed amalgams may also improve the bonding of these particles to the γ_1

Figure 21–8 η Cu-Sn rods embedded in γ_1 grains interlock γ_1 grains. (Courtesy of T. Okabe, R. J. Mitchell, M. B. Butts and C. W. Fairhurst.)

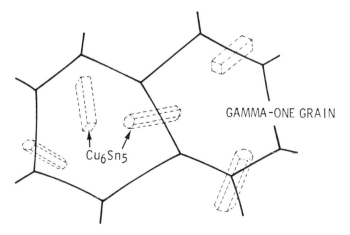

matrix. It is believed that such improved bonding will contribute to improved creep resistance of these systems.

The Effect of Manipulative Variables on Creep   The creep rate of an amalgam can be changed by altering the trituration time and the condensation pressure. For many amalgams, there is a trituration time which will produce a minimum creep rate.[33] Either undertrituration or overtrituration tends to increase the creep rate. If there is a delay between trituration and condensation, the creep rate increases.[34] However, increasing the condensation pressure decreases the creep rate.[33]

The mercury-alloy ratio can also affect this property. Those factors that tend to increase the final mercury content of an amalgam will increase its creep rate. For example, a delay between trituration and condensation will increase both the final mercury content and the creep rate. On the other hand, high condensation pressures express mercury, thereby lowering the final mercury content of the amalgam and decreasing its creep rate. The influence of final mercury content on creep rate is less significant for high copper amalgams, which inherently have low creep values and relatively low mercury contents.

However, for certain of these amalgams when the mercury content exceeds approximately 46 per cent, there is a sudden increase in creep and γ_2 begins to form.[35] As noted previously, other properties, e.g., strength, are also affected. Thus regardless of the alloy used, it is wise to utilize techniques that will provide an amalgam with a low mercury content. These factors will be covered in the next chapter.

References

1. Paffenbarger GC, Rupp NW, and Pater PR: Linear dimensional change of copper-rich dental amalgam. J Am Dent Assoc 99:468, 1979.
2. Espevik S: Effect of trituration dimensional changes of dental amalgam. Acta Odontol Scand 35:251, 1977.
3. Malhotra ML and Asgar K: Physical properties of dental silver-tin amalgams with high and low copper contents. J Am Dent Assoc 96:444, 1978.
4. Rhodes BF, Swartz ML, and Phillips RW: Physical properties of two high-copper amalgams and conventional amalgam. Oper Dent 4:71, 1979.
5. Fairhurst CW: Volume changes in the Ag-Sn-Hg reaction. IADR Program and Abstracts, No. M43, 1962.
6. Johnson LB: Dimensional change and pore development during hardening of Ag-Sn amalgams. Biomater Med Devices Artif Organs 1:329, 1973.
7. Schoonover IC, Souder W, and Beall JR: Excessive expansion of dental amalgam. J Am Dent Assoc 29:1825, 1942.
8. Fainsilber S, Moore BK, Swartz ML, and Phillips RW: Effects of saline contamination on zinc and zinc-free high copper amalgams. IADR Program and Abstracts, No. 107, 1980.
9. Macrae PD, Zacherl W, and Castaldi CR: A study of defects in class II dental amalgam restorations in deciduous molars. J Can Dent Assoc 28:491, 1962.
10. Goldberg J, Tanzer J, Munster E, Amara J, and Birkhed D: Clinical association of recurrent caries with marginal integrity and oral hygiene. IADR Program and Abstracts, No. 283, 1980.
11. Asgar K, Arfaei AH, and Mahler DB: Evaluation of amalgam tensile test methods. IADR Program and Abstracts, No. 140, 1977.
12. Nagai K, Ohashi M, Habu H, Makino K, Usui T, Matuso M, Hama M, and Kawamoto M: Studies on the tensile strength of dental amalgams by the application of diametral compression test. Part 2. Effects of manipulative variables. J Nihon Univ Sch Dent 13:21, 1971, B89.

13. Swartz ML and Phillips RW: Residual mercury content of amalgam restorations and its influence on compressive strength. J Dent Res 35:458, 1956.
14. Young FA, Wilsdorf HGF, and Paffenbarger GC: Some relationships between microstructure and strength of Ag_3Sn and dental amalgam. J Dent Res 52:281, 1973.
15. Vrijhoef MMA, Vermeersch AG, and Spanauf AJ: *Dental Amalgam.* Chicago, Quintessence Publ. Co., 1980.
16. Mahler DB: Behavior of three high-copper amalgams. J Biomed Mater Res 13:693, 1979.
17. Wing G: The condensation of dental amalgam. Dent Pract 16:52, 1965.
18. Mahler DB: Plasticity of amalgam mixes. J Dent Res 46:708, 1967.
19. Mahler DB, Van Eysden J, and Terkla LG: Relationship of creep to marginal fracture of amalgam. IADR Program and Abstracts, No. 553, 1975.
20. Letzel H, Aardening CJMW, Fick JM, and Vrijhoef MMA: Marginal breakdown of amalgam restorations versus creep. IADR Program and Abstracts, No. 245, 1977.
21. Osborne JW, Phillips RW, Gale EN, and Binon PP: Three-year clinical comparison of three amalgam alloy types emphasizing an appraisal of the evaluation methods used. J Am Dent Assoc 93:784, 1976.
22. Osborne JW, Cochran MA, and Gale EN: Marginal failure rate of high copper amalgams: A two-year report. IADR Program and Abstracts, No. 346, 1979.
23. Leinfelder KF, Strickland WD, Sockwell CL, and Eames WB: Two year clinical evaluation of high copper content amalgams. IADR Program and Abstracts, No. 425, 1979.
24. Mahler DB and Van Eysden J: Dynamic creep of dental amalgam. J Dent Res 48:501, 1969.
25. Mahler DB: Slow compressive strength test for amalgam. IADR Program and Abstracts, No. 29, 1969.
26. Vrijhoef MMA and Driessens FCM: The creep of dental amalgam. A factor determining the loss of an amalgam filling and its surrounding structure. Diorheology 11:191, 1974.
27. Espevik S and Sorensen SE: Creep of dental amalgam. Scand J Dent Res 83:245, 1975.
28. Mahler DB, Adey JD, and Marantz RL: Creep versus microstructure of γ_2-containing amalgams. J Dent Res 56:1493, 1977.
29. Espevik S: Creep of dental amalgam and its phases. Scand J Dent Res 85:492, 1977.
30. Winchell PG: Private communication, Purdue University, Indiana, 1976.
31. Okabe T, Butts MB, Mitchell RJ, and Fairhurst CW: Grain boundary sliding and creep in dental amalgams. IADR Program and Abstracts, No. 100, 1980.
32. Okabe T, Mitchell RJ, Butts MB, and Fairhurst CW: A study of high copper dental amalgams by scanning electron microscopy. *In* Microstructural Science (LeMay, Fallow, McCall eds.). New York, Elsevier North Holland, Inc., 1979, Vol. 7.
33. Osborne JW, Phillips RW, Swartz ML, and Norman RD: Static creep as affected by trituration time and condensation pressure. IADR Program and Abstracts, No. 30, 1974.
34. Spanauf AJ, Vrijhoef MMA, and Graff R: The influence of some manipulative factors on creep. Aust Dent J 22:203, 1977.
35. Mahler DB and Adey JD: The influence of final mercury content on the characteristics of a high-copper amalgam. J Biomed Mater Res 13:467, 1979.

22 DENTAL AMALGAM: TECHNICAL CONSIDERATIONS

A good modern dental amalgam alloy can be manipulated so that a restoration is obtained that is adequate in every respect. If the restoration is defective, in the great majority of cases the fault is with the dentist or auxiliary and not the material. As has been mentioned earlier, either the cavity preparation was poorly designed or the amalgam was not manipulated properly. The last factor will be discussed at length in reference to the influence of the technique on the physical properties and thus the clinical success of the amalgam.

SELECTION OF MATERIALS

There are certain criteria involved in the selection of an alloy. The weight of each will vary with the individual. Certainly, the first criterion is to make sure that it meets the requirements of the American Dental Association Specification no. 1 or a similar specification.

The manipulative characteristics are extremely important and a matter of subjective preference. Matters such as rate of hardening, smoothness of the mix, and ease of condensation and finishing vary with the alloy and the working speed and choice of the operator. For example, lathe-cut amalgams have an entirely different feel during condensation than do spherical amalgams, as has been noted. It is essential that the alloy selected be one with which the dentist and assistant feel comfortable. As was discussed, the operator variable is a major factor entering into the clinical lifetime of the restoration. Use of alloys and techniques that will encourage standardization in the manipulation and placement of the amalgam will enhance the quality of the service rendered.

Coincident with this is the delivery system provided by the manufacturer — its convenience, expediency, and capability to reduce human variables. As noted, the alloy may be purchased either in the form of a powder or a pellet. Also, preproportioned alloy and mercury in disposable capsules is another manner in which the alloy may be secured from many manufacturers. There are certain advantages and disadvantages to this concept, as will be discussed shortly. Nonetheless, the delivery system is an important consideration.

Obviously, the physical properties, as discussed in the previous chapter, should be reviewed in the light of claims made for superiority of one alloy over competing products. It should now be apparent that such an analysis of properties must be accompanied by a documented review of clinical performance in the form of well-controlled clinical studies. This is especially necessary for alloy formulations that depart from traditional compositions and in which an exact correlation between properties and performance has not as yet been established.

Alloys of conventional composition are still available, and acceptable amalgam restorations can be obtained from many of these. However, from the discussions in the previous chapters, it should be obvious that the newer high copper alloy system is now the one of choice. Improved physical properties, the elimination of the γ_2 phase, and the better corrosion resistance associated with these alloys generally lead to superior clinical performance.[1-3] A number of commercial products that are representative of the high copper alloys currently available are shown in Figure 22–1.

Lastly, owing to the escalation in the price of silver, the cost of the alloy has assumed a new importance. It is to be hoped that this criterion would not be given too much weight when balanced against the capability of the alloy to render maximum clinical service. However, if all other factors are equal, it is sensible to purchase the less expensive brand.

There is only one requisite for dental mercury and that is its purity. Common contaminating elements, such as arsenic, can lead to pulpal damage. Furthermore, a lack of purity may adversely affect the physical properties of the amalgam. Unfortunately, terms such as "pure," "redistilled," or "triple distilled" do not indicate the chemical quality of the mercury.

The designation "U.S.P." (United States Pharmacopeia) definitely insures a satisfactory purity. This designation indicates that the mercury has no surface contamination and that it contains less than 0.02 per cent nonvolatile residue. This requirement is encompassed in the American Dental Association Specification no. 6 for dental mercury. Consequently, the selection of a mercury that is guaranteed to meet this specification insures the necessary purity.

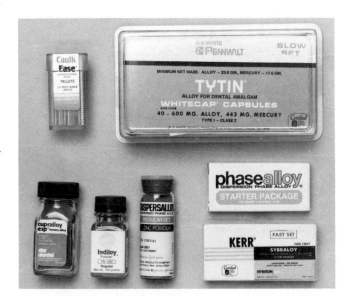

Figure 22–1 Commercial brands of representative high copper alloys.

MERCURY-ALLOY RATIO

In order to achieve amalgam mixes that were plastic and smooth, for many years it was necessary to use an amount of mercury considerably in excess of that desirable in the final restoration. Because of the deleterious effects of a high mercury content on the physical and mechanical properties of amalgam, it was mandatory to employ manipulative procedures that would reduce the amount of mercury left in the restoration to an acceptable level.

The techniques for achieving the reduction varied. However, basically, the removal of excess mercury was accomplished by squeezing or wringing the mixed amalgam in a squeeze cloth prior to insertion of the increments into the prepared cavity. Also, additional mercury-rich amalgam was worked to the top during condensation of each increment and was removed as the restoration was built up. One popular technique was to express mercury in increasing amounts from each successive increment, with each new increment serving somewhat as a blotter. This was referred to as the "increasing dryness technique." Although excellent restorations can be, and were, produced in this manner, it is obvious that the amount of mercury removed by the squeeze cloth and during condensation varied; thus there was considerable chance for error.

Of course, the most obvious method for reducing the mercury content of the restoration is to reduce the original mercury-alloy ratio. The present-day alloys are amenable to manipulation with reduced mercury-alloy ratios, and, in fact, are so designed. This method is known as the *minimal mercury* or the *Eames* technique, in recognition of the dentist who developed the concept.[4]

The technique is critical in that sufficient mercury must be present in the original mix to provide a coherent and plastic mass after trituration. On the other hand, it must be low enough that the mercury content of the restoration is at an acceptable level without the need to remove an appreciable amount during condensation. Thus the mercury content of the finished restoration essentially should be comparable to that of the original mercury-alloy ratio. This is usually in the order of 50 per cent, with lesser amounts being used with spherical alloys.

By eliminating the need to remove excess mercury from the original mix, via a squeeze cloth and condensation, the technique is standardized. Likewise, the possibility of a high mercury content in the final restoration, with its accompanying deleterious effects, is minimized. The technique also reduces contact of office personnel with metallic mercury and the contamination of the office environment.

Obviously, then, the method of choice for placement of amalgam restorations with today's alloys is the minimal mercury technique. However, as will be discussed, manipulative procedures are critical and the excellence of clinical restorations placed by this technique depends on proper manipulation. These include proportioning of the mercury and alloy. Since the recommended amount of mercury invariably is the minimum amount required to produce a useable mix, proportioning of the two components must be exact. Trituration and condensation of the amalgam must be done with equal care and attention to detail.

Proportioning   The amount of alloy and mercury to be used can be described as the *mercury-alloy* or *alloy-mercury ratio*. Either is correct and signifies the parts by weight of mercury and of alloy to be used for the particular technique employed. For example, a mercury-alloy ratio of 6:5 indicates that 6 parts of mercury are to be used with 5 parts of alloy by weight. Sometimes instead of a mercury-alloy ratio, manufacturers' instructions will specify the per cent of mercury by weight to be employed in the mix. A mix of amalgam prepared with a mercury-alloy ratio of 6:5 would contain 54.5 per cent mercury.

Of course, the recommended ratio will vary for different alloy compositions, particle size and shapes, and heat treatment. As intimated in the previous section, the particular manipulative and condensation technique favored by the dentist can also be a factor in selecting the desired ratio.

With the older alloys, mercury-alloy ratios in the order of 8:5 or 7:5 were the rule. The recommended mercury-alloy ratios for most modern lathe-cut alloys is in the realm of 1:1 or 50 per cent mercury, as noted earlier, although some may vary plus or minus a few per cent. With spherical alloys, the recommended amount of mercury may be closer to 40 per cent.

Regardless of the ratio, proportioning is particularly critical for the newer alloys, which make use of minimal mercury. If the mercury content is slightly low, the mix may be dry and grainy and insufficient matrix is present to cohesively bond the mass together. As can be seen in Figure 22–2, use of too little mercury in the mix impairs the strength of high-copper amalgams as much as does an inordinately high mercury content. Undoubtedly corrosion resistance is also reduced.

A wide variety of mercury and alloy dispensers, or proportioners, are available to the dental profession. They are of two general types. The most common type is the dispenser that is based on volumetric proportioning; the other measures by weight.

Most of the dispensers for alloy in powder form are relatively accurate if properly used. The chief objection is that in the volumetric devices the alloy tends to cling to the walls and corners of the dispensing well. Also, the usual objection to the measuring of a powder material by volume is relevant. As

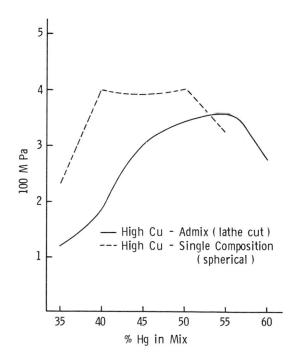

Figure 22–2 The effect of mercury-alloy ratio on the compressive strength of high copper amalgams prepared with a representative lathe-cut admix alloy and a representative spherical single composition alloy.

discussed in connection with gypsum products, the powder tends to pack in the container; thus, the weight is inaccurate from one measurement to the next. Also, any volumetric measurement for a specified weight of alloy depends upon the particle size of the alloy; the larger particle size requires a larger volume than does a small particle size in order to obtain the same weight. Consequently, the volume of the dispenser must be gauged for a given alloy and cannot be used for any other brand.

Probably the most convenient method for dispensing the alloy is to use pre-weighed pellets or tablets. The individual pellets in each bottle are quite uniform in weight, provided normal care is exercised in handling to avoid chipping of the pellet. Thus with pre-weighed pellets all that is required is an accurate mercury dispenser.

Because mercury is a liquid, it can be measured by volume without appreciable loss of accuracy. Standard deviations in weights of mercury as low as ±0.5 per cent may be attained with a number of commercial mercury dispensers.[5] However, even though the mercury dispenser may be well designed to provide reproducible spills of mercury, precautions must be exercised in its use. The dispenser should be held almost vertically to insure consistent spills of mercury. Tilting the bottle to a 45° angle results in unreliable mercury-alloy ratios. The dispenser should be at least half full when used. If the dispenser is one fourth or less full, the weight of mercury dispensed may be erratic. Finally, use of dirty mercury leads to entrapment of the contaminants in the reservoir and orifice of the device, preventing accurate delivery of the mercury.

If such variables are not controlled, variation in individual spills of mercury may be 3 or 4 per cent. With the use of low mercury-alloy ratios, variations of this magnitude result in a mix that is unusable.

In the case of pellets, if the amalgam alloy and mercury dispensers are not from the same manufacturer, the directions for use of the dispenser may not indicate the proper setting required to obtain the proper ratio for another product. Then it is necessary to weigh a pellet (e.g., on a pharmaceutical balance) and to calculate the amount of mercury required for the desired ratio. Increments of mercury may then be dispensed and weighed, and the desired adjustment of the dispenser established.

Disposable capsules containing pre-proportioned aliquots of mercury and alloy are now available. They contain alloy either in pellet form or as a pre-weighed portion of powder in conjunction with the appropriate quantity of mercury. To prevent any amalgamation from occurring during storage, the mercury and alloy are separated from each other by a plastic membrane. Before trituration, the membrane is ruptured and the mercury falls into the compartment with the alloy. Although more expensive, the pre-proportioned material is convenient and eliminates the chance of mercury spills during proportioning.

There are some disadvantages of pre-proportioned capsules other than expense. There is no opportunity to make minor adjustments in the mercury-alloy ratio to accommodate personal preference for a slightly drier or wetter mix. Likewise, there is no latitude in varying the size of the mix as supplied by the manufacturer.

Regardless of the method used, the proper amount of mercury and alloy always must be gauged before the start of trituration. The addition of mercury after trituration is contraindicated.

TRITURATION

Traditionally the alloy and mercury were mixed, or triturated, with a mortar and pestle. However, use of some form of mechanical device has now become almost universal. Mechanical amalgamation saves time and standardizes the procedure. In fact, it is difficult, if not impossible, to employ hand trituration for mixing amalgams prepared with low mercury-alloy ratios.

The object of trituration is to provide proper amalgamation of the mercury and alloy. The alloy particles are coated with a film of oxide which is difficult for the mercury to penetrate. This film must be rubbed off in some manner so that a clean surface of alloy can come in contact with the mercury. The oxide layer is removed by abrasion when the alloy particles and mercury are triturated in a mechanical amalgamator or by hand in a mortar and pestle.

Mechanical Trituration   A large number of commercial brands of amalgamators are available. Two representative ones are shown in Figure 22–3. The basic principle of operation is comparable for most of them. A capsule, which serves as a "mortar," can be seen between the arms on top of each machine. A cylindrical metal or plastic piston of smaller diameter than the capsule is inserted into the capsule and this serves as the "pestle."

The alloy and mercury are dispensed into the capsule. When the machine is activated, the arms holding the capsule oscillate at high speed; thus trituration is accomplished. There is an automatic timer for controlling the length of the mixing time, and most modern amalgamators have two or more operating speeds. Multiple speed amalgamators, such as those shown, are advantageous in that they provide greater versatility, often permitting the amalgamator to be used for mixing other pre-proportioned materials, i.e., cements and composite resins.

New amalgamators must have hoods that cover the reciprocating arms that hold the capsule, as shown in Figure 22–2. The purpose of the hood is to confine mercury that might be sprayed into the room during amalgamation from the use of a capsule with a poorly fitting lid.

Capsules are available with friction fit and with screw-cap lids. With either type it is important that the lid on the capsule fit tightly. If it does not, a fine mist of mercury will be sprayed out of the capsule by the vigorous shaking

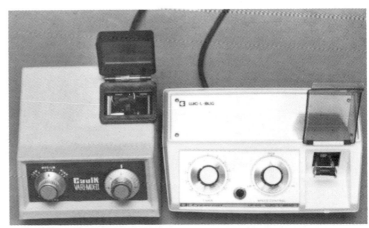

Figure 22–3   Two representative commercial mechanical amalgamators.

action of the amalgamator.[6] Loss of mercury can alter the mercury-alloy ratio to the extent that the mix is unusable. Even more important, an aerosol of mercury droplets is created that produces a potential risk of mercury inhalation. Capsule lids should be carefully checked prior to use and any that appear to be loose should be discarded. Also, with long use the fit may deteriorate as a result of wear.

A wide variety of capsule-pestle combinations are available. The size, shape, and weight of the pestles vary markedly. Some are made of plastic, while others are metal. They also vary in diameter and length. A most important consideration in selecting a capsule-pestle combination is the size of the pestle. The diameter and length of the pestle should be considerably less than the comparable dimensions of the capsule. For example, the capsule-pestle combination shown in Figure 22–4A is acceptable from this standpoint. If the pestle is too large, Figure 22–4B, the resultant mix may not be homogeneous. When the pellet form of alloy is used, the pellet or a piece of it may become wedged between the wall of the capsule and the pestle and not be completely broken up during mixing.

The pellets produced by different manufacturers differ to some extent in the ease with which they are reduced to powder. In instances when pellets are difficult to break, one should consider employing a small metal pestle rather than a plastic one of a lighter weight. Trituration of alloy in a capsule without a pestle should be limited to those alloys where that mode of manipulation is specifically recommended.

An amalgamator should be employed that operates at the speed recommended by the alloy manufacturer. Some older amalgamators do not operate at a sufficiently high rate of speed to properly amalgamate newer high copper alloys mixed with minimal mercury. Regardless of the alloy or amalgamator, no more than two pellets of alloy should be mixed in a capsule at one time.

The capsule should be clean and free of hardened alloy. Sometimes a portion of the mix may stick in a capsule. If undetected, it will harden. Although it may be possible to remove the hardened alloy by scraping it with an instrument, this usually produces scratches that merely compound the sticking problem in the future. In the long run it is probably just as well to discard the capsule.

The problem can often be avoided by the following procedure: At the end of amalgamation, quickly remove the pestle from the capsule, replace the lid, reinsert the capsule in the amalgamator and turn it on, then immediately off.

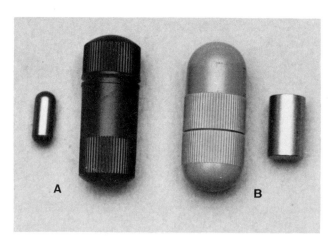

Figure 22–4 Capsule and pestle combinations demonstrating a satisfactory size relationship between the capsule and pestle (A) and an unsatisfactory pestle size (B).

A

B

This generally causes the mix to cohere so that the entire mass can be readily removed from the capsule.

No exact recommendations for mixing time can be given in view of the wide variety of amalgamators, which differ in speed, configuration of oscillating patterns, capsule designs, etc. In addition, the amount of work required for amalgamation of various alloys differs greatly from one to another; for example, spherical alloys usually require less amalgamation time than do lathe-cut alloys. Also, a larger mix requires slightly longer mixing time than does a smaller one.

Manufacturers' directions contain a time schedule for mixing the alloy. However, because of the variations in amalgamators, even of the same brand, this schedule should serve only as a rough guide. The very important factor, which must be decided by the dentist and assistant, is the optimum amalgamation time that is required to attain a mix of correct consistency — as will now be discussed. A general rule is that for a given alloy and mercury-alloy ratio, increased trituration time shortens the working and setting time.

Consistency of the Mix   It should now be evident that the proper combining of the alloy and mercury is one of the prime manipulative considerations. It is at this stage that the composition of the final amalgam is largely determined. In turn, this composition establishes the physical properties.

Provided that the same weight of alloy and mercury is used each time, and is triturated by the same amalgamator, attainment of a proper mix can be controlled by timing the trituration. The proper time can be determined by observing the consistency of the mix. For example, the somewhat grainy mix shown in Figure 22–5 is undertriturated. Not only will the amalgam restoration made from this mix be weak but also the rough surface left after the carving of the granular amalgam will decrease the tarnish resistance.

On the other hand, if the trituration is carried to the extent that the amalgam has the general appearance shown in Figure 22–6, the strength will be maximal and the smooth carved surface will retain its luster longer after polishing. Such an amalgam mix may be warm (not hot) when it is removed from the capsule. This will have no effect on the physical properties of the amalgam other than to shorten the working time somewhat.

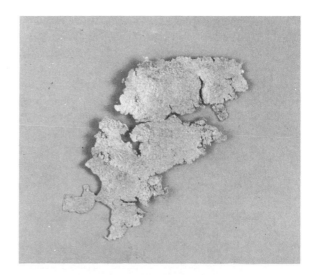

Figure 22–5 Undertriturated mix of amalgam. Such a mix has low strength and poor resistance to corrosion.

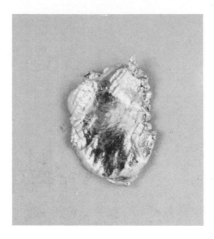

Figure 22-6   Properly triturated amalgam having maximum properties.

Thus, with experience the proper consistency can be recognized and the timing of the mix can be adjusted to attain such an appearance.

CONDENSATION

The purpose of condensation is to condense the unattacked gamma particles as closely together as possible and to force the amalgam into all parts of the cavity preparation and into an intimate adaptation to the cavity walls. Also, mercury-rich amalgam must be brought to the top of each increment as it is being condensed so that the increments bond one to the other. As previously noted, if excess mercury is present in the original mix, a major objective also is to remove the excess mercury from each increment as it is worked to the top by this condensing procedure. With the minimal mercury technique, removal of the soft plashy material during condensation of the alloy is, of course, less critical. Under proper conditions of trituration and condensation there is very little danger of removing too much mercury during condensation.

In summary, the goal of condensation is to compact the alloy into the prepared cavity so that the greatest possible density is attained, with sufficient mercury present to insure complete continuity of the matrix phase between the remaining alloy particles. If this goal is achieved, the strength of the amalgam is thereby increased and the creep is decreased.

After the mix is made, condensation of the amalgam into the prepared cavity should be promptly initiated. As can be seen in Figure 22-7, the longer the time lapse between mixing and condensation, the weaker will be the amalgam. In addition, the mercury content and creep of the amalgam are increased.[7] Although the permissible length of time between trituration and condensation varies to some degree with the alloy, a good rule is to discard amalgam that is 3 or 4 minutes old. Therefore, multiple mixes are required for a large restoration.

The reduction in strength resulting from delayed condensation is likely due to a combination of factors. It is probable that condensation of the partially set material fractures and breaks up the matrix that has already formed. Also, since the alloy has lost a considerable amount of plasticity, it is difficult to condense without producing internal voids and layering.[8]

The loss in strength incurred by allowing the amalgam mix to stand before condensation depends upon its hardening rate. A fast-setting amalgam, such as that obtained with alloy A in Figure 22–7, is affected to a greater extent than is the slower setting alloy B. Most modern alloys mixed with minimal amounts of mercury harden with considerable rapidity. Thus the working time is relatively short and the effects would be analogous to those observed with alloy A.

It follows, therefore, that the condensation should be as rapid as possible. In any event, a fresh mix of amalgam should be available if condensation takes longer than 3 or 4 minutes.

The field of operation must be kept absolutely dry during the condensation. The incorporation of the slightest moisture in a zinc-containing amalgam at this stage can result in a delayed expansion and other associated dyscrasia such as corrosion and loss of strength, as was discussed in Chapter 21. The ultimate result of moisture contamination is subsequent failure of the restoration.

Because of the nature of the operation, the condensation must always be accomplished within four walls and a floor; one or more walls may be a thin sheet of stainless steel, called a *matrix*. Condensation can be effected with either hand instruments or mechanical instruments.

Hand Condensation   The mix of amalgam should never be touched with the hands. The freshly mixed alloy contains free mercury and thus skin contact by dental personnel should be avoided. Secondly, there is moisture on the surface of the skin that would be source of moisture contamination of the amalgam. The increments of alloy should be carried to, and inserted in, the prepared cavity by means of instruments such as small forceps or an amalgam carrier designed for that purpose.

The condensing instrument generally is a contra-angle, and the working point is usually larger than that used in a gold foil condenser, as will be described in the next chapter.

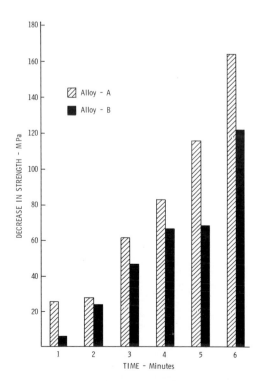

Figure 22–7 The effect of the elapsed time between trituration and condensation on the strength of the hardened amalgam. The greater the elapsed time, the less is the strength.

Once the increment of amalgam is inserted into the cavity preparation, it should immediately be condensed with heavy pressure to remove voids and to adapt the material to the walls. The condenser point or face is forced into the amalgam mass under hand pressure. Condensation is usually started at the center, and then the condenser point is stepped little by little toward the cavity walls.

Upon completion of condensation of the increment, the surface should be shiny in appearance. This indicates that there is sufficient mercury present at the surface to diffuse into the next increment so that each increment, as it is added, will bond to the preceding one. If this is not done and the increments do not bond, the restoration will be laminated. Such a restoration might be likened to a stack of bricks with no mortar cementing them together. It may subsequently fracture, probably when the matrix is removed. At best it would lack homogeneity and suffer severe corrosion.

Even with the minimal mercury techniques now in general use, it is probably desirable to remove some of the soft or plashy material that is brought to the surface of each increment. However, as was mentioned, this step is far less critical than when the per cent mercury recommended for the mix was far above the level acceptable in the clinical restoration.

This procedure of adding an increment, condensing it, adding another increment, etc., is continued until the cavity is overfilled. Any mercury-rich material at the surface of the last increment, constituting the overfill, will be removed when the restoration is carved.

Of course, if the cavity is a large one or if for some reason undue time is required to complete condensation, another mix should be made just before the original one is depleted or loses its plasticity. This can easily be accomplished, since mechanical mixing requires only a few seconds.

A well condensed amalgam restoration can be achieved only if the mix has a proper consistency. If it comes out of the mixing capsule dry and grainy (Fig. 22–5), either it has insufficient mercury due to loss of mercury from the capsule, incorrect proportioning of the mercury and alloy, or it is under-triturated. If the mix is coherent but hard and hot to the touch, it probably has been mixed too long and the setting reaction has progressed too far. In either case, condensation of the mix should not be attempted. Rather, a new mix should be prepared.

One of the most important factors in condensation is the size of the increments of amalgam that are carried into the cavity. The larger the piece, the more difficult it is to reduce the voids and adapt the alloy to the cavity walls.[9] Thus, relatively small increments of amalgam should be used throughout the condensation procedure in order to reduce void formation and obtain maximum adaptation to the cavity.

Likewise, heavy condensation pressure must be used to force the alloy particles together, reduce voids, and work mercury to the surface in order to achieve bonding between the increments.

Condensation Pressure   The area of the condenser point or face and the force exerted on it by the operator govern the condensation pressure. Obviously, when a given force is applied, the smaller the condenser the greater is the pressure exerted on the amalgam. For example, a thrust of 4.5 kg (10 lb) exerted on a circular condenser point 2 mm in diameter results in a condensation pressure of 140 kg/cm^2 (2000 psi). The same thrust applied to a 3.5 mm diameter condenser produces a condensation pressure of only 47 kg/cm^2 (670 psi).

The greater effectiveness of the smaller condenser is evident, provided that it is not unduly small and merely punches holes in the mass. On the other hand, if the condenser point is too large the operator cannot generate sufficient condensation pressure to adequately condense the amalgam and force it into retentive areas.

Although forces as great as 6.8 kg (15 lb) have been advocated for the thrust on the amalgam condenser, it is doubtful that forces of that magnitude are generally used. For example, the forces applied by 30 practitioners were measured by means of strain gauges cemented to amalgam condensers.[10] Forces in excess of 2.7 kg (6 lb) were seldom recorded, although forces as low as 0.45 kg (1 lb) were occasionally noted. Condensation forces in the general range of 1.4 to 1.8 kg (3 to 4 lb) appear to be a reasonable estimation of the average force employed. Certainly, in order to ensure maximum density and adpatation to the cavity walls, the condensation force should be as great as possible, consistent with patient comfort. It is doubtful that condenser points greater than 2 mm in diameter will provide adequate condensation of lathe-cut alloys.

One of the advantages of spherical amalgam alloys is that the strength properties tend to be less sensitive to condensation pressure. In fact, many of the spherical alloys have little "body" and thus offer only mild resistance to the condensation force. In many instances condensation becomes a matter of attaining good adaptation. When condensing these alloys, a large condenser can often be used.

The shape of the condenser points should conform to the area under condensation. For example, a round condenser point is ineffective adjacent to a corner or angle of a prepared cavity; a triangular or square point is indicated in such an area. Points of various shapes are, therefore, provided for the most effective condensation.

Mechanical Condensation   The procedures and principles of mechanical condensation are the same as those discussed for hand condensation, including the need to use small increments of amalgam. The only difference is that the condensation of the amalgam is essentially done by an automatic device. Various mechanisms are employed for these instruments. Some provide an impact type of force, while others use rapid vibration.

Whether the device is of the impact or vibratory type, less energy is needed than for hand condensation. Thus the operation may be less fatiguing to the dentist. Similar clinical results can be achieved using either hand or mechanical condensation; the selection is related to the preference of the dentist.

CARVING AND FINISHING

After the amalgam has been condensed into the prepared cavity, the restoration is carved to reproduce the proper tooth anatomy. The objective of carving is to simulate the anatomy, rather than to reproduce extremely fine detail. If the carving is too deep, the bulk of amalgam, particularly at the marginal areas, is reduced. If too thin, this area may fracture under masticatory stress.

If the proper technique is followed, the amalgam should be ready for carving soon after completion of the condensation; however, the carving should not be started until the amalgam is sufficiently hard to offer resistance to the carving instrument. A scraping or "ringing" sound should be heard when it is carved. If the carving is started too soon, the amalgam may be so plastic that it may be pulled away from the margins, even by the sharpest carving instrument.

After the carving, the surface of the restoration should be smoothed. This may be accomplished by judiciously *burnishing* the surface and margins of the restoration. If the alloy is a reasonably fast-setting one, it should have achieved sufficient strength by this time to support firm but not heavy rubbing pressure. Burnishing of the occlusal anatomy can be accomplished with a ball burnisher, and an instrument with rigid flat blade is best used on smooth surfaces. This can be followed by rubbing the surface with a moist cotton pellet or by lightly going over it with a rubber polishing cup and polishing paste.

This step of burnishing has been somewhat controversial with respect to its contribution to the long-term behavior of the restoration. The exact effect of burnishing on marginal adaptation and properties such as hardness is not well defined. However, there is ample evidence that amalgam surfaces that have been burnished, or burnished and then lightly polished, are much smoother than carved surfaces.[11] Clinical data on performance of restorations support the desirability of burnishing the fast-setting, high copper systems.[12] Burnishing of slow-setting alloys can damage the margins of the restoration.[13] Thus, when such an alloy is used, burnishing should not be done.

Certain precaution should be exercised in burnishing. Undue pressure should not be exerted and heat generation should be avoided. Any temperature above 60° C (140° F) causes release of mercury.[14] The mercury-rich condition thus created at the margins results in accelerated corrosion and/or fracture.

Regardless of alloy and the trituration and condensation technique, the carved surface of the restoration is rough. This is evidenced by the dull surface of the restorations at the left *(A)* of Figure 22–8. The surfaces are covered with scratches, pits, and irregularities. Even though the restoration surfaces have been carefully finished by burnishing and smoothing, they are rough at the microscopic level. If not removed by further finishing after the amalgam is completely set, these defects can result in concentration cell type corrosion.

The smooth surface on the restorations at the right *(B)* in Figure 22–8, produced by the final finishing procedure, is due to the reduction of the surface defects.

As stated above, the final finish of the restoration should not be done until

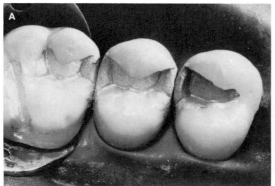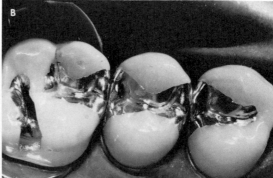

Figure 22–8 *A*, Amalgam restorations as they appear after carving. *B*, The same restorations after final finishing. (Courtesy of L. V. Hickey.)

the amalgam is fully set. It should be delayed for at least 24 hours after condensation and preferably longer. The need for extremely high luster is questionable. However, it is very important that the metal surface be smooth and uniform.

As just discussed, heat generation must be avoided. The use of dry polishing powders and discs can easily raise the surface temperature above the 60° C (140° F) danger point. Thus, a wet abrasive powder in a paste form is the agent of choice.

The technique of polishing is a matter of personal preference, and textbooks on operative dentistry should be consulted. The essential consideration is the use of diminishing grades of abrasives and to avoid producing heat.

As will be noted in the next section, the importance of finishing cannot be overemphasized. The restoration is not completed until its margins have been fully adjusted and its surfaces completely smooth.

TARNISH AND CORROSION

It is generally recognized that amalgam restorations often tarnish and corrode in the oral environment. The degree of tarnish, and the resulting discoloration, appear to be very dependent upon the individual's oral environment and to a certain extent upon the particular alloy employed. Electrochemical studies indicate that some passivation occurs as a result of the tarnish process which offers partial protection against further corrosion. Thus, a tendency toward tarnish, although perhaps unaesthetic, does not necessarily imply that active corrosion and early failure of a restoration will occur.

Active corrosion of a newly placed restoration occurs at the interface between the tooth and the restoration. The space between the alloy and the tooth permits the microleakage of electrolyte, and a classic concentration cell (crevice corrosion) process results. The buildup of corrosion products gradually seals this space, thus making dental amalgam a self-sealing restoration, as has been discussed.

The precise role of corrosion in the process of marginal breakdown has yet to be established. However, several theories have been developed relating the two. For conventional alloys there is indirect evidence that the γ_2 phase is implicated in both marginal failure and active corrosion. However, such a correlation is not possible for the high copper alloys.

Although black silver sulfide may be very evident in tarnish deposits, the most common corrosion products found with conventional amalgam alloys are oxides and chlorides of tin.[15] These are found both at the tooth-alloy interface and penetrating the bulk of old alloy restorations. In the case of high copper amalgams, corrosion products of copper are also seen, but the corrosion process is usually limited to the surfaces of the amalgam.

As noted, clinical data supporting the burnishing and polishing of amalgam restorations are not conclusive. However, theoretical considerations certainly indicate that every effort should be made to produce a smooth, homogeneous surface on a restoration in order to minimize tarnish and corrosion.

Whenever a gold restoration is placed in contact with an amalgam, corrosion of the amalgam can be expected as a result of the large differences in EMF of the two materials. The corrosion process liberates free mercury, which can contaminate and weaken the gold restoration. Biological effects (galvanism) can also result. Such a practice should be avoided.

A high copper amalgam is cathodic in respect to a conventional amalgam. Thus concern has been expressed that if new high copper amalgam restorations were placed in the same mouth with existing restorations of conventional amalgam, corrosion and failure would be accelerated in the latter. Although in vitro data support this concept,[16] clinical observations do not indicate that the corrosion is accelerated in such situations.[17] Laboratory models established to monitor corrosion in adjacent restorations suggest that the current flow paths are such that electrochemical interaction between the restorations is minimal.[18]

Since the γ_2 phase is the most anodic of those present in set amalgam alloys, the high copper amalgams, which virtually eliminate this phase, show improved laboratory corrosion behavior when compared with conventional amalgams. However, high mercury-alloy ratios can lead to the formation of γ_2 with even the high-copper alloys and thus promote corrosion. In a laboratory study, moisture contamination of amalgams during trituration has been shown to also increase the corrosion tendency of amalgams during the first 6 months.[19]

In general, high copper alloys show better corrosion behavior than do conventional alloys. Nevertheless, moisture contamination and high mercury-alloy ratios should be avoided. Everything should be done to minimize surface inhomogeneities and improve surface smoothness.

CLINICAL SIGNIFICANCE OF DIMENSIONAL CHANGE

Expansion   In one survey of the causes for failures of amalgam restorations, 16.6 per cent of a group of more than 1500 defective restorations failed because of excessive expansion.[20] As outlined in the previous chapter, there are two causes for excessive expansion of amalgam. One is insufficient trituration and condensation, and the other is the delayed expansion brought about by the contamination of the amalgam with moisture during trituration and condensation. The latter is unquestionably the principal cause for such failures.

According to the accepted theory, as discussed in Chapter 21, the delayed expansion is caused by the internal pressure exerted by the hydrogen that is one of the products of corrosion between the zinc in the amalgam and the incorporated moisture. The large expansion begins 4 to 5 days following condensation (Fig. 21–2).

Often such an expansion causes intense pain. Presumably, when an expansion of this magnitude occurs, the restoration may become wedged so tightly against the cavity walls that a pressure back toward the pulp chamber results. The pain is possibly the result of the existing trauma. Such pain may be experienced 10 to 12 days after the insertion of the restoration. If not removed, a contaminated amalgam restoration continues to expand and the final result may be similar to the protruding restoration shown in Figure 22–9. Undoubtedly, moisture was incorporated into the amalgam mix, from the hands of the operator and/or because the dry field of operation was not maintained. Excessive expansion and corrosion of the restoration has ensued and the restoration has extruded from the prepared cavity. Because the brittle amalgam margins are unsupported, they are susceptible to fracture, and marginal defects result. Leakage of the restoration then can produce a

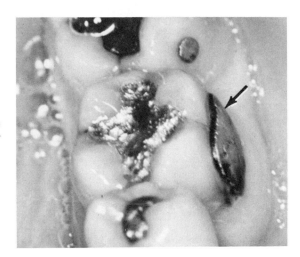

Figure 22–9 A Class V amalgam restoration (see arrow) that has failed because of excessive expansion. (Courtesy of J. Osborne.)

marginal discoloration with further corrosion and pitting caused by the concentration cells formed.

Another cause for the pitting of contaminated restorations is the escape of the hydrogen gas that collects near the surface. Some of the hydrogen may force its way through the surface of the amalgam and cause blisters. These are frequently seen in Class V restorations.

Pitting and corrosion, regardless of the cause, definitely reduce the strength of the amalgam restoration. If it proceeds far enough, the amalgam may become so pitted as to crumble under stress.

Delayed expansion occurring with moisture contamination of zinc-containing amalgams of either high or low copper content is illustrated in Figure 22–10. At 20 weeks, amalgam specimens prepared from both types of alloys (alloy A — low copper — and alloy B — high copper), when contaminated by moisture, expanded far in excess of the same uncontaminated amalgams. The expansion of the alloys at 20 days was also accompanied by a substantial reduction in strength (Fig. 22–11).[19]

It should be noted that the previous discussion has been concerned with moisture contamination during the manipulation and insertion of the amalgam. As stated in Chapter 21, after the restoration has been condensed no deleterious effects occur if saliva comes in contact with the external surface of the restoration during carving.

Contraction It has been pointed out that undertrituration results in reduced strength and possibly too great an expansion of the amalgam during hardening. It also is true that a slight contraction occurs with many modern amalgam alloys when they are properly triturated.

For many years it was believed that a slight expansion of the amalgam during setting would result in a restoration that would seal the cavity against ingress of oral fluids. Laboratory tests indicate no difference in the sealing properties of expanding and contracting alloys.[21] Likewise, observations on clinical restorations placed with thoroughly triturated amalgam that showed a contraction of 2 to 4 μm/cm failed to reveal a single example of marginal contraction after 2 years.[22] These restorations were actually superior in terms of surface condition and marginal adaptation. Still another study over a 3-year

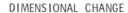

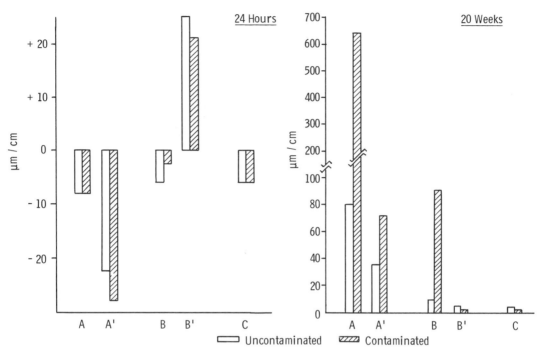

Figure 22–10   Effect of moisture contamination on the dimensional change of various types of amalgam alloys. A, zinc-containing low copper lathe-cut alloy; A′, zinc-free low copper lathe-cut alloy; B, zinc-containing high copper lathe-cut alloy; B′, zinc-free high copper lathe-cut alloy; C, zinc-free high copper spherical alloy.

period resulted in the same conclusion, even though the amalgam (from an alloy specially made for the purpose) contracted as much as 40 μm/cm.[23] This is double the amount of contraction permitted by the current American Dental Association specification.

It is very difficult to estimate whether an amalgam restoration in the mouth has contracted or expanded within the required 20 μm limits of such dimensional change. When it is recognized that the average human hair is 40 μm in diameter, it is virtually impossible to detect margins that may be open a few micrometers, either with the eye or with a dental instrument such as an explorer. It is for these reasons that through the years the American Dental Association specification has been broadened in terms of the permissible dimensional change on hardening, as measured on an unrestricted specimen.

It should be emphasized that these observations should not be construed as a recommendation for a contracting amalgam. They merely emphasize that small contractions during hardening as measured by laboratory methods do not appear to be clinically significant.

Zinc-Free Alloys   As might be expected, the deleterious effects of moisture spurred interest in the zinc-free alloys. Their use is certainly justified in those areas where it is virtually impossible to keep the operating region dry, such as the posterior teeth in the mouth of a child patient. In such cases if a zinc-containing alloy is used, the dentist must sacrifice normal condensation

COMPRESSIVE STRENGTH

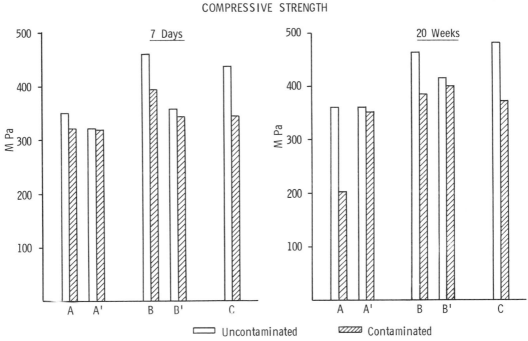

Figure 22–11 Effect of moisture contamination on the compressive strength of various types of amalgam alloys. A, zinc-containing low copper lathe-cut alloy; A', zinc-free low copper lathe-cut alloy; B, zinc-containing high copper lathe-cut alloy; B', zinc-free high copper lathe-cut alloy; C, zinc-free high copper spherical alloy.

procedures for the sake of speed. It is important that the restoration be placed before any moisture contamination occurs. For example, the condensation should be accomplished by filling the prepared cavity with a few large increments rather than with small increments, as previously recommended.

The use of zinc-free alloys provides some measure of safety in this regard, as can be seen in Figures 22–10 and 22–11. When contaminated by moisture, the expansion at 20 days of specimens of zinc-free alloys (A', B', and C) was not appreciably different from that of specimens prepared from the uncontaminated alloys. Also, at 20 weeks, contaminated zinc-free alloys A' and B' showed virtually no reduction in strength. However, the spherical single composition high copper alloy C, even though it contained no zinc, suffered a loss in strength both at 24 hours and 20 weeks when contaminated by moisture. Although the mechanism by which moisture reduces strength of alloys of this type has not been defined, it can be assumed that moisture present in the mix may interfere with the binding of the matrix.

The role of zinc in the manufacture of amalgam alloys was discussed in Chapter 20. So far as is known there are no great differences in the mechanical properties of the two types of alloys. In laboratory studies on electrochemical properties, amalgams prepared from zinc-containing and zinc-free alloys show no appreciable difference with respect to their tendency to corrode.[19]

The present trend is toward reduction of the zinc content of alloys. Many of the spherical, single composition, high copper alloys are zinc free. Although contaminated non-zinc alloys do not exhibit the high expansion, the strength of some is impaired (Fig. 22–11).

Regardless of composition, moisture is to be avoided in the manipulation and placement of amalgam restorations, or of any other restorative material.

THE EFFECT OF MERCURY

The amalgam restoration is possible only because of the unique characteristics of mercury. It is this metal that provides the plastic mass which can be inserted and finished in the teeth, and which then hardens to a structure that resists the rigors of the oral environment surprisingly well. However, it is also the element that so markedly influences the basic properties necessary to clinical success.

Toxicity   From the earliest use of this material, it has been asked whether mercury can produce local or systemic effects in the human. It is still occasionally conjectured that mercury toxicity from dental restorations is the cause for certain undiagnosed illnesses. It has been further suggested that a real hazard may exist for the dentist or dental assistant when mercury vapor is inhaled during mixing, thus producing an accumulative toxic effect. The matter has once again come to the foreground with the recent concern over mercury pollution of the environment.

Undoubtedly, mercury penetrates from the restoration into tooth structure. An analysis of dentin underlying amalgam restorations reveals the presence of mercury, which in part may account for a subsequent discoloration of the tooth. Use of radioactive mercury in silver amalgam has also revealed that some mercury might even reach the pulp.

However, the possibility of toxic reactions to the patient from these traces of mercury penetrating the tooth or sensitization from mercury salts dissolving from the surface of the amalgam is most remote. The danger has been evaluated in numerous studies. The patient's encounter with mercury vapor during insertion of the restoration is too brief and the total amount of mercury vapor too small to be injurious. Furthermore, any mercury leached from the amalgam is apparently not converted to the lethal form of methyl or ethyl mercury and is excreted rapidly by the body. The problem has been reviewed in detail, and the reader is referred to that literature.

What about dental office personnel? Dentists and their auxiliaries are exposed daily to the risk of mercury intoxication. Although metallic mercury can be absorbed through the skin or by ingestion, the primary risk to dental personnel is from inhalation.

The maximum level of exposure considered safe for occupational exposure is 50 micrograms of mercury per cubic meter of air. This is actually an average value to be calculated by averaging instantaneous exposures over a standard work day. Mercury is volatile at room temperature and has a vapor pressure of 20 milligrams per cubic meter of air, almost 400 times the maximum level considered acceptable. Mercury vapor has no color, odor, or taste and cannot be readily detected by simple means at levels near the maximum safe exposure. Since liquid mercury is almost 14 times more dense than water, in terms of volume a small spill can be significant. An eyedropper size drop of mercury contains enough mercury to saturate the air in a typical size operatory.

The American Dental Association estimates that one dental office in 10 exceeds the maximum safe exposure level for mercury. However, only a few cases of serious mercury intoxication due to dental exposure have been reported, and the potential hazard can be greatly reduced, if not eliminated, by attention to a few precautionary measures.

Obviously the operatory should be well ventilated. All excess mercury, including waste and amalgam removed during condensation, should be collected and stored in well-sealed containers. If spilled, it must be cleaned up as soon as possible. It is extremely difficult to remove mercury from carpeting. Ordinary vacuum cleaners merely disperse the mercury further through the exhaust. Mercury suppressant powders are helpful but should be considered temporary measures. If mercury comes in contact with the skin, the skin should be washed with soap and water.

As noted earlier, the capsule used with a mechanical amalgamator should have a tightly fitting cap to avoid mercury leakage. When grinding amalgam, a water spray and suction should be used; eye protection and a disposable mask are recommended.

The use of an ultrasonic condenser with amalgam is not recommended. A spray of small mercury droplets has been observed surrounding the condenser point during condensation.

More detailed recommendations can be obtained by consulting the most recent report of the American Dental Association Council on Dental Materials, Instruments, and Equipment.[24]

An important part of a hygiene program for handling toxic materials is periodic monitoring of actual exposure levels. Current recommendations suggest that this procedure be conducted at least on an annual basis. Several techniques are available. Instruments can be brought in to actually sample the air in the operatory and yield a time-weighted average for mercury exposure. Film badges are also available which can be worn by office personnel in a manner similar to radiation exposure badges. Or biological determinations can be performed on office staff to measure mercury levels in blood or urine.

The risk from mercury exposure to dental personnel cannot be ignored. However, close adherence to simple hygiene procedures will help insure a safe working environment.

Influence on the Restoration   Mercury is very important to the physical behavior of the amalgam restoration and an analysis of clinical restorations indicates a wide variation in their mercury content.

It is of particular interest that characteristically the mercury concentration is higher in the marginal areas. This observation is true regardless of the method of condensation or the "dryness" of the increments used to build the restoration. Whether hand or mechanical condensation was used, mercury analysis of a large number of restorations revealed that the mercury content of the marginal areas averaged between 2 to 3 per cent higher than that of the bulk of the restorations.[25] The higher mercury content at the margins is important because it is these areas that are critical in terms of corrosion, fracture, and secondary caries.

Restorations that have an unduly high mercury content have been judged to be clinically unsatisfactory by visual examination. Such a relationship is to be expected on the basis of the discussion in the previous chapter, in which it was shown that a marked decrease in the strength properties of traditional silver-tin amalgams occurred at a mercury content of approximately 55 per cent. When clinical restorations were placed with a low-copper alloy containing various quantities of mercury, those restorations containing mercury in excess of 55 per cent showed an appreciably higher incidence of marginal fracture and surface deterioration than did restorations that contained mercury in the 50 per cent range.[26] The higher the mercury content, the greater was the incidence and severity of dyscrasia that occurred as the restorations aged.

Since high mercury content has the same effect on the strength and creep[27] of high copper alloys as on the older low copper amalgams, it would be expected that high copper amalgam restorations with an excessively high mercury content would also exhibit a greater incidence of marginal degradation, etc. Certainly, if the mercury is too high then the weaker and corrosion-susceptible γ_2 phase will be formed.

MARGINAL DETERIORATION

As has been repeatedly mentioned, one of the most common types of amalgam failures is the so-called "ditched" restoration, such as the example shown in Figure 22–12. Although the ditching may not have progressed to the point at which secondary caries has developed, the restoration is unsightly, and further deterioration may be anticipated. Examination of clinical restorations has associated secondary caries with marginal discrepancies that exceeded 50 μm.[28]

Such failures are often attributed to a contraction of amalgam but, as explained, this is not likely. Marginal breakdown of amalgam restorations may be caused by, or related to, several factors.

Improper Cavity Preparation or Finishing   If unsupported enamel is left at the marginal areas of the cavity preparation, the tooth structure itself may in time fracture. Thus the "ditched" amalgam may involve fracture of adjacent enamel as well as the amalgam.

Improper carving and finishing of the restoration may leave a thin ledge of

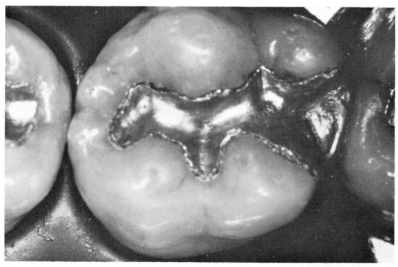

Figure 22–12   A typical "ditched" amalgam restoration. (Courtesy of H. W. Gilmore.)

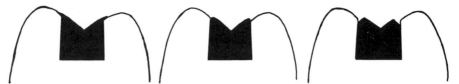

Figure 22–13   A common cause of marginal failure. If a feather ledge of the amalgam is left overlapping the enamel at the margin, it will fracture under masticatory stress. (Courtesy of G. M. Hollenback.)

amalgam extending over the enamel (Fig. 22–13). Such feather-like ledges are often difficult to detect and remove. One method mentioned was to touch the margins lightly with a soft prophylactic polishing cup and polishing paste. Probably a careful burnishing technique when a fast setting amalgam is used can be advantageous in eliminating some of these discrepancies.

Excess Mercury   The effect of a high final mercury content upon marginal deterioration has been discussed. Control of the mercury-alloy ratio, use of thorough trituration, and proper condensation reduce the possibility of such failures.

Creep   If the creep of the alloy is unduly high or if the manipulation is such that it tends to increase the creep, the potential for marginal breakdown is greatly enhanced. Certainly there is ample evidence that when other factors are controlled the alloy used for the restoration is a highly significant factor in incidence and severity of marginal failure of clinical restorations.

As was pointed out in Chapter 21, there appears to be little correlation between creep and marginal breakdown with alloys having creep values below the 1 per cent level. However, when the creep values are above this level, generally restorations of higher creep alloys experience greater marginal breakdown than do restorations of lower creep alloys.

There has been considerable speculation as to whether the property of creep per se is directly involved in the mechanics of marginal breakdown or whether it indirectly may identify alloys that possess other characteristics which make them vulnerable to this type of failure.

One theory that has been advanced is that the amalgam restoration is constrained by the walls of the cavity and anything that impinges upon the space, be it expansion of the amalgam or the build-up of corrosion products at the tooth-restoration interface, induces stresses in the amalgam and the surrounding tooth.[29] Under the constant stress the amalgam will plastically deform (creep) and, taking the path of least resistance, extrude from the cavity. When this occurs, the amalgam is no longer supported by the tooth structure. The unsupported edges are easily broken when stress is applied, such as during mastication, thus producing marginal breakdown or ditching. If this theory is correct, then obviously the higher the creep value, the less will be the plastic deformation. Thus, by better resistance to plastic deformation, the amount of extrusion from the cavity will be reduced and as a result so will the marginal breakdown.

Corrosion   Yet another theory suggests that the principal cause for this type of failure is fundamentally related to the degrading effect of the corrosion process.[30] The hypothesis is that the electropotential differences that exist between dissimilar metals in the oral cavity, or even between the various phases within the amalgam itself, initiate the corrosion process, as has been discussed. Oxidation is centered on the γ_2 phase, and apparently in time tin ions are released. These ions migrate to form corrosion products at the margins.

As the tin is released from the γ_2 phase, free mercury is left behind. This mercury can then diffuse back into the amalgam and react with the residual alloy particles to form additional γ_1 and γ_2 phases. A resulting unilateral expansion (referred to as "mercuroscopic expansion") in or near the amalgam-tooth interface produces a protrusion of the restoration from the cavity. Being unsupported and weakened by corrosion products, these margins may be easily fractured by occlusal stress.

Thus the sparsity or absence of the corrosion-susceptible γ_2 phase from the microstructure of high copper amalgams is suggested to be the factor underlying the superior resistance of these alloys to marginal breakdown. If this is correct, the property of creep would not be directly involved in the mechanism of marginal breakdown. It is true that amalgams that have little or no γ_2 generally have lower creep than alloys that form appreciable amounts of γ_2. Thus, on the basis of this theory, the creep test would serve primarily as a convenient means of identifying those amalgams that are most susceptible to corrosion and marginal failure.

Theoretically, expansion of the amalgam from moisture contamination of a zinc-containing alloy could also produce this type of failure.

Thus, it is obvious that several mechanisms, separately or working synergistically, may be identified with the frequently observed marginal degeneration of this restorative material. In fact, in one study an equation was derived to predict marginal fracture.[31] This calculation encompassed the creep of the alloy, its γ_2 and zinc content. It was found that the prediction equation produced an excellent fit to clinical data on a number of alloys.

At this time the exact mechanism of marginal breakdown and the specific property or properties is not known. However, it is prudent to select alloys that inherently have low creep and possess maximum resistance to corrosion.

Repaired Amalgam Restorations   Occasionally when an amalgam restoration fails, as from marginal fracture, it is repaired rather than replaced. A new mix of amalgam is condensed against the remaining part of the existing restoration. Such a restoration may be subjected to tensile and shear stresses. Therefore, the strength of the bond between the new and the old amalgam is important.

It has been shown that the bond strength of repaired amalgam, as measured by a transverse test, is less than one-half that of unrepaired amalgam.[32] The bond is a source of weakness. Factors such as corrosion and saliva contamination at the interface present formidable barriers that interfere with bonding of the old and new amalgam.[33] A technique of scraping the fractured amalgam surface with the edge of an amalgam condenser in the presence of mercury has been shown in vitro to markedly improve the bond strength of the repair.[34] The procedure is delicate, and whether it can be accomplished as effectively in the oral cavity as on the laboratory bench is not known.

Repair of amalgam restorations probably falls into the category of a hazardous procedure. Repair should be attempted only if the area involved is one that will not be subjected to high stresses.

References

1. Vrijhoef MMA, Vermeersch AG, and Spanauf AJ: Dental Amalgam. Chicago, Quintessence Publishing Co., Inc., 1980.
2. Leinfelder KF: Clinical performance of amalgams with high content of copper. Oper Dent 5:125, 1980.
3. Osborne JW, Phillips RW, Gale EN, and Binon PP: Three-year clinical comparison of three amalgam alloy types emphasizing an appraisal of the evaluation methods used. J Am Dent Assoc 93:784, 1976.
4. Eames WB: Preparation and condensation of amalgam with a low mercury-alloy ratio. J Am Dent Assoc 58:78, 1959.
5. Eames WB, Mack RM, and Auvenshine RC: Accuracy of mercury/alloy proportioning systems. J Am Dent Assoc 81:137, 1970.
6. Jorgensen KD and Okuda R: Mercury leakage of amalgam capsules. Acta Odontol Scand 29:461, 1971.
7. Rupp NW, Paffenbarger GC, and Patel PR: Effect of residual mercury content on creep in dental amalgam. J Am Dent Assoc 100:52, 1980.
8. Mahler DB: Plasticity of amalgam mixes. J Dent Res 18:137, 1970.
9. Eames WB: Factors influencing the marginal adaptation of amalgam. J Am Dent Assoc 75:629, 1967.
10. Mahler DB and Mitchum JC: Effect of precondensation mercury content on the physical properties of amalgam. J Am Dent Assoc 71:593, 1965.
11. Creaven PJ, Dennison JB, and Charbeneau GT: Surface roughness of two dental amalgams after various polishing techniques. J Prosthet Dent 43:289, 1980.
12. Leinfelder KF: Personal Communication.
13. Leinfelder KF, Strickland WD, Wall JT, and Taylor DF: Burnished amalgam restorations: A two year study. Oper Dent 3:2, 1978.
14. Mitchell JA, Dickson G, and Schoonover IC: X-ray diffraction studies of mercury diffusion and surface stability of dental amalgam. J Dent Res 34:744, 1955.
15. Marshall GW, Jackson B, and Marshall S: Copper-rich and conventional amalgam restorations after clinical use. J Am Dent Assoc 100:43, 1980.
16. Chen CP and Greener EH: A galvanic study of different amalgams. J Oral Rehabil 4:23, 1977.
17. Osborne JW, Phillips RW, Gale EN, and Norman RD: Clinical assessment of the marginal breakdown of conventional alloys adjacent to a dispersion alloy. J Dent Res 55:1140, 1976.
18. Marek M: Galvanic interactions between dental amalgam and other restorative materials. IADR Program and Abstracts, No. 133, 1980.
19. Fainsilber S, Moore BK, Swartz ML, and Phillips RW: Effects of saline contamination on zinc and zinc-free high copper amalgam alloys. IADR Program and Abstracts, No. 107, 1980.
20. Healey HJ and Phillips RW: A clinical study of amalgam failures. J Dent Res 28:439, 1949.
21. Swartz ML and Phillips RW: Influence of manipulative variables on the marginal adaptation of certain restorative materials. J Prosthet Dent 12:172, 1962.
22. Phillips RW, Boyd DA, Healey HJ, and Crawford WH: Clinical observations on amalgam with known physical properties, final report. J Am Dent Assoc 75:325, 1945.
23. McDonald RE and Phillips RW: Clinical observations on a contracting amalgam alloy. J Dent Res 29:482, 1950.
24. Report of Council on Dental Materials, Instruments and Devices: Recommendations in dental mercury hygiene — March, 1978. J Am Dent Assoc 96:487, 1978.
25. Wilson RT, Phillips RW, and Norman RD: Influence of certain condensation procedures upon the mercury content of amalgam restorations. J Dent Res 36:458, 1957.
26. Nadal R, Phillips RW, and Swartz ML: Clinical investigation on the relationship of mercury to the amalgam restoration: II. J Am Dent Assoc 63:488, 1961.
27. Mahler DB and Adey JD: The influence of mercury content on the characteristics of a high-copper amalgam. J Biomed Mater Res 13:467, 1979.
28. Jorgensen KD and Wakumoto S: Occlusal amalgam filling; marginal defects and secondary caries. Odontol Tidskr 76:43, 1968.

29. Osborne JW, Winchell PG, and Phillips RW: A hypothetical mechanism by which creep causes marginal failure of amalgam restorations. J Indiana Dent Assoc 57:16, 1978.
30. Jorgensen KD: The mechanism of marginal fracture of amalgam fillings. Acta Odontol Scand 23:347, 1965.
31. Mahler DB, Marantz RL, and Engle JH: A predictive model for the clinical marginal fracture of amalgam. J Dent Res 59:1420, 1980.
32. Terkla LG, Mahler DB, and Mitchum JC: Bond strength of repaired amalgam. J Prosthet Dent 11:942, 1961.
33. Consani R, Rhunke LA, and Stolf WL: Infiltration of a radioactive solution into joined silver amalgam. J Prosthet Dent 37:158, 1977.
34. Jorgensen KD and Saito T: Bond strength of repaired amalgam. Acta Odontol Scand 26:605, 1968.

23 DIRECT FILLING GOLD AND ITS MANIPULATION

Very few metals are used in the pure condition for dental restorative purposes, gold being the outstanding exception. One of the first materials used for dental restorations was pure gold and its popularity as a restorative material has increased somewhat in recent years. It is the most noble of metals, seldom tarnishing or corroding in the oral cavity. In this and certain other respects it is an almost ideal dental restorative material for permanently preserving tooth structure. Its chief disadvantages are its color, high coefficient of thermal conductivity, and difficulty of manipulation.

The presently available products may be divided into three categories, but all have certain characteristics in common. With one exception, they are all pure gold with purity in the 99.99 per cent, or better, range.

The Brinell hardness of pure gold is approximately 25. This extreme softness would seem to contraindicate its use in the mouth. However, its malleability and lack of oxide surface coating permit increments to be welded together readily in the cavity. In the process, the hardness and other properties are substantially increased. The ability to be welded at room temperature, provided the surface is free from adsorbed gases and other impurities, is a unique characteristic of gold. This characteristic makes possible the use of gold for placing restorations directly into the prepared cavity.*

Pieces of gold are placed in the prepared cavity and are welded together by a suitable condensing instrument. This process is referred to as *compaction* or condensing, and the gold restoration is built up into a coherent mass by this welding technique. The cohesion results from metallic bonding between the overlapped increments of gold under the pressure of compaction. This phenomenon is usually exhibited by metals and alloys only at a temperature considerably above that of the oral cavity.

---

*For this reason, gold foil may be referred to as a "direct filling material," as compared with gold alloys (Chapter 24), which are used to fabricate cast restorations in the dental laboratory. It will be recalled that in Chapter 14 the resins used for insertion directly into the prepared cavity were called "direct filling resins."

Although the dental profession sometimes refers to all direct filling golds as "foils," the present products might be described as

1. Foil
2. Electrolytic precipitate (mat gold)
3. Powder
4. Alloyed gold

Gold Foil   Because gold is the most malleable of metals, it is rolled for many applications to sheets 25 μm thick. It can be rolled even further, to approximately 15 μm, but to reduce it to the thicknesses used in dentistry, a beating operation is used. The product of this operation is called *gold foil*. The crystals of the original cast metal are deformed and elongated so that they have a fibrous structure. The surface texture, as seen in Figure 23–1, is a result of the surface against which the foil is formed.

Even though the original cast ingot may be as much as 15 mm thick, the gold is so malleable that only one softening (annealing) heat treatment is required in beating it to sub-micrometer thicknesses.

The gold foil is often supplied in flat square sheets of varying thickness. Standard foil comes in "No. 4" thickness, which weighs 4 grains (.259 gm) and is approximately .51 μm thick. The size of the sheets is standardized; therefore, this numbering system is actually a designation of thickness. Thus "No. 3" foil, used in most of the products described later, weighs 3 grains (.194 gm) and is approximately .38 μm thick.

The sheets may be cut into eighths, sixteenths, sixty-fourths, etc., and then compressed into pellets or cylinders. A number of sheets of foil may be placed on top of each other to form *laminated gold foil*, which can then be cut into pellets or formed into cylinders if desired. One of the original types of laminated foil was *platinum foil*, in which a sheet of pure platinum foil was sandwiched between two sheets of *pure gold foil*. Other forms of gold have almost completely replaced platinum foil.

The foil also can be made into ropes, or corrugated, by placing it between sheets of paper, which can be ignited in a closed container. This latter form of gold foil is of historical interest because it was an outcome of the great Chicago fire of 1871. A dental dealer had some books of gold foil in a safe. After the fire, the safe was opened, and it was found that the paper had charred, but the gold

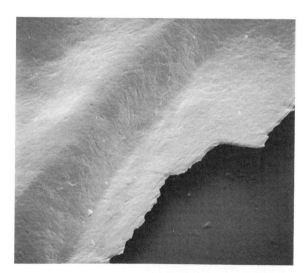

Figure 23–1   Scanning electron micrograph of the surface of gold foil. (750 ×) (Courtesy of C. E. Ingersoll.)

leaf itself was unharmed, except that it had become corrugated because of the shriveling of the paper while oxidizing in the air-tight safe. After the carbon was removed, it was found that the gold exhibited a superior welding property. Present preformed cylinders and ropes are made from this corrugated foil.

Whether the sheet is flat or is rolled into cylinders or ropes is immaterial. By definition, all of these various forms are foil. However, pure gold may be supplied to the dentist in forms other than as foil.

Electrolytic Gold   Another form of pure gold commonly used for dental restorations is *electrolytic gold,* or *mat gold.* This material is not actually a foil in the sense that it is a thin sheet prepared by rolling and beating. Rather it is a powder formed by electrolytic precipitation. The powder is then compressed into strips and heated to a temperature just below the melting point of gold, a process referred to as *sintering.* Sintering causes self-diffusion between the particles so that where the particles are in contact they will actually "grow" together. This self-diffusion of sintering is evidenced in Figure 23–2. However, a typical dendritic structure is still evident.

Mat gold is commonly supplied in small, thin strips that can be cut or formed by the dentist into the desired size. Mat gold is often preferred for its ease in building up the internal bulk of the restoration because it can be more easily compacted into, and adapted to, the retentive portions of the prepared cavity. However, gold foil is generally recommended for the external surface of the restoration. In other words, the mat gold is covered with a veneer of gold foil. The crystalline structure of the mat gold does not permit welding into as homogeneous a mass as does gold foil. Therefore, there is a greater tendency for surface pitting if it is used on the surface of the restoration.

The manufacturer may also supply pure gold in a form referred to as *mat foil.* In this case, a layer of mat gold is sandwiched between layers of gold foil.

Another form of electrolytic gold is available. This is an alloy of gold and calcium, the calcium content being 0.1 to 0.5 per cent by weight. For greater ease in handling, the alloy is sandwiched between two layers of gold foil. The intent of this formulation is to alter the crystalline structure so that hardness and strength will be increased.

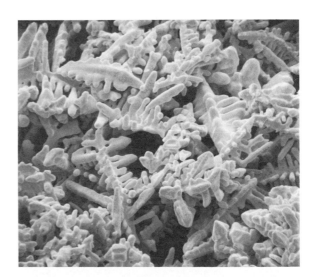

Figure 23–2 Scanning electron micrograph of mat gold. (750 ×) (Courtesy of C. E. Ingersoll.)

Powdered Gold   From time to time, gold powders have been available in agglomerated form.[1] These agglomerates were usually furnished with a liquid, such as an alcohol or dilute carbolic acid, to hold the agglomerate together until it was placed and compaction begun. The difficulties of using loose gold powder were resolved in the early 1960's by enclosing the powder in gold foil.

A very fine powder can be prepared either by atomizing the metal from its molten state or by chemical precipitation. The powder is a blend of gold particles varying in size up to a maximum of approximately 74 μm, with an average particle size of 15 μm.[2] Although these particles can be compressed by mild pressure into a loosely held mass, a pellet so formed tends to fall apart during handling and compaction. Consequently, the powder is formed into pellets of desirable size by mixing with a soft wax. The wax is subsequently burned off, as will be described. Each pellet is then wrapped with gold foil, rather than sintering the mass, as for mat gold. The foil forms an effective container for the powdered metal and acts as a matrix throughout the mass of gold as it is condensed. Figure 23–3 illustrates the construction of a typical pellet of powdered gold.

The powdered gold pellets have a cylindrical or irregular shape and a diameter of 1 to 2 mm. The ratio of foil to powder varies from approximately 1 to 3 for the smallest pellets to approximately 1 to 9 for the largest. Some operators believe that the use of pellets of powdered gold enhances cohesion during compaction and reduces the time required for placing the restoration, because each pellet contains approximately 10 times more metal by volume than a comparable sized pellet of gold foil.[3]

Cohesive and Noncohesive Gold   All of these forms of pure gold may be further classified as being cohesive, semicohesive, or noncohesive. As previously noted, the unique ability of gold to cohere or weld at oral temperature under pressure is dependent upon a clean surface that is free from impurities. Gold, like most metals, attracts gases, e.g., oxygen, to its surface, and any adsorbed gas film prevents cohesion of the individual increments of gold during their compaction. For this reason, the manufacturer usually supplies the gold to the dentist essentially free of surface contaminants and, therefore, inherently

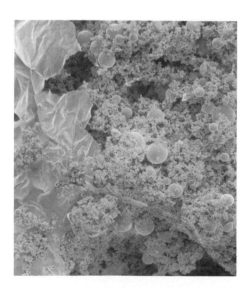

Figure 23–3 With the wax burned away, the spherical atomized particles can be seen. The finer and rougher surface particles are the chemically precipitated portion. (100 ×) (Courtesy of C. E. Ingersoll.)

cohesive. In this condition the material is referred to as cohesive gold foil, cohesive mat gold, or whatever the form may be. However, the manufacturer can subject the gold to a volatile agent such as ammonia, which is adsorbed on the surface of the gold. This volatile substance acts as a protective film to prevent adsorption of nonvolatile materials and the premature cohesion of pellets in their container. The volatile film is readily removed by heating in order to restore the cohesive character of the gold.

Noncohesive gold has a permanent nonvolatile agent adsorbed on its surface, such as an iron salt or an acidic gas (sulfur- or phosphorus-containing groups). It is rarely used today but may be employed to rapidly build up the bulk of a direct gold restoration. Noncohesive gold is supplied only as sheets of foil.

Removal of Surface Impurities With the exception of semicohesive and noncohesive gold foil, pure gold used for dental restorations is received by the dentist in a cohesive condition, with a minimum of surface contamination. In order to obtain the proper thickness of gold foil, the gold is subjected to three series of rollings and beatings. During this process the gold becomes strain hardened. In order to eliminate the hardening induced by this cold working and to permit further reduction in foil thickness, the foil is annealed. In addition, the "corrugating" operation is also an annealing process. Although the principal purpose of this annealing is to eliminate strain hardening, most of the surface impurities, such as oxygen, are volatilized at the same time.

Although the cohesive gold has invariably been so treated by the manufacturer, it is customary for the dentist or dental assistant to heat the foil or pellet immediately before it is carried into the prepared cavity. This step is commonly referred to as "annealing" or "heat treatment." Although it is possible that a certain amount of further recrystallization or stress relief may occur during such a treatment, the conceivable metallographic changes are not the primary objective of the heating. Rather, the foil is heated as a precautionary measure to volatilize any remaining surface gases and ensure a totally clean surface. Consequently, the term "annealing" is a misnomer. It is suggested that the term *degassing* is more appropriate for this procedure and it will be referred to as such in subsequent discussions.

Degassing is definitely essential. A number of surface gases may be present, particularly if the dentist does not keep the foil container closed when it is not in use. Gold atoms hold oxygen by secondary bonding forces. Moisture may collect on the foil. Sulfur dioxide may also be a contaminant because it is usually present in the urban atmosphere, particularly in the dental office where certain sulfur-containing compounds may be used during dental treatment.

Apropos of such a possibility of contamination, it is important that the cohesive gold foil be stored in a tightly sealed bottle or container and exposed to the atmosphere for as short a time as possible before use. Even under these conditions, oxygen from the bottle can be adsorbed by the gold. If the dentist forms the foil into pellets or ropes, it is advisable that chamois finger tips be worn in order to protect the gold from contamination. A totally dry cavity is mandatory throughout the compaction process in order to ensure complete cohesion.

From the foregoing, it is obvious that decontamination of the gold surface is essential in order to attain cohesion and to ensure maximal physical properties in the compacted restoration. Proper degassing is, therefore, a matter of heating the gold long enough, at a given temperature, to volatilize all gases and moisture, yet at the same time avoiding injury to the foil in the process. Underheating during the decontamination procedure should be avoided because it leaves impurities on the foil that prevent thorough welding and results in flaking and a pitted surface. On the other hand, overheating is equally injurious. Heating at too high a temperature can cause impurities from the heating tray and/or handling instruments to be incorporated into the gold. Heating for too long a time can cause embrittlement, both by incorporation of impurities and by grain growth in the case of foil, and oversintering in electrolytic or powder products.

In an attempt to determine the optimal temperature required to remove surface impurities, specimens were uniformly compacted from gold foil that had been heated for 5 minutes at various temperatures.[4] The Brinell hardness numbers of specimens so compacted are shown in Figure 23–4. The data indicate that temperatures below 315° C (600° F) are not adequate to attain the optimal hardness of the compacted gold. The values were not significantly different in the temperature range between 315° C (600° F) and 760° C (1400° F).

It is not known whether these data are typical of other physical properties or for all of the various forms of pure gold filling materials that are commercially available. The amount of surface contamination present can possibly influence the temperature and the time that is needed to clean the surface.

Aside from the purification of the surface of the foil, the total result of this heating is not entirely known. In light of the considerable strain hardening of the foil during manufacture, if the foil was not recrystallized completely beforehand and if a change in grain structure occurred during degassing, such a change might be a factor in the effectiveness of compaction. Owing to the thinness of the foil, the use of ordinary metallographic techniques to study this phenomenon is impractical. Consequently, little is known about the recrystallization temperature or the possibility of subsequent grain growth if the foil is overheated.

Studies have been made on the recrystallization of gold metal (not foil). For example, it has been shown that the recrystallization temperature of severely cold-worked gold is 200° C (390° F).[5] In another study in which pure

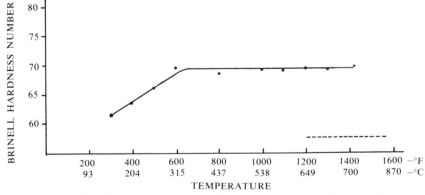

Figure 23–4 Brinell hardness number of specimens prepared from gold foil that was heated to various temperatures for surface decontamination. The dotted line indicates the general temperature range produced by an open alcohol flame. (Adapted from Hollenback and Collard, J South Calif State Dent Assoc, Sept., 1961.)

gold (99.990% pure) was used, the recrystallization temperature was found to be 150° C (302° F).[6] Obviously such a difference is not of concern in the present discussion, but by analogy the values may help in estimating the recrystallization of the gold foil. It is interesting to note that the usual degassing temperatures are higher than either of these values. From the evidence thus far presented, it appears that the recrystallization temperature of the foil possibly may not influence the physical properties of the compacted mass to any extent, although further study is needed. As previously noted, probably the sole purpose of degassing is to remove surface impurities.

Direct filling golds may be heated by one of two methods: in bulk on a tray, heated by either a gas flame or electricity, or piece by piece in an open flame. Electrical heating is probably best for products other than the gold powder wrapped in foil because it is more uniform, it is easier to control, and there is less chance of contamination.

In practice, when heated in bulk, the ropes or pellets of pure gold are placed on a mica tray. Care should be taken to handle the pieces only with stainless steel tweezers or similar instruments which will not contaminate the foil. Excessive amounts should be avoided, since the difficulties of prolonged heating, referred to earlier, can arise from repeated heating as well.

The electric "annealer" is maintained at a temperature between approximately 343° C (650° F) and 371° C (700° F). The time required to volatilize the moisture and gases varies from 5 to 20 minutes, depending upon the particular temperature employed.

The method of degassing the gold piece by piece in an open flame consists of picking up each piece of gold individually, heating it directly in an open flame, and placing it into the prepared cavity. The fuel for the flame may be alcohol or gas, but alcohol is preferred as there is less danger of contamination.

Alcohol, however, should be pure methanol or ethanol without colorants or other additives. Denatured alcohol can be used if the denaturant is known to be methanol. Some denaturants may be solids, which can contaminate, or higher alcohols, which produce free carbon caused by incomplete burning.

There are certain advantages and disadvantages to electric or flame heating. The problems associated with the use of electric annealing are as follows: (1) the pellets may stick together if the tray is moved; (2) air currents may affect the uniformity of heating; (3) it is difficult to anneal appropriate amounts of gold; (4) with prolonged heating there is a danger of overannealing; (5) the size selection among the pieces of degassed gold is limited; and (6) there is a greater chance of contamination if the gold is not used immediately.

On the other hand, there are distinct advantages to the use of a flame, such as: (1) ability to select a piece of gold of the desired size; (2) can degas only the quantity of gold needed; (3) less danger of overannealing; and (4) less chance of contamination of gold between the time of degassing and use.

Compaction of Cohesive Gold Foil   The compaction technique for gold foil illustrates the procedure generally employed for other forms of direct filling golds. Originally, compaction of gold foil was accomplished entirely by impact with a mallet. Each piece of foil was compacted by a special instrument, known as a condenser, the face of which was placed against the foil, and the other end struck sharply with a small mallet. Current techniques make wide use of mechanical devices for applying the pressures required to weld the foil. A detailed account of the technique for the insertion of a gold foil restoration is not within the scope of this text.

In brief, starting points are cut in the prepared cavity and the first pieces of foil are wedged into these areas. Subsequently, additional foil is welded to these pieces. In this manner, the compaction is continued and the prepared cavity is gradually filled. The original foil condensers had a single pyramid-shaped face but the present instruments have a series of small pyramids or serrations on the face. These act as swagers, exerting lateral force on their inclines, in addition to providing direct compressive forces as the load is applied to the condenser.

Although acceptable in terms of the physical properties of the compacted foil, the use of a hand condenser with a mallet is tedious for both the dentist and patient. Each piece of foil must be carefully "stepped" by placing the condenser point against the rope or pellet in successive adjacent positions as the instrument is struck with the mallet. The stepping may be more readily accomplished and standardized by a mechanical condenser.

The mechanical gold foil condensers consist of points activated by comparatively light blows that are repeated with frequencies that range from 360 to 3600 per minute. In other words, a vibratory type of motion is employed, with the vibrations being produced either pneumatically or electrically. The intensity of the blow itself may also be regulated. Thus, frequency and intensity may be altered to provide proper compaction in different parts of the prepared cavity. Compaction with such mechanical devices is quite rapid and is accomplished with greater comfort for the patient.

Whatever the method employed, each piece of foil should be compacted over its entire length so that voids are not bridged. The most dense structure occurs directly under the face of the condenser, with the compacted layers arranged at right angles to the direction of compaction, as shown in Figure 23–5. Loose or moderately compacted layers lie adjacent to, or below, these areas of greatest density. Thus, as nearly as possible, the condenser should traverse the entire surface of each foil increment.

Density   The direct gold restoration is characterized by dense masses, associated with adjacent areas containing void spaces (Fig. 23–5). As previously stated, the dense layers are oriented at right angles to the direction at which the compaction force is applied. It is evident from this figure that deformation of either mat gold or gold foil is limited to short distances, confined to the immediate area of the face of the condenser. Porosities are present below these areas because of incomplete contact and welding between the individual layers or particles of the gold.

The greatest strength of compacted gold, as measured by the ultimate tensile strength, lies within the entangled masses of gold.[7] The weakest part is in the porous areas between the layers of the closely compacted increments. Thus, the maximal strength throughout the restoration is attained by minimizing the internal voids.

Voids on the surface of the restoration increase the susceptibility to electrolytic corrosion. Furthermore, in a direct gold restoration, voids at the restoration-tooth interface may be present to the extent that gross leakage occurs which invites secondary caries. However, one of the merits of the properly compacted gold restoration is the small amount of microleakage that does take place.

Apparently, voids are inevitable but they should be kept to a minimum, a

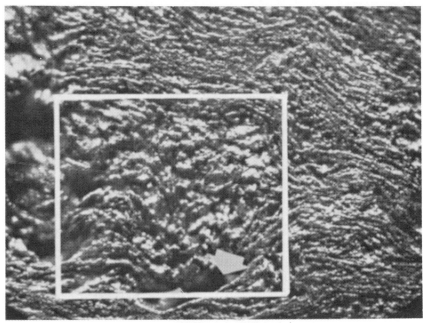

Figure 23–5 A cross section of compacted gold foil. A portion of loosely compacted foil is outlined by the rectangle and the arrow indicates a void. The dense layers above the rectangle show good compaction directly under the face of the condenser. (From Hodson, Dent Progr, Oct., 1961.)

factor that depends upon the skill of the operator. The size and shape of the condenser face, the dimensions of the prepared cavity, and the dynamics of the compacting system all influence the density of the compacted gold restoration.

The number of voids and the corresponding apparent density in a direct gold restoration may be estimated by the specific gravity of the compacted gold. It can be assumed that the specific gravity of the restoration should be approximately that of pure gold (19.32). A survey of the specific gravity of restorations compacted from the various forms of direct gold materials, placed by different operators and with varying techniques, indicates that the values range from 16 to 19. These results suggest that the theoretical ideal of a dense and solid gold restoration is never achieved, regardless of the form of gold or the technique used.

Size of the Condenser Point The diameter of the condenser point is an important factor in determining the effectiveness of the welding. Assuming the condenser point to be circular, its surface area is directly proportional to the square of its diameter. The energy distribution of the impact onto the foil depends upon the area of the condenser point. For example, a given amount of energy is distributed over four times as much area of foil with a condenser point 2 mm in diameter than with a similar point 1 mm in diameter. In other words, the *concentration* of the energy, and consequently the strain hardening of the gold, should be four times as great with the 1-mm condenser as with the larger condenser.

It follows, therefore, that small condenser points are indicated for use with direct filling gold in order to provide effective energy distribution without increasing the impact energy to an extent that the oral structures are damaged. The surface area of the points in use may vary between equivalent circular areas with diameters 0.5 to 1 mm. It should be understood that the points can be of any contour desired provided their surface areas are within the limits specified. The lower limit for the point diameter is established on the basis of a possible penetration of the foil by the point.

Physical Properties of Compacted Gold   The physical properties of the various forms of direct filling gold, and the influence of various methods of compacting, have been tested extensively. Unfortunately, it is difficult to compare the data from these studies because each investigation involves somewhat different experimental conditions. However, the results summarized in Table 23–1 are probably representative.[8]

The strength is determined by measuring the transverse strength because most of the strength characteristics of a dental restoration can be evaluated by means of this test.[9] Transverse strength is a reflection of all three types of stress — compressive, tensile, and shear (Chapter 3). Fracture in bending is propagated from regions of maximal tensile strength and, because of the relationship of tensile strength to cohesion, bending strength does in part measure cohesion.

Hardness, per se, may not be a critical factor in evaluating the effectiveness of a particular restoration in carrying out its intended purpose of preserving the tooth. The more important aspect is that this property is indicative of the overall quality of the compacted gold. In other words, the better the control of the variables involved in preparing the gold and compacting it into the prepared cavity, the greater is the hardness, and vice versa.

It is of academic interest that the quotients of the strength and hardness values (Table 23–1) are approximately 500, the factor by which BHN values for gold alloys are multiplied to obtain their tensile strength, as indicated in the next chapter. This is possibly indicative of the importance of tensile stress in the determination of transverse strength, as previously noted.

In this study, the density values in Table 23–1 are not the true density or

Table 23–1.   *Representative Physical Properties of Direct Filling Golds**

MATERIAL AND TECHNIQUE	TRANSVERSE STRENGTH (MPa)	(psi)	KHN	APPARENT DENSITY† (gm/cm³)
Mat gold				
Hand	161	23,000	52	14.3
Mechanical	169	24,100	62	14.7
Combined	169	24,100	53	14.5
Powdered gold				
Hand	165	23,600	55	14.4
Mechanical	155	22,200	64	14.5
Combined	190	27,100	58	14.9
Gold foil				
Hand	296	42,300	69	15.9
Mechanical	265	37,900	69	15.8
Combined	273	39,000	69	15.8
Mat gold and gold foil				
Hand	196	28,000	70	15.0
Mechanical	206	29,400	71	15.1
Combined	227	32,400	75	15.0

*From Richter and Cantwell, J Prosthet Dent July–Aug., 1965.
†Density measured by dividing the weight of the specimen by its volume.

specific gravity because they were determined by linear measurement. Such values include all blebs, pores, and other surface irregularities and should be called the *apparent density*. If such porosities and voids are not present, one would expect the density to be that of gold (19.3 gm/cm³). It is evident from the fifth column of Table 23–1 that the true density is not even approached.

The transverse strength, hardness, and density are apparently somewhat greater when gold foil or the combinations of mat gold and gold foil are employed, as compared with when powdered gold or mat gold is used alone. Such data would imply a somewhat better cohesion during compaction, as would be expected on the basis of the nature of each form of gold. Gold foil offers the maximal opportunity to reduce internal porosities owing to its inherently dense, laminated structure. Although these results are in general agreement with most investigations, others have not found such a wide difference in the physical properties of specimens compacted with the various forms of direct golds. It is likely that the differences in data from these studies are due to the particular experimental conditions present and the individual operative technique employed.

Although all three methods of condensation produce specimens that are comparable in transverse strength and density, the use of the mechanical condenser improves the hardness somewhat when mat gold and powdered gold are employed.

There is no evidence that the differences in the physical properties among the various forms of gold, including the gold-calcium alloy, or the method of compaction, as shown in Table 23–1 and in other studies,[10, 11] are clinically significant. The physical properties of the restoration are probably more greatly influenced by the competence of the operator in manipulating and placing the direct gold.

Unfortunately, the restorations made with the direct filling golds do not exhibit as much overall strength and resilience as do those made with the dental gold alloys to be discussed in the next chapter. Consequently, they cannot be used to encompass a tooth, e.g., as a cast crown, nor can they withstand masticatory stresses if used to restore a cusp. Therefore, the use of direct filling golds is generally limited to areas where they simply "fill" rather than veneer or reconstruct the tooth. Thus, they are utilized principally in the Class III or Class V restoration.

Metallography The effect of compaction upon the metallurgy and the physical properties of the direct gold can be related to the phenomena that have been discussed in previous chapters. The space lattice of pure gold is face-centered cubic. The close-packed orientation of the atoms accounts for the inherently high density of gold.

However, for several reasons the theoretical ideal of solid density is never achieved.[12] As previously explained, porosity is produced by incomplete contact between the increments of gold that lie outside the area covered by the point of the condenser. Furthermore, although slip planes make possible the malleability of the gold, strain hardening, and crystal fracture in the case of mat gold, eventually makes the structure so disorganized that further slip is impossible. Brittle fracture then results. Although the effect of strain hardening on the physical properties of gold foil has not been fully determined, measurements made on wrought gold can possibly be related to the compaction of gold foil.[13] When a specimen of wrought, annealed gold is reduced in thickness by 60 per cent, through cold work, the tensile strength increases from 134 MPa (19,000 psi) to 225 MPa (32,000 psi), the yield strength increases from practically 0 to 211 MPa (30,000 psi), and the Brinell hardness number increases from 25 to 58. The strength properties of direct filling gold can probably be influenced similarly.

The Direct Gold Restoration   There can be no doubt that a properly inserted direct gold restoration is unsurpassed from the standpoint of service. With the variety of forms of direct gold that are now available and the modern equipment for manipulating and compacting the gold, the time involved in placing the restoration has been reduced.[14] The concern of some for the possible damaging effect on the pulp by the trauma produced by the forces of compaction has been disputed.[15] Apparently direct gold compacted properly into sound tooth structure produces only a minimal pulpal response.

However, it should be emphasized that the technical skill of the dentist is of paramount importance to the success of the direct gold restoration. A direct gold restoration of poor quality can prove to be one of the most inferior of all clinical restorations.

The proper insertion of a direct gold restoration challenges the technical proficiency of the dentist as does no other type of restoration. If not able to meet this challenge, then the dentist should employ some other type of restoration.

References

1. Baum L: Tooth Filling Material. US Patent No. 3,191,303 (June 29), 1965.
2. Lund MR and Baum L: Powdered gold as a restorative material. J Prosthet Dent 13:1151, 1963.
3. Baum L: Gold foil (filling golds) in dental practice. Dent Clin North Am, March, 1965, pp. 199–212.
4. Hollenback GM and Collard EW: An evaluation of the physical properties of cohesive gold. J South Calif Dent Assoc 29:280, 1961.
5. Williams RS and Homerberg VO: Principles of Metallography. 5th ed. New York, McGraw-Hill Book Co., Inc., 1948, pp. 52 and 72.
6. Rose TK: On the annealing of gold. J Inst Metals 10:150, 1913.
7. Mahan J and Charbeneau GT: A study of certain mechanical properties and the density of condensed specimens made from various forms of pure gold. J Am Acad Gold Foil Oper 8:6, 1965.
8. Richter WA and Cantwell KR: A study of cohesive gold. J Prosthet Dent 15:722, 1965.
9. Mahler DB and Terkla LG: Analysis of stress in dental stuctures. Dent Clin North Am, pp 789–798, Nov., 1958.
10. Xhonga F: Direct golds, Part I. J Am Acad Gold Foil Oper 13:17, 1970.
11. Xhonga F: Direct golds, Part II. J Am Acad Gold Foil Oper, 14:5, 1971.
12. Hodson JT: Structure and properties of gold foil and mat gold. J Dent Res 42:575, 1963.
13. Roeser WF: Gold (99.99 + Air). *In* Lyman T: Metals Handbook. 7th ed., Metals Park, Ohio, American Society for Metals, 1954, pp. 1116–1117.
14. Desautels P: A comparative study on the physical properties of three gold restorative materials. Thesis, Indiana University, 1971.
15. Thomas JJ, Stanley HR, and Gilmore HW: Effect of gold foil condensation on human dental pulp. J Am Dent Assoc 78:788, 1969.

24 NOBLE METAL DENTAL CASTING ALLOYS

Casting is one of the most widely used methods for the fabrication of metallic restorations outside of the mouth. A pattern of the lost tooth structure or the dental appliance to be reproduced in metal is constructed in wax. The wax is surrounded by an investment which is essentially a mixture of a binder such as the α-hemihydrate of gypsum or a phosphate and silica which is mixed with water in the usual manner. After the investment has hardened, the wax is removed and the molten metal is forced into the space or mold left by the wax. The resulting structure is a remarkably accurate duplication of the pattern if proper technique is employed. A complete description of the casting procedure will be presented in the following four chapters.

Many of the technical considerations of the procedure are dependent upon a knowledge of the casting alloy itself. Therefore, it is necessary to discuss this phase of the subject before the details of the casting process are presented. According to the discussion in Chapter 19 of the oral cavity as a severe corrosion environment, it is not surprising that the metals that have been used most extensively for dental castings are noble metal alloys. In this chapter the characteristics of dental casting alloys involving the noble metals will be discussed. The base metal alloys used for this purpose are covered in Chapter 34.

History A brief description of the evolution of the present alloys is appropriate in order to understand the rationale employed in arriving at the current formulations.

The history of the noble metal dental alloys has been influenced by three major factors: the technological changes in dental prostheses, metallurgical advancements, and price changes of the metals (particularly since 1968).

In 1907, Taggart introduced the technique of cast inlay restorations.[1] He made use of the ancient lost wax process and developed an air pressure device for forcing a small amount of pure gold into the investment mold.

This inlay technique was an instant success and it soon burgeoned into the casting of complex inlays (such as MOD's), crowns, bridges, and partials. As pure gold did not have the properties essential for these types of restorations and appliances, existing jewelry alloys were quickly adopted. These were gold alloys strengthened with copper and silver. In that era the dental profession, not so concerned with precious metal value, also found that platinum was a potent strengthener. In 1932 the dental materials group at the National

Table 24–1. *Classification of Casting Gold Alloys*

Type	Gold and Platinum Group Metals (Minimum %)	VHN* (Softened)	
I (Soft)	83	50	90
II (Medium)	78	90	120
III (Hard)	78	120	150
IV (Extra hard)	75	150	...

*Vickers Hardness Number.

Bureau of Standards surveyed the alloys that had begun to emerge and roughly classified them as seen in Table 24–1.

What is interesting about these first dental golds is that gold and platinum were considered the only noble metals that could provide chemical stability in the oral environment. If these same alloys were tested today, using present standards to predict tarnish resistance, they would be found to tarnish rather badly. At that time some tarnish tests were conducted and the results suggested that alloys with a gold content below 65 to 75 per cent tarnished too readily for dental usage.[2] In fact, it was recommended that a standard for tarnish resistance should be established. Thus dentists must have been experiencing tarnish problems.

Subsequently, several patents were issued for dental gold alloys that contained palladium as a substitute for platinum.[3, 4] One of those also included indium in the composition.[3] The predominance of the palladium produced a white alloy. Since the price of palladium at that time was higher than that of gold, these alloys did not appear on the market as dental alloys.

However, by 1948, there appeared the listing of the compositions of dental noble metal alloys shown in Table 24–2. With these alloys, the tarnishing tendency of the original platinum-containing alloys had apparently disappeared. Today we know why. In gold alloys palladium is a specific for making silver non-tarnishing. These alloys then became the mainstay of the dental alloys of that day.

In the late 1950's, a technological breakthrough occurred in dental technique that was to dramatically change the fabrication of dental prostheses.[5] This was an invention that covered a method for obtaining a compatible combination of a dental alloy and dental porcelain. As dental porcelain had a distinctly lower coefficient of thermal expansion than gold alloys, it had not been possible to secure a bond between the two. Soda and potash were added to raise the coefficient of the porcelain but that was not enough. However, by adding platinum and palladium to the gold, the coefficient of the alloy was lowered to just the right amount for compatibility. By serendipity the melting

Table 24–2. *Composition Limits of Dental Casting Gold Alloys (Gold Color)* *

Type	Gold (%)	Silver (%)	Copper (%)	Palladium (%)	Platinum (%)	Zinc (%)
A	79–92.5	3–12	2–4.5	0–0.5	0–0.5	0–0.5
B	75–78	12–14.5	7–10	1–4	0–1	0.5
C	62–78	8–26	8–11	2–4	0–3	1
D	60–71.5	4.5–20	11–16	0–5	0–3.5	1–2

*Metals Handbook, 1948 edition.

range of the alloy was raised sufficiently to permit firing of the porcelain onto the gold alloy at 1030° C (1900° F).

The metal-porcelain restoration that now became possible through this development will be covered in detail in Chapter 31. However, a brief description of it will be useful to the student at this time, since the following discussion will include the noble metal alloys used for this purpose.

Metal-Ceramics The chief objection to the use of porcelain as a restorative material, either in prosthetic or crown and bridge procedures, is its lack of strength, particularly tensile and shear strength. Although it can resist compressive stress with reasonable success, the necessary design factors usually do not permit shapes in which the compressive stress is the principal force.

A method by which this disadvantage may be minimized is to fuse the porcelain directly to a cast alloy crown shell that fits the prepared tooth. If a strong bond is effected between the porcelain veneer and the metal, and with proper design and physical properties of the porcelain and metal, the porcelain is reinforced so that brittle fracture can be avoided or, at least, minimized. This is often referred to as a *porcelain fused to metal* restoration. A more proper term is a *metal-ceramic* restoration. Alloys to be used for this application will be referred to as metal-ceramic alloys.

When porcelains or glasses are used in this manner, they are called *ceramic enamels,* although the distinction is more or less arbitrary. The technique, in brief, is as follows: a thin metal "thimble" for the veneered crown, pontic, or other structure, is cast essentially as described in Chapters 27 and 28. The porcelain or enamel is then fused as a veneer over the metal crown. First a layer of opaque porcelain is fused onto the casting, and then the tooth contour is built up by fusing an overlay of translucent "enamel" porcelain. The final veneered structure is then cemented on the prepared tooth as usual.

Commercially, such an enameling process is very old. Enameled pans and cooking utensils with the enamel baked on steel or other metals have been in use for many years. Enameled bathtubs, water tanks, metal "tiles," and many other applications of ceramic enamels are common in modern life. The rationale and technique for such uses of ceramic enamels are very similar to their dental applications.

Now let us return to the alloy whose development made the metal-ceramic restoration a reality. It contained 88 per cent gold, but was much too soft for stress-bearing restorations such as bridges. Also, since there was no evidence that any chemical bond existed between the metal and ceramic, mechanical retention and undercuts were advocated to avoid porcelain separation.

At this time a stress bond test was developed in which the stress was concentrated at the interface.[6] Using this test it was found that when porcelain was baked to this new alloy, the bond strength was less than the cohesive strength of the porcelain. This meant that if failure occurred in the metal-ceramic restoration, it would most likely occur at the interface. By adding less than 1 per cent of such oxide forming elements as iron, indium, and tin to the alloy the bond strength was improved by a factor of 3.

This 1 per cent addition of base metals to the gold, palladium, and platinum alloy was all that was needed to obtain a slight oxide film on the surface of the metal in order to achieve a bond strength superior to the strength of the porcelain itself. This type of alloy then became the standard for the metal-ceramic restoration. In time, base metal alloys (Chapter 34) were also developed for this purpose.

MODERN NOBLE METAL ALLOYS

Grain Refined Alloys   Perhaps the true era of the modern noble metal alloys began with the improvement made in refining the grain size from approximately 150 μm down to 50 μm.

Figure 24–1 shows two etched full crown castings still attached to the sprue. The difference in grain size between the coarse grain alloy (approximately 300 μm) and the fine grain alloy (approximately 60 μm) is easily seen. Methods of controlling grain size were previously discussed in Chapters 15 and 17.

Iridium proved to be a particularly powerful grain refiner, requiring only 20 to 50 ppm to initiate grain refining.[7] The importance of this refining was far reaching. It raised the yield strength and, somewhat paradoxically, also the elongation. It reduced the large dendrites of the coarse grain structure to produce a more homogeneous casting having better tarnish resistance. Also, production lots of the alloy varied less in properties from melt to melt. Fine grain dental alloys have become universal.

Lower Gold Content Alloys   Simultaneously, different alloy manufacturers began to increase the palladium content of the 99 per cent noble metal-ceramic alloy for two reasons: a significant palladium increase gave a much stiffer and stronger alloy and it lowered the density of the alloy, yielding more cast dental units per ounce of metal.[8, 9] The gold color disappeared with such alloying but this was no longer important in the metal-ceramic technique. Shortly after this alloy was introduced, gold in the United States was placed on the free market and after a slow rise began to climb rapidly in price, well above the price of palladium. The new white metal-ceramic alloys, containing as much as 35 per cent palladium, became attractive not only for their increased strength but also for their lower cost. There was one minor but insidious problem, those alloys containing appreciable amounts of silver tended to tinge the porcelain veneer green at the edges.

Also, just prior to the gold price climb, a crown and bridge yellow gold alloy was developed with markedly reduced gold content as compared with conventional dental golds.[10] This alloy was the result of research to determine

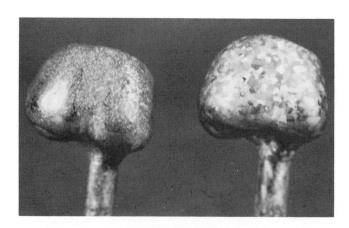

Figure 24–1 Two etched full crown castings. The larger grain size of the alloy on the right is evident. (Courtesy of J. Tuccillo.)

the lower limit of gold content necessary for tarnish resistant dental alloys. This research produced two discoveries.

1. Palladium was specific in rendering the silver in gold alloys tarnish resistant. It had been determined that silver rather than the copper induced tarnish in the oral cavity in the customary dental golds. For the low gold compositions, about 1 per cent palladium was needed for every 3 per cent silver to offset the tarnish propensity of the silver. It is now clear why palladium was creeping into the dental golds, as indicated by the 1948 ASM Handbook (Table 24–2).

2. The silver-copper ratio had to be carefully balanced to yield a low silver-rich phase in the microstructure.[11] The new alloy contained as low as 42 per cent gold, with 25 per cent silver and 9 per cent palladium. This alloy was tested in vitro and in a clinical study and was found to tarnish less than a 75 per cent gold alloy containing no palladium.[12] This resulted in numerous alloys being introduced into the market in the low gold range of 42 to 50 per cent.

By 1978 the price of gold began to climb so rapidly that a severe requirement was imposed on the noble metal dental alloys — to reduce the precious metal content to a minimum yet still retain the advantages of the noble metals for dental use. Thus a new set of alloys came to the forefront in dental usage, as will be discussed.

The Noble Metals   As has been pointed out, the noble metals have traditionally been the basis for the inlay alloys and crown and bridge alloys by virtue of their chemical stability in the oral cavity. The term noble metal is somewhat relative. As seen in Chapter 19, the lower the position of a metal in the standard EMF series, the more active is the metal, i.e., the higher a metal is in the series, the more inert it is, and hence the greater is its nobility. Table 15–1, the periodic table of the elements, indicates the metals that are usually considered to be noble. These are gold, platinum, the platinum group metals (palladium, rhodium, ruthenium, iridium, and osmium), and silver.

The Precious Metals   The eight elements above also compose the so-called precious metals, a term that might be considered definitive and official, in that these eight metals are so defined by the major metallurgical societies and the federal government agencies, e.g., the National Bureau of Standards and the National Materials Advisory Board. Of these eight elements, four are currently of major importance in dental casting: gold, palladium, platinum, and silver. The first three are inert in the oral cavity. Silver, provided that it is alloyed with substantial amounts of palladium, also resists corrosion. Iridium and ruthenium might be mentioned as having a minor role as trace elements for grain refining gold and palladium-based dental alloys.

A chart of some of the fundamental properties of the four major noble metals is given in Table 24–3.

These four noble metals have a face-centered cubic crystal structure. All are white except gold, which has the well known yellow "gold" color. Silver is sometimes described as the "whitest" of the metals. Gold and silver are relatively low in melting point and elastic modulus, whereas palladium and platinum are relatively high in these properties. Those properties play an important functional role in dental alloys. For example, gold and silver based alloys are preferred because of their ease in melting and casting. The thermal expansion coefficient tends to follow the reciprocal relationship, i.e., the higher the melting point, the lower the coefficient. The metal-ceramic alloys make effective use of this property, as has been seen.

Table 24–3. *Some Fundamental Properties of Four Noble Metals Used in Dentistry*

	SILVER	GOLD	PALLADIUM	PLATINUM
Density gm/cc	10.40	19.3	12.02	21.45
Melting point °C (°F)	961 (1761)	1063 (1945)	1552 (2826)	1769 (3217)
Therm. exp. coef. $\times 10^{-6}/°C$ $(10^{-6}/°F)$	19.7 (10.9)	14.2 (7.9)	11.1 (6.2)	8.9 (4.9)
Young's modulus MPa $(10^6$ psi)	71,000 (10.3)	80,000 (11.6)	112,400 (16.3)	147,000 (21.3)

Karat and Fineness Traditionally, the gold content of a dental alloy has been specified according to its *karat* or *fineness*. The karat of an alloy is the parts of pure gold in the alloy in 24 parts of alloy. For example, 24 karat gold is pure gold; 22 karat gold is an alloy containing 22 parts pure gold with the remaining 2 parts composed of other metals. Similarly, 18 karat gold consists of 18 parts pure gold in 24 parts; and so on.

A more practical rating is by the fineness of the alloy. The fineness of a gold alloy is the parts per thousand of pure gold. Pure gold is 1000 fine. Thus, if three-fourths of the alloy is pure gold, it is said to be 750 fine. The fineness rating is 10 times the percentage gold composition of the alloy.

The use of both karat and fineness for the gold content is decreasing in favor of the percentage composition. Since 1977 it has been an American Dental Association requirement for the dental alloy manufacturers to specify the percentage gold, palladium, and platinum content on all packets containing dental alloy. Noble metal alloys are usually packaged and priced in 1, 2, and 20 dwt* lots.

Material Cost Per Dental Unit Increases and fluctuations in the free market prices of precious metals have generated considerable concern about the cost per pennyweight of different alternative alloy systems. However, it should be emphasized that in evaluating the cost of different alloys for a specific dental appliance the invariant quantity is the total volume of the dental casting. Differences in alloy properties may allow for slight changes in design for a given application, but, in general, the volume of a casting is fixed irrespective of the choice of alloy.

The net materials cost in a dental casting is calculated by multiplying the volume by the density of the alloy by the cost of the alloy per unit weight. Thus the role of alloy density is equal to that of alloy cost per unit weight in determining the materials cost in a particular dental casting.

Referring to Table 24–3, the densities of palladium and silver are approximately half those of gold and platinum. Alloys containing appreciable amounts of palladium and silver offer a double advantage over high gold and platinum alloys if materials cost is the principal concern.

Nomenclature Reference was made in Table 24–1 to Types I to IV dental alloys and in the history section to yellow golds, white golds, low golds, etc. The

*1 dwt is a pennyweight = 1/20th troy oz, = 1.555 grams.

following is the current nomenclature practice for the noble metal dental alloys.

Types by Function   In 1927 the Bureau of Standards established gold casting alloys Types I through IV according to dental function, with hardness increasing from Type I to Type IV.[13] In 1960 the metal-ceramic alloys emerged; thus the following categories can now be defined:

Type I (soft) — small inlays — easily burnished and subject to very slight stress.

Type II (medium) — inlays subject to moderate stress; thick ¾ crowns, abutments, pontics, full crowns, and sometimes soft saddles.

Type III (hard) — inlays subject to high stress; thin ¾ crowns, thin cast backings, abutments, pontics, full crowns and saddles, short span bridges. Type III alloys usually can be age hardened.

Type IV (extra hard) — inlays subject to very high stresses, saddle bars and clasps, partial frameworks, and long span bridges. (Full crowns are often made of this type.) These alloys can be age hardened by an appropriate heat treatment.

Metal-Ceramic (hard and extra hard) — Compatible for veneering with dental porcelain, copings, thin-walled crowns, short span bridges with the hard type, long span bridges with the extra hard type.

Types by Alloy Description   There has been psychological preference for the yellow color over white metal for dental prostheses where metal is exposed. However, with the wide acceptance of acrylic and porcelain veneers, little metal is customarily visible in modern dental restorations. So the yellow color is no longer as important. With the sharp rise in the price of gold, there has been a notable trend toward the white dental alloys.

The *white golds* are alloys that are predominantly gold in composition, but are whitened with palladium, or palladium and silver. *Low golds* are crown and bridge alloys with gold content below the Type III and Type IV compositions. Yellow-colored alloys as low as 42 per cent gold have been used successfully as dental alloys. White precious metal alloys are usually palladium-dominant alloys. Palladium-silver alloys are, as the name implies, palladium-silver based, with or without a small gold content. These are frequently termed "semi-precious" alloys. This term is confusing. There is no accepted dividing line in terms of composition that delineates "precious" from "semi-precious" alloys. In general the term semi-precious alloy should be avoided.

A list of these subcategories can be summarized as follows:

Color and principal element (or elements) —

Yellow golds — yellow colored by virtue of gold present, greater than 60 per cent gold content.

White golds — white colored but with more than 50 per cent gold content.

Low golds or economy golds — usually yellow colored but with gold content below 60 per cent, and generally in the 42–55 per cent range.

Silver-palladium — white colored, predominantly silver in composition but with substantial amounts of palladium to provide nobility and render the silver tarnish resistant. May or may not contain small amounts of gold. Casting temperatures are in the range of the yellow gold alloys.

Palladium-silver — white colored palladium-based metal-ceramic alloy. Softening temperatures are high enough to permit the fusing of porcelain.

Thus in dental practice one is apt to refer to a "yellow gold Type II alloy," "low gold Type III," or "metal-ceramic white gold," etc. Types I and II are frequently referred to as inlay golds, with Type II for the inlays subject to extra stress. Development of modern direct filling materials has considerably reduced the use of Type I and II alloys. There is a tendency to lump the Type III and IV alloys together, simply calling them crown and bridge alloys, recognizing that Type IV alloy is used for the more demanding crown and bridge prostheses that are subject to conditions of higher stress.

Composition and Properties of the Modern Noble Metal Alloys

The three factors that primarily influenced the development of the noble metal dental alloys were described in the history section of this chapter. The pressure of the increasing precious metal prices was the most recent factor dominating these developments, yielding the current alloys.

Composition, General Features   In Table 24–4 can be seen a listing of 11 alloys that could be considered representative of the modern dental alloys. These representative alloys do not, of course, exhaust the alloy varieties that are available, but they are by far the most popular. Different manufacturers have alloys that vary somewhat in gold, copper, silver, platinum, and palladium content. However, the major differences occur in the minor additions, and these details are usually proprietary.

Of the minor additions, indicated in Table 24–4, zinc is added primarily as an oxygen scavenger. The presence of silver in an alloy, without the addition of a small amount of zinc, causes absorption of oxygen from the atmosphere during melting; the oxygen is then rejected during solidification, thus tending to produce gas porosity in the casting.

Indium, tin, and iron are additions that harden the metal-ceramic gold-palladium alloys, iron being the most effective (especially when platinum is also present). Gallium is added principally to compensate for the decreased thermal expansion coefficient that results from making the metal-ceramic alloys silver-free. The elimination of silver from these alloys markedly decreases the propensity for the green stain at the margins of the metal-porcelain interface.

It should be mentioned that all modern noble dental alloys are generally fine grain. This is accomplished by additions of very small quantities of

Table 24–4. *Typical Compositions of Some Modern Noble Metal Dental Alloys*

		Per Cent Au	Per Cent Cu	Per Cent Ag	Per Cent Pd	(In, Sn, Fe, Zn, Ga)
Type I	(yellow gold)	83	6	10	0.5	Bal.
Type II	(yellow gold)	77	7	14	1	"
Type III	(yellow gold)	75	9	11	3.5	"
Type III	(low gold)	46	8	39	6	"
Type III	(silver-palladium)			70	25	"
Type IV	(yellow-gold)	69	10	12.5	3.5(+3.0 Pt)	"
Type IV	(low gold)	56	14	25	4	"
Type IV	(silver-palladium)	15	14	45	25	"
Metal-ceramic (white gold)		52			38	"
Metal-ceramic (palladium-silver)				30	60	"
Metal-ceramic (yellow gold)		88		1	6.5(+4.0 Pt)	"

iridium, ruthenium, or rhenium (about 100–150 ppm), as has been discussed.

Gold, silver, and palladium are all soluble in each other in the solid state, and all are face-centered cubic; therefore, the alloys are all face-centered cubic. Copper is also face-centered cubic but, as noted in Chapter 17, it induces an intermediate ordered face-centered tetragonal phase with gold or palladium, and with silver it has quite limited solubility in the solid state. Thus copper is the principal hardener. Copper in excessive amounts tends to redden the yellow alloys and reduces resistance to tarnish and corrosion. Silver helps to minimize the reddening effect of copper.

Palladium has been substituted extensively for platinum in most of the yellow gold Types I to IV alloys. It serves to harden the alloy but also whitens it. It raises the fusion temperature if appreciable amounts are added. The introduction of palladium as a major alloy component has made possible alternative noble metal casting alloys with substantially reduced materials cost per unit casting, as has already been noted.

In Table 24–4 it can be seen that the Types I and II alloys differ very little from the original ones published by the Bureau of Standards (Table 24–1), except that there is some palladium present to render the silver tarnish resistant.

The Types III and IV *yellow gold* alloys in Table 24–4 are conventional American Dental Association type high gold alloys whose compositions probably date back to the 1940's. Although the use of these alloys is decreasing as a result of economic pressures, their use is still significant. More importantly, these alloys have been developed and tested over a long time interval. Their handling characteristics and clinical performances are well established. Thus they serve as a benchmark against which the characteristics and performance of the more recently developed alternative alloy systems can, and should, be compared. Hence their inclusion in Table 24–4 is warranted even though they are not actually new developments.

A major difference between the Type II silver-palladium white alloys and the Type IV silver-palladium white alloys is that the latter can be significantly age hardened by heat treating because of its gold and copper content. This alloy is one of the few cases in dental metallurgy where gold is added not so much for its nobility and color but for its age hardening effect.

Note that the metal ceramic alloys do not contain copper owing to its strong tendency to "green" the porcelain. The absence of copper means that other strengthening mechanisms have to be developed and that these alloys are not, in general, age hardenable, as will be discussed later.

Physical Properties   Table 24–5 gives the more important physical properties of the set of alloys shown in Table 24–4. Similar listings of properties are generally available for the alloys of any particular manufacturer.

The melting range sets the basis for the casting temperature. The upper limit of the range is the liquidus. To this should be added 75 to 150° C (150–300° F) in order to obtain the proper casting temperature. The lower limit of the melting range can similarly be used to estimate maximum soldering temperatures.

The metal-ceramic alloys must have a high melting range so that the metal is solid well above the porcelain baking temperature to minimize distortion (*sag*) of the casting during porcelain application. On the other hand,

Table 24–5.   *Physical Properties of Some Modern Noble Metal Dental Alloys*

		MELTING RANGE	DENSITY (gm/cc)	YIELD STRENGTH MPa	YIELD STRENGTH (psi)	HARDNESS (VHN)	PER CENT ELONGATION
Type I	(yellow gold)	943–960° C (1730–1760° F)	16.6	103	(15,000)	80	36
Type II	(yellow gold)	924–960° C (1695–1760° F)	15.9	186	(27,000)	101	38
Type III	(yellow gold)	932–960° C (1710–1760° F)	15.5	207 H275	(30,000) (H40,000)	121 H182	39 H19
Type III	(low gold)	843–916° C (1550–1680° F)	12.8	241 H586	(35,000) (H85,000)	138 H231	30 H13
Type III	(silver-palladium)	1021–1099° C (1870–2010° F)	10.6	262 H323	(38,000) (H47,000)	143 H154	10 H 8
Type IV	(yellow gold)	921–943° C (1690–1720° F)	15.2	275 H493	(40,000) (H71,500)	149 H264	35 H 7
Type IV	(low gold)	871–932° C (1600–1710° F)	13.6	372 H720	(54,000) (H104,500)	186 H254	38 H 2
Type IV	(silver-palladium)	930–1021° C (1705–1870° F)	11.3	434 H586	(63,000) (H85,000)	180 H270	10 H 6
Metal-ceramic (white gold)		1271–1304° C (2320–2380° F)	13.5	572	(83,000)	220	20
Metal-ceramic (palladium-silver)		1232–1304° C (2250–2380° F)	10.7	462	(67,000)	189	20
Metal-ceramic (yellow gold)		1149–1177° C (2100–2150° F)	18.3	450	(65,300)	182	5

H = Age hardened condition. Other values are for the quenched (softened) condition.

the Types I to IV alloys must have considerably lower fusion temperatures if they are to be cast with conventional equipment and if gypsum investments are used. The width of the melting range is also of interest. As was pointed out in Chapter 17, the wider the melting range, the greater is the tendency for coring during solidification.

The density (gm/cc), or rather, the reciprocal of this, called the specific volume (cc/gm), is an indication of the number of average dental units that can be cast from a unit weight of the metal. The ratio of the extreme densities in the table, for example from 10.7 to 18.3 for the metal-ceramic alloys, indicates that more equivalent castings can be cast from the lower density alloy than from the one with higher density (in this example, 70 per cent more). Such wide density variations may influence casting techniques, especially if centrifugal type casting machines are used, as will be seen in subsequent chapters.

Before considering the other properties listed in Table 24–5, some consideration needs to be given to the effects of heat treatment on the noble metal alloys.

Heat Treatment of Noble Metal Alloys   As previously discussed in Chapters 17 and 18, gold alloys can be significantly hardened if the alloy contains a sufficient amount of copper. Types I and II alloys usually do not harden, or harden to a lesser degree than do the Types III and IV alloys. The actual mechanism of hardening is probably the result of several different solid-solid transformations. Although the precise mechanism may be in doubt, the criteria for successful hardening are not: they are time and temperature.

Alloys that can be hardened can, of course, also be softened. In metallurgical terminology the *softening heat treatment* is referred to as solution heat treatment. The *hardening heat treatment* is termed age hardening.

Softening Heat Treatment   The casting is placed in an electric furnace for 10 minutes at a temperature of 700° C (1292° F), and then it is quenched in water. During this period, all intermediate phases are presumably changed to a disordered solid solution, and the rapid quenching prevents ordering from occurring during cooling. The tensile strength, proportional limit, and hardness are reduced by such a treatment, but the ductility is increased.

The softening heat treatment is indicated for structures that are to be ground, shaped, or otherwise cold worked, either in or out of the mouth.

While 700° C is a good average softening temperature, each alloy has its optimum temperature, and the manufacturer should specify the most favorable temperature and time.

Hardening Heat Treatment   The age hardening or hardening heat treatment of dental alloys can be accomplished in several ways.

One of the most practical hardening treatments is by "soaking" or aging the casting at a specific temperature for a definite time, usually 15 to 30 minutes, before it is water quenched. The aging temperature depends on the alloy composition but is generally between 200° C (400° F) and 450° C (840° F). The proper time and temperature are specified by the manufacturer.

Ideally, before the alloy is given an age hardening treatment, it should be subjected to a softening heat treatment to relieve all strain hardening, if present, and to start the hardening treatment with the alloy as a disordered solid solution. Otherwise, there would not be a proper control of the hardening process, since the increase in strength, proportional limit, and hardness and the reduction in ductility are controlled by the amount of solid-solid transformations allowed. The transformations, in turn, are controlled by the temperature and time of the age hardening treatment.

Because the proportional limit is increased during age hardening, a considerable increase in the modulus of resilience can be expected. The hardening heat treatment is indicated for metallic partial dentures, saddles, bridges, and other similar structures. For small structures, such as inlays, a hardening treatment is not usually employed.

Returning to Table 24–5, pairs of mechanical property values appear for the Type III and Type IV alloys. Those values tagged with an "H" refer to the age hardened condition. The corresponding value in each pair is for the quenched, softened, single phase state. Pairs of values are not given for the Type I, Type II, and metal-ceramic alloys, since these are not significantly age hardenable.

The *yield strength,* the proportional limit, and the elastic limit are all measures of essentially the same property, as was seen in Chapter 3. This property reflects the capacity of an alloy (and hence the cast prosthesis) to withstand mechanical stresses without permanent deformation. In general, the yield strengths increase when progressing from Type I to Type IV alloys. Age hardening substantially increases the yield strength (in one case by nearly 100 per cent).

The *hardness* values for noble metal alloys correlate quite well with the yield strengths. Traditionally, hardness has been used for indicating the suitability of an alloy for a given type of clinical application.

The *elongation* is a measure of ductility or the degree of plastic deformation an alloy can undergo prior to fracture. A reasonable amount of elongation is essential if the clinical application will require deformation of the "as cast" structure (i.e., clasp and margin adjustment and burnishing). Age hardening reduces the elongation, in some cases very significantly. Alloys with low elongation are brittle materials and fracture readily if deformed.

One property not included in Table 24–5 is the ultimate tensile strength. Manufacturers often stress this property; however, it has little clinical significance. From a practical point of view, a cast prosthesis that has undergone plastic deformation in service has failed whether or not actual fracture has occurred.

Functional Characteristics   The following are important functional characteristics for dental casting alloys.

Stiffness. It will be recalled that stiffness is the resistance to elastic deformation and is determined by the elastic modulus. This property is quite important in applications such as long span bridges and partial denture frameworks. The palladium-based alloys have higher stiffness than do the gold-based alloys.

Resilience — the capacity to absorb mechanical energy without plastic deformation. For the metal-ceramic alloys, it is important that the deflection under stress be small, thereby acting to support the brittle porcelain veneer. As was stated in Chapter 2, the modulus of resilience is given by the square of the yield strength divided by twice the elastic modulus.

Compatibility to porcelain — the elastic modulus, thermal expansion coefficient, and heat conductivity are properties that contribute to porcelain compatibility, but in a rather complex manner. The metal must form surface oxides to allow bonding to occur, as was noted. However, components of the alloy must not discolor the porcelain.

Tarnish resistance is a fundamental requirement of all dental alloys. The metal must not dissolve in the mouth fluids or liberate toxic corrosion products. Allowing for some passivating effect, the metal must arrive at an inert state and maintain that condition.

Fatigue resistance is the ability of a metal to withstand repeated deformation in the elastic region. It can be measured only by cyclical stress tests. Testing should be done in mouth fluid conditions because fatigue failure differs for different corrosive environments, as pointed out in Chapter 19.

Sag resistance is the ability of a dental alloy to resist plastic and creep flow under its own weight during porcelain firing and soldering.

Fit is the ability of a casting to faithfully reproduce the pattern from which it is constructed. It is especially important with large fixed prostheses. Both the metal and the casting conditions are involved. One of the biggest alloy related factors which influence fit is casting shrinkage.

Casting Shrinkage. As noted in a previous chapter, most metals and alloys, including gold and the noble metal alloys, shrink when they change from the liquid to the solid state.

Such a consideration is of importance in the dental casting procedure. For example, if a mold for an inlay is an accurate reproduction of the missing tooth structure, the gold inlay after casting is too small by the amount of its casting shrinkage.

The shrinkage occurs in three stages: (1) the thermal contraction of the liquid metal between the temperature to which it is heated and the liquidus temperature; (2) the contraction of the metal inherent in its change from the liquid to the solid state; and (3) the thermal contraction of the solid metal which occurs down to room temperature.

The first-mentioned contraction is probably of no consequence, because as

Table 24–6. *Percentage Linear Thermal Contraction of Gold Alloys and Gold from Their Melting Points (Solidi)* *

METAL	THERMAL CONTRACTION FROM MELTING POINT TO 25°C (77°F) (%)
Gold (100%)	1.76
Gold (90%), silver (10%)	2.03
Gold (90%), copper (10%)	1.62
Gold (90%), nickel (10%)	1.91

*From Coleman, *National Bureau of Standards Research Paper No. 32.*

the liquid metal contracts in the mold, more molten metal can flow into the mold to compensate for such a shrinkage. The casting technique, to be described in subsequent chapters, allows for such a flow of molten metal.

The thermal contraction of a number of dental alloys and gold has been measured, and the results are presented in Table 24–6.

A determination[14] of the casting shrinkage of smooth, cylindrical castings, 6.35 mm (¼ in) in diameter and 25.4 mm (1 in) in length, resulted in the values given in Table 24–7. The last three alloys listed were typical casting gold alloys with compositions in the range given in Table 24–2.

The values for the casting shrinkage differ for the various alloys, presumably because of differences in their composition. It has been shown, for example, that platinum, palladium, and copper are all effective in reducing the casting shrinkage of an alloy. It is of interest that the value for the casting shrinkage of pure gold (Table 24–7) closely approaches that of its maximal linear thermal contraction (Table 24–6).

In general, it is apparent that the values obtained for the casting shrinkage are less than the linear thermal shrinkage values given in Table 24–6, even though the casting shrinkages as obtained included both the solidification shrinkage and the thermal shrinkage.

This seemingly anomalous condition can be accounted for by two logical assumptions: (1) When the mold becomes filled with molten metal, the metal starts to solidify at the walls of the mold because the temperature of the mold is less than that of the molten metal. (2) During the initial cooling, the first layer of metal to solidify against the walls of the mold is weak, and it tends to adhere to the mold until it gains sufficient strength as it cools to pull away. When it is sufficiently strong to contract independently of the mold, it shrinks thermally until it reaches room temperature.

The important consideration is that the thermal shrinkage of the first weak, solidified layer is initially prevented by its mechanical adhesion to the walls of the mold. During this period, it is actually stretched because of its

Table 24–7. *Linear Casting Shrinkage of Inlay Casting Gold Alloys*

METAL	CASTING SHRINKAGE (%)
Gold (100%)	1.67
22-karat alloy*	1.50
Type I	1.56
Type II	1.37
Type III	1.42

*Approximate composition: gold, 91.6%; silver, 4.2%; copper, 4.2%.

interlocking with the investment material. Thus, any contraction occurring during solidification can be eliminated. Also, part of the total thermal contraction can be eliminated, with the result that the observed casting shrinkage is less than might be expected on the basis of the possible stages of the shrinkage.

Because the thermal contraction as the alloy cools to room temperature dominates the casting shrinkage, the higher melting alloys will tend to exhibit greater shrinkage. This must be compensated for in the casting technique if good fit is to be obtained.

Working Characteristics

Ease of casting — the alloy must be easily melted in current casting machines, with a minimum of slag formation on the melt. Most precious metals satisfy this requirement. Also, the liquid metal must possess sufficient fluidity to rapidly fill the mold.

Ease of soldering — most noble metal alloys pass this test well. The liquid solder must wet the alloy surface readily and form a true adhesive bond. The metal-ceramic alloys can be soldered at two steps in the porcelain technique: presoldering, before, and postsoldering, after the porcelain has been applied. It is an important feature of the noble metal dental alloys that both soldering techniques work well.

Ease of burnishability — an important requirement of inlays and crowns is that the margins can be manipulated with the dentist's burnishing tool. One measure of burnishability is the elongation value divided by the hardness or yield strength. Precious metals with high gold or high palladium content generally exhibit this characteristic.

Recycling Noble Metal Casting Alloys As will be seen in subsequent chapters, there is always surplus metal that is detached from the casting during the process of finishing the casting before placement in the mouth. Owing to the intrinsic value of the previous metals contained in the alloy, the net materials cost of the casting can be substantially reduced if such scrap can be recycled. One obvious alternative is to collect such scrap and return it to the alloy supplier for credit.

However, the noble metal casting alloys are sufficiently stable that they can be recast two or three times without appreciable changes in composition. The only elements likely to be lost are the more volatile base metals, such as zinc, indium, and the iron in metal-ceramic alloys.[15] This assumes that the alloy is not abused by substantial overheating. Compositional losses can be remedied by the addition of at least equal amounts of new alloy to the scrap when recasting. Alloy scrap should be carefully cleaned and foreign material removed before reuse.

Because of the large number of different alloy types and variations in composition among different alloy manufacturers, it should be obvious that alloy scrap should be segregated by type and manufacturer if it is to be recast. Indiscriminate combining of any alloy scrap results in an alloy of unknown composition and properties and is definitely contraindicated.

References

1. Taggart WH: A new and accurate method of making gold inlays. Dent Cosmos 49:1117, 1907.

2. Souder W: Standards for dental materials. J Am Dent Assoc 22:1873, 1935.
3. U.S. Patent No. 1,987,451, NO Taylor, 1935.
4. U.S. Patent No. 2,050,077, EM Wise, 1936.
5. U.S. Patent Nos. 3,052,982 and 3,052,983, M Weinstein, A Weinstein, and S Katz, 1962.
6. Shell JS and Nielsen JP: Study of the bond between gold alloys and porcelain. J Dent Res 41:1424, 1962.
7. Nielsen JP and Tuccillo JJ: Grain size in cast gold alloys. J Dent Res 45:964, 1963.
8. U.S. Patent No. 3,819,366, M Katz, 1974.
9. U.S. Patent Nos. 3,961,420 and 3,981,723, JJ Tuccillo, 1976.
10. U.S. Patent Nos. 3,424,577 and 3,767,391, JJ Tuccillo and JP Nielsen, 1969 and 1973.
11. Tuccillo JJ and Nielsen JP: Observations of the onset of sulfide tarnish on gold base alloys. J Prosthet Dent 25:629, 1971.
12. Burse AB, Swartz ML, Phillips RW, and Dykema RW: Comparison of the in vivo and in vitro tarnish of three gold alloys. J Biomed Mater Res 6:267, 1972.
13. Coleman RL Jr: Physical properties of dental materials. IV. Cast-gold alloys. Dent Cosmos 69:1007, 1927.
14. Hollenback GM and Skinner, EW: Shrinkage during casting of gold and gold alloys J Am Dent Assoc 33:1391, 1946.
15. Tuccillo JJ, Liehtenberger H, and Nielsen JP: Composition stability of gold base dental alloys for different melting techniques. J Dent Res 53:1127, 1974.

25 INLAY CASTING WAX

The first procedure in the casting of an inlay or crown is the preparation of a wax pattern. The cavity is prepared in the tooth and the pattern is carved, either directly in the tooth or on a die that is a reproduction of the tooth and the prepared cavity. If the pattern is made in the tooth itself, it is said to be prepared by the *direct technique*. If it is prepared on a die, the procedure is called the *indirect technique*. There are modifications of the techniques, but these two classifications are sufficient for the present purpose.

American Dental Association Specification no. 4 divides dental inlay casting waxes into three types: Type A, a hard or low-flow wax that is rarely used except in some indirect techniques; Type B, a medium wax employed in direct techniques; and Type C, a soft wax used for indirect techniques for construction of inlays and crowns. Somewhat different properties are required for the various types, as will be discussed.

However the pattern is prepared, it should be an accurate reproduction of the missing tooth structure. The wax pattern forms the outline of the mold into which the gold alloy is cast. Consequently, the casting can be no more accurate than the wax pattern, regardless of the care observed in subsequent procedures. Therefore, the pattern should be well adapted to the prepared cavity, properly carved, and the distortion minimized. After the pattern is removed from the prepared cavity, it is surrounded by a gypsum-containing, or other type, material known as *investment*. This process is called *investing the pattern*. Investments and investing procedures are discussed in Chapters 26 and 27.

Wax patterns are used in the casting of many complex restorations other than inlays and crowns, but the present discussion will be limited to the construction of restorations employed in operative dentistry.

Composition A number of formulas for inlay wax have been published, some of which are quite complex. The essential ingredients of a successful inlay wax are paraffin wax, gum dammar, and carnauba wax, with some coloring material. All of these substances are of natural origin, derived from mineral or vegetable sources.

Paraffin wax is generally the main ingredient, usually in a concentration of 40 to 60 per cent. Paraffin is derived from the high-boiling fractions of petroleum. It is composed mainly of a complex mixture of hydrocarbons of the methane series, together with a minor amount of amorphous or microcrystalline phases. The wax can be obtained in a wide melting or softening range, depending upon the molecular weight and distribution of the constituents. The melting range can be determined by a time-temperature cooling curve as shown in Figure 25–1 for an inlay paraffin wax. The time-temperature relationship during cooling indicates the successive solidification of progressively lower molecular weight fractions. Such a condition is desirable from a dental standpoint because it imparts a moldability to the wax below its temperature of liquefaction. Since paraffin can be obtained with almost any desired melting point, it is evident that the paraffin used for Type B waxes will have a higher melting point than will the paraffin used for Type C waxes.

Unfortunately, the paraffin wax is likely to flake when it is trimmed, and it does not present a smooth, glossy surface, which is a desirable requisite for an inlay wax. Consequently, other waxes and natural resins are added as modifying agents.

Gum dammar, or dammar resin, is a natural resin derived from a certain variety of pine tree. It is added to the paraffin to improve the smoothness in molding, and to render it more resistant to cracking and flaking. It also increases the toughness of the wax, and it enhances the smoothness and luster of the surface.

Carnauba wax occurs as a fine powder on the leaves of certain tropical palms. This wax is quite hard, and it has a relatively high melting point. It is combined with the paraffin to decrease the flow at mouth temperature. It has an agreeable odor, and it also contributes to the glossiness of the wax surface even more than does the dammar resin.

Candelilla wax can also be added to replace partially or entirely the carnauba wax. The candelilla wax contributes the same general qualities as

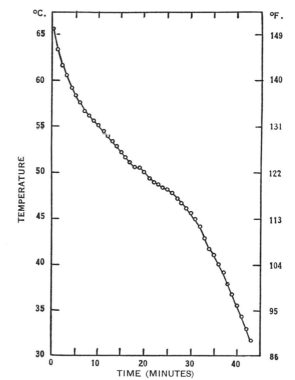

Figure 25–1 Time-temperature cooling curve for a Type B inlay wax.

the carnauba wax, but its melting point is lower, and it is not as hard as carnauba wax. Ceresin may replace part of the paraffin in order to modify the toughness and carving characteristics of the wax.

In modern inlay waxes, the carnauba wax is often replaced in part with certain synthetic waxes that are compatible with paraffin wax. At least two waxes of this type can be used. One is a complex nitrogen derivative of the higher fatty acids and the other is composed of esters of acids derived from montan wax, a petroleum derivative. As in impression compound, a synthetic wax is preferable to a natural wax because it has greater uniformity. Because of the high melting point of the synthetic waxes, more paraffin can be incorporated and the general working qualities of the product are improved.

Control of the properties of the wax is accomplished by a combination of factors. These include the amount of carnauba wax, the melting range of the hydrocarbon wax, and the presence of resin.[1]

Desirable Properties   Some of the properties that are desirable for an inlay wax can be summarized as follows:

1. When softened, the wax should be uniform. In other words, it should be compounded with ingredients that will blend with each other so that there will be no graininess or hard spots in the plastic material.

2. The color should be such that it will contrast with the die material. It is necessary to carve the wax margins close to the die; therefore, a definite contrast in color facilitates proper finishing of the margins.

3. There should be no flakiness or similar surface roughening when the wax is bent and molded after softening. Such flakiness is likely to be present in paraffin wax, and this is one of the reasons modifiers are added.

4. After the wax pattern has solidified, it is necessary to carve the original tooth anatomy in the wax and, as stated before, to carve the wax at the margins so that the pattern conforms exactly to the surface of the die. The latter procedure sometimes requires that the wax be carved to a very thin layer. If the wax pulls with the carving instrument or chips as it is carved, such precision cannot be attained.

5. As previously noted, after the mold has been formed, the wax is eliminated from the mold. Elimination is usually accomplished by heating the mold so as to ignite the wax. If, after burning, the wax leaves a residue that might provide an impervious coating on the walls of the mold, the final cast inlay may be adversely affected, as will be described in a later section. Consequently, the wax should burn out, forming carbon, which is later eliminated by oxidation to volatile gases. American Dental Association Specification no. 4 requires that the melted wax, when vaporized at 500° C (932° F) shall leave no solid residue in excess of 0.10 per cent of the original weight of the specimen.

6. Ideally, the wax pattern should be completely rigid and dimensionally stable at all times until it is eliminated. The wax pattern is subject to flow unless it is handled very carefully. It will also be shown that it is subject to relaxation, a factor which must be taken into consideration in its manipulation.

Flow   One of the desirable properties of the Type B inlay wax is that it exhibits a marked plasticity or flow at a temperature slightly above that of the mouth. The temperatures at which the wax is plastic are indicated by the time-temperature cooling curve for a typical Type B wax shown in Figure

25–1. The interpretation of this curve is the same as for its counterpart — a typical time-temperature cooling curve for a solid solution alloy. The wax begins to harden at approximately 56° C (133° F), the point at which the curve first departs from a straight line, and it is solid below approximately 40° C (104° F), when it again cools at a constant rate.

Inlay waxes do not solidify with a space lattice, as does a metal. Instead the structure is more likely to be a combination of crystalline and amorphous materials, displaying limited ordering of the molecules. The wax lacks rigidity and may flow under stress even at room temperature.

American Dental Association Specification no. 4 provides certain requirements for the flow properties of inlay waxes at specific temperatures. The flow is measured by subjecting cylindrical specimens to a designated load at the stated temperature and measuring the percentage shortening in length. The flow properties of three waxes obtained by this method are shown in Figure 25–2. The maximal flow permitted for Type B waxes at 37° C (98° F) is 1 per cent. The low flow at this temperature permits carving and removal of the pattern from the prepared cavity at oral temperature without distortion. In addition, both Type B and Type C waxes must have a minimal flow of 70 per cent at 45° C (113° F).

At approximately this temperature the wax is inserted into the prepared cavity. If the wax does not have sufficient plasticity, it does not flow into all of the areas in the preparation and reproduce the required detail.

For example, wax No. 2 in Figure 25–2 exhibits a flow of 73 per cent at a temperature of 45° C (113° F). However, at a temperature only 8° C (14° F) lower, the flow is slight.

Wax No. 1 in Figure 25–2 might be satisfactory for use in the indirect technique, but it would be too soft at oral temperature to be removed from the tooth without distortion. On the other hand, wax No. 3 softens at too high a temperature for use in forming an inlay pattern with either technique.

Thermal Properties   As previously noted, the inlay waxes are softened with heat, forced into the prepared cavity in either the tooth or the die, and cooled.

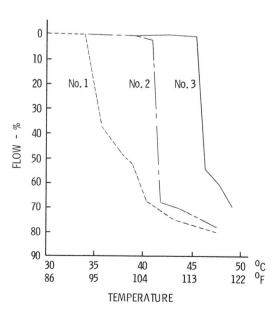

Figure 25–2   Flow of a soft (No. 1), a medium (No. 2), and a hard (No. 3) inlay wax, tested according to the method described in American Dental Association Specification no. 4. (Adapted from Souder and Paffenbarger, National Bureau of Standards Circular C433.)

The thermal conductivity of the waxes is low, and time is required both to heat them uniformly throughout and to cool them to body or room temperature.

Another thermal characteristic of inlay waxes is their high coefficient of thermal expansion. As can be noted from Figure 25–3, the wax may expand linearly as much as 0.7 per cent with an increase in temperature of 20° C (36° F) or contract as much as 0.35 per cent when cooled from 37 to 25° C (99 to 77° F). The average linear coefficient of thermal expansion over such a temperature range is 350×10^{-6} per °C.

A comparison with the coefficient of thermal expansion of dental materials given in Table 3–2 indicates that inlay wax expands and contracts thermally more per degree temperature change than any other dental material. This is one of the disadvantages inherent in waxes, when used in the direct technique.

This property is less significant when the wax is used in the indirect technique because the pattern is not subjected to a change from mouth to room temperature. In fact, American Dental Association Specification no. 4 contains no requirements for thermal expansion for Type C waxes. A maximum of 0.6 per cent linear change in dimension when heated from 25 to 37° C (77 to 99° F) is permitted for Type B waxes.

The amount of the thermal dimensional change may be affected by the previous treatment of the wax. Curve A in Figure 25–3 represents the thermal expansion of an inlay wax that had been previously cooled under pressure. As can be observed, the expansion rate increases abruptly above approximately 35° C (95° F). The temperature at which the change in rate occurs is the glass transition temperature. Some constituents of the wax probably change crystalline form at this temperature, and the wax is more plastic at higher temperatures. Not all waxes exhibit transition temperatures; the transition point shown in Figure 25–3 appears to be characteristic of a paraffin wax.

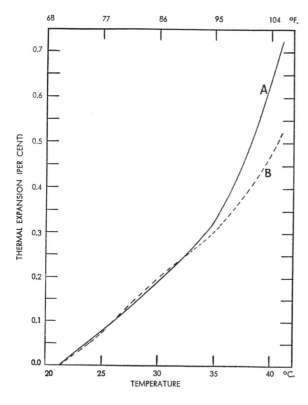

Figure 25–3 Thermal expansion of an inlay wax. Curve A represents the thermal expansion when the wax was held under pressure while it was cooling from the liquid state. When the same wax was allowed to cool without pressure and again heated, curve B resulted.

It is of interest to note that if the wax is allowed to cool without being placed under pressure, the transition temperature is not so pronounced when it is reheated, nor is the change in the linear coefficient of thermal expansion so great, as shown in curve B, Figure 25–3.

There is another possible explanation for the difference in behavior, upon reheating, of a wax cooled under pressure and the same wax cooled without applied pressure. It is related to the behavior of dissolved or occluded air or solvents. Certain waxes have a phenomenal capacity for gas and solvent retention, which may often remain undetected. The gas trapped within the wax expands upon reheating, causing a pronounced expansion as the wax becomes sufficiently plastic to flow.

Other factors, such as the temperature of the die and the method used for applying pressure to the wax as it solidifies, also influence the coefficient of thermal expansion.[2] However, this property of inlay waxes is probably not a serious problem when used in the indirect technique, provided no marked variation in temperature occurs after the removal of the pattern from the die.

Many of these properties have been reported for natural, commercial, and dental waxes.[1, 3, 4] Likewise, the stress-strain properties have been measured.[5]

Wax Distortion   Distortion is probably the most serious problem faced when forming the pattern and removing it from the mouth or die. Such distortion arises from thermal changes and from the release of the stress inherent in the pattern. These stresses are induced from the natural tendency of the wax to contract upon cooling, from occluded gas bubbles, from the change in shape of the wax during molding, and from the manipulative variables, such as carving, pooling, and removal. The amount of residual stress and resulting distortion are, therefore, governed by the method of forming the pattern, its handling, and the length of time and the temperature at which it is stored. All of these factors will be discussed in the following sections.

The change in dimension, or distortion, of a wax pattern during relaxation, as with any thermoplastic material, may be considerable as the stress unavoidably induced in the wax during manipulation is released. Such distortion can be demonstrated by a simple experiment. A piece of inlay wax can be softened over a Bunsen burner, bent into a horseshoe shape, and chilled in this position. It is now floated in a pan of water at room temperature, as shown in Figure 25–4A. If it is permitted to remain in this position for a number of hours, it may appear as in Figure 25–4B. The marked opening of the horseshoe is due to the release of stress.

The condition is similar to but more critical than that in impression compounds. In impression compound, as it is used for the impression of an edentulous mouth, the soft tissues might compensate for slight errors in the denture base, caused by the relaxation of the compound. In an inlay wax, however, any warpage of the pattern, even though slight, results in the misfit of the rigid metallic inlay on the unyielding, hard tissue of the tooth.

In all probability, the effect of pressure on the thermal expansion of the wax, as indicated in Figure 25–3, is not a basic phenomenon caused by a molecular change, but rather a "uniform distortion" caused by relaxation. For example, if the wax represented by curve A is held under pressure while cooling from above its glass transition temperature, the intermolecular distances might be reduced slightly so that the average distance is less than that

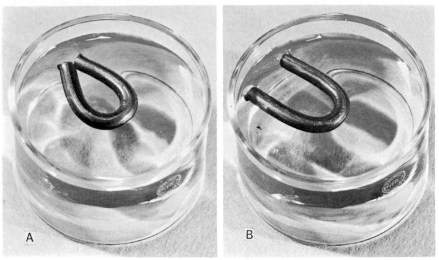

Figure 25–4   *A*, A stick of inlay wax is bent into the shape of a horseshoe and floated on water at room temperature. *B*, After 24 hours the same stick of wax may appear as shown.

under equilibrium conditions. If the wax is reheated, the expansion due to the relaxation is added to the normal thermal expansion, thus apparently increasing the latter. Also, as explained, the influence of entrapped gases cannot be ignored in the relaxation phenomenon.

It should be recalled that such changes by diffusion occur readily in waxes because of their low internal energy. In fact, similar changes probably occur in the wax specimens shown in Figure 25–4 without change in temperature. For example, when the wax is bent above its transition temperature the average intermolecular distance is increased on the outside of the bend because of the tensile stresses. On the other hand, the average intermolecular distance is decreased on the inner surface because the total distance is decreased. After chilling in this position, the stresses are relieved gradually at room temperature, and the wax specimen tends to straighten (Fig. 25–4*B*).

Causes of Distortion   According to the current theory of the causes of distortion, any method of manipulation that creates a structural inhomogeneity of the wax, involving localized variations in intermolecular distance, may result in a distortion of the pattern. Such a distortion occurs during the restoration of ambient equilibrium conditions. In other words, the internal energy of the mass is not uniform, and a change in shape by relaxation occurs as the energy equalizes either with time or with change in temperature.

In practice, when the wax is softened and molded to the form of the cavity, and then carved, stresses are inadvertently introduced and the pattern is likely to be distorted for the same reason as was the stick of inlay wax in Figure 25–4.

There are a number of factors that may cause distortion and that are under the control of the operator, but they cannot be entirely eliminated. For example, if the wax is not at the same temperature throughout when it is adapted to the cavity, some parts of the wax pattern may thermally contract more than others and stresses be introduced. If the wax is not held under uniform pressure during cooling, it is possible for some of the molecules to be compressed more closely together than others. Here again, when relaxation

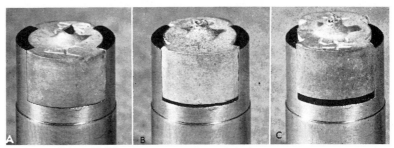

Figure 25–5 Castings made from patterns prepared with melted wax, cooled under pressure. *A*, Pattern invested immediately. *B*, Pattern stored for two hours before investing. *C*, Pattern stored for 12 hours before investing.

occurs, a distortion may take place. If wax has to be melted and added to the pattern in order to repair some parts that were not accurately obtained or to repair a damaged area, the added wax will introduce stresses during cooling. During the carving operation, some of the molecules of the wax will undoubtedly be disturbed, and a stress will result.

It may be necessary to perform all of these operations during fabrication of the pattern. If a technique can be used by which the amount of carving, the amount of change in temperature, and similar factors can be minimized, the less will be the subsequent relaxation and warpage of the pattern.

Once the pattern is obtained, the entire effect can be minimized if the temperature of the pattern is not changed and if it is surrounded by the hard investment as soon as possible after being removed from the die. It should always be the rule to invest the pattern as soon as possible after it has been prepared. Once the pattern is surrounded by the hardened investment, no further distortion can occur. The wax may be eliminated and the casting made at any time that is convenient.

The possible effect of storing the wax pattern is shown in Figure 25–5. Note that the casting fits best when the pattern is invested immediately after it has been obtained.

Wax distortion may appear to be relatively unimportant when the indirect technique is employed and the pattern is stored on the die. The die confines the pattern and thereby aids in preventing distortion. However, relaxation of stress may still take place in directions away from the die, such as the marginal areas or a surface that is not enclosed by the die. For this reason, the margins of the wax pattern should always be checked just before it is removed from the die. Any minute distortion that may have occurred during the time that the pattern was on the die can be detected. The wax can then be readapted to its correct contour and fit.

Naturally, the configuration of the prepared cavity influences the degree of distortion. Although a slight amount of dimensional change does not greatly interfere with the visible fit of a casting made from a simple two-surfaced pattern, a corresponding distortion of the long, nearly parallel walls of an MOD (mesio-occluso-distal) pattern results in a gross inaccuracy of the casting. It should be a paramount rule that, regardless of its type, the pattern should be invested as soon as possible after removal from the die.

Reduction of Distortion   Regardless of the method employed, some relaxation and pattern distortion occur. The distortion probably cannot be eliminated completely, but it can be reduced to a point that it is not of clinical importance.

There are a number of methods for minimizing such distortion, some of which are more effective than others:

1. Only those waxes that are guaranteed to meet American Dental Association Specification no. 4 for dental inlay wax should be used. Furthermore, the proper wax should be selected according to the technique to be employed.

2. If the indirect technique is used, melting the wax into the matrix band on the die helps to increase the homogeneity, particularly if the wax is held under pressure equal from all sides while it solidifies. Because the pressure is hydrostatic, i.e., equal in all directions, it is presumed that the reduction in the intermolecular distances is uniform. Therefore, the relaxation that occurs after the pressure and the matrix band are removed should also be uniform. In other words, a uniform expansion should occur.

The method of choice might be to dip the die repeatedly in the molten wax. Thus, layers are formed until the wax becomes sufficiently thick to carve the pattern. Presumably, each layer of wax anneals each partially solidified layer. Another technique is to carry the wax onto the die by means of a spatula, building it in increments. However, the wax has a tendency to pull away from the die as it solidifies. Also, the die lubricant tends to prevent intimate adaptation. This may be overcome by repeated application of finger pressure as the "core" wax is laid down.

3. The weakness of these methods is that further stresses are probably introduced during any subsequent pattern repair or carving. If the distortion of the final pattern is to be reduced to its lowest degree, ideally it should be swaged on the die.

For example, the die and pattern can be mounted in a closed vessel fitted with a piston and containing water, preferably at approximately 38° C (100° F). If a force is applied to the piston, a hydrostatic pressure is applied to the pattern somewhat as described in the first method except, in this case, the final pattern is involved. Any subsequent distortion is immeasurably small and of no consequence. The theory is the same as discussed in (2). In certain types of patterns, at least with techniques such as these, the stress may be minimal.[6]

4. Probably the most practical and quickest method for avoiding distortion of the pattern is to invest it immediately after removal from the mouth. As was previously noted, the shape and bulk of the pattern vary according to the prepared cavity. Therefore, the time required for relaxation of various patterns is unknown. Consequently, the safest method is to invest it at once. When the investment hardens, there will be no further distortion of the pattern. As will be discussed in a subsequent chapter, the mold may distort during subsequent manipulations, but the pattern per se does not change.

Manipulation of Inlay Wax   The wax is generally softened with "dry heat." The greatest danger from the use of a water bath is probably not the leaching out of water extractable materials, at least for most wax compositions and with conventional heating techniques. The hazard would likely be from inadvertent inclusion of droplets of water into the pattern. This could conceivably cause several problems: (1) spattering upon flaming, (2) smearing of the wax surface upon polishing, and (3) distortion of the pattern upon thermal changes. Because dry heat precludes these problems it is generally recommended. In any event, some inlay waxes become crumbly and unmanageable after they have been softened in warm water for any length of time.

If the wax is softened over a flame, care should be taken not to volatilize any of the constituents. The safest method is to hold a stick of wax above the visible flame, and to rotate it rapidly until it becomes plastic. The wax is then kneaded and shaped approximately to the form of the prepared cavity. Direct patterns should be formed at the minimum temperature needed to give adequate plasticity. American Dental Association Specification no. 4 ensures adequate plasticity in a temperature range that can be safely tolerated by the pulp.

After the wax is inserted into the prepared cavity it is held under pressure while it solidifies. Pressure may be applied either with the finger or by the patient biting on the wax. It is not necessary to chill the pattern with water, but if water is used, low temperatures should be avoided. The best procedure is to allow the pattern to cool gradually by itself to mouth temperature.

Considerable care should be observed in the removal of the pattern from the prepared cavity so that it is not distorted. Under no circumstance should it be hooked with an explorer point and rotated out of the prepared cavity. A complicated pattern, such as for an MOD cavity, can best be removed by luting a staple to the pattern so that each prong is fastened above a corresponding step portion. The pattern can then be removed with dental tape looped through the staple. In this manner, the pattern can be withdrawn in a direction parallel to the axial walls with a minimum of distortion.

However it is removed, the pattern should be touched as little as possible with the hands because such a procedure introduces an additional and unnecessary temperature change. Unnecessary temperature changes should be avoided in order to minimize the relaxation. Such precautions are necessary whether the direct or indirect technique is employed.

For fabricating the indirect pattern, the die is first lubricated to prevent the wax from sticking. A wetting agent should be applied to the pattern in a film of minimal thickness; any excess may prevent intimate adaptation of the wax to the die. The melted wax may then be added in layers with a wax spatula, or painted on with a camel's-hair brush. In the case of a full cast crown, the die may be dipped repeatedly into the liquid wax, as previously described.

The prepared cavity is overfilled, and the wax is then carved to the proper contour. When the margins are being carved, extreme care should be taken to avoid abrading any surface of the stone die. A silk cloth may be used for a final polishing of the pattern, rubbing toward the margins.

The type and amount of relaxation are dependent upon factors not always under the control of the operator; therefore, for reasons previously noted, the best procedure is to invest the pattern as soon as possible after it has been removed from the mouth or die.

OTHER DENTAL WAXES

There are a number of other types of waxes employed for somewhat different purposes than the inlay waxes described. The composition of each type is adjusted for the particular requirements called for. One of the most common is *baseplate* wax.

As the name suggests, baseplate wax is used principally to establish the initial arch form in the construction of complete dentures. Supplied in 1 to 2 mm thick red or pink sheets, the wax is approximately 75 per cent paraffin or ceresin, with additions of beeswax and other resins or waxes. American Dental Specification no. 24 includes Type I, II, and III, also designated as soft, medium, and hard. The differentiation from one to another is by the percentage flow of each type at room temperature, at mouth temperature, and at 45° C (113° F). The harder the wax, the less is the flow at a given temperature. The difference in flow of the three types is advantageous in the particular usage. Type I, a soft wax, is used for building veneers; Type II, a medium wax, is designed for patterns to be tried in the mouth in normal climatic conditions; Type III, a hard wax, is for trial in the mouth in tropical climates.

Because residual stress is present within the wax from contouring and manipulating the wax, the finished denture pattern should be flasked as soon as possible after completion.

Another group of dental waxes is composed of the impression waxes, also referred to as "bite" or "corrective" waxes. They will distort if withdrawn from undercut areas, and therefore are limited to use in edentulous portions of the mouth. Although corrective waxes are quite soft at mouth temperature, they do have sufficient body to register the detail of soft tissue, and they are rigid at room temperature.

Other waxes include the "sticky" waxes, which are quite tacky when melted but firm and brittle when cooled. These waxes are used to join and temporarily stabilize the components of a bridge before soldering or the pieces of a broken denture prior to the repair. "Boxing" wax is yet another useful material for enclosing an impression before the plaster or stone cast is poured.

References

1. Craig RG, Powers JM, and Peyton FA: Thermogravimetric analysis of waxes. J Dent Res 50:450, 1971.
2. Hollenback GM and Rhoads JE: Thermal expansion of pattern wax, Part III. J South Calif Dent Assoc 28:6, 1960.
3. Craig RG, Eick JD, and Peyton FA: Flow of binary and tertiary mixtures of waxes. J Dent Res 45:397, 1966.
4. Ohashi M and Paffenbarger GC: Melting, flow and thermal expansion characteristics of some dental and commercial waxes. J Am Dent Assoc 72:1141, 1966.
5. Craig RG, Eick JD, and Peyton FA: Strength properties of waxes at various temperatures and their practical application. J Dent Res 46:300, 1967.
6. Hollenback GM, Baum L, and Lund MR: A study of the stability of pattern wax. J South Calif Dent Assoc 29:210, 1961.

26 INVESTMENTS FOR SMALL CASTINGS

After the wax pattern has been obtained, a *sprue former* or *sprue pin* is attached to it and it is surrounded with *investment*. It is mixed in the same manner as plaster or dental stone, placed around the pattern, and allowed to set. After the investment hardens, the sprue former is removed, the wax is also removed, and the molten metal is forced into the mold cavity left by the wax, through the *sprue* or *ingate* formed by the sprue former. These procedures will be described in detail in the next two chapters.

The following discussion deals with the investments used for the fabrication of small dental castings, i.e., inlays, onlays, and crowns. Generally two types are employed, depending on the melting range of the alloy and the preference of the individual. They are the *gypsum-bonded* and *phosphate-bonded* investments. The gypsum-based materials are the older type traditionally used for conventional gold alloys. The phosphate-based investments are designed primarily for alloys used in the metal-ceramic restoration. (This restoration is discussed in Chapters 24 and 31.)

A third type is the *silica-bonded* investment, which is used principally in the casting of base metal alloy partial dentures. That investment will be discussed in Chapter 35.

GYPSUM-BONDED INVESTMENTS

American Dental Association Specification no. 2 for casting investments for dental gold alloys encompasses three types of investments. The various types are based upon the appliance to be fabricated, whether it is fixed or removable, and the method of obtaining the expansion required to compensate for the contraction of the gold alloy. Type I investments are those employed for the casting of inlays or crowns and when the alloy casting shrinkage compensation is accomplished principally by thermal expansion of the investment. Type II investments are also used for the casting of inlays or crowns, but the major mode of compensation is by the hygroscopic expansion of the investment. Type

III investments are utilized in the construction of partial dentures with gold alloys. This chapter will be concerned only with Types I and II investments.

Composition   As already noted, the essential ingredients of the dental inlay investment employed with the conventional gold casting alloys are a hemihydrate of gypsum and a form of silica. Most investments now contain α-hemihydrate because greater strength is obtained. This gypsum product serves as a binder to hold the other ingredients together and to provide rigidity. The strength of the investment is dependent upon the amount of binder present. The investment may contain 25 to 45 per cent of the gypsum product. Investments with binders other than gypsum will be discussed in a subsequent chapter.

Gypsum   As noted, the α-hemihydrate form is generally the binder for investments used in casting gold-containing alloys with melting ranges below 1000° C (1800° F). Unfortunately, when this material is heated to the temperatures required for complete dehydration and sufficiently high to ensure complete castings, it shrinks considerably and frequently fractures.

The thermal expansion curves of the three common forms of gypsum products are shown in Figure 26–1. All forms shrink considerably after dehydration of from 200 to 400° C (400–750° F). A slight expansion then occurs, to approximately 700° C (1300° F), and then a tremendous contraction

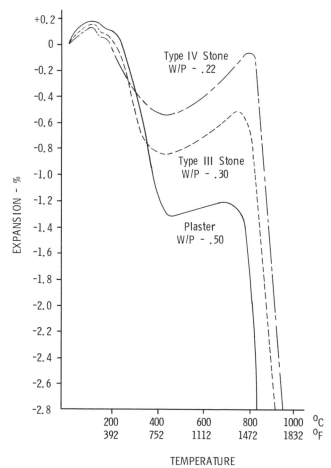

Figure 26–1 Dimensional change of three forms of gypsum when heated. (Courtesy of R. Neiman, Whip-Mix Corp.)

occurs. This latter shrinkage is most likely due to decomposition, and sulfur gases (e.g., sulfur dioxide) are emitted. This decomposition not only causes shrinkage but also contaminates the castings with the sulfides of the non-noble alloying elements, such as silver and copper. Thus it is imperative that gypsum investments should not be heated above 700° C (1300° F). Even safer, especially with those products containing carbon, is to avoid exceeding 650° C (1200° F). In this way, proper fit as well as uncontaminated alloys will be obtained.

Needless to mention, castings, even if successfully made in pure gypsum molds, will be extremely undersized. Obviously, the α-hemihydrate, which requires less mixing water and shrinks less, as shown in Figure 26-1, is now the obvious choice as a binder.

Silica   Silica, SiO_2, is added to provide a refractory during the heating of the investment, and to regulate the thermal expansion. Usually, the wax pattern is eliminated from the mold by heat. During the heating, the investment is expected to expand thermally to compensate partially or totally for the casting shrinkage of the gold alloy. Gypsum, regardless of whether it is set plaster or stone, shrinks considerably when it is heated, as was seen in Figure 26-1.

If the proper form of silica is employed in the investment, such a contraction can be eliminated and changed to an expansion during heating. Silica exists in at least four allotropic forms: quartz, tridymite, cristobalite, and fused quartz. The first and third are of particular dental interest.

When either quartz, tridymite, or cristobalite is heated, a change in crystalline form occurs at a transition temperature characteristic of the particular form of silica. For example, when quartz is heated, it inverts from a "low" form, known as α-quartz, to a "high" form, called β-quartz, at a temperature of 575° C (1067° F). In a similar manner, cristobalite undergoes an analogous transition between 200° C (392° F) and 270° C (518° F) from "low" or α-cristobalite to "high" or β-cristobalite. Two inversions of tridymite occur at 117° C (243° F) and 163° C (325° F), respectively. The β-allotropic forms are stable only above the transition temperature noted, and an inversion to the lower or α-form occurs upon cooling in each case. In powdered form the inversions occur over a range of temperature rather than instantaneously.

The density decreases as the α-form changes to the β-form, with a resulting increase in volume that is evidenced by a rapid increase in the linear expansion as indicated in Figure 26-2. Consequently, the shrinkage of gypsum shown in Figure 26-1 can be counterbalanced by the inclusion of one or more of the crystalline silicas.

Fused quartz is amorphous and glasslike in character, and it exhibits no inversion at any temperature below its fusion point. It has a very low linear coefficient of thermal expansion and is of little use in dental investments.

Quartz, cristobalite, or a combination may be used in a dental investment. Both are now available in pure form. Tridymite is no longer an expected impurity in cristobalite.

On the basis of the type of silica principally employed, dental investments are often classified as *quartz investments* or *cristobalite investments*.

Modifiers   In addition to silica, certain modifying agents, coloring matter, and reducing agents, such as carbon or powdered copper, are present. The reducing agents are used in some investments in an attempt to provide a non-oxidizing atmosphere in the mold when the gold alloy is cast.

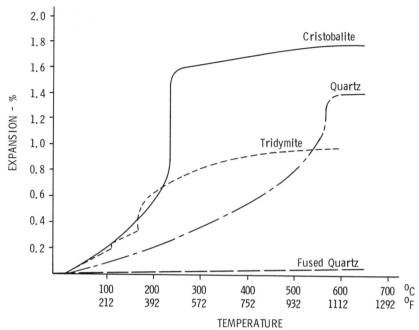

Figure 26–2 Thermal expansion curves of four forms of silica. (Courtesy of R. Neiman, Whip-Mix Corp.)

Unlike the dental stones, a setting expansion is usually desirable in an investment to assist in compensating for the contraction of the gold alloy. Some of the added modifiers, such as boric acid and sodium chloride, not only regulate the setting expansion and the setting time but also prevent most of the shrinkage of gypsum when it is heated above 300° C (572° F), as will be discussed. In some cases, the modifiers are limited to the usual "balancing" agents to regulate the setting time and setting expansion, as was described for the dental stones.

The microstructure of a set gypsum-bonded investment can be seen in Figure 26–3.

Setting Time   The setting time of an investment can be measured in the same manner as for plaster. Furthermore, it can be controlled in the same manner.

According to American Dental Association Specification no. 2 for dental inlay casting investment, the setting time should not be less than 5 minutes, nor more than 25 minutes. Usually the modern inlay investments set initially in 9 to 18 minutes. Sufficient time should be allowed for mixing and investing the pattern before the investment sets.

Normal Setting Expansion   A mixture of silica and gypsum hemihydrate results in setting expansion greater than that of the gypsum product when it is used alone. The silica particles probably interfere with the intermeshing and interlocking of the crystals as they form. Thus, the thrust of the crystals is outward during growth and therefore more effective in the production of an expansion.

Generally, the resulting setting expansion in such a case is high. American Dental Association Specification no. 2 for Type I investment permits a maximal setting expansion *in air* of only 0.5 per cent. The setting expansion of

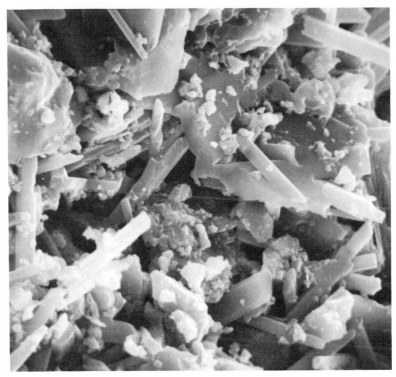

Figure 26-3 Microstructure of surface of fractured specimen of a set gypsum-bonded investment. The elongated, rod-like particles are gypsum and the larger, irregular particles are the silica refractory. (Original magnification 4200 ×)

such modern investments is approximately 0.4 per cent. It can be regulated by retarders and accelerators, as described previously.

The purpose of the setting expansion is to aid in enlarging the mold to compensate partially for the casting shrinkage of the gold. There is some doubt that all of the setting expansion is effective in expanding the wax pattern. The *normal setting expansion* of investment has traditionally been determined in a manner similar to that for dental plaster, in which the expansion is measured as the linear dimensional change that occurs as the investment sets in a V-shaped trough. Thus, the normal setting expansion can occur essentially unrestricted. However, the trough technique does not accurately measure the actual or *effective setting expansion* of the investment while it is setting under the conditions of practical usage.

For example, the effectiveness of the setting expansion in enlarging the mold containing the wax pattern may be related to the thermal expansion of the pattern caused by the heat of reaction that occurs coincidentally with the setting of the investment. It follows from such a theory that the setting expansion is effective only to the extent that the exothermic heat is transmitted to the pattern. The amount of heat present depends upon the gypsum content of the investment; therefore, the setting expansion of an investment with a comparatively high gypsum content is more effective in enlarging the mold than is a product with a lower gypsum content. Likewise, manipulative conditions that increase the exothermic heat increase the effective setting expansion, e.g., the lower the water/powder ratio for the investment, the greater is the effective setting expansion.

Variables other than the exothermic heat of reaction also influence the effective setting expansion. As the investment sets it eventually gains sufficient strength to produce a dimensional change in the wax pattern as setting expansion occurs. The inner core of the investment within a MOD wax pattern can actually force the proximal walls outward to a certain extent. If the pattern has a thin wall, then the effective setting expansion is somewhat greater than for a pattern with thicker walls because the investment can move the thinner wall more readily.[1] Also, the softer the wax, the greater is the effective setting expansion because the softer wax is more readily moved by the expanding investment. If a wax softer than a Type B inlay wax is used, the setting expansion may cause a serious distortion of the pattern.[2]

Hygroscopic Setting Expansion   The theory of the hygroscopic setting expansion was previously described in connection with the setting of dental plaster and stone. It was pointed out that the hygroscopic setting expansion differs from the normal setting expansion in that it occurs when the gypsum product is allowed to set under or in contact with water and that it is greater in magnitude than the normal setting expansion.

The hygroscopic setting expansion was first discovered in connection with an investigation of the dimensional changes of a dental investment during setting.[3] As illustrated in Figure 26–4, the hygroscopic setting expansion may be six or more times the normal setting expansion of a dental investment. As a matter of fact, when it is measured on a mercury bath, it may be as high as 5 per cent linear. As will be shown in the next chapter, the hygroscopic setting

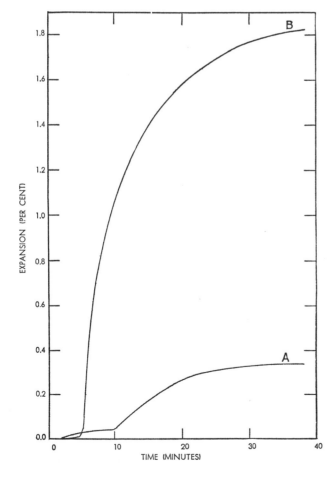

Figure 26–4 Curve A, normal setting expansion of dental investment. Curve B, hygroscopic setting expansion; water was added five minutes after the beginning of mixing. W/P ratio — 0.30.

expansion is one of the methods for expanding the casting mold to compensate for the casting shrinkage of the gold alloy.

Different commercial investments exhibit different amounts of hygroscopic expansion. Although all investments appear to be subject to hygroscopic expansion, the expansion in some cases is not as great as in others. For this reason, certain investments are specially formulated to provide a substantial hygroscopic expansion when the investment is permitted to set in contact with water. American Dental Association Specification no. 2 for such Type II investments requires a minimal setting expansion in water of 1.2 per cent; the maximal expansion permitted is 2.2 per cent.

A number of factors are important in the control of the hygroscopic expansion:

Effect of Composition   The magnitude of the hygroscopic setting expansion of a dental investment is generally proportional to the silica content of the investment, other factors being equal. The finer the particle size of the silica, the greater is the hygroscopic expansion. In general, the α-hemihydrate is apt to produce a greater hygroscopic expansion in the presence of silica than is the β-hemihydrate, particularly when the expansion is unrestricted. As previously stated in Chapter 4, the hygroscopic expansion of the stone or plaster alone is very slight.

A dental investment should have enough hemihydrate binder with the silica to provide sufficient strength after hygroscopic expansion. Otherwise, a shrinkage occurs during the subsequent drying of the set investment. At least 15 per cent of binder is necessary to prevent a drying shrinkage.

Effect of the W/P Ratio   The higher the W/P ratio of the original investment-water mixture, the less is the hygroscopic setting expansion. This effect is more marked in some commercially available investments than in others.

Effect of Spatulation   With most investments, the shorter the mixing time, the less is the hygroscopic expansion. It should be noted that this factor is important in connection with the control of the effective setting expansion as well.

Shelf Life of the Investment   The older the investment, the less is its hygroscopic expansion. Consequently, the amount of investment purchased at one time should be limited.

Effect of Time of Immersion   The greatest amount of hygroscopic setting expansion is observed if the immersion takes place before the initial set. The longer the immersion of the investment in the water bath is delayed beyond the time of the initial set of the investment, the less is the hygroscopic expansion.

Effect of Confinement   Both the normal and hygroscopic setting expansions are confined by opposing forces, such as the walls of the container in which the investment is placed or the walls of a wax pattern. However, the confining effect on the hygroscopic expansion is much more pronounced than the similar effect on the normal setting expansion. The effective hygroscopic setting expansion is, therefore, likely to be less in proportion to the expected expansion than is the normal setting expansion.

When the dimensional change in the wax pattern itself is measured after investing, the increase in the effective setting expansion when the investment is immersed in a 38° C (100° F) water bath is apparently not the result of hygroscopic expansion per se. Rather, it is due mainly to the softening of the wax pattern at the water bath temperature permitting an increase in effective setting expansion.[4] The latter results from a combination of thermal expansion of the wax pattern plus the softened condition of the wax, reducing its confining effect on the expansion of the setting investment.

Effect of the Amount of Added Water   In the previous discussions, it has been assumed that the investment was immersed in a water bath, and that it could sorb as much water as necessary to effect the expansion. However, the magnitude of the hygroscopic setting expansion can be controlled by the amount of water that is added to the setting investment.

It has been proved that the magnitude of the hygroscopic expansion is in direct ratio to the amount of water added during the setting period until a maximal expansion occurs. No further expansion is evident regardless of any amount of water added.

The effect of some of the factors previously discussed (W/P ratio, mixing, and shelf life) on the maximal hygroscopic setting expansion is illustrated in Figure 26–5 in reference to the amount of water added. As can be noted, the effect of these factors on the maximal expansion is as predicted.

The important consideration to be noted in Figure 26–5 is that, within the limits of the investigation, below the maximal expansion the magnitude of the hygroscopic setting expansion is *dependent only on the amount of water added,* and is independent of the W/P ratio, the amount of mixing, and the age or shelf life of the investment. This finding is the basis for a mold expansion technique to be described in the next chapter.

Theory of Hygroscopic Setting Expansion   As discussed in connection with the hygroscopic expansion of gypsum products (Chapter 4), the hygroscopic setting expansion is a continuation of the ordinary setting expansion because the immersion water replaces the water of hydration and, thus, prevents the confinement of the growing crystals by the surface tension of the excess water.[5] Owing to the diluent effect of the quartz particles, the hygroscopic setting expansion in these investments is greater than when the

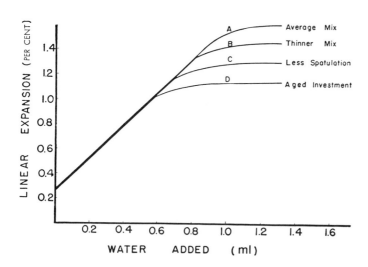

Figure 26–5 Graphic representation of the relation of the linear hygroscopic setting expansion and the amount of water added as influenced by certain manipulative factors. (From Asgar, Mahler, and Peyton, J Prosthet Dent, Sept., 1955.)

gypsum binder is used alone. This effect is the same as previously described for normal setting expansion.

It should be emphasized that the phenomenon is purely physical. The hemihydrate binder is not necessary for the hygroscopic expansion because investments with other binders exhibit a similar expansion when allowed to set under water. As a matter of fact, an expansion can be detected when water is poured into a vessel containing only small, smooth quartz particles. The water is attracted between the particles by capillary action and thus causes the particles to separate, creating an expansion. The effect is not permanent, of course, after the water is evaporated, unless a binder is present.

Any water insoluble powder that can be wetted can be mixed with the gypsum hemihydrate, and hygroscopic expansion results. Consequently, the quartz per se is not a factor.

The influence of all of the factors previously described can be related to the theory presented. The greater the amount of the silica or the inert filler, the more easily the added water can diffuse through the setting material and the greater is the expansion, for the same reason as described for the normal setting expansion of investment. The W/P ratio affects the hygroscopic expansion for the same reason that it affects the normal setting expansion. Once setting starts, the later the water is added to the investment, the less is the hygroscopic setting expansion because part of the crystallization has already started in a "normal" fashion. Some of the crystals have intermeshed and inhibit further crystal growth after the water is added. On the same basis, the less water added, the lower is the expansion, i.e., there is less counteraction of the surface tension action.

Finally, it should be noted that the term "hygroscopic" in its strict sense is a misnomer. Although the added water may be drawn into the setting material by capillary action, the effect is not related to hygroscopy. Furthermore, on the basis of the theory, the hygroscopic setting expansion is as "normal" a phenomenon as that which occurs during what is designated as "normal setting expansion." However, the terms have gained general acceptance by usage even though they may be inaccurate on the basis of theoretical considerations.

Thermal Expansion   As noted in a previous section, the thermal expansion of the gypsum-bonded investment is directly related to the amount of silica present and to the type of silica employed.

A considerable amount of quartz is necessary to counterbalance the contraction of the gypsum during heating. Even when the quartz content of the investment is increased to 60 per cent, with the balance being hemihydrate binder, the initial contraction of the latter is not eliminated.

The contraction of the gypsum is entirely balanced when the quartz content is increased to 75 per cent (Fig. 26-6). If a sufficient amount of setting expansion had been present, the casting made at 700° C (1292° F) would probably have fit the die reasonably well. The thermal expansion curves of quartz investments will be influenced by the particle size of the quartz, the type of gypsum binder, and the resultant W/P ratio necessary to provide a workable mix.[6]

The effect of cristobalite as compared with that of quartz is strikingly demonstrated in Figure 26-7. Owing to the much greater expansion that occurs during the inversion of the cristobalite, the normal contraction of the gypsum during heating is easily eliminated. Furthermore, the expansion

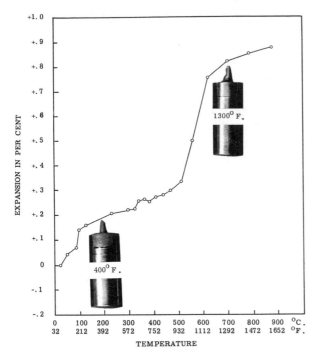

Figure 26–6 Thermal expansion of an investment that contains 25 per cent plaster of Paris and 75 per cent quartz. (Courtesy of G. C. Paffenbarger.)

occurs at a lower temperature because of the lower inversion temperature of the cristobalite in comparison with that of quartz. As can be noted (Fig. 26–7), a reasonably good fit of the castings is obtained when the gold alloy is cast into the mold at temperatures of 500° C (932° F) and above.

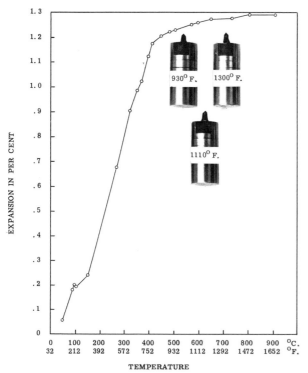

Figure 26–7 Thermal expansion of an investment that contains cristobalite instead of quartz. (Courtesy of G. C. Paffenbarger.)

The thermal expansion curves of an investment give some idea of the form of the silica that is present. As can be seen from Figures 26–6 and 26–7, the investments containing cristobalite expand earlier and to a greater extent than those containing quartz. Some of the modern investments probably contain both quartz and cristobalite.

The desirable magnitude of the thermal expansion of a dental investment depends upon its use. If the hygroscopic expansion is to be relied upon to compensate for the contraction of the gold alloy, as for the Type II investments, American Dental Association Specification no. 2 requires that the thermal expansion be between 0.0 and 0.6 per cent. However, for the Type I investments, which rely principally upon thermal expansion for compensation, the thermal expansion must be not less than 1.0 nor greater than 2.0 per cent. In addition, the specification establishes minimal and maximal values for the combined setting or hygroscopic expansion, whichever the case may be, and the respective thermal expansion.

Another desirable feature of an inlay investment is that its maximal thermal expansion be attained at a temperature not greater than 700° C (1292° F). This temperature is normally the mold temperature in the casting of gold alloy when a thermal expansion technique is employed. As noted earlier and as will be shown later, the gold alloys are apt to be contaminated at a mold temperature higher than 700° C (1292° F).

Effect of the W/P Ratio   The magnitude of thermal expansion is related to the amount of solids present. Therefore, it is to be expected that the more water

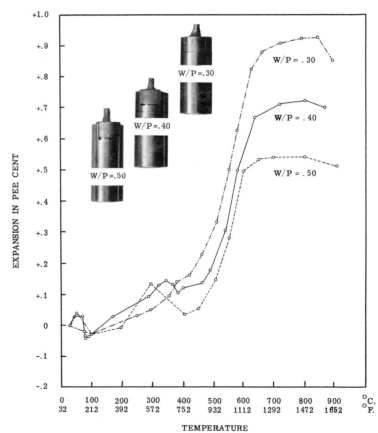

Figure 26–8   Effect of the water/powder ratio on the thermal expansion of an investment that contains 20 per cent plaster of Paris and 80 per cent quartz. (Courtesy of G. C. Paffenbarger.)

used in mixing the investment, the less is the thermal expansion. This effect is demonstrated by the curves shown in Figure 26–8. Although the variations in the W/P ratios shown are rather extreme, the curves indicate that it is imperative to measure the water and powder accurately if the proper compensation is to be realized.

Effect of Chemical Modifiers   A disadvantage of an investment that contains sufficient silica to prevent any contraction during heating is that the weakening effect of the silica in such quantities is apt to be too great. The addition of small amounts of the chlorides of sodium, potassium, or lithium to the investment eliminates the contraction caused by the gypsum and increases the expansion without the presence of an excessive amount of silica.[7]

Boric acid has somewhat the same effect. It also hardens the set investment. However, it apparently disintegrates during the heating of the investment and a roughened surface on the casting may result. Silicas do not prevent the gypsum shrinkage but counterbalance it, whereas chlorides actually reduce gypsum shrinkage below temperatures of approximately 700° C (1292° F).

Thermal Contraction   When an investment is allowed to cool from 700° C, its contraction curve follows the expansion curve during the inversion of the β-quartz or cristobalite to its stable form at room temperature. Actually, the investment contracts to less than its original dimension. This contraction below the original dimension is not related to any property of the silica; it occurs because of the shrinkage of gypsum when first heated.

If the investment is reheated, it expands thermally to the same maximum reached when first heated. However, in practice the investment should not be heated a second time because internal cracks may develop.

Strength   The strength of the investment must be adequate to prevent fracture or chipping of the mold during heating and casting of the gold alloy.

Although a certain minimal strength is necessary to prevent fracture of the investment mold during casting, surprisingly it has been postulated that the compressive strength should not be unduly high.[8] In several studies on the fit of castings made by various techniques, it has been found that all castings for the Bureau of Standards MOD die showed a constant pattern of distortion.[9, 10] The distortion apparently results from a directional restraint by the investment to the thermal contraction of the casting as the alloy cools to room temperature.

Although the total thermal contraction of the investment is similar to that of the gold alloy from the casting temperature down to room temperature, the contraction of the investment is fairly constant until it cools to below 550° C (1022° F). Thus when the alloy is still quite hot and weak the investment can resist alloy shrinkage by virtue of its strength and constant dimension. This then can cause distortion and even fracture in the casting if the hot strength of the alloy is low. While this is rarely a factor with gypsum-bonded investments, it can be with other types of investments to be discussed later in the chapter.

Thus, it is theorized, the compressive strength of the investment mold could be a factor to be considered, in addition to the expansion, when evaluating the dimensional accuracy of dental castings.[8] Ideally, the investment would have sufficient expansion to compensate for all of the thermal contraction of the alloy. However, after burn-out of the mold, the strength should be no greater than that required to resist the impact of the metal entering the mold.

The strength of an investment is usually measured under compressive stress. The compressive strength is increased according to the amount and the type of the gypsum binder present. For example, the use of α-hemihydrate instead of plaster definitely increases the compressive strength of the investment. The use of chemical modifiers as described in the previous section also aids in increasing the strength because more of the binder can be used without a marked reduction in the thermal expansion.

According to American Dental Association Specification no. 2, the compressive strength for the inlay investments should not be less than 2.5 MPa (360 psi) when tested 2 hours after setting. Any investment that meets this requirement should possess adequate strength for the casting of an inlay. However, when larger, complicated castings are made, a greater strength is necessary, as required for the Type III partial denture investment.

The strength of the investment is affected by the W/P ratio in the same manner as any other gypsum product; the more water employed in mixing, the lower is the compressive strength. Heating the investment to 700° C (1292° F) may increase or decrease the strength as much as 65 per cent, depending on the composition.[8] The greatest reduction in strength upon heating is found in investments containing sodium chloride. After the investment has cooled to room temperature, its strength decreases considerably, presumably because of fine cracks that form during cooling.

Fineness   The fineness of the investment may affect its setting time, the surface roughness of the casting, and other properties. It was previously noted that a fine silica results in a higher hygroscopic expansion than when a coarse silica is present. A fine particle size is preferable to a coarse one. The finer the investment, the smaller will be the surface irregularities on the casting.

Porosity   During the casting, the molten metal is forced into the mold under pressure. As the molten metal enters the mold, the air must be forced out ahead of it. If the air is not completely eliminated, a so-called *back pressure* builds up to prevent the gold alloy from completely filling the mold. The common method for venting the mold is through the pores of the investment.

In general, the more gypsum crystals present in the set investment, the less is its porosity. It follows, therefore, that the less the hemihydrate content and the greater the amount of gauging water used to mix the investment, the more porous it is.

The particle size of the investment is also a factor. The more uniform the particle size, the greater is its porosity. This factor is of greater importance than is the actual particle size. A mixture of coarse and fine particles exhibits less porosity than an investment composed of a uniform particle size.

Technical Considerations   The same precautions for storage of an investment should be observed as for plaster or dental stone. Under conditions of high relative humidity, the setting time may change for the reasons given in connection with the storage of plaster and stone. Under such conditions, the setting expansion and the hygroscopic expansion may be altered so that the entire casting procedure may be adversely affected. The investments should, therefore, be stored in airtight and moisture-proof containers. During use, the containers should be opened for as short a time as possible.

As has been explained, all investments are composed of a number of ingredients, each of which possesses a different specific gravity. There is a tendency for these components to separate, according to their specific gravities, under the normal vibration that occurs in the dental laboratory. Under certain conditions this separation may influence the setting time, and other properties, of the investment. For this reason, as well as the danger of accidental moisture contamination, it is advisable to purchase the investment in relatively small quantities.

The selection of an investment is largely a matter of preference. Some investments are formulated for casting inlays and crowns employing thermal expansion as the main factor for casting shrinkage compensation, and some for use with hygroscopic setting expansion. Consequently, the choice is dependent in part upon the specific techniques for which the investment is designed. Acceptable castings for the range of typical dental cavity preparations can be made with a number of investments and techniques.[11]

As previously noted, the investment should be weighed and the water should be measured in the proportioning of the investment mix. Only in this manner can one expect to control the setting or the thermal expansion, in relation to the compensation needed for the casting shrinkage, and other important properties.

Some dental manufacturers supply their investment in pre-weighed packages so that one need only measure the gauging water.

The mixing and subsequent manipulations of the investment will be described in the next chapter.

The rapid growth in use of the metal-ceramic restoration and the increased use of higher melting alloys have resulted in an increased use of phosphate- or silica-bonded investments. Although these investments are somewhat harder to remove from castings than gypsum investments, even that problem has been reduced recently and they will produce satisfactory results with conventional gold alloys. The phosphate-bonded materials are discussed in the following section. Since the silica-bonded investments are used primarily for constructing base metal alloy partial dentures, they are covered in Chapter 34.

PHOSPHATE-BONDED INVESTMENTS

In introducing an expanded section on phosphate investments, it is most appropriate to quote from the late Eugene Skinner, whose name appears in the title of this text.[12] In 1963 he stated: "The definite advantage of this type of investment is that there is less chance for the contamination of the gold alloy during casting. . . . So far as is known at present, such contamination is avoided with phosphate-bonded investments. On this basis, I am inclined to predict that the dental investment of the future may be phosphate-bonded and not gypsum-bonded."

As predicted, the phosphate investments enjoy a popularity possibly even greater than that of the gypsum-bonded materials. The tremendous increase in the use of metal-ceramic restorations necessitated the use of higher melting gold alloys that did not cast well into gypsum investments. Likewise, the present trend is toward the use of more inexpensive alloys, all of which require phosphate investments.

Composition These investments, like the gypsum investments, consist of refractory fillers and a binder. The filler is silica, in the form of cristobalite, quartz, or a mixture of the two and in a concentration of approximately 80 per cent. The purpose of the filler is to provide refractoriness and a high thermal expansion. The particle size will vary from sub-micron to that of a fine sand. The seemingly sandy feel does not necessarily relate to casting smoothness or affect the ease of removing the casting from the investment.

The binder consists of magnesium oxide (basic) and a phosphate that is acid in nature. Originally phosphoric acid was used but mono-ammonium phosphate has replaced it, since it can be incorporated into the powdered investment. Using phosphoric acid would be cumbersome, as most phosphate investments already utilize one liquid, the powder being mixed with an aqueous colloidal silica suspension.

Since the newer gold-containing alloys and other alloys used in metal-ceramic restorations have higher melting temperatures than traditional gold alloys, it usually follows that their contraction during solidification is also greater. This necessitates a greater expansion in the investment. Fortunately, the colloidal silica suspensions just mentioned became available in time for use with the phosphate investments.

In order to simplify the procedure and to facilitate shipping, since colloidal silica solutions freeze in cold weather, some phosphate investments have been produced in which water may be used as the gauging liquid.

Carbon is often added to the powder to help produce clean castings and facilitate the "dig-out" of the casting. This addition is appropriate when the casting alloy is gold, but there is disagreement regarding the effects of carbon in phosphate investments used for casting silver-palladium and/or base metal alloys. It has been suggested that it embrittles the alloys, even though the investment is heated to temperatures that burn out the carbon. The latest evidence indicates that palladium does not react with carbon at temperatures below 1504° C (2740° F).[13] Thus, if the casting temperature of a high palladium alloy exceeds this critical point, a phosphate investment without carbon should be used. Also, a carbon crucible should not be employed for melting the alloy. Generally, even gold alloys used with porcelain should not be premelted or fluxed on charcoal blocks because trace elements that provide high strength are in effect removed, or reduced below the desired level.

Setting Reactions The chemical reaction for the binder system that causes the investment to set and harden is generally written as follows:

$$NH_4H_2PO_4 + MgO + 5H_2O \rightarrow NH_4MgPO_4 \cdot 6H_2O$$

However, phosphates are quite complex and the reaction is not as simple as thus indicated. One version is that the magnesium ammonium phosphate formed is polymeric.[14] While the stoichiometric quantities are equal molecules of magnesia and mono-ammonium phosphate, an excess of magnesia is usually present and some of it is never fully reacted. What is thus formed is a predominantly colloidal multimolecular $(NH_4MgPO_4 \cdot 6H_2O)_n$ coagulating around excess MgO and fillers.

Upon heating, the binder of the set investment undergoes thermal reactions as suggested in the following way:[14]

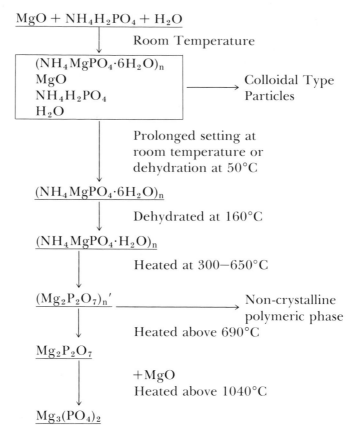

$$MgO + NH_4H_2PO_4 + H_2O$$

Room Temperature

$(NH_4MgPO_4 \cdot 6H_2O)_n$
MgO
$NH_4H_2PO_4$
H_2O $\longrightarrow$ Colloidal Type Particles

Prolonged setting at room temperature or dehydration at 50°C

$(NH_4MgPO_4 \cdot 6H_2O)_n$

Dehydrated at 160°C

$(NH_4MgPO_4 \cdot H_2O)_n$

Heated at 300–650°C

$(Mg_2P_2O_7)_n{}'$ $\longrightarrow$ Non-crystalline polymeric phase

Heated above 690°C

$Mg_2P_2O_7$

$+MgO$
Heated above 1040°C

$Mg_3(PO_4)_2$

The final products are crystalline $Mg_2P_2O_7$ and some excess MgO, along with essentially unchanged quartz and/or cristobalite. Some $Mg_3(PO_4)_2$ may be formed if the investment is grossly overheated or when the molten metal contacts the mold cavity surfaces.

Setting and Thermal Expansion   Theoretically the reaction should entail a shrinkage, as in gypsum products, but in practice there is a slight expansion and this can be increased considerably by using a colloidal silica solution instead of water. This latter substitution gives phosphate investments an unusual advantage in that the expansion can be controlled from a shrinkage to a significant expansion. Figure 26–9 shows the effect of the concentration of a typical liquid, essentially colloidal silica in aqueous suspension, in increasing the setting and thermal expansion.

Figure 26–10 illustrates the thermal expansion of a typical phosphate investment when mixed with water, as compared with the same investment mixed with its accompanying special liquid. It is most interesting that phosphate investments, when mixed with water, have a shrinkage in essentially the same temperature range as gypsum-bonded investments (200–400° C [400–750° F]). This contraction is practically eliminated when a colloidal silica solution replaces the water.

Some users of a phosphate-bonded investment prefer to decrease expansion by increasing the liquid/powder ratio rather than by decreasing the

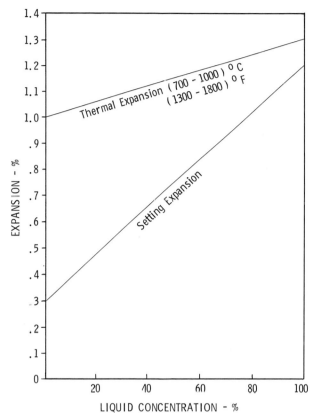

Figure 26–9 The influence of liquid concentration on the setting and thermal expansion of a phosphate-bonded investment. (Courtesy of R. Neiman, Whip-Mix Corp.)

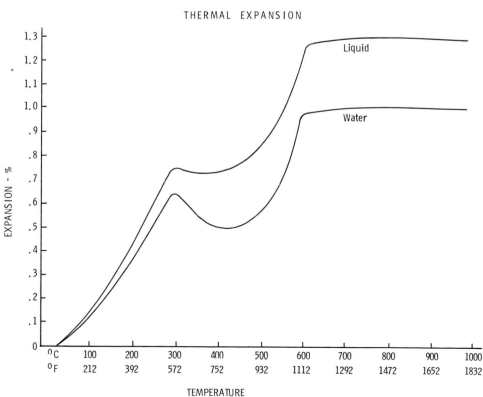

Figure 26–10 Thermal expansion of a phosphate-bonded investment mixed with water as compared with the special liquid. (Courtesy of R. Neiman, Whip-Mix Corp.)

concentration of the special liquid. Or they may use a combination of these two methods.

The thermal shrinkage in phosphate investments is due to the decomposition of the binder, magnesium ammonium phosphate, and is accompanied by evolution of ammonia, which is readily apparent by its odor. (In gypsum investments the shrinkage is due to the transformation of the calcium sulfate from the hexagonal to the rhombic configuration, as has been noted.) However, some of the shrinkage is masked because of the expansion of the refractory filler, especially in the case of cristobalite.

Working and Setting Time   Unlike gypsum investments, phosphate investments are markedly affected by temperature. The warmer the mix, the faster it will set. The setting reaction itself gives off heat, and this further accelerates the rate of setting. Increased mixing time and mixing efficiency, as determined by the type of mixer and speed of mixing, result in a faster set and a greater rise in temperature. In general, the more efficient the mixing, the better is the casting in terms of smoothness and accuracy. The ideal technique is to mix as long as possible yet have just enough time for investing. Mechanical mixing under vacuum is preferred.

A third variable that has a considerable effect upon the working and setting time is the liquid/powder ratio, which is often varied considerably depending upon user preference. An increase in the liquid/powder ratio will increase the working time, which can be very short (2 minutes or even less) when the investment is mixed at the manufacturer's recommended liquid/powder ratio and at high speed (1750 rpm) for the recommended time. This is especially true if the laboratory is warm and the liquid has not been chilled.

Miscellaneous Properties   At one time, detail reproduction and surface smoothness of a metal-ceramic gold alloy restoration cast in a phosphate-bonded investment were generally considered inferior to those characteristic of a conventional gold alloy cast in a gypsum-bonded investment. Increasing the special liquid/water ratio used for the mix markedly enhances casting surface smoothness, but can lead to oversized extracoronal castings. However, improvement in the technique, and also perhaps the investment, now makes it possible to fabricate castings having very few surface imperfections when the phosphate-bonded investment is used with either a low or a high fusing gold alloy.

Additional considerations in the use of such investments will be discussed in Chapter 28.

References

1. Van Aken J: Distortion of wax patterns as influenced by hygroscopic expansion of the investment. Tschr Tandhelk 68:583, 1961.
2. Mahler DB and Ady AB: The influence of various factors on the effective setting expansion of casting investments. J Prosthet Dent 13:365, 1963.
3. Scheu CH: A new precision casting technic. J Am Dent Assoc 19:630, 1932.
4. Mahler DB and Ady AB: The effect of the water bath in hygroscopic casting techniques. J Prosthet Dent 15:1115, 1965.
5. Mahler DB and Ady AB: An explanation for the hygroscopic setting expansion of dental gypsum products. J Dent Res 39:578, 1960.

6. Jones DW: Thermal behavior of silica and its application to dental investments. Br Dent J 122:489, 1967.

7. Earnshaw R: The effects of additives on the thermal behaviour of gypsum-bonded casting investments. Part I. Aust Dent J 20:27, 1975.

8. Earnshaw R: The compressive strength of gypsum-bonded investments at high temperatures. Aust Dent J 14:264, 1969.

9. Teteruck WR and Mumford G: The fit of certain dental casting alloys using different investing materials and techniques. J Prosthet Dent 16:910, 1966.

10. Jenkins CBG: An Evaluation of Five Gold Inlay Investing Techniques and the Effects of Certain Variables in the Procedure. Thesis, Indiana University, 1968.

11. Jenkins CBG and Phillips RW: An evaluation of five inlay investing techniques employed with different types of wax patterns. J Prosthet Dent 25:211, 1971.

12. Skinner EW: Some recent technical advances in dental materials. J Am Dent Assoc 66:176, 1963.

13. JF Jelenko Co.: Thermotrol Technician, 34:No. 1, Winter, 1980.

14. Neiman R and Sarma AC: Setting and thermal reactions of phosphate investments. J Dent Res 9:1478, 1980.

27

NOBLE METAL ALLOY CASTING PROCEDURES: THEORETICAL CONSIDERATIONS. INVESTMENT EXPANSION TECHNIQUES. INVESTING PROCEDURES

Although dental castings of any size from a denture base to the smallest inlay can be made, only the procedure employed for the construction of a small restoration, e.g., a crown, will be discussed. The fundamental principles are the same, regardless of the size of the casting, and the techniques differ only in minor details.

Theoretical Considerations   The sole objective of the casting procedure is to provide a metallic duplication of missing tooth structure, with as great an accuracy as possible. The tolerance limits for the dental inlay are not known. In a clinical study, 10 experienced dentists were asked to evaluate the marginal adaptation of a group of inlays, using an explorer and roentgenograms.[1] After grading the cemented restorations, they microscopically measured the marginal openings at various areas. For "acceptable" restorations, the mean opening at the occlusal surface was 21 μm, but it was 74 μm at the gingival region, which is not as accessible visually. These 10 dentists were not able to evaluate consistently the marginal openings of some areas, either by explorer or roentgenogram. The difficulty in detecting small discrepancies at the margins of cemented restorations is evidenced by examination of Figure 27–1. A magnification of the cross section of the tip of an unused explorer is reproduced adjacent to a human hair. The picture poses the question of how readily one can detect a hairline gap by running an explorer over the margins of the restoration.

Therefore, it is obvious that the accuracy of the inlay or crown should be greater than can be detected by the eye or by the conventional methods of clinical testing. At the margins of the cemented restoration, a thin line of cement is always present, even though it may not be readily visible. The present dental cements are soluble and deteriorate in the oral cavity, as will be discussed in Chapter 29. Thus, the less accurate the casting and the greater the amount of cement exposed, the more likely is the restoration to fail. Certainly, absolute accuracy of fit cannot be realized continuously under oral conditions because of the differential thermal dimensional changes between the tooth and the gold restoration and other factors. It stands to reason, however, that the more accurate the fit of the casting in the prepared cavity, the less is the likelihood of leakage and the recurrence of caries.

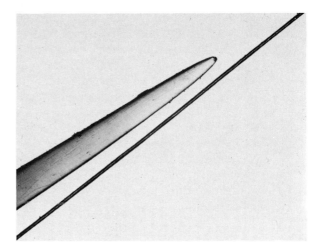

Figure 27–1 Metallographic cross section of an unused explorer tip (top) and a 60 μm hair. (25 ×) (From McLean and Von Fraunhofer, Br Dent J, Aug. 3, 1971.)

Assuming that the wax pattern is satisfactory, the procedure then becomes a matter of enlarging the mold uniformly and sufficiently to compensate for the casting shrinkage of the gold alloy.

Theoretically, if the shrinkages of the wax and the gold alloy are known, the mold can be expanded an amount equal to such a shrinkage, and the problem is solved. Unfortunately, there are variables in the behavior of the materials involved, especially the wax, that cannot be rigidly controlled. The overall dimensional accuracy possible with current techniques has never been clearly defined. Although minimal deviations of approximately 0.1 per cent have been reported, there may be variations as high as 1.0 per cent.[2] Thus, neither the allowable tolerance of accuracy in the fit of the casting nor that obtainable during the casting procedure is known. In the last analysis, the casting procedure is partly empirical and a matter of routine procedure, which should be rigidly followed.

There are, however, many steps in the procedure concerning which a considerable number of facts are known; their application will be discussed in subsequent sections. There are also certain ramifications of the techniques here described which produce equally satisfactory results. However, any technique involves strict adherence to certain fundamentals that are common to all. It is these fundamentals which will be stressed.

Compensation Techniques The compensation for the shrinkages inherent in the technique may be obtained by any one, or combinations of, the following three methods:

1. Thermal expansion of the wax pattern.
2. Setting expansion or hygroscopic expansion of the investment.
3. Thermal expansion of the investment.

The thermal expansion of the wax pattern can be obtained by maintaining the temperature of the water-investment mixture at approximately 40 to 42° C (104 to 108° F) after the pattern has been invested, before the investment sets. As might be predicted from the discussion of wax distortion, such a treatment produces a relaxation of the wax and a consequent distortion. For this reason, this technique is no longer employed.

The two casting techniques currently employed are *thermal expansion* and *hygroscopic expansion*. As can be deduced from their names, the principal mold compensation in the first technique is by the thermal expansion of the investment from room temperature to a high temperature, 650–700° C (1200–1300° F), at which the casting is made. In the second technique, the main mold compensation is realized by the hygroscopic expansion of the investment; the mold is heated between only 482 and 510° C (900 and 950° F). Although 482° C is generally preferred, some investments give better results at 565 to 593° C (1050 to 1100° F). On the basis of their respective mold temperatures at the time of casting, the two methods are often designated as *high heat* and *low heat* casting technique, respectively.

Aside from the differences mentioned, the operations involved are quite similar and the two techniques will be described simultaneously. If no differentiation is made, it can be assumed that the procedures described are common to both.

PREPARATION OF THE DIE

The most commonly used die material is a Type IV gypsum. This material is relatively inexpensive, is easy to use, and is generally compatible with all impression materials. Its reproduction of detail and dimensional accuracy are considered to be adequate, the setting expansion being 0.1 per cent or less. Also it is possible to reproduce a line less than 20 μm in width when the impression material is a non-aqueous elastomer. However, gypsum dies are sometimes modified to (1) make them more abrasion resistant, (2) change the dimensions of the dies, (3) increase the refractoriness of the dies, or (4) produce a combination of these effects.

The chief disadvantage of the Type IV gypsum die is its susceptibility to abrasion during carving of the wax pattern. Several means are used to increase the abrasion resistance. However, each may also increase the die dimensions, thus reducing accuracy.

So-called *gypsum hardeners,* such as aqueous colloidal silica or soluble resin solutions, can be used instead of water when mixing the stone. Although there may be no significant increase in hardness, the abrasion resistance is increased by approximately 100 per cent,[3] as is the fluidity of the mix.

A possible disadvantage is the slightly increased setting expansion. However, as can be seen in Table 27–1, in most cases the increase is small and has little clinical significance. The figures represent the dimensions of the stone die at the occlusal and cervical areas, as compared with those of an aged silicone impression taken of the original cavity preparation. The use of hardener A increased the expansion of a Type IV gypsum 0.1 per cent at the

Table 27–1. *Dimensional Change in Dies of Various Materials as Compared to Original Silicone Impression**

| | PER CENT DIMENSIONAL CHANGE | |
MATERIAL	Occlusal	Cervical
Type IV stone	0.06	0.00
Type IV stone + gypsum hardener A	0.16	0.08
Type IV stone + gypsum hardener B	0.10	0.10
Silica-filled epoxy resin	−0.15	−0.26
Aluminum-filled epoxy resin	−0.14	−0.19
Electroformed silver die	−0.10	−0.20

*From Toreskog, Phillips, and Schnell, J Prosthet Dent, 16:119, 1966.

occlusal, while hardener B caused an increased expansion of only 0.04 per cent. The dimensional changes at the cervical were of the same order of magnitude.

The abrasion resistance of the gypsum die can also be enhanced by treating the surface of the set gypsum with a resin, such as epoxy, acrylic, styrene, or cyanoacrylate. The mixed but uncured resin is applied to the stone die, either in a concentrated form or diluted with an agent such as acetone. Dilution enhances penetration of the resin into the stone and reduces the tendency of the resin to increase the die dimensions. After the resin has been allowed to penetrate the stone, it polymerizes. Also, thermoplastic polymers, dissolved in volatile solvents to form a solution, may be used.

Such resin treatment can produce a moderate increase in strength and hardness of the gypsum, the increase being directly proportional to the W/P ratio of the stone mix and, therefore, the porosity of the set gypsum. The increase in abrasion resistance is much more pronounced than is the increase in strength and hardness. For example, when one dry Type III gypsum was treated with a diluted epoxy resin, the abrasion resistance increased 35 times.[4] For a Type IV gypsum, using a lower W/P ratio, the increase would be less. Thus these resins, which fill the spaces between the calcium sulfate dihydrate crystals, are most effective when the stone is dried before application of the resin.

The disadvantage of treating the set gypsum with such an agent is that the resin can form a surface layer 10 μm or more thick, if not handled correctly.

Methods for Altering Die Dimensions   If the user desires a die stone that has less setting expansion than about 0.1 per cent, additional accelerator (potassium sulfate) and retarder (borax) can be added to the gauging water. By this method a mean setting expansion of 0.01 per cent can be achieved when using some Type IV gypsum products.[5]

At other times a die slightly larger than the prepared tooth is desired, either to aid in compensating for the casting shrinkage of the alloy or to provide additional space between the tooth and the casting during cementation. Colloidal silica can be added to the gauging liquid. Also, the surface application of resins can be used to deliberately increase die dimensions, as well as having a side effect in a die hardening technique as just noted.

Another rather unique technique has been developed to increase gypsum die dimensions in order to reduce or eliminate the distortion of the wax pattern that accompanies the setting expansion of a gypsum-bonded investment.[6] The die is dipped first in benzoyl peroxide and then in a BIS-GMA/TEGMA monomer containing a tertiary amine. Under standardized conditions the polymerized resin coats the die surface to a depth of 30 μm. The wax pattern can then be fabricated on this enlarged die and invested in an investment that has essentially no setting expansion and insufficient thermal expansion to compensate fully for the casting shrinkage of the alloy.

Die spacers may also be used in conjunction with the stone die. The purpose is to prevent the layer of cement from interfering with the complete seating of an otherwise precisely fitting casting.[7] The most common die spacer is made by coating the gypsum die with a resin to within about 0.5 mm of the margin. Special proprietary paint-on liquids can be used, as well as model paint, colored nail polish, or thermoplastic polymers dissolved in volatile solvents.

Die Stone-Investment Combination   There is yet another technique that has been developed, in which the die material and the investing medium have a comparable composition. A commercial gypsum-bonded material, called Divestment, is mixed with a colloidal silica liquid. The die is made from this mix and the wax pattern constructed on it. Then the entire assembly (die and pattern) is invested in the Divestment, thereby eliminating the possibility of distortion of the pattern upon removal from the die or during the setting of the investment. The setting expansion of the material is 0.9 per cent and thermal expansion 0.6 per cent when heated to 677° C (1250° F).

Since Divestment is a gypsum-bound material, it is not recommended for high fusing alloys, as used in the metal-ceramic restoration. However, it is a highly accurate technique for use with conventional gold alloys, especially for extra-coronal preparations.[8]

Other Die Materials   With the inelastic impression materials, such as compound, amalgam may be condensed into the impression to form the die.

Other non-gypsum die materials are also available, such as acrylic, polyester, and epoxy resins. These materials are limited in their compatibility with impression materials, which would ordinarily be non-aqueous elastomers rather than hydrocolloid or compound. Compatibility is very specific and germane only to the particular brand rather than to chemical types of impression materials. Moreover, in the case of filled autopolymerizing acrylic resins, the curing contraction is excessive (0.6 per cent linear for one material). Therefore, acrylic resin cannot be used when an accurate die is required. The same may be said for polyester resin materials.

Various epoxy die materials do appear to be reliable in respect to dimensional change upon polymerization, this change being a linear contraction of about 0.1 to 0.2 per cent (Table 27–1). Even though epoxy dies are generally undersize in comparison with the prepared tooth,[9] especially in the axial direction, they are said to be used successfully by some commercial dental laboratories.[10]

In all fairness, it should be noted that in some cases the resin die will be no more undersize than the stone die is oversize. However, this must be taken into consideration, as it may be necessary to adjust the investing and casting technique accordingly. A casting fabricated on the slightly undersize resin die will fit back on the tooth differently than will one made on the slightly large stone die.

All factors considered, the Type IV gypsums appear to be the most successful die materials available. With care, abrasion during carving of the wax pattern can be avoided. However, in the construction of a porcelain jacket crown a platinum matrix is generally swaged on a die of the preparation. Gypsum dies are readily damaged, so a less brittle material, such as resin or metal, is preferred.

Electroformed Dies   The metal dies that are produced when an impression material is electroplated have high strength, hardness, and abrasion resistance. Detail reproduction of a line 4 μm or less in width is readily attainable when a non-aqueous elastomeric impression material is used. Currently, the more popular impression-metal material combinations are (1) compound plated with copper and (2) polysulfide polymer plated with silver.

Data for addition polymerizing silicone-copper dies are very limited as yet, but this combination should become more popular if silver plating solutions continue to be in short supply. The copper plating bath and anode are less expensive than the silver cyanide electrolyte and silver anode, but greater technical difficulty in electroforming may be encountered. Accuracy will depend to a great extent upon the degree of tensile stress that develops in the electroform during deposition and to what extent this stress can be controlled. Other promising impression-die combinations are polyether-silver, polyether-nickel, and condensation silicone-nickel.[11]

The popularity of copper plated compound dies began in the early 1930's. There are several modifications of the fabrication technique, but the following description is typical:

The first step in the procedure is to treat the surface of the impression material so that it conducts electricity. This process is referred to as *metalizing*. A thin layer of metal is deposited on the compound or wax. This metal layer determines to a large extent the surface character of the finished die. Various metalizing agents are available, including bronzing powder suspended in oil of almonds and aqueous suspensions of silver powder and powdered graphite, both as separate agents or in combination with one another.

These agents can be burnished on the surface of the impression with a camel's hair brush. Chemical deposition of silver from a silver nitrate solution can be employed if greater surface detail reproduction is desired.

The electroplating bath itself is primarily an acid solution of copper sulfate containing certain other ingredients. For example, phenol and ethyl alcohol tend to increase the hardness and ductility of the electrodeposited copper. The greater the concentration of the copper sulfate, the faster the copper is deposited, whereas the acid content increases the *throwing power,* a term which refers to the ionic penetration of the electric field in a concave structure, such as an impression for a full crown. Impressions of teeth generally have walls with long depth relative to the occlusal area. A considerable amount of throwing power is, therefore, desirable.

A compromise is usually effected between the rate of the electrodeposition and the throwing power by regulating the composition of the electroplating bath. The composition presented in Table 27–2 is workable. The solution should be allowed to stand for several days after mixing before it is used.

An electrical contact is made between the copper matrix band or the metal tray and the metalized surface of the impression, which is the cathode in the electroplating bath. A plate of copper is used for the anode. All parts not to be electroplated are insulated with wax or a similar nonconductor. A direct current of 0.1 ampere per square centimeter of surface is applied for approximately 10 hours, following an initial electrodeposition at half that current density.

Hydrocolloid impressions are difficult to electroplate, and the process is not feasible for dental use. The electroformed die made from the polysulfide rubber impression is clinically acceptable when a silver cyanide bath is used,

Table 27–2. *Composition of an Electroplating Bath for Wax or Compound Impressions*

Copper sulfate, anhydrous	225–250 gm
Sulfuric acid, concentrated	75 ml
Phenol	10 ml
Ethyl alcohol	25–50 ml
Distilled water	1000 ml

Table 27–3. *Composition of a Silver Cyanide Bath for Electroplating Polysulfide Rubber Impressions*

Silver cyanide	36 gm
Potassium cyanide	60 gm
Potassium carbonate	40 gm
Distilled water	1000 ml

although it is generally slightly less accurate than a properly constructed stone die.

In addition to the dimensional change in the elastomer induced from the continuing polymerization during electroplating, distortion is inherent in the electroforming process itself. The electrodeposited metal tends to contract during deposition. Flat surfaces tend to become curved and sharp angles rounded, for example. If the electroformed metal does not adhere tenaciously to the impression material, as is often the case for silicone impression materials, the distortion is even greater.

The polysulfide rubber impression is cleaned thoroughly and dried. It is then metalized with a fine silver powder. Although other metalizing agents can be used, the silver powder results in a superior surface on the electroformed die.

A silver cyanide bath is preferred to an acid copper bath. The reliability and throwing power of the silver bath appear to be better. Also, it is possible that the dimensional stability of the polysulfide rubber is better in the alkaline silver cyanide bath than in the acid copper sulfate medium.

A formula for a satisfactory silver cyanide bath is given in Table 27–3. Special care should be observed so that acid or other chemicals do not inadvertently contact this solution. Acids in particular may produce fumes of the extremely toxic hydrocyanic acid. As a precaution, the bath should be kept in a well-ventilated environment.

An anode of pure silver, at least twice the size of the area to be plated, is employed and the electroplating is carried out as before for approximately 10 hours using 5 to 10 milliamperes per square centimeter of cathode surface.

Whatever the plating method, the electroformed die is filled with dental stone. When the stone hardens, it is mechanically locked to the rough interior of the electroformed metal shell. The impression material is then removed to provide a die with greater surface hardness and resistance to abrasion than one of gypsum. Acrylic resin or a low fusing alloy that contracts during solidification should not be used to fill the electroplated impression. Shrinkage of these materials will distort the electroform.

THE SPRUE FORMER

The purpose of the sprue former or sprue pin, as it is usually called, is to provide an ingate or sprue in the investment through which the molten alloy can reach the mold after the wax has been eliminated. It is usually constructed of metal, although a wax or a resin may be employed. If the metal sprue former is covered with a thin layer of soft wax, the warmed pin may be more safely removed without marring the walls of the investment.

The size of the sprue former depends to a considerable extent on the type and size of the pattern, the type of the casting machine to be used, and the dimensions of the flask or ring in which the casting is to be made.

The diameter of the average sprue pin may vary between Brown and

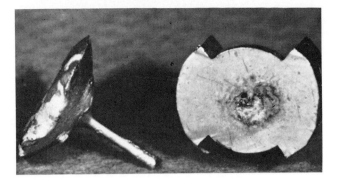

Figure 27–2 Localized shrinkage caused by using a sprue of improper diameter.

Sharpe gauge No. 10 and No. 16, 2.6 and 1.29 mm (0.10 and 0.05 inch). If the pattern is small, the sprue pin itself must be small (e.g., 1.25 mm) because a large sprue former attached to a thin, delicate pattern would cause a distortion. Likewise, if the gold is to be melted directly above the sprue or ingate, as in the air pressure casting machine to be described in the next chapter, the use of extremely large sprues is to be avoided in order to prevent the molten gold from flowing into the ingate under its own weight, before the pressure is applied. The largest sprue size is 2.1 mm in this case. If the gold is to be melted in a separate crucible, as in a centrifugal casting machine, then any diameter compatible with the size of the pattern may be used.

Generally, however, for the average size pattern, sprue formers smaller in diameter than approximately 1.5 mm are contraindicated. If the sprue is too small, the molten metal freezes completely in this area first and localized shrinkage porosity results, as shown in Figure 27–2.

In Table 27–4 can be seen the wire gauge numbers and corresponding diameters which cover the general range of sprue sizes used in dental castings.

A *reservoir* can be used as an added precaution. The reservoir is a piece of wax attached to the sprue former approximately 1 mm from the pattern. The purpose of the reservoir is, of course, to prevent localized shrinkage porosity. When the molten gold alloy flows into the mold, the fused metal in the reservoir should be the last to solidify so that any voids in the mold caused by shrinkage are immediately filled from the reservoir. Thus, the importance of providing a greater bulk of gold in the reservoir than in the thickest cross section of the casting becomes evident, as does the necessity for placing the reservoir as close to the pattern as possible so that the alloy in the connecting ingate does not solidify first.

Table 27–4. *American (Brown & Sharpe) Wire Gauge Numbers and Wire Diameter*

Gauge No. B & S	Diameter	
	cm	*inches*
6	0.4115	0.1620
8	0.3264	0.1285
10	0.2588	0.1019
12	0.2053	0.08081
14	0.1628	0.06408
16	0.1291	0.05082
18	0.1024	0.04030

From *Handbook of Chemistry and Physics*, 58th ed., Cleveland, CRC Press, Inc., 1977–1978, p. F-16.

A reservoir is a necessity only with sprue formers of very small diameter. If an ample size sprue pin is used, a reservoir is usually unnecessary.

Localized shrinkage porosity generally occurs at the point of sprue attachment, as seen in Figure 27–2. However, under certain circumstances it may develop in an area removed from the sprue, even when a sprue of proper diameter is employed. On occasion, the wax pattern for a MOD cavity preparation may involve two normal or bulky proximal walls connected by a thin occlusal isthmus. In such a case, if the sprue is attached to one of the contact points on a proximal surface, the molten metal solidifes first in the thin occlusal portion of the mold. Shrinkage porosity then develops in that area and possibly in the proximal surface that is opposite the point of sprue attachment. A double sprue attached to both proximal surfaces prevents such a failure because it provides molten metal that can enter all areas of the mold before solidification occurs at the occlusal surface.

The sprue pin is usually heated and attached to the pattern by a localized melting of the wax. Care must be exercised to avoid overheating the pattern and thus distorting an adjacent margin. A hollow sprue pin is especially good from this standpoint because its heat capacity is lower than that of a solid sprue. It is also helpful to attach a drop of wax to the pattern and attach the sprue pin to this added wax (Fig. 27–3). Pliable sticky wax is especially helpful with vacuum investing techniques.

When attached, wax should be used to build up the sprue pin at this point so that it flares out slightly in the direction of the pattern. The sprue former should never taper toward this area so that the movement of the entering metal is restricted.[12] Flaring of the sprue former may act in much the same way as a reservoir, and it facilitates the flow of molten metal into the cavity.

The position of the sprue former attachment is often a matter of individual judgment in relation to the shape and form of the wax pattern. Some prefer the occlusal surface, others wish to preserve the anatomy of the pattern; thus they may attach the sprue on the proximal wall. As a general rule, it is desirable to attach it at the point of greatest bulk in the pattern. In that case, there is less chance of distortion upon attaching the sprue, and the molten metal is more apt to remain liquid in this area until the entire mold is filled.

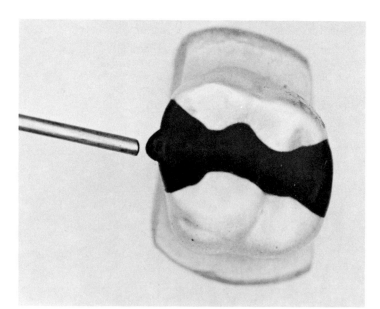

Figure 27–3 Attaching sprue former to a wax pattern. Sprue is attached to the drop of wax.

The direction of the sprue former is also important. It should never point directly toward a thin or delicate part of the mold because the molten metal, as it rushes in, may abrade or fracture the investment in this area and a casting failure may result.

Even if the sprue pin is the right size, it is important that it not be attached at a right angle to a broad flat surface of the mold. The entering hot metal impinges the mold surface at this point to cause a *hot spot,* producing a localized lingering of molten metal after the casting as a whole has solidified. This in turn creates a shrinkage void, or suck-back porosity, as will be described in the next chapter. This effect is illustrated in Figure 27–4A. Fortunately, the flaring of the sprue prevents the localized shrinkage from occurring in a critical area. When the same pattern is sprued at an angle of 45 degrees to the proximal wall, a satisfactory casting is obtained as presented in Figure 27–4B.

The length of the sprue former depends upon the length of the casting ring. If the sprue is too short, the mold may be so far removed from the end of the casting ring that it is difficult for the gases to be vented so that the metal fills the mold completely. If the gases are not completely eliminated, a type of porosity referred to as "back pressure" porosity develops. This effect will also be discussed in greater detail in the following chapter. A good rule to follow is to adjust the sprue length so that the portion of the wax pattern farthest from the sprue pin is within 6.5 mm (¼ inch) of the open end of the ring. In the next chapter it will be noted that the expansion of the investment is not uniform throughout the ring. Thus, in order to minimize distortion and establish reproducibility of casting accuracy, some manufacturers recommend placement of the pattern as close to the center of the ring as possible.

The material of which the sprue former is made is important. A carbon

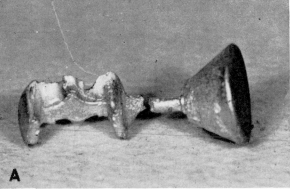

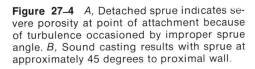

Figure 27–4 *A,* Detached sprue indicates severe porosity at point of attachment because of turbulence occasioned by improper sprue angle. *B,* Sound casting results with sprue at approximately 45 degrees to proximal wall.

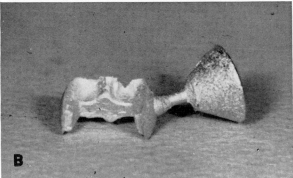

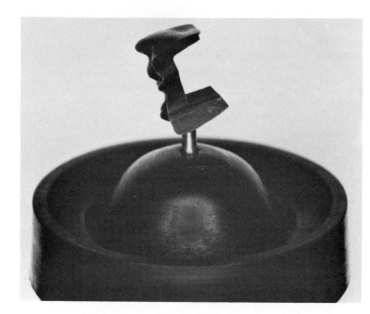

Figure 27–5 Sprue former attached to wax pattern and crucible former.

steel or iron sprue pin in contact with the wet investment is apt to rust. When withdrawn, iron rust is likely to cling to the walls of the ingate, later to contaminate the gold alloy. Plastic sprues, especially if solid, soften above the melting point of inlay waxes. This may prevent expansion and/or outflow of the wax, causing possible distortion or cracking of the mold. Therefore, if a metal sprue pin is used it should be stainless steel or brass. If resin, then it should be hollow.

The metal sprue former should be heated as little as possible before it is attached to the pattern. However, care should be taken that it is firmly held by the pattern so that it does not pull loose during the investing procedure. A hollow sprue pin is especially recommended because of its greater retention to the pattern.

The sprue pin is best attached to the pattern while the latter is in position on the die or in the tooth, provided that it can be attached so that the pattern can be removed directly in line with the principal axis of the tooth or the prepared cavity. In such a case, any visible distortion of the pattern can be detected and repaired. If the direction of the sprue pin after attachment is such that the pattern cannot be removed from the prepared cavity without a tipping or a twisting, the pattern should be removed with a sharp explorer point or a U-shaped staple as previously described, and the sprue former should be carefully attached to the pattern after it has been laid on the bench or table.

The sprue former with the pattern is then attached to the *sprue base* or *crucible former,* which may be made of metal, rubber, or some type of resin. A typical crucible former, with the wax pattern attached, can be seen in Figure 27–5.

THE LINER

Provision must be made for the setting expansion of the investment. The solid metal ring or casting flask inhibits the setting expansion. In fact, the mold may become smaller rather than larger because of the reverse pressure resulting from the confinement of the setting expansion. This disadvantage can be overcome by the use of a three-part split ring or by the use of very flexible rubber rings, either of which can be increased in volume by the force of the setting expansion.

Possibly the most widely used means of preventing the confinement of the setting expansion is to line the casting ring with a sheet of asbestos, or comparable material, to form a cushion for the setting expansion. The liner also prevents the restriction of the investment thermal expansion by the metal ring. In order to prevent possible folding of the liner during vacuum investing, it is desirable to line the ring with dry liner and tack it to the ring with pliable sticky wax at the junctions. The lined ring is then immersed in water for a time to permit full sorption of the water. The excess water is merely shaken off. Squeezing the liner will remove the water in a variable manner.

Not only does the liner afford greater normal setting expansion in the investment but also the absorbed water causes a semihygroscopic expansion as it is drawn into the investment during setting, as shown in the curves in Figure 27–6. The use of one liner (C) produces an increase in excess of the normal setting expansion. Thicker material or two layers (D) provide even greater semihydroscopic expansion and also affords a more unrestricted normal setting expansion of the investment. This observation can be taken advantage of in order to increase the expansion modestly if desired, by using two liners instead of one. In any case the thickness of the liner should not be less than approximately 1 mm.

The desired length of the liner remains a matter of controversy. If the length of the liner is somewhat shorter than the ring itself, the investment is confined at the ends of the ring. The longitudinal setting and hygroscopic

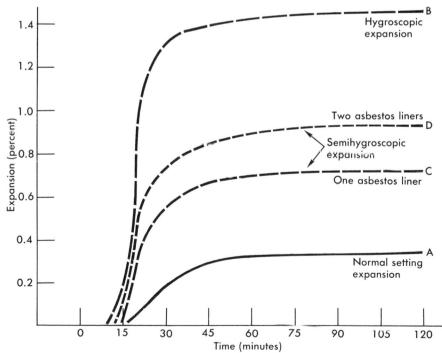

Figure 27–6   Normal setting (A) and hygroscopic expansion (B) of an investment as compared to the somewhat restricted expansion that occurs in an inlay ring lined with one (C) and two (D) asbestos liners. (From R. Neiman, Whip-Mix Corp.)

expansion are thereby restricted, as compared with using a liner that is flush with the ends of the ring.

However, the expansion of the investment is always greater in the unrestricted direction, i.e., longitudinally, than in the lateral direction, toward the ring itself. It is, therefore, desirable to reduce the expansion in the longitudinal direction. Placing the liner somewhat short of the ends of the ring, 3 mm (⅛ inch), tends to produce a more uniform expansion, and there is less chance for distortion of the wax pattern and the mold.

In recent years there has been concern that asbestos might be a health hazard, in light of its carcinogenic potential if inhaled in the form of micrometer size particles. However, the type used for lining rings, as described, has a good binder. There is no evidence that with careful use it poses any danger.

Nonetheless, it is possible that asbestos could become unavailable in the foreseeable future. Therefore, manufacturers have been providing substitutes. These are of two general types. One consists of an organic cellulose material that has the same water sorption as asbestos and provides a comparable setting expansion of the investment. However, it does burn away during burnout. This could permit the investment mold to slide out of the ring when lifted out of the furnace. Thus it is essential that such liners be approximately 3 mm (⅛ inch) short of both ends of the ring.

The other substitute consists of a silica-alumina fiber paper. The water sorption of this type of liner is very low but it does have a marked "cushioning" effect and permits some setting expansion and complete thermal expansion of the investment. It also must be kept short of the ends of the ring.

INVESTING

The wax pattern should be cleansed of any surface dirt and the separating medium. A number of commercial products are available, or a diluted synthetic detergent may be used. The pattern is then rinsed with room temperature water and gently air-dried, or a little of the cleaner may be left on the pattern to act as a wetting agent.

The investment and water should be proportioned accurately for the reasons outlined in the previous chapter. The same precautions should be observed in mixing the water and investment as were outlined for the mixing of plaster or stone. The investment powder should be sifted into the water so that the least possible amount of air is introduced at this stage. The mixture can then be vibrated to remove any large air bubbles. If the mixing is done by hand, the mixture should not be whipped during the process.

The use of a mechanical mixer, either hand or motor driven, is recommended. The revolution of the paddle is so rapid that any air bubbles are broken up to the extent that their effect on the surface roughness of the casting is minimized. The investment is then vibrated a second time after it has been mixed.

In general, there are two methods for investing the wax pattern. The most common is to attach the sprued pattern to the crucible former, which in turn is attached to the lined casting ring. Under mild vibration the investment is flowed around it to fill the ring. In the second method the lined casting ring is first filled with investment, and then the crucible former with the attached pattern is gently forced, with slight agitation, into the investment until the crucible former and ring are in contact. The investment may be allowed to set with the ring supporting the crucible former, or the unit may be turned over so that the crucible former supports the ring.

In either technique, and especially the second, the wax pattern may be painted with a layer of investment before it is forced into the investment filled ring. Also, it is generally advantageous to coat the wax pattern with a surface tension reducing agent before painting on the investment. Since such a surfactant retards the setting of gypsum, the excess wetting agent should be removed from the pattern with a damp sable brush or a gentle air stream before applying the investment.

If the hygroscopic technique is employed, the casting ring, with the crucible former end down, is immediately immersed in a water bath at a temperature of 37 to 38° C (98.6 to 100° F). For the thermal expansion technique, the investment is allowed to harden in the ring placed on the bench. In either case, the wax elimination described in the next chapter is not started for at least one hour after investing the pattern.

Control of the Shrinkage Compensation   On occasion, it may be desirable to increase or reduce the mold dimensions. For example, a greater compensation for the casting shrinkage may be required for the MOD inlay or full cast crown than for a simple occlusal inlay. In the former case, even a slightly undersized casting does not seat completely because of the friction between the casting and the cavity walls, which are generally long and parallel. Furthermore, the configuration of the pattern may also influence the effective setting or hygroscopic expansion. The proximal walls of a thin, delicate pattern offer less resistance and are more readily moved during the setting of the investment than walls that are bulky or continuous as in the full cast crown.

A number of factors influence the dimensions of the casting. As previously discussed, two liners allow more setting and thermal expansion than does a single liner.

The direction at which the sprue former is attached to the wax pattern influences the dimensions of the casting to a certain extent. For example, if the MOD pattern shown in Figure 27–3 had been sprued on the occlusal surface, the mesio-distal expansion would be restricted somewhat by the metal ring, even when a liner is employed. The inadequate expansion in this direction could prevent a complete seating of the casting. Under certain conditions a somewhat different fit of the casting might result if the sprue is attached to a proximal surface of the pattern, as shown in Figure 27–3, so that the mesio-distal expansion is in a direction toward the open ends of the ring.

The setting, hygroscopic, and thermal expansions of investments can be controlled to a certain extent by varying the W/P ratio. The less the W/P ratio, the greater is the shrinkage compensation, and the converse is true. For example, one experiment demonstrates that a difference in the fit of a casting can be detected when the gauging water is changed only 0.5 ml.[13] With some investments the effect of the W/P ratio is less significant.

However, there is a limit to which the W/P ratio can be reduced. If the mix is too thick, it cannot be applied to the wax pattern without a likelihood of distorting the pattern and of producing air voids during the investing. There is also a practical limitation on how much the W/P ratio can be increased in order to reduce the expansion. If the water-investment mixture is too thin, a rough surface on the casting results.

The problem of too much expansion of the mold in the thermal expansion technique using cristobalite investment may be important. As can be noted from Figure 26–7, a thermal expansion of 1.3 per cent may take place with such an investment. If an effective setting expansion of 0.3 to 0.4 per cent is added to such a thermal expansion, a total linear expansion as high as 1.7 per cent may be obtained. Such an expansion is definitely higher than the average casting shrinkage of the gold alloy and, as a result, the casting may be too large.

In addition to control of the hygroscopic expansion by the W/P ratio, the hygroscopic expansion can be regulated either by reducing the time of immersion of the setting investment or by controlling the amount of water to be added during the setting. The longer the delay before the investment is immersed in the water bath, the less is the hygroscopic expansion.

The modern hygroscopic investment technique generally provides correct expansion for most types of patterns. However, some may require a variation in expansion. A popular method is to vary the W/P ratio. Use of a softer wax will provide greater expansion than if a hard wax was employed.[14] Increasing the burnout temperature and the water bath temperature will also increase the expansion, and decreasing these temperatures will decrease expansion. None of these methods should be carried to an extreme, however.

In one technique the shrinkage compensation is controlled by the addition of water during the setting of the investment, as described in the preceding chapter. This method is usually referred to as the *controlled water added technique.*

Controlled Water Added Technique   As shown in Figure 26–5, the linear hygroscopic expansion increases directly with the amount of water added until a maximal expansion is attained. The investments for use with the water added hygroscopic casting technique are so composed that their maximal expansion during immersion in water exceeds the desired mold compensation. The desired amount of hygroscopic expansion is then obtained by adding only enough water to the investment to provide the desired expansion.

A soft, flexible rubber ring is employed instead of the usual asbestos-lined metal ring. The pattern is invested as usual. A specified amount of water is then added on the top of the investment in the rubber ring and the investment is allowed to set, usually at room temperature. The crucible former, the sprue former, and the rubber ring are removed prior to the elimination of the wax.

The confining effect of the wax pattern may be reduced by a softening of the occlusal portion of the wax pattern. This can be done by placing the setting investment in a water bath at 38° C (100° F) but keeping the water level below the top of the ring, or by using a softer wax at the occlusal and in conjunction with a bench set of the investment.[15]

Vacuum Investing   One of the defects of a casting is likely to be the presence of nodules on its surface, caused by the collection of air bubbles during the investing. If the precautions previously outlined are observed, there is no reason why an excellent surface on the casting cannot be obtained routinely, particularly after a certain degree of skill and experience has been acquired.

However, if the personal equation in this regard is to be eliminated, the logical solution is to subject the water-investment mixture to a vacuum during the investing procedure, in order to remove the air bubbles. A representative dental vacuum investing device is shown in Figure 27–7. The unit illustrated utilizes a vacuum both for mixing and investing.

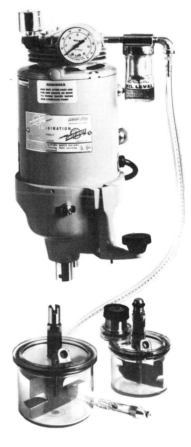

Figure 27–7   A combination motor driven mixer-investor and vacuum pump. The direct-drive chuck, when viewed from above, turns counterclockwise at 1750 rpm. The gear driven chuck, nearest the viewer, rotates clockwise at 425 rpm and is used to drive the shaft and blades of vacuum mixers, such as the 500 ml unit in the foreground. The 200 ml investor, right, is driven by the direct drive chuck. (Courtesy of R. Neiman, Whip-Mix Corp.)

The porosity of the investment is definitely reduced by vacuum investing, presumably because of the increased density obtained. As a result, the texture of the surface of the casting is somewhat smoother, with better reproduction of fine detail. The compressive strength of the investment is increased slightly by the vacuum investing.

Not all of the air is removed under the vacuum treatment. The amount removed depends somewhat upon the consistency of the mix. The more viscous the mix, the more air bubbles remain in the investment. However, a thick mix is usually necessary because of the desired shrinkage compensation, and because of the poor surface texture that is obtained with a thin mix.

Apparently, air bubbles can be entrapped on flat or concave surfaces facing away from the direction of the air evacuation. In order to minimize this effect, the pattern should be tilted whenever possible so that the water vapor bubbles can stream across all of the surfaces of the pattern as they rise to the top, and thus remove any clinging air bubbles. Vibration will cause any air in the investment to rise and will free the upper surfaces of the pattern from air bubbles. However, it will enhance the chance for bubbles to collect on the bottom surfaces. As mentioned, tilting of the pattern is helpful.

If vibration is excessive, it may even cause solids in the investment to settle and leave free water against the surface of the pattern, resulting in roughness.

As previously stated, equally good results can be obtained with hand investing as with vacuum investing. However, the latter method is probably more dependable in the prevention of surface nodules. In a comparison of the two methods, a study indicated that 95 per cent of the vacuum-invested castings made were free from nodules, whereas only 17 per cent of the castings made from hand-invested patterns by the same operators were entirely free from nodules.[16] Freedom from surface imperfections is highly important, as even a tiny nodule on a casting may damage a frail enamel margin when the casting is tried in the prepared cavity. The finished casting should always be checked under magnification for such defects.

References

1. Christensen GJ: Marginal fit of gold inlay castings. J Prosthet Dent 16:297, 1966.
2. Suffert LW and Mahler DB: Reproducibility of gold castings made by present day dental casting technics. J Am Dent Assoc 50:1, 1955.
3. Toreskog S, Phillips RW, and Schnell RJ: Properties of die materials. A comparative study. J Prosthet Dent 16:119, 1966.
4. Sanad MEE, Combe EC, and Grant AA: Hardening of model and die materials by an epoxy resin. J Dent 8:158, 1980.
5. Finger W: Effect of the setting expansion of dental stone upon the die precision. Scand J Dent Res 88:159, 1980.
6. Jorgensen KD and Finger W: Die-spacing technique by diffusion precipitation. Scand J Dent Res 87:73, 1979.
7. Eames WB, O'Neal SJ, Monteiro J, Miller C, Roan JD, and Cohen KS: Techniques to improve the seating of castings. J Am Dent Assoc 96:432, 1978.
8. Baum L, Phillips RW, and Lund MR: Textbook of Operative Dentistry, Philadelphia, W. B. Saunders Co., 1981.
9. Nomura GT, Reisbick MH, and Preston JD: An investigation of epoxy resin dies. J. Prosthet Dent 44:45, 1980.
10. Moser JB, Stone DG, and Willoughby GM: Properties and characteristics of a resin die material. J Prosthet Dent 34:297, 1975.
11. Stackhouse JA: Linear dimensions of electrodeposits and impression material substrates. IADR Program and Abstracts, No. 195, 1979.
12. Asgar K and Peyton FA: Pits on inner surfaces of cast gold crowns. J Prosthet Dent 9:448, 1959.
13. Martin KH: An investigation of the effect of the water/powder ratio on the accuracy of the fit of gold alloy castings. Aust Dent J 1:202, 1956.
14. Mahler DB and Ady AB: The effect of the water bath in hygroscopic casting techniques. J Prosthet Dent 15:1115, 1965.
15. Cecconi BT and Asgar K: Modified hygroscopic gold casting technique. J Prosthet Dent 33:216, 1975.
16. Lyon HW, Dickson G, and Schoonover IC: Effectiveness of vacuum investing in the elimination of surface defects of gold castings. J Am Dent Assoc 46:197, 1953.

28 NOBLE METAL ALLOY CASTING PROCEDURES (CONTINUED): WAX ELIMINATION AND CASTING.

The fundamentals associated with the casting procedure itself are common to both gypsum and phosphate-bonded investments. Thus, although the following discussion is focused upon gypsum investments, most of it is germane to the other type. However, later in the chapter a section is devoted to special considerations for the phosphate investments.

After the investment has hardened for at least one hour, the wax elimination and heating of the investment to the casting temperature can be started. The crucible former is removed carefully so that the metal or plastic sprue former remains in the investment. Any loosely attached investment around the edge of the ring is removed as shown in Figure 28–1. Unless it is wax or hollow plastic, the sprue former is then carefully removed so that the surface around the ingate is not chipped. The ring should then be inverted and any small particles of investment in the area of the ingate removed with a camel's hair brush. As an added precaution, the inverted ring should be rapped sharply on the top of the laboratory bench to remove any particles that may have fallen into the ingate.

Wax Elimination and Heating There are at least two methods by which the wax can be removed from the mold. One is to remove it by flushing the mold with boiling water. A disadvantage of the method is that some of the very fine detail of the mold may be lost by a solution or a disintegration of the gypsum binder.

In most of the techniques under discussion, the wax pattern is eliminated by heat. In the thermal expansion technique, the casting ring containing the invested pattern is heated slowly to the temperature at which the maximal thermal expansion of the investment is obtained, usually 700° C (1292° F).

For all practical purposes, some investments attain their maximum expansion at 650° C (1200° F). With those materials, heating the mold to this temperature only is preferred, for it minimizes the chance for investment decomposition, as will be described.

Some of the melted wax is absorbed by the investment and the residual carbon from the ignition becomes trapped in the investment. If the thermal expansion technique is employed, the mold is heated sufficiently so that a great deal of the carbon is removed in the form of carbon monoxide or dioxide.

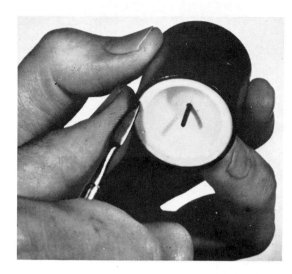

Figure 28–1 Any loose pieces of investment around the edge of the ring should be carefully removed as shown.

It is best to start the burnout while the mold is still wet. The water in the pores of the investment reduces the absorption of the wax, and as the water boils, it tends to flush the wax out. This is facilitated by placing the ring with the sprue hole down. For these reasons, if the mold must be stored overnight, it should be kept in a humidor or in water.

In the hygroscopic technique, the ring is heated no higher than 480° C (900° F) because an appreciable thermal expansion of the investment is not desired. Even though the mold is usually held at this temperature for 60 to 90 minutes, sufficient residual fine carbon may be retained to reduce the venting of the mold. Because of this, back pressure porosity is a greater hazard in the low heat technique than in the high heat technique. Likewise, the investments generally employed with the low heat technique may be more dense.

Muffle furnaces are often so airtight that burnout takes place in a reducing atmosphere, preventing complete oxidation of the wax residues. Keeping the door open slightly permits air to enter and provides enough oxygen for elimination of the wax. This is particularly important for the hygroscopic expansion technique when a lower burnout temperature is used.

The rate at which the investment is heated is a factor in producing a smooth surface on the casting. If heating is too rapid at the start, the steam resulting from the elimination of the free water and water of crystallization may cause the walls of the mold to flake off as the steam emerges from the investment. In extreme cases, the steam pressure may build up within the investment to such an extent that an explosion may occur. In such a case, the entire mold may fracture or disintegrate.

Too rapid heating may also cause cracking in the investment. In such a case, the outside layer of the investment becomes heated before the center portions. Consequently, the outside layer starts to expand thermally, resulting in compressive stress in the outside layer counteracting tensile stresses in the middle regions of the mold. Such a stress distribution causes the brittle investment to crack from the interior outwardly in the form of radial cracks. These cracks in turn will produce a casting with fins or spines similar to those shown in Figure 28–2. This condition is especially likely to be present after a too rapid heating of a cristobalite investment. The comparatively low inversion

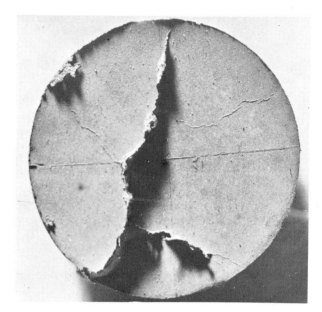

Figure 28–2 Fins on the surface of a casting which formed as a result of cracks in the investment.

temperature of the cristobalite, and the rapid rate of expansion during the inversion, makes it especially important to heat the investment slowly.

A safe heating period for any inlay investment is not less than 60 minutes and preferably longer. The amount of thermal expansion does apparently vary somewhat with the rate of heating, although the exact effect is still controversial and may vary for the type of investment. Several studies have shown that fast heating produces an additional expansion for a quartz investment but merely alters the shape of the expansion curve for a cristobalite investment.[1, 2] On the other hand, another investigation found that when a certain quartz investment was heated to 700° C (1292° F) in 3 hours, its linear thermal expansion was 1.15 per cent. When the same investment was heated to that same temperature in only 9 minutes, the expansion was only 0.89 per cent.[3]

Nevertheless, it is apparent that the rate of heating may alter the size of the casting, at least of those produced by a quartz investment. For this reason the heat rate and time prescribed should be followed.

In the thermal expansion technique, the ring is placed in a furnace at room temperature. In the low heat technique, the ring can be placed in an oven preheated to 480° C (900° F) without fear of the investment cracking during the wax elimination.

Although a gas furnace can be used if special care is observed in regulating the heat, an electric furnace is more easily controlled. The ring is inverted when placed into the furnace so that the crucible end is in contact with the bottom of the muffle. This position permits some of the wax to drain out of the sprue. It also prevents any small fragments of investment that may become dislodged during the wax elimination from falling down into the mold. If the ring is resting directly on the surface of the furnace muffle, the position of the ring should be reversed near the end of the burnout period. With the sprue hole facing upward, oxygen can more readily contact the wax and ensure a complete elimination. Sometimes the ring is placed on perforated or slotted ceramic trays. In such a case, the circulation of air beneath the ring is adequate and it is not necessary to invert the ring.

With the thermal expansion technique, the heating is continued until a temperature of 700° C (1292° F) is reached, as indicated by a pyrometer. However, as mentioned earlier, a temperature of 650° C (1200° F) is usually adequate and much safer. At this temperature, the sprue is cherry red when it is viewed in a shadow. In direct light this color is an indication of a much higher temperature. If the investment is heated to a too high temperature, a rough casting results, as well as a possible contamination of the gold alloy with sulfur, because of the chemical disintegration of the investment.

Contamination of the gold alloy and resulting brittleness in the casting, because of a breakdown of dental investments, is probably more common than generally realized. Sulfur gases are given off by gypsum investments when heated above 700° C. The mechanism of this investment decomposition and alloy contamination is related to a chemical reaction between the residual carbon and the calcium sulfate binder.[4]

Calcium sulfate *per se* does not decompose unless heated to about 1000° C (1832° F). However, the reduction of calcium sulfate by carbon takes place rapidly above 700° C in accordance with the following reactions:

$$CaSO_4 + 4C \rightarrow CaS + 4CO$$
$$3CaSO_4 + CaS \rightarrow 4CaO + 4SO_2$$

Thus, this reaction takes place whenever gypsum investments are heated above 700° C in the presence of carbon. The sulfur dioxide as a product of this reaction contaminates gold castings and makes them extremely brittle. This fact places emphasis, then, upon completely eliminating the wax and avoiding burnout temperatures above 700° C, particularly if the investment contains graphite.

Consequently, the furnace should be equipped with an accurate pyrometer and thermocouple. Furthermore, after the casting temperature has been obtained, the casting should be made immediately. A maintenance of the high casting temperature for any considerable period may result in a sulfur

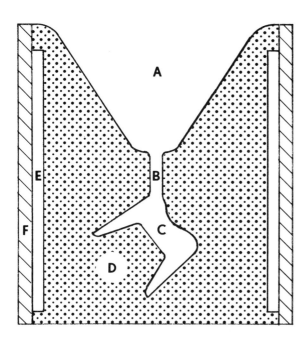

Figure 28–3 A diagrammatic representation of a dental casting mold: A, crucible former; B, sprue; C, wax pattern; D, investment; E, liner; F, casting ring. (Courtesy of A. Steinbock, Whip-Mix Corp.)

contamination of the casting as indicated and also in a rough surface on the casting owing to the disintegration of the investment.

Obviously, with a mold temperature of 480° C (900° F), as is employed with the low heat technique, the danger of contamination of the gold alloy because of the disintegration of the investment is nonexistent despite any excessive amount of carbon present. Furthermore, with quartz investments the rate of heating is less critical with this technique because the quartz inversion occurs above this temperature.

Because the wax is eliminated less rapidly in the low heat technique, the ring should be held at the casting temperature of 480° C (900° F) for a minimum of 45 minutes in order to insure complete wax elimination.

A diagrammatic representation of a longitudinal section of the mold as it should appear after elimination of the wax is shown in Figure 28–3. The entire mold, including the ingate, is filled with molten alloy, with sufficient metal left over in the crucible to form the *button*. Before the casting is placed in the mouth, the sprue portion is cut through close to the casting, and the excess metal is saved for recasting.

Time Allowable for Casting   As noted in Chapter 26, the investment contracts thermally as it cools. When the thermal expansion or high heat technique is used, it can be expected that after the heated ring is removed from the furnace the investment loses heat, and the mold contracts. Owing to the presence of the asbestos liner, and to the low thermal conductivity of the investment, a short period can elapse before the temperature of the mold is appreciably affected. Under average conditions of casting, approximately one minute can pass without a noticeable loss in dimension.

In the low heat casting technique, the temperature gradient between the investment mold and the room is not so great as that employed with the high heat technique. Also, the thermal expansion of the investment is not so important to the shrinkage compensation. However, the burnout temperature lies on a fairly steep portion of the thermal expansion curve rather than on a plateau portion as in the high heat technique. Therefore, in the low heat casting technique the alloy should also be cast soon after removal of the ring from the oven.

Casting Machines   There are several types of casting machines: (1) the alloy is melted in situ in the crucible hollow of the ring, followed by an applied air pressure on the melt (Fig. 28–4); (2) the alloy is melted in a separate crucible and the metal cast into the mold by centrifugal force (Fig. 28–5); (3) the alloy is melted electrically by a resistance or induction furnace, then cast into the mold centrifugally by motor or spring action. A representative casting machine of this type is shown in Figure 28–6; (4) the alloy is melted as in (3) but cast by air pressure and/or vacuum assist.

The general procedure for each is described below, with certain advantages and disadvantages cited. However, it is important to follow the manufacturer's directions precisely.

1. Although the alloy is melted in the hollow left by the crucible former, the high surface tension of the liquid metal prevents it from falling down into the sprue channel. Once the metal has been melted to the casting temperature, the airtight piston is applied with 10 to 15 psi air pressure to force the metal into the mold. In a thin-walled crown the mold will fill in less than a second with solidification of the metal beginning in about 1 second and completed in

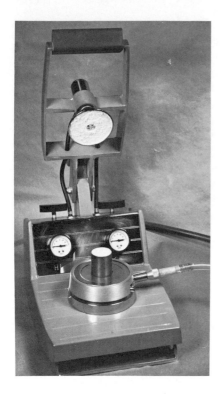

Figure 28–4 An air pressure casting machine with the ring in position. The gold alloy is melted directly in the crucible formed in the investment. Above the ring can be seen the piston through which the air pressure is applied, forcing the molten alloy into the mold. The table below the ring may be connected to a source of vacuum which is activated just before the pressure starts.

approximately 5 seconds. With larger castings, these time intervals may be doubled.

The pressure gradient along the sprue axis and casting is almost nil, with the pressure in the liquid metal being essentially that applied by the air

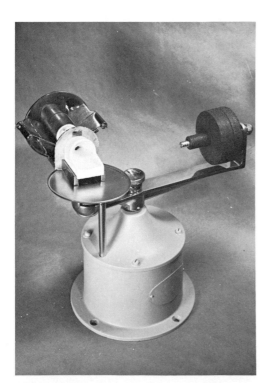

Figure 28–5 A centrifugal casting machine.

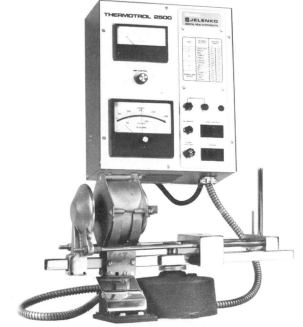

Figure 28–6 A spring wound electrical resistance melting furnace casting machine. (Courtesy of J. Tuccillo, Jelenko Co.)

pressure. This means that the heat loss in the metal is mostly dependent upon the thickness in different parts of the casting; the thinner the section, the faster is the solidification. The button being the thickest section, and also in the region where the casting ring was additionally heated during melting, ensures that the solidification essentially progresses from the tip end of the casting to the button.

2. Here the casting machine spring is first wound from 2 to 5 turns (depending upon the particular machine and the speed of casting rotation desired). The metal is melted by a blowpipe in a ceramic crucible attached to one of the arms of the casting machine. The other arm usually has a "broken arm" feature that assists in speeding the molten metal into the mold. Once the metal has reached the casting temperature, the machine is released and the spring triggers the rotational motion. The peak speed is reached in less than 1 second, gradually slowing down in approximately a minute. The spring should be such that the peak rotation speed is from 5 to 8 rps, maintaining this rotational speed for the 5 seconds or so while the metal freezes.

Once the metal fills the mold there is a hydrostatic pressure gradient developed along the length of the casting. The four factors that contribute to this pressure gradient are: (a) rotational speed; (b) the geometry of the casting machine (the radial distance from the casting to the rotation axis being the key value); (c) the geometry of the casting and sprue; the longer the distance from the button to the tip of the casting, the greater is the pressure at the tip and; (d) the metal density.[5]

The pressure gradient from the tip of the casting to the button surface is quite sharp and parabolic in function, coming to zero at the button surface. Ordinarily the pressure gradient at the moment before freezing begins reaches about 30–40 psi at the tip of the casting. Because of this gradient, there is also a gradient in the heat transfer rate such that the greatest rate of heat transfer to the mold is at the high pressure end of the gradient, i.e., the tip of the casting. Since this end is also frequently the sharp edge of the margin of a crown, there is a double assurance that the solidification progresses from the tip to the button surface.

3. In this case there is an automatic melting of the metal in a graphite crucible in a furnace rather than by use of a blow pipe. This is an advantage, especially for certain alloys, such as those used for metal-ceramic restorations, which are delicately alloyed with trace base metals that tend to oxidize on overheating. Another advantage is that the crucible in the furnace is located flush against the casting ring. Therefore, the button remains molten slightly longer, again ensuring that solidification progresses completely from the tip of the casting to the button surface. However, as noted in Chapter 26, a carbon crucible should not be used in the melting of high palladium alloys, where the temperature exceeds 1504° C (2740° F). Carbon crucibles should also not be used with base metal alloys.

4. With this unit, the metal is melted, either by electrical resistance or induction, in a graphite crucible integral with the casting machine. Once it reaches the casting temperature, the metal is forced into the mold by air pressure and/or vacuum at the other end of the ring. The device has become very popular in the casting of jewelry but to date has not been used as much as the other three for dental castings. Here, again, there is no pressure gradient except for a slight gravity head from the surface of the button to the tip of the casting.

So far as is known, there is little practical difference in the properties or accuracy of castings made with any of the four types. The choice is a matter of personal preference.

Fusing the Noble Metal Alloy   The alloy is best melted by placing it on the side of the crucible. In this position, the operator can better observe the progress of the melting, and there is a greater opportunity for any gases in the flame to be reflected from the surface of the metal rather than to be absorbed.

The fuel employed in most cases is a mixture of natural or artificial gas and air, although oxygen-air and acetylene can also be used. The temperature of the gas-air flame is greatly influenced by the nature of the gas and the proportions of gas and air in the mixture. Considerable care should be taken to obtain a nonluminous brush flame, with the different combustion zones clearly differentiated.

Two types of flame that can be obtained with the gas-air blowpipe are shown in Figure 28–7. The air supply for the lower flame is excessive, and

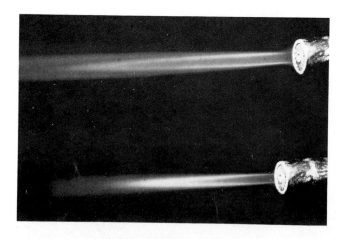

Figure 28–7 Two types of nonluminous flame showing combustion areas. The upper flame should be employed for fusing the noble metal alloy. The lower flame results from too much air in the mixture.

incomplete combustion and a lower temperature result. This type of flame is likely to be favored by the beginner because the roaring sound that accompanies this flame adjustment "sounds hot." The upper brush flame indicates the proper adjustment for maximal efficiency and temperature.

The parts of the flame can be identified by the conical areas. The first long cone emanating directly from the nozzle is the zone in which the air and gas are mixed before combustion. No heat is present in this zone. The next cone, which is green and immediately surrounding the inner cone, is known as the *combustion zone*. Here, the gas and air are in partial combustion. This zone is definitely oxidizing and it should always be kept away from the metal during fusion.

The next zone, dimly blue, is the *reducing zone*. It is the hottest part of the flame and is just beyond the tip of the green combustion zone. This area should be kept constantly on the metal during fusion. The outer cone (*oxidizing zone*) is the area in which combustion occurs with the oxygen in the air. Under no circumstances should this portion of the flame be employed to fuse the alloy. Not only is its temperature lower than that of the reducing zone, but also it causes oxidation of the metal.

With a little practice, the proper zone in contact with the metal can be readily detected by the condition of the metal surface. When the reducing zone is in contact, the surface of the alloy is bright and mirror-like, as indicated in Figure 28-8A. When the oxidizing portion of the flame is in contact with the metal there is a dull film of "dross" developed over the surface, as seen in Figure 28-8B.

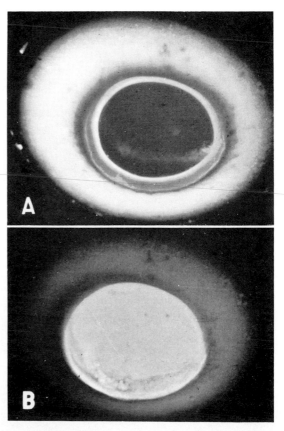

Figure 28–8 *A,* Mirror-like surface of the metal indicates proper fusion. *B,* Cloudy surface indicates surface oxidation by blowpipe flame.

Although care should be taken not to overheat the alloy, there is generally more likelihood of underheating when the gas-air flame is used. The alloy first appears to be spongy, and then small globules of fused metal appear. A gradual spheroiding of the bulk of the alloy occurs as indicated in Figure 28–8A. At the proper casting temperature, the molten alloy is light orange and tends to spin or follow the flame when the latter is moved slightly. Ideally at this point, the metal should be approximately 38 to 66° C (100 to 150° F) above its liquidus temperature. The casting should be made immediately when the proper temperature is reached.

As previously discussed, there are also various devices available for melting the alloy electrically.

It is desirable to use a flux to aid in minimizing porosity. When properly employed, the flux increases the fluidity of the metal and the film of flux formed on the surface of the molten alloy helps to prevent oxidation. Reducing fluxes containing powdered charcoal are often used, but small bits of carbon may be carried into the mold and cause a deficiency at a critical margin. Although such reducing fluxes are excellent for cleaning old metal, a better flux for the casting procedure itself may be made from equal parts of fused borax powder ground with boric acid powder. The boric acid aids in retaining the borax on the surface of the metal. The flux is added when the alloy is completely melted and should be used with both old and new metal.

Old sprues and buttons from the same alloy may be recast if they are not contaminated or have not been unduly abused, as was noted in Chapter 24. The metal is placed on a charcoal block, melted, and adequately fluxed, in this case with a reducing flux containing powdered charcoal (Fig. 28–9). A common mistake is to remove the blowpipe prematurely, which permits the molten metal to absorb gas from the atmosphere, with a resulting oxidation of the metal. Proper procedure is to turn the air off and allow the luminous gas flame to protect the surface until the solidification is complete (Fig. 28–10).

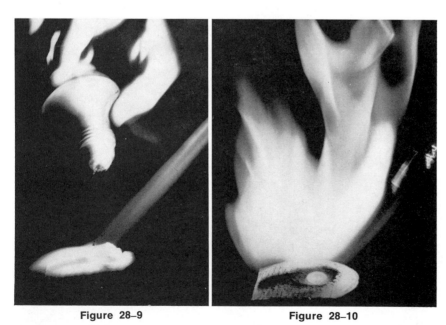

Figure 28–9   **Figure 28–10**

Figure 28–9 Melting "scrap gold" on a charcoal block. An adequate amount of reducing flux is used.

Figure 28–10 After the "scrap gold" has been fused, it should be cooled in a luminous gas flame to prevent oxidation and gas occlusion.

Cleaning the Casting   After the casting has been completed, the ring is removed and quenched in water as soon as the button emits a dull red glow. Two advantages are gained in quenching: (1) The noble metal alloy is left in an annealed condition for burnishing, polishing, and similar procedures. (2) When the water contacts the hot investment, a violent reaction ensues. The investment becomes soft and granular, and the casting is more easily cleaned.

Often the surface of the casting appears dark with oxides and tarnish. Such a surface film can be removed by a process known as *pickling,* which consists of heating the discolored casting in an acid. Probably the best pickling solution for gypsum-bonded investments is a 50 per cent hydrochloric acid solution. The hydrochloric acid aids in the removal of any clinging investment as well as of the oxide coating. The disadvantage of the use of hydrochloric acid is that the fumes from the acid are likely to corrode office and laboratory metal furnishings. A similar solution of sulfuric acid is more advantageous in this respect. Ultrasonic devices are also available for cleaning the casting, as are commercial pickling agents of solutions of acid salts.

The best method for pickling is to place the casting in a test tube or dish and to pour the acid over it. It may be necessary to heat the acid, but boiling should be avoided because of the considerable amount of acid fumes evolved. After pickling, the acid is poured off and the casting is removed. The pickling solution should be renewed frequently, as it is likely to become contaminated with use.

In no case should the casting be held with steel tongs so that both the casting and the tongs come into contact with the pickling solution. If this is done, the casting may become contaminated. The pickling solution usually contains small amounts of copper dissolved from previous castings. When the steel tongs contact this electrolyte, a small galvanic cell is created and copper is deposited on the casting at the point where the tongs grip it. This copper deposition extends into the metal and is a future source for discoloration in the area.

It is a common practice to heat the casting and then to drop it into the pickling solution. The disadvantage of this method is that a delicate margin may be melted in the flame or the casting may be distorted by the sudden thermal shock when plunged into the acid.

After the pickling, the casting should be washed thoroughly in running water to insure that the acid is completely removed.

Technical Considerations for Phosphate-Bonded Investments   When investing a wax pattern in a phosphate-bonded investment, the procedure is essentially the same as for a gypsum-bonded investment. As previously mentioned, the working time can vary depending upon the liquid/powder ratio, temperature, mixing time and rate, and operator skill and experience.

When phosphate investments found their way into dental laboratories that were also using gypsum investments, some problems arose with faulty setting of the investments and imperfect castings. Specifically, castings made in gypsum investments, following the use of phosphate investments, were inferior. It was learned that traces of phosphate investments posed difficulties in the setting of gypsum investments. Any residual investment particles left in the mixing bowls, even after thorough washing, are sufficient to influence the behavior of the gypsum materials. Manufacturers now caution users to use separate mixing bowls for the two different types of investment.

As with any investment having a high thermal expansion and with marked changes in expansion occurring, or even an actual contraction, it is necessary to use slow heating during burnout in order to prevent possible cracking or spalling. Some furnaces have means for slowing the rate of heating. With those that do not, it is advisable to use a two stage burnout, holding at 200–300° C (400–500° F) for at least 30 minutes before completing the burnout.

Although phosphate investments appear very strong, they are still subject to a number of disrupting influences during burnout. At first the wax softens and then expands much more than does the investment. When investing, it is desirable to leave 3–6 mm of investment around each pattern and to stagger the patterns if several are placed in the same ring. A number of patterns in one plane can exert tremendous pressure and fracture almost any investment but particularly the phosphate-bonded materials. The rapid expansion of the cristobalite at approximately 300° C (600° F) requires slow heating to prevent fracture. After the temperature reaches 400° C (800° F), the rate of heating can be safely increased.

After burnout, usually at a final temperature of 700–900° C (1300–1650° F) depending upon the alloy melting range, the casting is made. As previously mentioned, the permeability of the phosphate investment is low in relation to that of a gypsum-bonded investment. Therefore, the required casting pressure should be greater than for a gypsum mold.

Recovery and cleaning of the casting is more difficult when a phosphate-bonded investment is used because such materials do not contain the soft gypsum products. Also, the particles usually include large grains of quartz. In some cases, such as with gold-containing alloys, the investment will break away cleanly on the exterior surfaces. With other alloys the investment will adhere rather tenaciously, usually requiring cleansing in an ultrasonic cleaner. Neither the phosphate binder nor the silica refractory is soluble in hydrochloric or sulphuric acid. Cold hydrofluoric acid will dissolve the silica refractory quite well without damage to a gold-palladium-silver alloy but must be used with caution when the alloy is silver-palladium based. In fact HF acid should not be used unless the student is familiar with first aid techniques and the necessary neutralizing solutions are immediately at hand.

Base metal alloys require a light grit-blasting, usually with fine aluminum oxide. Chromium-based partials are usually sand-blasted to remove the investment. The nature of the adhering films of investment and their reaction with base metal alloys have been studied.[6] Acid should never be used for cleaning base metal alloys.

When handled with care, phosphate investments perform quite well. Because they are refractory and do not readily decompose to form a corrosive atmosphere when heated, they are also suitable for use as soldering investments.

CAUSES FOR DEFECTIVE CASTINGS

An unsuccessful casting may result in considerable trouble and loss of time. In almost all cases, defects in castings can be avoided by strict observance of procedures governed by certain fundamental rules and principles. Seldom is a defect in a casting attributable to other factors than the carelessness or ignorance of the operator. With present techniques, casting failures should be the exception, not the rule.

Defects in castings can be classified under four headings: (1) distortion, (2) surface roughness and irregularities, (3) porosity, and (4) incomplete or missing detail. Some of these factors have been discussed in connection with some of the phases of the casting techniques. The subject will now be summarized and analyzed in some detail.

Distortion   Any marked distortion of the casting is probably related to a distortion of the wax pattern, as described in Chapter 25. This type of distortion can be minimized or prevented by proper manipulation of the wax and handling of the pattern.

Unquestionably, some distortion of the wax pattern occurs as the investment hardens around it. The setting and hygroscopic expansions of the investment may produce an uneven movement of the walls of the pattern.

The occurrence of this type of distortion comes in part from the movement of the proximal walls outward unevenly in the three-surface restoration. The gingival margins are forced apart by the mold expansion, whereas the solid occlusal bar of wax resists expansion during the early stages of setting. The configuration of the pattern, type of wax, and thickness all influence the distortion that occurs, as has been discussed. For example, it increases as the thickness of the pattern decreases. As would be expected, the less the setting expansion of the investment, the less is the distortion.

Unfortunately, there is probably not a great deal that can be done to control this phenomenon. Generally, it is not a serious problem except that it accounts for some of the unexplained inaccuracies that may occur in small castings. It is possible that the greater the amount of residual stress present in the pattern, the greater might be the distortion upon setting of the investment.

Evidence has been presented that a further distortion of the mold may occur during the thermal expansion of the investment in the high heat technique.[7] Consequently, although the distortion during the hygroscopic expansion may be greater than that which occurs during normal setting expansion, the overall distortion may be of somewhat the same magnitude in both the low heat and the high heat techniques. This is assuming, of course, that a 38° C (100° F) water bath is used. The wax pattern is softened sufficiently to follow the expanding investment more evenly. In any event, this type of distortion is small and its effect can be generally disregarded as a cause when it is necessary to remake a casting because of a gross distortion.

Surface Roughness, Irregularities, and Discoloration   The surface of a dental casting should be an accurate reproduction of the surface of the wax pattern from which it is made. Excessive roughness or irregularities on the outer surface of the casting necessitate additional finishing and polishing, whereas irregularities on the cavity surface prevent a proper seating of an otherwise accurate casting.

Surface roughness should not be confused with surface irregularities. Surface roughness is defined as relatively finely spaced surface irregularities whose height, width, and direction establish the predominant surface pattern.[8] Surface irregularities refer to isolated imperfections, such as nodules, that do not characterize the total surface area.

Even under optimal conditions, the surface roughness of the dental casting is invariably somewhat greater than that of the wax pattern from which it is made. The difference is probably related to the particle size of the investment and its ability to reproduce the wax pattern in microscopic detail. Under proper manipulative techniques, the normal increased roughness in the casting should not be a major factor in dimensional accuracy. However, an improper technique can lead to a marked increase in surface roughness, as well as to the formation of surface irregularities.

Air Bubbles   Small nodules on a casting are caused by air bubbles that become attached to the pattern during or subsequent to the investing procedure. Such nodules can sometimes be removed if they are not in a critical area. However, on margins or on tissue surfaces, as the nodules at A in Figure 28–11, removal of these irregularities might alter the fit of the casting. As previously noted, the best method to avoid air bubbles is to use the vacuum investing technique.

If a manual method is used, various precautions can be observed to eliminate air from the investment mix before the investing. As previously outlined, the use of a mechanical mixer, and vibration both before and after mixing, should be practiced routinely. However, the vibration should not be too great, as the particles of the investment will settle and produce a thin mixture or water film at the surface of the mixed investment.

A wetting agent may be helpful in preventing the collection of air bubbles on the surface of the pattern, but it is by no means a certain remedy. As previously discussed, it is important that the wetting agent be applied in a thin layer. It is best to air dry the wetting agent, as any excess will dilute the investment, possibly producing surface irregularities on the casting.

Although a slight vibration during the painting of the pattern may be of aid in the elimination of air bubbles, it may cause water bubbles to form. A better method is to paint the pattern as described in the previous chapter.

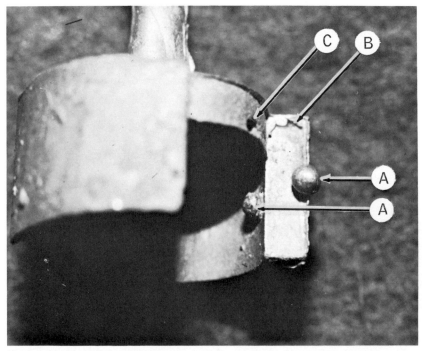

Figure 28–11   Surface irregularities on an experimental casting caused by: A, air bubbles; B, water film; C, inclusion of foreign body. (Courtesy of D. Vieira.)

After the pattern has been inserted in the ring, any vibration causes the bubbles present to circulate in the viscous investment mix, and some of them are almost sure to cling to the pattern.

Water Films   Wax is repellent to water, and if the investment becomes separated from the wax pattern in some manner, a water film may form irregularly over the surface. Occasionally, this type of surface irregularity appears as minute ridges or veins on the surface, as shown in Figure 28–11.

If the pattern is moved slightly, jarred, or vibrated after investing, or if the painting procedure does not result in an intimate contact of the investment with the pattern, such a condition may result. A wetting agent is of aid in the prevention of such a type of irregularity. Too high a W/P ratio may also produce this effect.

Too Rapid Heating   This factor has been discussed in a previous section. It results in fins or spines on the casting similar to those shown in Figure 28–2. Or, a characteristic surface roughness may be evident owing to a flaking of the investment when the water or steam pours into the mold. Furthermore, such a surge of steam or water may carry some of the salts used as modifiers into the mold, which are left as deposits on the walls after the water evaporates. As previously mentioned, the mold should be heated gradually. At least 60 minutes should elapse during the heating of the investment-filled ring from room temperature to 700°C. The greater the bulk of the investment, the more slowly it should be heated.

Underheating   Incomplete elimination of the wax residues may occur if the heating time is too short or if there is insufficient air available in the furnace. These factors are particularly important with the low temperature investment techniques. Voids or porosity may occur in the casting from the gases formed when the hot gold alloy comes in contact with the carbonaceous residues. Occasionally the gold may be covered with a tenacious carbon coating that is virtually impossible to remove by pickling.

A faulty pyrometer may also account for underheating, or overheating for that matter, of the mold. It is not unusual to find that the pyrometer reading may be inaccurate by as much as 100° C. It should be checked periodically. Dental manufacturers supply small templets of chemicals that melt at a specific temperature. When placed into the furnace the pellet melts, and at that time the pyrometer setting may be adjusted correctly.

W/P Ratio   The higher the W/P ratio, the rougher is the casting. However, if too little water is used, the investment may be unmanageably thick, so that it cannot be properly applied to the pattern. Or, in vacuum investing, the air may not be sufficiently removed. In either case, a rough surface on the casting may result. As is so often emphasized, the amount of water and investment should be measured accurately.

Prolonged Heating   When the high heat casting technique is used, a prolonged heating of the mold at the casting temperature is likely to cause a disintegration of the investment, and the walls of the mold are roughened as a result. Furthermore, the products of decomposition are sulfur compounds that may contaminate the gold alloy to the extent that the surface texture is affected. Such contamination possibly is the reason why the surface of the casting sometimes does not respond to pickling. When the thermal expansion technique is employed, the mold should be heated to the casting temperature, never higher than 700° C (1292° F), and the casting should be made immediately.

Temperature of the Gold Alloy   If the noble metal alloy is heated to too high a temperature before casting, the surface of the investment is likely to be attacked, and a surface roughness of the type described in the previous section may result. As previously noted, in all probability the alloy is not overheated with a gas-air blowpipe when used with the gas supplied in most localities. If other fuel is used, special care should be observed that the color emitted by the molten gold alloy is no lighter than a light orange.

Casting Pressure   Too high a pressure during casting produces a rough surface on the casting. A gauge pressure of .10 to .14 MPa (15 to 20 psi) in an air pressure casting machine or three to four turns of the spring in an average type of centrifugal casting machine is sufficient for small castings.

Composition of the Investment   The ratio of the binder to the quartz influences the surface texture of the casting. Also, a coarse silica causes a surface roughness. If the investment meets American Dental Association Specification no. 2, the composition is probably not a factor in the surface roughness.

Foreign Bodies   When foreign substances get into the mold, a surface roughness may be produced. For example, a rough crucible former, with investment clinging to it, may roughen the investment upon its removal so that bits of investment are carried into the mold with the molten alloy. Carelessness in the removal of the sprue former may be a similar cause.

Usually, contamination results not only in surface roughness but also in incomplete areas or surface voids. An example may be seen at C in Figure 28–11. Any casting that shows sharp, well-defined deficiencies indicates the presence of some foreign particles in the mold, such as pieces of investment or bits of carbon from the flux. Bright appearing concavities may be the result of flux being carried into the mold with the metal.

Surface discoloration and roughness can result from sulfur contamination, either from investment breakdown at elevated temperatures or from a high sulfur content of the blowpipe flame. Black castings that are brittle and do not clean readily during pickling result.

Impact of Molten Alloy   It was pointed out that the direction of the sprue former should be such that the molten gold alloy does not strike a weak portion of the mold surface. Occasionally, the molten gold may fracture or abrade the mold surface as it strikes it, regardless of its bulk. Unfortunately, sometimes the abraded area is smooth so that it cannot be detected on the surface of the casting. Such a depression in the mold is reflected as a raised area on the casting, often too slight to be noticed yet sufficiently large to prevent the seating of the casting. This type of surface roughness or irregularity can be avoided by proper spruing so as to prevent the direct impact of the molten metal at an angle of 90 degrees with the investment surface. A glancing impact is likely to be less damaging, and at the same time an undesirable turbulence is avoided.

Pattern Position If several patterns are invested in the same ring they should not be placed too close together. Likewise, too many patterns positioned in the same plane in the mold should be avoided. The expansion of wax is much greater than that of the investment, causing breakdown or cracking of the investment if a thickness of several millimeters is not present.

Other Causes There are certain surface discolorations and roughness which may not be evident when the casting is completed, but which may appear during service. For example, various gold alloys, such as solders, bits of wire, or various types of casting alloys should never be melted together and re-used. The resulting mixture would not possess the proper physical properties, and might form eutectic or similar alloys with low corrosion resistance. Later discoloration and corrosion generally result during service.

Contamination with copper during improper pickling may be a factor in future surface change.

A source of discoloration often overlooked is the surface contamination of a gold alloy restoration with mercury. Mercury penetrates rapidly into the alloy and causes a marked loss in ductility and a greater susceptibility to corrosion. Completed castings should never be placed in contact with amalgam dies or on a bracket table where amalgam scrap may be lying. As stated in Chapter 19, it is not a good practice to place gold alloy restorations in contact with amalgam restorations for this and other reasons.

Porosity Porosity may occur both internally and externally. The latter is a factor in surface roughness, but also it is generally a manifestation of internal porosity. Not only does the internal porosity weaken the casting but also, if it appears on the surface, it may be a cause for discoloration. If severe, it can produce leakage at the tooth-restoration interface, and secondary caries may result. Although the porosity in a casting cannot be prevented entirely, it can be definitely minimized by a proper technique. There are numerous causes for porosity, and some of them will be discussed in detail.

Porosities in noble metal alloy castings may be classified as follows:
1. Those caused by solidification shrinkage
   a. Localized shrinkage porosity
   b. Microporosity
2. Those caused by gas
   a. Pinhole porosity
   b. Gas inclusions
   c. Subsurface porosity
3. Those caused by entrapped air in the mold

1a. Porosity due to localized shrinkage is generally caused by incomplete feeding of molten metal during solidification. As noted in Chapter 24, the linear contraction of noble metal alloys in changing from a liquid to a solid is at least 1.25 per cent. Therefore, there must be continual feeding of molten metal through the sprue to make up for the shrinkage of metal volume during solidification. If the sprue freezes in its cross-section before this feeding is completed to the casting proper, a localized shrinkage void will occur in the last portion of the casting that solidifies, as shown in Figure 28–12(a).

Localized shrinkage generally occurs near the sprue-casting junction, but it may occur anywhere between dendrites, as shown in Figure 28–13*C,* where the last part of the casting that solidified was in the low melting metal that

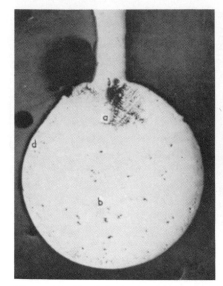
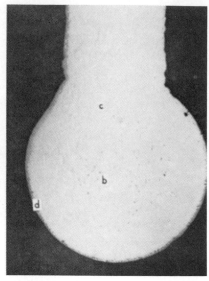

Figure 28–12   Spherical gold alloy casting showing localized shrinkage porosity (a), microporosity (b), pinhole porosity (c), and subsurface porosity (d). (From Ryge, Kozak, and Fairhurst, J Am Dent Assoc, June, 1957.)

lingers as the dendrite branches develop. This latter type occurs particularly in coarse grained alloy castings.

This type of void may also occur externally, usually in the interior of a crown near the area of the sprue, if a hot spot has been created by the hot metal impinging from the sprue channel on a point of the mold wall. This hot spot will cause the local region to freeze last and result in what is called *suck-back* porosity,[9] as shown in Figure 28–14, left.

Such voids can be eliminated by (1) flaring the point of sprue attachment, as noted in Chapter 27, and (2) reducing the mold-melt temperature differential, i.e., lowering the casting temperature by about 30° C.

lb. Microporosity also occurs from solidification shrinkage but is generally present in fine grain alloy castings when the solidification is too rapid for the microvoids to segregate to the liquid pool. This premature solidification causes the porosity shown in Figure 28–12(b) and portions of Figure 28–13A in the form of small irregular voids.

Such phenomena can occur from the unduly rapid solidification if the mold or casting temperature is too low. Unfortunately, this type of defect is not

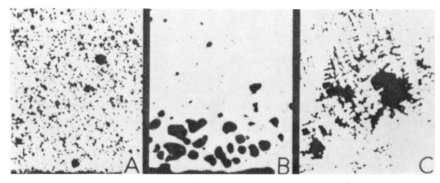

Figure 28–13   *A,* Microporosity, pinhole porosity, and gas inclusions. (Microporosity voids are irregular in shape, whereas the other two types tend to be spherical; the largest spherical voids are gas inclusions.) *B,* Subsurface porosity. *C,* Localized shrinkage porosity. (Courtesy of G. Ryge.)

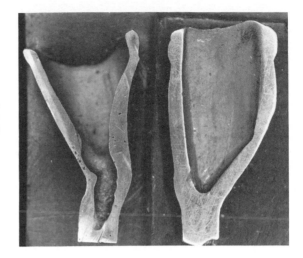

Figure 28–14 A demonstration of suck-back porosity. The coping at left was cast at 1370° C (2500° F), while the one at the right was cast at 1340° C (2450° F). (Courtesy of J. Nielsen.)

detectable unless the casting is sectioned. In any case, it is generally not a serious defect.

The effects of various factors involved in formation of microporosity, and other types, are summarized in Table 28–1.

2a and b. The pinhole and gas inclusion porosities are both related to the entrapment of gas during solidification. They are both characterized by a spherical contour but they are decidedly different in size. The gas inclusion porosities are usually much larger than the other type, as indicated in Figure 28–13A.

Many metals dissolve or occlude gases while they are molten. For example, both copper and silver dissolve oxygen in large amounts in the liquid state. Molten platinum and palladium have a strong affinity for hydrogen as well as oxygen. Upon solidification, the absorbed gases are expelled and the pinhole porosity results. The larger voids (Fig. 28–13A) may also result from the same cause, but it seems more logical to assume that such voids may be caused by gas mechanically trapped by the molten metal in the mold or else carried in during the casting procedure.

All castings probably contain a certain amount of porosity, as exemplified by the photomicrograph shown in Figure 28–15B. However, the porosity should be kept to a minimum because it may affect the physical properties of the casting deleteriously.

Oxygen is dissolved by some of the metals, such as silver, in the alloy while they are in the molten state. During solidification, the gas is expelled to form blebs and pores in the metal. As was pointed out earlier, this type of porosity may be attributed to abuse of the metal. Castings severely contami-

Table 28–1. *Effects of Technical Factors on the Porosity Resulting from Metal Solidification**

TYPE OF POROSITY	INCREASED SPRUE THICKNESS	INCREASED SPRUE LENGTH	INCREASED MELT TEMPERATURE	INCREASED MOLD TEMPERATURE
Localized shrinkage porosity	Decreased	Increased	Decreased	Decreased
Subsurface porosity	Increased	Decreased	Increased	Increased
Microporosity	No effect	No effect	Decreased	Decreased

*From Ryge, Kozak, and Fairhurst, J Am Dent Assoc, June, 1957.

A

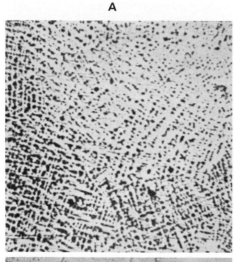

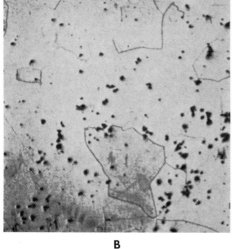

B

Figure 28-15 *A,* Grain structure of a Type III noble metal alloy as cast. *B,* Same alloy after homogenizing at 725° C (1337° F) for 70 minutes. Pin hole porosity can be noted in *B.* (Courtesy of B. Hedegard.)

nated with gases are usually black when they are removed from the investment and do not clean easily on pickling (Fig. 28–16). The porosity that extends to the surface is usually in the form of small pinpoint holes (Figs. 28–12[c] and 28–13A). When they are polished out, others appear.

Larger spherical porosities can be caused by gas occluded from a poorly

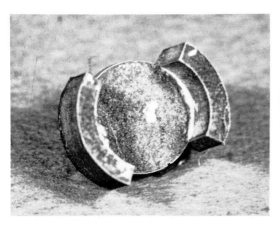

Figure 28-16 A black-coated noble metal alloy casting resulting from sulfur contamination or oxidation during melting of the alloy.

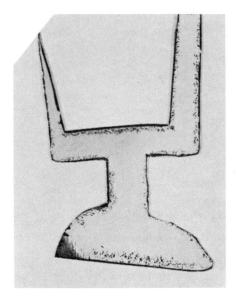

Figure 28–17 Subsurface porosity seen around the entire periphery of a casting. (From Ryge, Kozak, and Fairhurst, J Am Dent Assoc, June, 1957.)

adjusted blowpipe flame, or if the reducing zone of the flame is not used (Fig. 28–13*A*).

These types of porosity can be minimized by premelting the gold alloy on a charcoal block if the alloy has been used before, and by correctly adjusting and positioning the blowpipe flame during melting.

2c. Subsurface porosity occurs on occasion as is shown in Figures 28–12(d) and 28–13*B*. At other times it may be particularly evident, as seen in Figure 28–17. The reasons for the presence of such voids have not been completely established. It may be due to the simultaneous nucleation of solid grains and gas bubbles at the first moment that the metal freezes at the mold walls. As has been explained, this type of porosity can be diminished by controlling the rate at which the molten metal enters the mold.

3. Entrapped air on the inner surface of the casting, sometimes referred to as "back pressure" porosity, can produce dyscrasias such as those seen in Figure 28–18. This is caused by the inability of the air in the mold escaping through the pores in the investment, or by the pressure gradient pushing the air pocket out via the molten sprue and button.

The entrapment is frequently found in a "pocket" at the cavity surface of a crown or MOD (Fig. 28–18). Occasionally it is even found on the outside surface of the casting when the casting temperature or mold temperature is so low that solidification occurs before the entrapped air can escape. It is

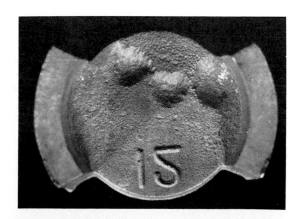

Figure 28–18 Surface irregularity on cavity side of casting due to back pressure porosity.

aggravated by the modern dense investments, the increase in mold density effected by vacuum investing, and the tendency for the mold to clog with residual carbon when the low heat technique is used. All of these factors tend to slow down the venting of gases from the mold during casting.

Proper burnout, an adequate mold and casting temperature, and a sufficiently high W/P ratio all help to eliminate this phenomenon. It is good practice to make sure that the thickness of investment between the tip of the pattern and the end of the ring not be greater than approximately 6.5 mm (1/4 inch). The use of vent rods does not seem to help this condition.

Incomplete Casting   Occasionally, only a partially complete casting, or perhaps no casting at all, is found. The obvious cause is that the molten alloy has been prevented, in some manner, from completely filling the mold. At least two factors that might inhibit the ingress of the liquefied metal are insufficient venting of the mold and high viscosity of the fused metal.

The first consideration, i.e., insufficient venting, is directly related to the back pressure exerted by the air in the mold. If the air cannot be vented with sufficient rapidity, the molten alloy does not fill the mold before it solidifies.

In such a case, the magnitude of the casting pressure should be suspected. If insufficient casting pressure is employed, the back pressure cannot be overcome. Furthermore, the pressure should be applied for at least four seconds. The mold is filled and the metal is solidified in approximately one second or less, yet it is very soft during the early stages. Therefore, the pressure should be maintained for a few seconds beyond this point. An example of an incomplete casting because of insufficient casting pressure is seen in Figure 28–19. These failures are usually exemplified in rounded, incomplete margins.

A second common cause for an incomplete casting is incomplete elimination of the mold. If too many products of combustion remain in the mold, the pores in the investment may become filled so that the air cannot be vented. If moisture or actual particles of wax remain, when the molten alloy contacts either of these foreign substances an explosion may occur which may produce sufficient back pressure to prevent the mold from being filled. An example of a casting failure because of incomplete wax elimination can be seen in Figure 28–20. Although similar to the incomplete casting in Figure 28–19, it can be noted that the rounded margins are quite shiny rather than dull. This shiny condition of the metal is due to the strong reducing atmosphere created by the carbon monoxide left by the residual wax.

The possible influence of the W/P ratio of the investment has already been discussed. The lower the W/P ratio, the less is the porosity of the investment. Greater pressure during casting is indicated in such a case.

Different gold alloy compositions probably exhibit varying viscosities in the molten state, depending on composition and temperature. However, both the surface tension and the viscosity of a molten alloy are decreased with an increase in temperature; so far as is known, an incomplete gold alloy casting resulting from too great a viscosity of the casting metal can be attributed to insufficient heating. The temperature of the alloy should be raised higher than its liquidus temperature so that its viscosity and surface tension are lowered, and so that it does not solidify prematurely as it enters the mold. Such premature solidification may account for the greater susceptibility of the white gold alloys to porosity because their liquidi are higher. Thus, they are more difficult to melt with gas-air fuel.

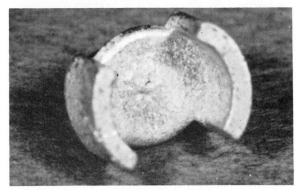

Figure 28–19 Rounded, incomplete margins are evidence of insufficient casting pressure.

Figure 28–20 Incomplete casting resulting from incomplete wax elimination is characterized by rounded margins and shiny appearance.

Figure 28–19

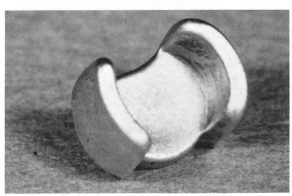

Figure 28–20

The surface tension is also important, inasmuch as a high surface tension may cause rounded margins on a casting that might otherwise be satisfactory. Such defects can be remedied by heating the gold alloy to a higher temperature before casting.

References

1. Macasaet AA and Dickson G: Some Factors Affecting the Dimensional Changes of Gold-Alloy Investments. National Bureau of Standards Report 7574. Washington, DC, U.S. Government Printing Office (June 30), 1962.
2. Jenkins CBG: An evaluation of five gold inlay investing techniques and the effects of certain variables in the procedure. Thesis, Indiana University School of Dentistry, 1968.
3. Osborne J and Skinner EW: Physical properties of gypsum model investments. J Am Dent Assoc 59:708, 1959.
4. O'Brien WJ and Nielsen JP: Decomposition of gypsum investments in the presence of carbon. J Dent Res 28:541, 1959.
5. Nielsen JP: Pressure distribution in centrifugal dental casting. J Dent Res 57:261, 1978.
6. Allen FC and Asgar K: Reaction of cobalt-chromium casting alloy with investment. J Dent Res 45:1516, 1966.
7. Mumford GM and Phillips RW: Measurements of thermal expansion of cristobalite type investments in the inlay ring — preliminary report. J Prosthet Dent 8:860, 1958.
8. American Standard Surface Roughness, Waviness and Lay. American Standards Association B46.1, 1955.
9. Nielsen JP and Ollerman R: Suck-back porosity. Quintessence of Dental Technology, No. 1, Report 007, p. 61, 1976.

29 DENTAL CEMENTS FOR LUTING

Dental cements are materials of comparatively low strength, but they are used extensively in dentistry when strength is not a prime consideration. With two possible exceptions, they are not truly adhesive to enamel or dentin. Except for the resin cement they dissolve and erode in oral fluids. Such defects are likely to make them impermanent.

However, regardless of certain inferior properties, they possess so many desirable characteristics that they are used in 40 to 60 per cent of all restorations. They are employed as cementing (referred to as *luting*) agents for fixed cast restorations or orthodontic bands, as thermal insulators under metallic restorations, for temporary or permanent restorations, as root canal sealants, and for pulp capping. It should be reemphasized that as a group their chemical and physical properties leave much to be desired, and the manipulative techniques must be designed to provide the optimal behavior.

Classification of Dental Cements Dental cements are generally classified according to their composition, as presented in Table 29–1. Representative products used as luting cements are shown in Figure 29–1. With the exception of calcium hydroxide and resin materials, the setting reactions are those of an acid and a base.[1] The liquids act as the acid and the powders as the base.

The American Dental Association specifications for the various cements further classify certain of the cements as Type I and Type II on the basis of their properties, and thus their intended use. For example, a Type I zinc phosphate cement is a "fine grain" cement (small particle size intended for cementation of precision fitting castings). The Type II zinc phosphate cement is a "medium grain" cement and is recommended for all other uses, i.e., thermal insulating bases and cementation of orthodontic bands. As would be expected, certain requirements, e.g., film thickness, are more stringent for the Type I cement than for the Type II.

Zinc silicophosphate cements are available in Types I and II. They are somewhat translucent. Therefore, from an esthetic standpoint they have been particularly applicable for the cementation of porcelain restorations, i.e., jacket crowns.

Copper, silver, and mercury salts are sometimes added to the cements to render them bacteriostatic or bactericidal. Copper oxide may also be used in place of zinc oxide for this reason. The effectiveness of such antibacterial agents in preventing dental caries, including such cements, is controversial.

Table 29–1. *Classification and Uses of Dental Cements*

CEMENT	PRINCIPAL USES	SECONDARY USES
Zinc phosphate	Luting agent for restorations and orthodontic appliances	Intermediate restorations Thermal insulating bases Root canal restorations
Zinc phosphate with silver or copper salts	Intermediate restorations	
Copper phosphate (red or black)	Intermediate restorations	
Zinc oxide–eugenol	Temporary and intermediate restorations Temporary and permanent luting agent for restorations Thermal insulating bases Pulp capping agent	Root canal restorations Periodontic bandage
Polycarboxylate	Luting agent for restorations Thermal insulating bases	Luting agent for orthodontic appliances Intermediate restorations
Silicate	Anterior restorations	
Silicophosphate	Luting agent for restorations	Intermediate restorations Luting agent for orthodontic appliances
Glass ionomer	Coating for eroded areas Luting agent for restorations	Pit and fissure sealant Anterior restorations Thermal insulating bases
Resin	Luting agent for restorations	Temporary restorations
Calcium hydroxide	Pulp capping agent Thermal insulating bases	

Furthermore, they are more irritating to the pulp than are other cements. For this reason they are rarely used today, and are generally confined to non-vital teeth or on rare occasions to the cementation of orthodontic appliances.

When the prepared cavity approaches the pulp, a cement base is employed to protect the pulp against mechanical and thermal trauma. Any of the cements can be used for this purpose except the silicate, resin, and copper cements, all of which are considered to be too irritating.

Zinc phosphate cement, as well as most of the other commonly used cavity base materials, is an excellent thermal insulator. It can be seen from Table 29–2 that the thermal conductivity values of various base materials are in the same general range as other recognized insulators, such as asbestos and cork. Dentin itself, of course, has very low thermal conductivity (Table 3–1) and therefore is a good insulator from temperature changes in the mouth and from that generated during the setting of restorative materials.

The zinc oxide–eugenol cements are popular as base materials, and some are formulated for permanent cementation of gold restorations. They have a palliative action on the pulp and, as noted, are good thermal insulators.

The polycarboxylate cements are a relatively recent innovation in this field. There is evidence that this type of cement develops a certain amount of adhesion to tooth structure. Such cements are used primarily as luting agents

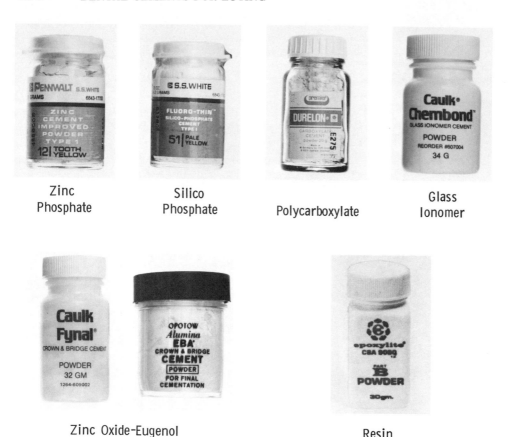

| Zinc Phosphate | Silico Phosphate | Polycarboxylate | Glass Ionomer |

| Zinc Oxide-Eugenol | | Resin |

Figure 29–1   Commercial products representative of the various types of cements used for luting purposes.

for cast restorations. Because of this adhesive characteristic, they are also employed to a certain extent for the direct bonding of orthodontic brackets, thereby eliminating the need for banding the teeth. Since their biological characteristics are comparable to zinc oxide–eugenol cement, they are also frequently used as a base material.

The newest of the cements is the glass ionomer cement. The cement is translucent and thus it is used for restoration of anterior teeth (Type II). Glass ionomer cement, as polycarboxylate cement, has some potential for adhesion to tooth structure and is kind to the pulp. Because of their adhesive properties, the glass ionomer cements are employed for restoration of eroded gingival areas without use of a cavity preparation for retention. There is a Type I glass ionomer cement that is used for cementation of cast metal and porcelain restorations. The cement also has been advocated as a pit and fissure sealant.

Table 29–2.   *Thermal Conductivity of Various Cement Base Materials as Compared to Two Commonly Recognized Insulators*

MATERIAL	THERMAL CONDUCTIVITY $[cal.\ sec^{-1}\ cm^{-2}(°C./cm)^{-1}] \times 10^{-4}$
Zinc phosphate cement (dry)	3.11
Zinc phosphate cement (wet)	3.88
Zinc oxide–eugenol	3.98
Asbestos fiber	1.90
Cork	7.00

Because the cement is relatively kind to the pulp it is applicable for use as a thermal insulating base beneath other types of restorations.

Resin cements have had only limited use for cementation of restorations; however, resins are being used quite extensively for direct attachment of orthodontic brackets to teeth.

The silicate cements are used almost exclusively as permanent filling materials. They possess reasonably good esthetic properties when they are first inserted in the tooth. Unfortunately, they gradually disintegrate in the oral fluids, and they may stain and craze. Thus, they should not be called permanent in comparison with the metallic filling materials, for example. Since the introduction of composite resin systems, the popularity of silicate cement has steadily declined. It will be discussed in the next chapter.

ZINC PHOSPHATE CEMENT

As zinc phosphate is the oldest of the luting cements and thus is the one that has the longest "track record," it serves as a standard with which newer systems can be compared. Furthermore, much of the basic information discussed in the following sections is directly applicable to other types of cement.

Composition   The basic constituent of zinc phosphate powder is zinc oxide. The principal modifier is magnesium oxide, usually in a concentration of approximately 10 per cent. In addition, the powder may contain small amounts of other oxides, e.g., bismuth and silica.

The liquids are essentially phosphoric acid, water, aluminum phosphate, and, in some cases, zinc phosphate. The metallic salts are added to reduce the reaction rate of the liquid with the powder. The water content of most liquids is 33 ± 5 per cent. The amount of water present is a factor in the control of the ionization of the liquid, and it is an important ingredient, since it influences the rate and type of the powder-liquid reaction.

Although the compositions of the liquids of various brands of cement are similar, generally the liquids cannot be interchanged for use with the various powders. The composition of the liquid is critical, and the manufacturer employs special care in compounding it.

Chemistry of Setting   When a zinc oxide powder is mixed with phosphoric acid, a solid substance is rapidly formed with considerable evolution of heat. However, the zinc oxide is heat treated so as to reduce its activity.

The exact nature of the product of this reaction is not certain. In the past it has been supposed that the tertiary zinc phosphate $[Zn_3(PO_4)_2 \cdot 4H_2O]$ (hopeite) is the final product. However, recent studies have refined this model.[2-4] Zinc oxide powders that have not been deactivated do react to form hopeite, but the crystalline mass that is formed is not cohesive. Properly deactivated zinc oxide powder, such as that in dental cement powder, reacts with the liquid initially to form an amorphous cement matrix of zinc orthophosphate, apparently without the intermediate formation of acid phosphates. After a few minutes, crystallites of hopeite develop, but only on the surface of the cement. Thus the set cement consists of a matrix of amorphous zinc phosphate which binds unreacted zinc oxide particles together, with crystallites of hopeite developing at the surface of the cement mass. The final result is a cored structure as seen in Figure 29–2.

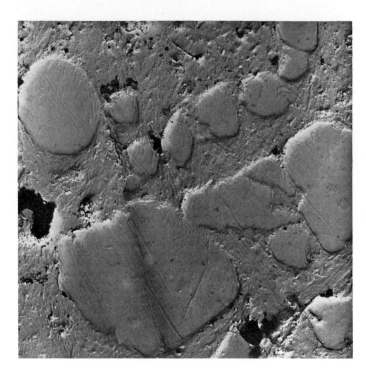

Figure 29–2 Electron micrograph of a set zinc phosphate cement. The core is the undissolved zinc oxide powder and the matrix is tertiary zinc phosphate. 40,000 ×. (Courtesy of Alan A. Grant.)

In the dental cement, the reaction is modified by the addition of aluminum and zinc to the liquid. The aluminum appears to be the most important additive, as it forms aluminophosphoric acid complexes with phosphoric acid. These complexes apparently moderate the reaction and help prevent the cement paste from forming undesirable crystallites. The reactivity of the powder is reduced by sintering the ingredients at temperatures between 1000 and 1400° C (1830 – 2550° F) into a cake, which is ground and sifted to a fine powder. Magnesium oxide plays an important role by aiding the sintering of the zinc oxide powder.

It should be mentioned that a zinc phosphate cement has been developed that uses water as the liquid rather than a phosphoric acid solution. The powder of such a cement generally is composed of zinc oxide, monozinc or monomanganese phosphate, and tertiary zinc phosphate. Calcium monophosphate may also be used. Since all contain acid phosphate salts, the pH level of the cement mix is the same as that of a conventional zinc phosphate cement. Also, the physical properties tend to be inferior. Since the *water-settable* zinc phosphate cements afford no discernible advantage over the conventional cements, they have not been popular.

Properties   The physical and mechanical properties of Type I zinc phosphate cement, along with the requirements set forth in the American Dental Association specification for zinc phosphate cement, are listed in Table 29–3.

The values for all of the cements listed in this table are taken from a variety of sources; therefore, they are representative of a typical cement. Naturally, some variation occurs in properties from one brand to another. However, it should be emphasized that the differences induced by manipulative variables are usually much greater than are those inherent between brands.

Following is a discussion of the properties of zinc phosphate cement, the

Table 29-3. *Properties of Luting Cements*

MATERIAL	TIME OF SETTING Min	COMPRESSIVE STRENGTH-24 HR. MPa	psi	FILM THICKNESS μm	SOLUBILITY AND DISINTEGRATION (BY WEIGHT) %	DIAMETRAL TENSILE STRENGTH-24 HR. MPa	psi	PULP RESPONSE
ADA Spec. No. 8 Type I (cementing)	5 min 9 max	68.7	9956	25 max	0.2 max	No specification		*
Zinc Phosphate	5.5	103.5	15000	18	0.06	5.5	800	Moderate
ZOE	4–10	27.6	4000	25	0.04	–	–	Mild
ZOE + EBA and alumina	9.5	55.2	8000	25	0.05	4.1	600	Mild
ZOE + polymer	6–10	48.3	7000	32	0.08	4.1	600	Mild
Silicophosphate	3½–4	144.8	21000	25	0.4	7.6	1100	Moderate
Resin cement	4–10	65.5	9500	10–60	0.6–0.1	Not available		Severe
Polycarboxylate	5.5	55.2	8000	21	0.06	6.2	900	Mild
Glass Ionomer	6.5	86.2	12500	24	1.25	6.2	900	Mild

*Based on comparison with silicate cement — *severe* irritant.

factors that influence these properties, and ultimately the clinical usage and behavior of the cement.

Control of the Setting Time   The setting time of the cement must be accurately controlled. If the cement sets too fast, the viscosity increases so rapidly that it is impossible to seat the casting fully. This effect of increased viscosity on the ability to seat the casting is illustrated in Figure 29–3. The crown in Figure 29–3A, which was cemented 2.5 minutes after start of the cement mix, is properly seated on the prepared tooth. However, owing to the increased viscosity of the cement, the crown that was cemented at 5 minutes (Fig. 29–3B) failed to seat completely. A thick layer of cement is exposed at the cervical margin.

It is obvious that matrix formation must be sufficiently slow that adequate working time is provided. However, if the setting time is too long, chairtime would be prolonged unduly. A reasonable setting time at oral temperature for a zinc phosphate cement is between 5 and 9 minutes.

The setting time is usually measured with 1 pound Gillmore needle at a temperature of 37° C (98.6° F) and a relative humidity of 100 per cent. It is defined as the time elapsing from the start of mixing until the point of the needle no longer penetrates the surface of the cement when the needle is gently lowered onto it.

The setting time, as influenced by the manufacturing process, is affected as follows:

1. The composition and the sintering temperature of the powder undoubtedly are factors in control of the setting time. The higher the sintering temperature, the more slowly the cement sets.

2. The composition of the liquid, as already described, is a factor because

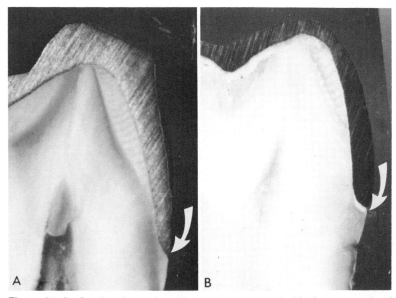

Figure 29–3   Section through gold crowns cemented with the same mix of zinc phosphate cement. The crown shown in *A* was cemented 2.5 minutes after the start of the mix, while that shown in *B* was cemented at 5 minutes. Because of the increase in viscosity of the cement with time, the casting in *B* failed to seat completely, leaving a thick layer of cement exposed at the margins (arrow).

the salts, particularly those of aluminum, and the water definitely influence the setting time.

3. The larger the particle size of the powder, the less rapid is the reaction because of the decreased surface contact of the powder with the liquid.

In a sense, when the powder and liquid are mixed, the manufacturing process is continued. The factors under the control of the dental assistant and dentist are as follows:

A. The lower the temperature during mixing, the longer is the setting time. The temperature can be controlled by cooling the mixing slab.

B. In some cases, the rate at which the powder is added to the liquid may influence the setting time markedly. Generally, the more slowly the powder is added, the longer is the setting time. A slow addition of the powder prolongs the mixing time and, therefore, delays the setting time.

C. The longer the mixing time, within practical limits, the longer is the setting time. It should be noted that this effect is directly the reverse of the similar situation with plaster. The matrix forms after the mixing is completed. Any such formation during mixing is broken up.

D. The more liquid employed in ratio to the powder, the slower is the setting rate. This effect arises from the peritectic nature of the reaction.

The best method for the control of the setting time is to regulate the temperature of the mixing slab. Generally, it is desirable to increase the setting time to be certain that sufficient time is available for the manipulation of the cement, and so that the maximal amount of powder can be incorporated until the desired consistency is reached. For this reason, the mixing slab is cooled. It is usually recommended that the slab not be cooled below the dew point of the environment; otherwise, moisture collects on the slab, and, as will be discussed, the properties may be lessened.[5]

However, recent research suggests that when the slab is cooled below the dew point the chemical reaction (matrix formation) is slowed to such a degree that additional powder may be incorporated into the mix without an inordinate increase in viscosity. Apparently the increased amount of powder offsets, at least to some degree, the deleterious effects of the water contamination on the properties of the cement.[6]

Lengthening the setting time by the use of a lower powder-liquid ratio is to be avoided because of the adverse effect on the strength and solubility.

The rate at which the powder is added to the liquid also is an effective means by which the setting time may be controlled. Addition of the powder in small amounts, with thorough mixing of each increment, can extend the setting time.

Water Content of the Liquid   As previously noted, the water content of the liquid is established by the manufacturer and it should be maintained; otherwise. the chemical equilibrium may be disturbed. Erratic behavior of the cement may often be traced to improper care of the liquid.

The effect of small changes in the water content of the liquid on the setting time of zinc phosphate cement is not a marked one. However, either loss or gain of water from the liquid does impair the physical and mechanical properties of the resultant cement. Cements prepared with liquids as received from the manufacturer are considerably stronger and less soluble than cements prepared from liquids to which water had been added or removed by evaporation.[5]

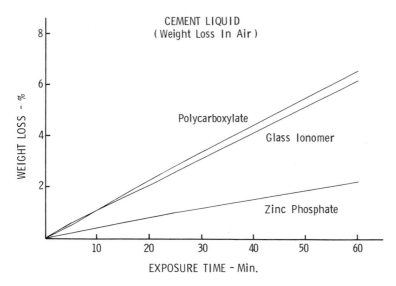

Figure 29–4 Loss of water from cement liquids when exposed to air.

With repeated opening of the bottle over a period of time the water-acid ratio of the remaining liquid may be altered. Insufficient water in the liquid is often evidenced by formation of crystals on the walls of the bottle, or a general cloudiness of the liquid. Such a condition is the result of the precipitation of buffering salts. Unfortunately, if water is absorbed by the liquid no change in appearance can be observed. However, with the air conditioned offices of today evaporation of water is more likely to occur than is imbibition.

If the cement liquid is left on the slab for any length of time, evaporation of water occurs, as shown in Figure 29–4. The liquid should not be dispensed until just prior to initiation of mixing. As will be noted, this is good practice to follow with all types of cements.

Consistency   The consistency of the initial mixture of powder and liquid is of considerable importance. From the standpoint of the physical properties, a mix of thick consistency is desirable. However, in the seating of an inlay or crown in a prepared cavity, an extremely viscous mix is not indicated because the mix will not flow readily from beneath the casting; thus the restoration would not seat properly.

The consistency of the cement is definitely related to the liquid-powder ratio. Under a given set of conditions, the more powder incorporated into the liquid, the thicker is the mix. However, as stated previously, the temperature of the mixing slab also governs the viscosity of the mix by accelerating or retarding the setting reaction, as shown in Figure 29–5.

Two mixes of cement were prepared with the manufacturer's recommended powder-liquid ratio, employing identical manipulative procedures. The only variable was the difference in the temperature of the mixing slabs. The mix of cement prepared on the cool slab (Fig. 29–5A) is suitable for cementation of cast restorations; the mix made on the warm slab (Fig. 29–5B) is much too viscous for use with precision fitting castings.

Thus, the cement must be mixed on a cool slab in order to permit the maximum amount of powder to be incorporated and, hence, to attain maximum properties and maintain a usable consistency.

Some manufacturers supply the powder and liquid preproportioned into capsules, in the same manner as was noted with alloy and mercury for

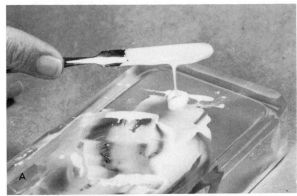

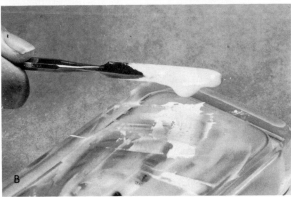

Figure 29–5 Two mixes of cement prepared with identical powder-liquid ratios. The temperature of the mixing slab in *A* was 18° C (66° F); the temperature of the slab in *B* was 29.5° C (85° F). (From Phillips RW, Swartz ML, and Norman RD, Materials for the Practicing Dentist, St. Louis, CV Mosby Co., 1969.)

amalgam. Mixing of the encapsulated material is accomplished with high speed amalgamators. Cooling of the capsules in a refrigerator will reduce the viscosity and extend the working time of the cement mix to some extent.

Owing to the difference among brands of cement, the powder-liquid ratio to produce the proper consistency usually varies from one product to another. The manufacturer should specify the proper powder-liquid ratio to provide the desired consistency.

Film Thickness For an inlay or crown to be seated properly, the film of cement should be sufficiently thin so that it does not interfere with the fit of the restoration. On the other hand, the thickness of the cement film and the fit of the restoration are determined to an extent by the cementation pressure, the viscosity and temperature of the cement, and the taper of the walls of the prepared cavity.[7]

In order to facilitate complete seating of cemented restorations of certain designs (e.g., full cast crowns with long parallel walls), it is often desirable to provide an escape route for the excess cement. One technique is referred to as "venting" the casting. Venting is accomplished by drilling a small hole in the occlusal surface of the cast gold crown. When the crown is cemented on the tooth, the excess cement can escape through the hole. The hole is subsequently filled either by condensation of gold foil or with a previously prepared cast gold plug.

The minimal thickness of the film is logically related to the particle size of the powder employed. However, the actual film thickness can be less than that of the maximal particle dimension. Undoubtedly, the size of the original particle is reduced by its solution in the liquid during mixing. It may also be crushed during mixing and by the pressure exerted on the casting when it is seated. For instance, it has been determined that a cement made from a powder having one or more particles 75 μm in one dimension possessed a film thickness as low as 35 μm.[8]

Nevertheless, the particles that are squeezed between the walls of the restoration and the tooth are eventually able to withstand the pressure exerted by the dentist in seating the restoration. The size of these particles has been termed the *effective grain size* of the cement.[9] Generally, the finer the original particles, the smaller is the effective grain size and the lower is the film thickness.

The test employed for film thickness is that described in American Dental Association Specification no. 8 for zinc phosphate cement. A cement mix of standard consistency is placed between two glass plates, under a given load, for 10 minutes. According to the specification, the increase in thickness of the two plates caused by the cement film should not be greater than 25 μm for a Type I cement (Table 29–3) and 40 μm for a Type II cement.

Contact with Moisture   In the light of the previous discussion of the critical nature of the water content of the cement, it is evident that the area near the cement must be kept dry while the powder-liquid mixture is being prepared and inserted in the tooth, and during hardening. If the cement is allowed to harden under a film of saliva, some of the phosphoric acid is leached out, and the surface of the cement is dull, soft, and easily dissolved by oral fluids.

The effect of time of exposure to moisture on the solubility of zinc phosphate cement is illustrated by the graph in Figure 29–6.[10] One group of cement specimens was placed in contact with water 10 minutes after preparation. This would approximate the time at which the cement might be exposed to saliva under clinical conditions. The remaining specimens were protected from water for the time intervals indicated.

The solubility of specimens exposed to water at 10 minutes was appreciably greater than that of specimens protected for longer periods. The degrading effects of early exposure to water indicate that exposed surfaces of cement should be protected from oral fluids for as long a period as possible. A coat of cavity varnish (to be discussed in Chapter 30) applied to the margins of newly cemented restorations and orthodontic bands should assist in providing this protection.

However, it should not be inferred from the foregoing that a condition of complete desiccation need or should exist. For example, if the walls of a prepared cavity are dried with alcohol and hot air, it is possible that more phosphoric acid may be absorbed from the cement liquid into the dentinal tubules, and the pulp may be injured.

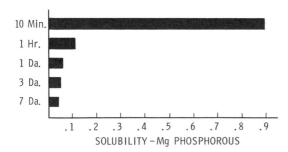

Figure 29–6 Effect on solubility of time at which specimens of zinc phosphate are exposed to water following mixing. The longer the cement is protected from water, the less is the solubility.

After the cement has set, it should not be allowed to dry out; this causes a shrinkage and crazing of the surface that inevitably results in its disintegration. The coating of cavity varnish should minimize dehydration as well as prevent premature contact with oral fluids.

Retention   As discussed in Chapter 2, adhesion refers to a bonding between unlike molecules. There is no adhesion between the zinc phosphate cement and tooth structure or any of the restorative materials with which it is employed.

However, there undoubtedly is a mechanical interlocking, such as a gluing action in paper or wood joints, which provides a certain amount of retention of the restoration. Whenever a casting is seated in the prepared cavity, the surfaces of both the casting and the tooth structure have slight roughnesses and irregularities into which the plastic cement is forced. After the cement hardens, such extensions, many of which are undercut, assist in providing retention of the inlay. The mechanism is diagrammed in Figure 29–7. For this reason, highly polished surfaces do not exhibit as great a retention when they are united with dental cement as do slightly roughened surfaces. This mechanical bonding mechanism is similar to that attained by acid etching techniques used with restorative resins (Chapter 14).

It should be re-emphasized that this retention as is formed with this and most other dental cements is mechanical, and does not provide a truly adhesive joint. Furthermore, the retention of the restoration is controlled principally by the mechanics of the cavity design and not by the adhesive characteristics of the cements.

The thickness of the film between the casting and the tooth also is a factor in the retention. The thinner the film, the better is the cementing action. This effect is probably the result of a number of factors, one of which is that the cement itself is subject to internal flaws, such as air spaces and structural defects in bulk, which are minimized in a thin film. Other factors that play a role are related to surface chemistry, surface tension, and similar phenomena.

There are, however, other inherent properties that influence the cement

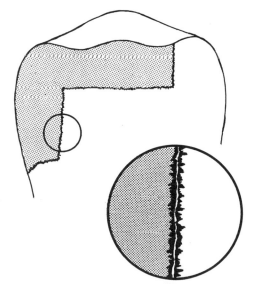

Figure 29–7 A diagram of the suggested mechanism whereby a dental cement provides mechanical retention of a gold inlay. The cement penetrates into irregularities in the tooth structure and the casting, and upon hardening aids in holding the restoration in place. The enlargement shows fracture of these tiny cement projections and loss of retention, possibly resulting in dislodgement of the inlay. (From Phillips RW, Swartz ML, and Norman RD, Materials for the Practicing Dentist, St. Louis, C. V. Mosby Co., 1969.)

bond besides film thickness. For example, if most of these extensions of cement fractured, the restoration would no longer be mechanically locked to the tooth (Fig. 29–7). Therefore, the greater the strength of the cement, the less should be the tendency for fracture of these cement extensions. It has been shown that generally greater tensile or shear forces are required to unseat appliances cemented with luting agents that have a high compressive strength than with cements of low compressive strength.[11] However, the stresses developed during mastication are exceedingly complex. Undoubtedly properties other than compressive strength are involved. These include toughness, the tensile and shear strength of the cement, film thickness, and other properties previously discussed.

The mechanical retention is also dependent upon the dimensional changes occurring in the cement during setting, as a result of the water gain or loss, or as a result of the differences in the coefficient of thermal expansion of the tooth, of the structure luted, and of the cement itself.

Strength   The strength of dental cements is generally determined by inducing a compressive stress. According to American Dental Association Specification no. 8, the 24-hour compressive strength of a zinc phosphate cement should not be less than 68.7 MPa (9956 psi) (Table 29–3).

As previously stated, the strength of the cement is dependent upon the powder-liquid ratio. This dependence is illustrated in Figure 29–8. As can be noted, the compressive strength increases rapidly as the amount of powder is increased. The mixture for a standard consistency of this particular cement is 2.8 (1.4 gm of powder to 0.5 ml of liquid). The strength obtained by increasing the powder above this amount is relatively small, particularly when compared to the decrease in strength when less powder is used.

The set cement gains its maximal strength, for all practical purposes, within the first day. In fact it attains approximately 75 per cent of its maximal strength during the first hour.

When zinc phosphate cements are placed in contact with water for long periods of time, there is a gradual decrease in strength, probably because of

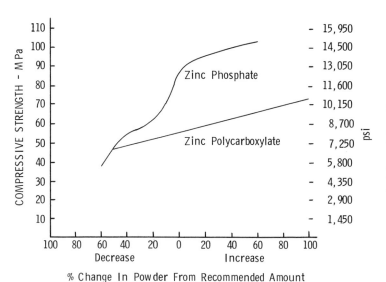

Figure 29–8 Effect of powder-liquid ratio on the strength of two cements. Cement specimens were prepared with greater and lesser amounts of powder (higher and lower powder-liquid ratios) than recommended by the manufacturers, which is represented by 0.

slow dissolution of the material, similar to that which takes place in the mouth.

The strength of a zinc phosphate cement is probably sufficient when it is placed under an inlay or crown. However, when it is exposed to the oral forces, as in a temporary filling material, its brittleness and relatively low strength cause fractures and disintegration under such conditions of stress and erosion.

Solubility and Disintegration   Probably the property of greatest clinical significance is the solubility and disintegration of the cement. In fact, this property is one of the most important considerations in the use and selection of any dental material. In the cemented cast restoration, solubility of the cement is of utmost significance. A thin line of cement is always exposed to oral fluids at the margins even though this *cement line* may not be readily visible to the naked eye. It has been estimated that visual acuity under oral conditions is approximately 50μm.[12, 13] Thus, whenever any cement line is visible in the mouth, it is probably thicker than 50 μm. However, as previously discussed, marginal discrepancies several times this magnitude often go undetected, particularly in the cervical region of the restoration. This exposed layer of cement gradually dissolves so that the restoration eventually may loosen and secondary caries develop.

Other than errors in cavity preparation, cement solubility is probably the main factor contributing to caries around the inlay or crown. Every precaution must be taken to produce an accurately fitting restoration that minimizes the layer of exposed cement and then to handle the material in such a manner that its solubility is as low as possible.

The solubility is usually measured by immersion of a cement disk in distilled water for 24 hours, in accordance with American Dental Association Specification no. 8. The specimen is then removed, the water evaporated, and the weight of the non-volatile solubility products determined. In this test the maximum allowable solubility is 0.2 per cent (Table 29–3). When tested in this manner many products show considerably lower values.

If the cement is immersed in dilute organic acids, the solubility is much higher than in distilled water. The fact is evidenced in Figure 29–9, in which solubility has been measured in lactic, acetic, and citric acids as well as in distilled water. It is obvious that the solubility in the organic acids is greater than in distilled water. Likewise, the solubility increases when the pH of the medium is lowered. The increase in solubility with reduced pH is probably due to the greater solubility of the zinc oxide component of the cement and also, but to a lesser extent, the increased solubility of the phosphate matrix.

In the oral cavity, deleterious agents such as organic acids are present in varying concentrations, depending upon the flora and nutrients available. For

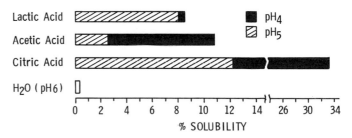

Figure 29–9   Solubility of a typical zinc phosphate cement when immersed in pH 4 and pH 5 dilute organic acid solutions and in water for a period of 1 week. The solutions were changed daily.

example, after ingestion of certain foods, plaque on the surface of the tooth or restoration may be acidic for an hour or longer. Acetic and other organic acids have been associated with the lowered pH.

The data in Figure 29–9 suggest that durability of the cement is basically related to the type and pH of the acids to which it is exposed. Thus the solubility in such media is indicative of the dangers inherent when the zinc phosphate cements are exposed to oral fluids.

It must be emphasized that the type of test by which these values were obtained must be regarded as a simple screening test. Such a test is undoubtedly useful for examining the relative vulnerability of cements of the same type (i.e., one zinc phosphate cement to another zinc phosphate cement) and the influence of certain variables, such as pH, on the solubility rate of the particular species of cement.

However, no laboratory test will accurately predict the in vivo disintegration rate of one cement system as compared with a different one. Recent in vivo solubility and disintegration studies have been conducted in which the cement samples were inserted in wells in crowns, bridge pontics, and denture bases and exposed to the oral environment.[14-16] There was no correlation between the relative loss of different types of cements in vivo and the comparable solubility levels of these same cements as determined by laboratory tests (e.g., zinc phosphate cement as compared with a silicophosphate cement and/or a zinc oxide–eugenol).

The development of a single laboratory test for comparison of the various types of cements with respect to their relative durability in the mouth is complicated by the complex make-up of the oral environment and the difference in the chemical make-up and disintegration mechanisms of the various kinds of cement.[17]

Biological Properties As might be expected from the presence of the phosphoric acid, the acidity of the cements is quite high at the time they are inserted in the tooth.

Three minutes after the start of the mixing, the pH of zinc phosphate cement is approximately 3.5, as indicated in Table 29–4. The pH then increases rapidly, approaching neutrality in 24 to 48 hours. The pH is lower and remains lower for a longer period of time when thin mixes are employed. Both the initial and the 28-day pH of thin mixes of zinc phosphate cement are somewhat lower than those recorded with the thicker mixes.[18]

From these data it is evident that any damage to the pulp from acid attack by zinc phosphate cement occurs during the first few hours after insertion. However, studies with zinc phosphate cements prepared with liquids containing radioactive phosphoric acid indicate that in some teeth the acid from the cement can penetrate a thickness of dentin as great as 1.5 mm.[19] Thus, if the

Table 29–4. *The pH of Dental Cements at Various Time Intervals after Mixing**

Cement	3 Min.	1 Hr.	24 Hrs.	48 Hrs.	7 Days	28 Days
Zinc phosphate	3.5	5.9	6.6	6.8	6.9	6.9
Silicophosphate	3.2	5.4	6.1	6.3	6.5	6.7
Silicate	2.8	3.7	5.0	5.2	5.2	5.2
Type I copper	0.8	3.0	4.7	5.1	5.2	5.3

*A standard consistency mix was used and the pH was determined by means of microantimony electrodes.

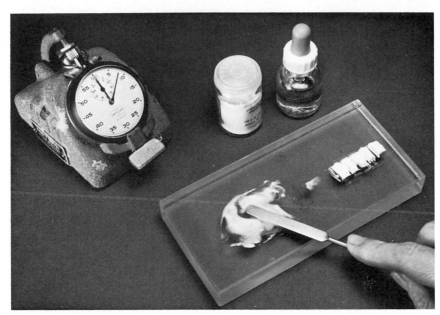

Figure 29-10 When mixing zinc phosphate cement, a small amount of powder is used at the start. A rotary motion is used with the spatula, covering a large portion of the slab.

underlying dentin is not protected against the infiltration of this acid, pulpal injury may occur.

Manipulation   In summary, the following points should be observed in the manipulation of zinc phosphate cements.

1. It is probably not necessary to use a measuring device for proportioning the powder and liquid, as the desired consistency may vary according to the clinical conditions. However, the maximal amount of powder possible for the operation at hand should be used in order to ensure minimum solubility and maximum strength.

2. A cool mixing slab should be employed. The cool slab delays the setting and allows the operator to incorporate the maximum amount of powder before the matrix formation proceeds to a point at which the mixture stiffens.

3. Mixing is initiated by the addition of a small amount of powder, as shown in Figure 29-10. Small quantities are incorporated at a time, using brisk spatulation. A considerable portion of the mixing slab is used. A good rule to follow is to spatulate for 15 or 20 seconds before adding another increment. The mixing time is not unduly critical and completion of the mix usually requires approximately one and a half minutes.

As stated previously, the appropriate consistency varies with the purpose for which the cement is to be used. However the desired consistency is always attained by the addition of more powder and never by allowing a thin mix to stiffen.

4. The casting should be seated immediately, before cement matrix formation occurs. After the casting has been seated, it should be held under pressure until the cement sets in order to minimize the air spaces. The field of operation should be kept dry during the entire procedure.

5. The cement liquid should be stored in a stoppered bottle. It should be exposed to the air as little as possible. If the liquid becomes cloudy, it should not be used.

ZINC SILICOPHOSPHATE CEMENT

Zinc silicophosphate cements are a combination of silicate and zinc phosphate cements. The powder contains both silicate and zinc oxide powder, and the liquid is phosphoric acid. The properties of a Type I cement are listed in Table 29–3. Since such a cement is recommended for cementation of precision castings, obviously it must meet the same requirement as does zinc phosphate cement with respect to maximum film thickness (25 μm). The values for the remaining properties of the silicophosphate cement fall between those of zinc phosphate and of silicate cement. The pH tends to be only slightly lower than that of zinc phosphate cement (Table 29–4).

The composition and manipulation will be discussed in Chapter 30. At this point it is sufficient to say that the outstanding features of zinc silicophosphate cement are that it is somewhat translucent and it possesses some anticariogenic properties by virtue of the fluoride contained in the powder.

COPPER CEMENTS

Silver salts or copper oxides are sometimes added to the powders of the zinc phosphate cements supposedly to increase their antibacterial properties. The cement may be white, black, or red depending on the type of oxide added to the powder. Copper cements have been classified according to the percentage of the copper oxide that is used as a replacement for the zinc oxide.

The chemistry of the copper cements is very similar to that of the zinc phosphate cements, and they should be manipulated in the same manner. They have been used primarily as temporary restorative materials, particularly in children's dentistry. However, they are seldom used anymore because of their poor biological characteristics. They rank high on the list of pulp irritants, which is readily understood when the pH of the set cement is noted (Table 29–4).

ZINC OXIDE–EUGENOL CEMENT

These cements are usually dispensed in the form of a powder and liquid or sometimes as two pastes. The components are mixed together in much the same manner as zinc phosphate cement. A wide variety of zinc oxide–eugenol (ZOE) formulations are available for use as temporary cements and restorations, permanent cements, intermediate restorations, and thermal insulating bases. They also serve as root canal sealants and periodontal dressings. The pH is approximately 7 at the time they are inserted into the tooth. Thus they are one of the least irritating of all dental materials.

The various formulations and uses are reflected in American Dental Association Specification no. 30 for zinc oxide–eugenol restorative materials, which lists four types of materials. Type I ZOE preparations are those designed for temporary cementation. Type II are designed for permanent cementation of restorations or appliances fabricated outside the mouth. A Type III cement is for use as a temporary filling material and thermal insulating base, whereas Type IV is used for cavity liners. The latter implies the use of the material as a coating on the pulpal wall in order to provide protection from chemical insult from the restorative material. However, the thickness would not be adequate to provide thermal protection to the pulp.

In this chapter only those cements used for temporary and permanent cementation are discussed. Those formulations used for temporary restorations, bases, and liners will be discussed in the next chapter.

Composition and Chemistry   The basic components of the cements are zinc oxide and eugenol, hence the setting reaction and microstructure arc essentially the same as those of the impression pastes discussed in Chapter 7. However, there are numerous means by which the handling characteristics and physical properties of zinc oxide-eugenol preparations can be altered. As a result, cements suitable for a wide range of uses are produced.

As with the impression pastes, different types of zinc oxide produce different reaction rates. The most active zinc oxide powders are those formed by decomposing zinc hydroxide, zinc carbonate, or some similar zinc salt by heating to approximately 300° C (570° F). Particle size also affects setting rate. If everything is equal, cements prepared from smaller particles of zinc oxide powder will set more rapidly than ones prepared with larger particles.

Many salts accelerate the setting reaction, but zinc compounds such as zinc acetate, zinc proprionate, and zinc succinate are especially useful. As noted in Chapter 7, alcohol, glacial acetic acid, and small amounts of water are commonly employed to accelerate the set of zinc oxide–eugenol preparations. The fact that water is necessary in order to initiate the setting reaction has been discussed. As with the impression pastes, the set can be retarded with glycol or glycerine.

Properties   The powder-liquid ratio, just as with zinc phosphate cement, affects the setting time. The higher the powder-liquid ratio, the faster is the set. Cooling the mixing slab slows the setting reaction unless the temperature is below the dew point so that the condensate is incorporated into the mix. In the latter instance the setting reaction would of course be accelerated.

Additions such as rosin and small amounts of dicalcium phosphate or mica enhance the smoothness of the mix.

The particle size of the zinc oxide also affects strength.[20] In general, the smaller the particles, the stronger is the cement. However, the specific effect of particle size on strength depends upon the particular additives that are present. For example, the influence of particle size on strength is far more pronounced on formulations that contain ortho-ethoxybenzoic acid (EBA) than on other zinc oxide-eugenol materials. The addition of alumina or of fused silica to the powder also improves strength.

An appreciable increase in strength can be achieved by substitution of EBA for a portion of the eugenol. However, this addition increases the solubility of the cement unless hydrogenated rosin is included in the formulation. Another means of substantially increasing strength is by the discrete incorporation of polymers in the eugenol.

The mechanics by which additives enhance strength of zinc oxide–eugenol cements is not entirely understood. Perhaps the ortho-ethoxybenzoic acid acts as a chelating agent to form zinc carboxylate. Other additives may segregate in the matrix that surrounds the zinc oxide core, in essence to form a composite structure.

Type I   As noted previously, ZOE has a pH of 7 and is exceedingly biocompatible with the pulp. In addition it seals the cavity surprisingly well against the ingress of oral fluids, at least for a short time; hence, irritation from microleakage is minimized. Although the physical and mechanical properties generally are inferior, the material is excellent from a biological standpoint. For this reason it has long been used for temporary restorations and as a palliative dressing in sensitive teeth prior to insertion of the permanent restoration.

Temporary bridges and crowns of resin or metal are often constructed for the purpose of maintaining tooth position and to provide coverage for the prepared teeth while the permanent appliances are being fabricated. On other occasions it is necessary to temporarily cement the permanent castings. Temporary cementation is accomplished with the Type I ZOE cements. Once the problem has been ameliorated the restorations are removed and recemented with a permanent luting agent.

The strength of a temporary cement must be low in order to permit removal of the restoration without trauma to the teeth and, in the case of a permanent restoration, without damage to the casting. Actually, these cements are available in a relatively wide range of strengths. The specification for compressive strength of temporary cements ranges from no requirement (not applicable) for materials classified as *non-setting* to a maximum of 31 MPa (4500 psi) for materials that attain a "hard set." The properties of one such hard setting cement are listed in Table 29-3. However, in order to facilitate removal of the restorations, it is generally desirable to employ a formulation that is in the lower strength range.

Type II   The biological properties that make ZOE so useful as a temporary restoration also make it attractive as a permanent cement. However, a limiting factor has been the comparatively low physical properties, strength in particular. The upgrading of the strength properties has been accomplished via the addition of alumina or some other inorganic filler to the powder and EBA to the liquid. Also, polymers may be added for this purpose. The end results are the so-called "improved" ZOE cements for permanent cementation (Type II).

In order to qualify as a Type II cement the compressive strength must be at least 31 MPa (4500 psi). The properties of a typical EBA cement and of a polymer reinforced ZOE material can be seen in Table 29-3. Obviously, both of these cements are inferior to zinc phosphate cement in terms of compressive strength. In general, the higher the strength of the cement, the greater is the retention of the cemented restoration, as has been discussed earlier.

However, other properties such as toughness and the ability of the cement to wet the tooth and flow into small discrepancies undoubtedly play a role. When the tensile force required to remove occlusal inlays cemented with various commercial Type II ZOE cements was measured (Fig. 29-11), there was considerable difference in the retention afforded by the various materials. Despite the fact that the ZOE cements had appreciably lower compressive strength, virtually the same amount of tensile force was required to remove

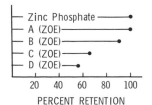

PERCENT RETENTION

Figure 29-11   Relative retention of Class I inlays cemented with four reinforced zinc oxide–eugenol commercial cements, as compared with the retention of the same inlays cemented with a representative zinc phosphate cement. Retention was measured by application of a tensile stress.

inlays cemented with ZOE cements A and B as was required to dislodge inlays cemented with zinc phosphate cement. Furthermore although the compressive strengths of ZOE materials B, C, and D were similar, the retentive ability of C and D was inferior to that of B.

The minimal requirements for permanent luting agents in terms of the strength needed for retention have not been specifically defined, but a minimal value of 31 MPa (4500 psi) has been suggested. However, the demands imposed upon the cement itself undoubtedly vary with the particular clinical situation, e.g., the mechanical design of the cavity and the stress imposed on the restoration. Probably in many situations the reduced retention, as evidenced by some ZOE preparations, would not pose problems. For example, in a full crown restoration adequate retention is usually afforded by virtue of the cavity design, and minimal demands are placed upon the cement itself. However, in certain other restorations, such as a three-quarter crown serving as a bridge abutment, considerable stress may be placed upon the cement-tooth or cement-casting interface.

The solubility of Type II ZOE cements (Table 29–3) is in the same range as that of zinc phosphate cement when determined by the conventional short term tests using gravimetric analysis of nonvolatile solubility products. Some of the shortcomings of this test have been discussed previously. Research on the solubility and disintegration of ZOE cements in an aqueous environment indicates the mechanism of breakdown to be one of hydrolysis of the zinc eugenolate matrix to form zinc hydroxide and eugenol.[21, 22] These products would not be detected by this laboratory test procedure. The eugenol is volatilized during evaporation of the storage medium, whereas the zinc hydroxide is relatively insoluble and tends to cling to the specimen surface.

It will be noted from Table 29–3 that the film thickness of some of these cements may slightly exceed the film thickness requirement.

It is obvious that while the ZOE cements are superior to zinc phosphate cement with respect to biological characteristics, they are inferior overall in terms of certain physical properties.

ZINC POLYCARBOXYLATE CEMENT

Polycarboxylate, or *polyacrylate*, cement was the first system developed with a potential for adhesion to tooth structure.[23, 24]

Composition and Chemistry The polycarboxylate cements are powder-liquid systems. The liquid is an aqueous solution of polyacrylic acid and copolymers. The powder is similar in composition to that used with zinc phosphate cement — principally zinc oxide with some magnesium oxide. Stannic oxide may be substituted for magnesium oxide. It may also contain small quantities of stannous fluoride, and of other salts that modify the setting time and enhance the manipulative characteristics. The most important additive is stannous fluoride, which increases the strength of the cement and also acts as a source of fluoride, which well may impart anticariogenic properties to the cement. This matter will be discussed in the next chapter.

When the powder and liquid are combined, the cement-forming mechanism is thought to be a reaction of zinc ions with the polyacrylic acid via the carboxyl groups. The zinc can also react with the carboxyl groups of adjacent polyacrylic acid chains so that an ionically cross-linked structure is formed.

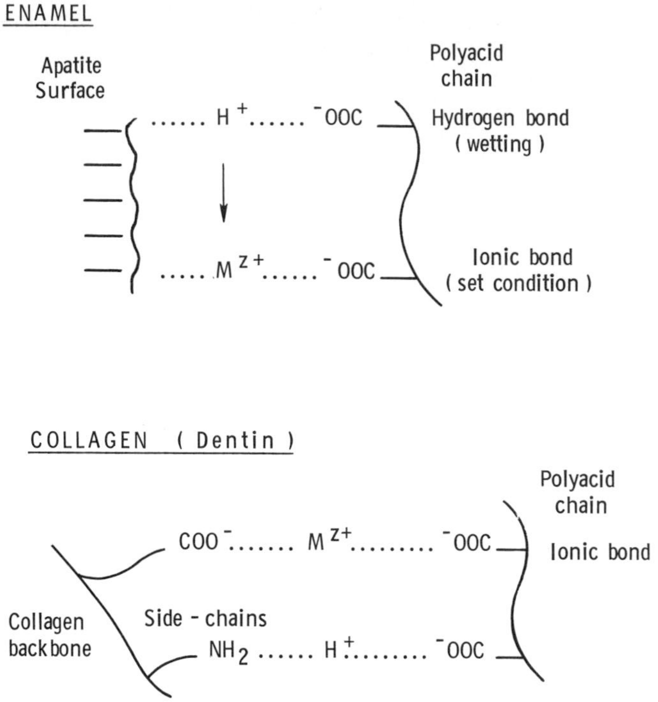

ENAMEL

Apatite
Surface

Polyacid
chain

— { ...... H $^+$ ...... $^-$OOC — Hydrogen bond
— }   (wetting)
— {   ↓
— }
— { ..... M $^{z+}$ ...... $^-$OOC — Ionic bond
                                    (set condition)

COLLAGEN (Dentin)

Polyacid
chain

COO $^-$ .... M $^{z+}$ .... $^-$OOC — Ionic bond

Collagen   Side - chains
backbone   — NH $_2$ ...... H $^+$ .... $^-$OOC —

Figure 29–12 The diagram illustrates postulate mechanisms for the adhesion of polycarboxylate and glass-ionomer cement to enamel and dentin as suggested by Wilson, AD, *in* Aspects of Adhesion-8, Transcription Books, pp. 285–306, 1975. The upper diagram shows a suggested mechanism whereby the fresh, mobile cement paste wets and adheres to the enamel apatite surface by hydrogen bonds provided by free carboxylic acid groups. As the cement reaction proceeds, most of these hydrogen bonds, as represented by the arrow, are replaced by metal ions to give metal ion bridges that provide adhesion for the cement to the enamel.

The lower diagram illustrates possible mechanisms of adhesion between those cements and dentin. Collagen contains some branch chains that terminate in carboxylic acid groups and others that terminate in amino groups. The former can link to the cement mass by metal ion bridging, while the latter groups bond by hydrogen bridges. (By permission of A. D. Wilson, Laboratory of the Government Chemist, Crown Copyright.)

Thus, the hardened cement consists of zinc oxide particles dispersed in a structureless matrix of zinc polycarboxylate.

The exact mechanism of the adhesion to the calcium in tooth structure is not entirely known and remains a subject for speculation. The suggested method of bonding is shown in Figure 29–12. Initially the cement paste adheres to the apatite by hydrogen bonding, but as the cement sets the hydrogen bonds are replaced by metal ions producing a metal ion bridge. There is some evidence that the cement also may bond to the collagen of the dentin. As shown in Figure 29–12, it is postulated that adhesion to collagen may involve both hydrogen and ionic bonding.

Recently several polycarboxylate cements have been marketed as a single component system, consisting of a powder that is mixed with water. The polyacrylic acid is dried and the powdered acid is mixed in with the traditional cement powder. When this powder is mixed with water, the polyacrylic acid goes into solution and the setting reaction proceeds, as described for the conventional powder-liquid system.

Properties   The properties of polycarboxylate cement, when manipulated to produce a consistency suitable for cementation, are seen in Table 29–3. As with all materials, properties differ to some degree with the product and testing procedure. The values shown are representative.

The compressive strength of the polycarboxylate cements falls into the range of the reinforced zinc oxide–eugenol cements but is inferior to the zinc phosphate cement. However, the strength of polycarboxylate cement appears to be less sensitive than zinc phosphate cement to small fluctuations in powder-liquid ratio. This is shown in Figure 29–8, where the strengths of a zinc phosphate and a polycarboxylate cement, as related to the amount of powder present in the mix, are compared. Reducing the recommended amount of powder in the mix of polycarboxylate cement by one-third reduced the strength by approximately 5 MPa (700 psi), or about 9 per cent. On the other hand, a comparable reduction in the amount of powder incorporated into a mix of zinc phosphate cement reduced the strength by about 35 per cent as compared with that attained with the recommended ratio.

The tensile strengths of polycarboxylate, zinc phosphate, and the reinforced zinc oxide–eugenol cements are comparable. Higher strengths are obtained for all cements with the diametral test, as compared with the uniaxial test.

The solubility of the polycarboxylate cements in distilled water is in the same range as that of zinc phosphate cements (Table 29–3). This system, as do the zinc phosphate and zinc oxide–eugenol cements, has a considerably higher disintegration rate in organic acids. However, it should be reiterated that caution should be observed in using in vitro solubility data on different types of cement to extrapolate predictions on longevity in the oral cavity. Even in vivo studies on the disintegration of specimens of cements inserted in various dental appliances have not as yet fully solved this problem.[14-16] In one such study zinc polycarboxylate cements exhibited a slightly lower rate of disintegration than did zinc phosphate cement, but in other investigations it was somewhat higher.

Although a polycarboxylate cement mix prepared with the correct powder-liquid ratio and proper manipulation appears to be very thick and viscous, as compared with corresponding mixes of zinc phosphate cement, it will form a film of 25 μm or less. Hence it meets the requirement that has been established for the cementation of precision fitting castings. The viscous appearance of the cement is misleading in that it is no more difficult to seat a precise fitting casting with polycarboxylate cement than it is with zinc phosphate cement. This phenomenon is related to the rheological properties of the cement. Polycarboxylate cement behaves as a pseudoplastic material and zinc phosphate as a newtonian liquid (Chapter 3).

Adhesion to Tooth Structure   As discussed, there is considerable evidence that this type of cement does adhesively bond to tooth structure. A rather wide range of bond strengths to enamel and dentin has been reported. Again, the differences may be attributed to the individual test methods. However, regardless of the exact values reported in individual studies, the relative results are in agreement. Representative data are seen in Figure 29–13.[25]

In this study the bond strength was evaluated by measuring the tensile stress required to separate a cylinder of cement from enamel and dentin surfaces. The superiority of the bond attained with the polycarboxylate cement on both enamel and dentin, as compared with that of zinc phosphate cement, is obvious. It should be pointed out that the values for enamel where no thermal cycling was involved do not represent the true bond strength. It is actually higher than this figure, since most of the specimens failed in cohesion rather than in adhesion at the enamel–cement interface, i.e., the strength of the bond to enamel exceeded the tensile strength of the cement under the axial loading used in this test.

When specimens were thermal stressed by cycling between water baths having a 40° C (70° F) temperature differential, the bond strength between the polycarboxylate cement and tooth structure decreased. However, the degrading effect was not so great as for zinc phosphate cement. When zinc phosphate cement specimens were subjected to temperature stressing, the cement invari-

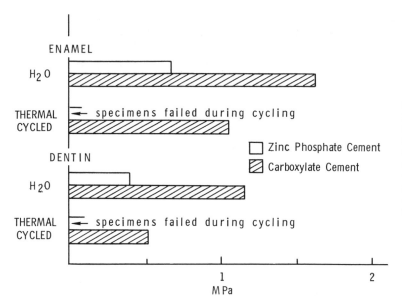

Figure 29–13 The tensile strength required to separate specimens of a polycarboxylate cement, as compared with zinc phosphate cement, from enamel and dentin surfaces after storage in water for 1 week. Thermal stressed specimens were subjected to 2500 cycles between water baths maintained at 10 and 50° C.

ably separated cleanly from the tooth during the cycling operation. The fact that the strength of the bond of polycarboxylate cement to enamel is greater than to dentin would support the theory of calcium bonding, since there is a higher apatite concentration in enamel than in dentin.

pH and Biological Considerations   The pH of the cement liquid is approximately 1.7. However, the liquid is rapidly neutralized by the powder. Thus, the pH of the mix rises rapidly as the setting reaction proceeds. The pH of a polycarboxylate cement is comparable to that of a zinc phosphate cement at various time intervals.

Despite the initial acidic nature of the polycarboxylate cements, they produce minimal irritation to the pulp. They are in the same realm as the zinc oxide–eugenol cements.[26]

Several theories have been advanced to explain the difference in the reaction of the dental pulp to polycarboxylate and zinc phosphate cements, even though the pH values of the cements are comparable. It is possible that the large size of the polyacrylic acid molecule and/or its tendency to complex with protein may limit its diffusion through the dentinal tubules.

A major factor in the popularity of this cement system is this excellent biocompatibility to the pulp. As for the zinc oxide–eugenol cements, postoperative sensitivity is negligible when the polycarboxylate cement is used as a luting agent or base.

Clinical Considerations   As is true for all newer materials, a correlation of the properties of this cement to clinical behavior awaits long-term studies. However, based on current information, a number of observations can be made.

The working time with these cements is relatively short. If satisfactory results are to be obtained, mixing and cementing operations must be carried out with dispatch.

Despite the adhesion of the cement to tooth structure, polycarboxylate cements may not be superior to zinc phosphate or some of the reinforced zinc oxide–eugenol cements with respect to retention of cast gold restorations. A comparable force is required to remove gold inlays cemented either with zinc phosphate cement or with a polycarboxylate cement. The difference seems to be in the mode of failure. With zinc phosphate cement, failure usually occurs at the cement-tooth interface. In the case of the polycarboxylate cements, the failure usually occurs cohesively or at the cement-metal interface, not adhesively at the tooth-cement interface. The cement is unable to bond to the metal in the chemically dirty "as cast" or "pickled" condition.

Thus it is essential that this chemically dirty surface on the cavity side of the casting be removed in order to provide a mechanical bond at the cement-metal interface. The surface can be carefully abraded with a small stone, for example. Also, there are a number of devices available that make use of an airborne abrasive. It has been suggested that adhesive bonding might be attained by electroplating the casting with tin and thereby obtain a bond through the reaction of the carboxyl groups in the cement and the tin.[27] However, there is need for further research to determine the validity of that hypothesis.

Regardless of the technique used, it is imperative that the pickled surface of the casting be removed.

Manipulation Since this type of cement affords an opportunity to obtain adhesion to at least one component of tooth structure, a meticulously clean surface is necessary in order to provide intimate contact and interaction between the cement and the tooth. Various media may be safely employed for cleaning the cavity preparation of debris left from instrumentation or remnants of a temporary restorative material. These include water, a dilute solution of hydrogen peroxide (1–3 per cent) or the cement liquid itself. At least one manufacturer supplies a solution for that purpose.

After cleansing, the cavity is isolated to prevent further contamination from the oral fluids. Blotting the surface prior to cementation is considered to be sufficient drying.

The cement liquids are quite viscous. The viscosity of the liquid is dependent upon the concentration and molecular weight of the polyacrylic acid. Thus, within limits, it is possible for manufacturers to prepare cements of varying viscosities for particular uses. The powder-liquid ratios required to produce a cement of suitable cementing consistency vary among different brands, but they are in the general range of 1.5 parts of powder to 1 part of liquid by weight.

The material should be mixed on a surface that will not absorb liquid. A glass slab may afford some advantage over the treated paper pad that is generally supplied because it can be cooled. Cooling slows the chemical reaction to some extent and thus provides a somewhat longer working time.

Also, the working time may be extended to some degree if the powder is cooled in a refrigerator. Under no circumstances should the liquid be cooled, since the viscosity of the liquid increases when the temperature is decreased. Polyacrylic acid is unstable at either high or low temperatures.

The liquid should not be dispensed prior to the time when the mix is to be made. It loses water to the atmosphere very rapidly, as shown in Figure 29–4. The loss of water from the liquid results in a very marked increase in its viscosity. In fact, if the liquid is left on the slab for only a minute or two its viscosity may be significantly increased.

The powder is rapidly incorporated into the liquid in large quantities. The mix should be completed within 30 or 40 seconds in order to provide sufficient working time to carry out the cementing operation. Although the mix appears to be quite thick as compared with a similar mix of zinc phosphate cement, as noted previously polycarboxylate cements will flow readily into a thin film when placed under pressure.

However, it is esential that the cement be used while the surface is still glossy. Loss of luster and a dull, stringy, rubber consistency indicate that the setting reaction has progressed to the extent that a satisfactory film thickness and proper wetting of the tooth surface by the cement can no longer be attained. This change in consistency is illustrated in Figure 29–14A, where the

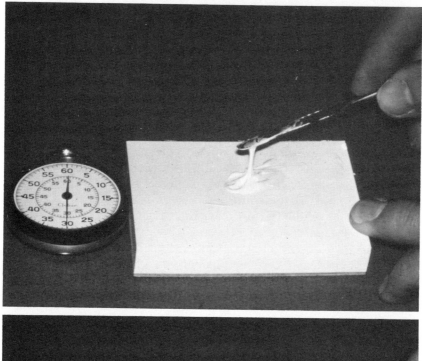

A

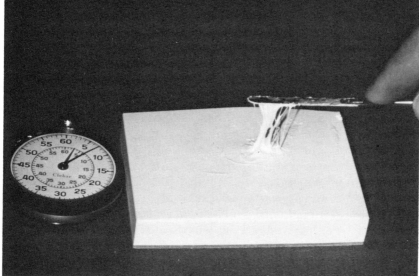

B

Figure 29–14 *A,* Consistency of mix of polycarboxylate cement upon completion of 30 second mix. *B,* If mixing time is prolonged or the mix allowed to remain on the slab, the cement becomes dull in appearance and the consistency tacky. (Courtesy of M. Jendresen)

consistency of the cement is shown immediately after completion of the 30 second mix as compared with the consistency after an additional time on the mixing slab (Fig. 29–14B).

During setting, the cement passes through a rubbery stage. The excess cement that has extruded at the margins of the casting should not be removed while the cement is in this stage, since there is danger that some of the cement may be pulled out from beneath the margins. Excess is not removed until the cement becomes hard.

GLASS IONOMER

The Type I versions of the glass ionomer cements are fine grained and hence are suitable for cementation of castings. They are dispensed as a powder and liquid. The powder is an aluminosilicate glass, similar to that of silicate cements. The liquid basically is an aqueous solution of a copolymer of a polyacrylic acid and other organic acids, analogous to the liquid of polycarboxylate cement but generally somewhat less viscous. The complete chemistry and properties of the glass ionomer cements will be deferred to the next chapter where Type II glass ionomer cements, in reference to their use as restorative materials, are discussed.

The properties of a representative Type I glass ionomer cement are seen in Table 29–3. For the most part, the mechanical properties are in the range of those for zinc phosphate. This cement appears to be somewhat stronger in compression than is the polycarboxylate cement. The 24-hour solubility in water, and also the in vivo data, fall into the range of the zinc silicophosphate cement. This would be anticipated, since silica glass is a constituent of both cement powders. The cement is relatively translucent and resembles tooth structure.

The glass ionomer cements adhere to tooth structure by virtue of the polyacrylic acid in the liquid. The chemical adhesion to tooth structure is the same as was described for the polycarboxylate cements (Fig. 29–12). As with polycarboxylate cements, the adhesion to enamel is superior to the bond to dentin.[28]

The glass ionomer cement is kind to the pulp, eliciting a response comparable to that of polycarboxylate cement, as would be anticipated on the basis of composition. In addition, the cement possesses the potential for inhibiting or reducing secondary caries by virtue of the release of the fluoride that is a constituent of the silicate glass powder, as will be discussed in Chapter 30.

Manipulation   The prepared tooth structure should be meticulously cleaned and dried in order to attain adhesion of the cement. Likewise, the retention of the casting can be improved if the inside surface is cleaned, as described for the polycarboxylate cement. The mixing procedure is similar to that described for zinc polycarboxylate cement. The powder is introduced into the liquid in large increments and spatulated rapidly for 45 seconds. As with all cements, the properties of a Type I glass ionomer cement are markedly influenced by manipulative factors. The recommended powder-liquid ratio varies with different brands, but it is in the range of 1.25 to 1.5 gm of powder per 1 gm of liquid.

Cementation should be done before the cement loses its shiny appearance. This cement, like zinc phosphate cement, becomes brittle once it has set. When the cement hardens, the excess or "flash" can be removed by flicking or breaking the cement away at the margins.

This new cement is particularly susceptible to attack by water during its setting. Therefore, it is necessary to coat all of the accessible margins of the restoration to protect the cement from premature exposure to moisture. It is possible that newer formulations may be more resistant to the aqueous environment.

RESIN CEMENT

Currently there are two types of resin cements on the market for cementation of castings. Basically the compositions are that of chemically activated direct-filling resins, poly (methyl methacrylate) and BIS-GMA. Both contain fine particle fillers to reduce the coefficient of thermal expansion and polymerization shrinkage.

From the standpoint of properties, the principal advantage of these cements is that they are virtually insoluble in water. In other respects they are inferior to other cementing media. They are somewhat irritating to the pulp. Thus it is essential that the pulpal wall be protected by a layer of $Ca(OH)_2$. Like other resins they do not adhere to tooth structure. Thus, in time water may penetrate the tooth-cement interface.

The manipulative characteristics are somewhat inferior to most other types of cements. With some resin cements, the film thickness is high and difficulty has been encountered in obtaining complete seating of the casting. Also the time at which the excess cement (flash) is removed is critical. The flash should be removed immediately upon seating of the casting. If done while the cement is in a rubbery stage, some of the cement may be pulled out from under the casting. The resulting void at the margins then increases the susceptibility to secondary caries. Removal of the flash is difficult if delayed until polymerization of the cement is completed. For such reasons, the resin cements have not been widely used for cementation of precision castings.

However, the advent of the enamel acid etching technique for retention of direct filling resin restorations has led to the use of resins for bonding orthodontic brackets directly to the tooth surface.[29] In this way the need for banding teeth is eliminated.

Resin materials designed for this procedure, either BIS-GMA or poly (methyl methacrylate) are commercially available. The enamel surface is etched with a phosphoric acid solution in the area where the bracket is to be placed. The technique of etching and the precautions to be observed are the same as was described in Chapter 14 for direct filling resins. The mixed resin is then applied and the bracket is held in position on the tooth until the resin polymerizes. Plastic brackets to which the resin will bond are available for this purpose. Use of clear plastic brackets is mandatory if the resin employed for attachment is a light-cured material. However, metal brackets are more popular. Since the resin does not bond to metal, the brackets must be designed to provide a means of mechanical retention. This is generally accomplished by attaching some sort of metal mesh or screen to the back of the bracket. The fluid resin flows through the mesh and polymerizes, thus providing a mechanical lock.

References

1. Wilson AD: The chemistry of dental cements. Chem Soc Rev 7:265, 1978.
2. Wilson AD, Kent BE, and Lewis BG: Zinc phosphate cements: Chemical study of in vitro durability. J Dent Res 49:1049, 1970.
3. Servais GE and Cartz L: Structure of zinc phosphate cement. J Dent Res 50:613, 1971.
4. Crisp S, O'Neill IK, Prosser HJ, Stuart B, and Wilson AD: Infrared spectroscopic studies on the development of crystallinity in dental zinc phosphate cements. J Dent Res 57:245, 1978.
5. Norman RD, Swartz ML, Phillips RW, and Sears CR: Properties of cements mixed from liquids with altered water content. J Prosthet Dent 24:410, 1970.
6. Kendzior GM, Leinfelder KF, and Hershey HG: The effect of cold temperature mixing on the properties of zinc phosphate cement. Angle Orthodont 46:345, 1976.
7. Jørgensen KD: Factors affecting the film thickness of zinc phosphate cements. Acta Odontol Scand 18:479, 1960.
8. Souder W and Paffenbarger GC: Physical Properties of Dental Materials. National Bureau of Standards Circular C433, Washington, D.C., U.S. Government Printing Office, 1942.
9. Jørgensen KD and Petersen GF: The grain size of zinc phosphate cements. Acta Odontol Scand 21:255, 1963.
10. Swartz ML, Sears CR, and Phillips RW: Solubility of cement as related to time of exposure in water. J Prosthet Dent 26:501, 1971.
11. Oldham DF, Swartz ML, and Phillips RW: Retentive properties of dental cements. J Prosthet Dent 14:760, 1964.
12. Nelsen RJ, Wolcott RB, and Paffenbarger GC: Fluid exchange at the margins of dental restorations. J Am Dent Assoc 44:288, 1952.
13. Christensen GJ: Marginal fit of gold inlay castings. J Prosthet Dent 16:297, 1966.
14. Osborne JW, Swartz ML, Goodacre CJ, Phillips RW, and Gale EN: A method for assessing the clinical solubility and disintegration of luting agents. J Prosthet Dent 40:413, 1978.
15. Mitchem JC and Gronas DG: Clinical evaluation of cement solubility. J Prosthet Dent 40:453, 1978.
16. Richter WA and Ueno H: Clinical evaluation of dental cement durability. J Prosthet Dent 33:294, 1975.
17. Wilson AD: Specification test for the solubility and disintegration of dental cements: A critical evaluation of its meaning. J Dent Res 55:721, 1976.
18. Norman RD, Swartz ML, and Phillips RW: Direct pH determinations of setting cements. Parts I and II. J Dent Res 45:136 and 1214, 1966.
19. Swartz ML, Niblack BF, Alter EA, Norman RD, and Phillips RW: In vivo studies on the penetration of dentin by constituents of silicate cement. J Am Dent Assoc 76:573, 1968.
20. Norman RD, Phillips RW, Swartz ML, and Frankiewicz T: The effect of particle size on the physical properties of zinc oxide-eugenol mixtures. J Dent Res 43:252, 1964.
21. Wilson AD and Batchelor RF: Zinc oxide-eugenol cements: II. Study of erosion and disintegration. J Dent Res 49:593, 1970.
22. Wilson AD, Clinton DJ, and Miller RP: Zinc oxide-eugenol cements. IV. Microstructure and hydrolysis. J Dent Res 52:253, 1973.
23. Smith DC: A review of the zinc polycarboxylate cements. J Can Dent Assoc 37:22, 1971.
24. Smith DC: Dental cements. Dent Clin North Am 15:3, 1971.
25. Phillips RW, Swartz ML, and Rhodes B: An evaluation of a carboxylate adhesive cement. J Am Dent Assoc 81:1353, 1970.
26. Truelove EL, Mitchell DF, and Phillips RW: Biologic evaluation of a carboxylate cement. J Dent Res 50:166, 1971.
27. McLean JW: A new method of bonding dental cements and porcelain to metal surfaces. Oper Dent 2:130, 1977.
28. Maldonado A, Swartz ML, and Phillips RW: An in vitro study of certain properties of a glass ionomer cement. J Am Dent Assoc 96:785, 1978.
29. Betteridge MA: Bonding of orthodontic attachments: Its use and technique. Br Dent J 147:162, 1979.

30 CEMENTS FOR RESTORATIONS. CAVITY VARNISHES, LINERS AND BASES.

Cements are employed for temporary and intermediate restorations and for the esthetic restoration of anterior teeth. Currently there are two types, silicate and glass ionomer, that are designed for that purpose. Both are translucent and resemble porcelain in appearance. Since these cements are attacked by oral fluids and in time degrade, they are not considered permanent in the same sense as are metallic restorations, such as amalgam. For example, the average life of a silicate restoration has been estimated at 4 years. Although some restorations may last as long as 25 years, others may require replacement in a year or even less. As will be seen, this erratic behavior is probably due to variations in technique and/or differences in the oral environment. Less is known concerning the longevity of glass ionomer restorations, since this cement is quite new and long term clinical observations are lacking.

The use of silicate cements has diminished markedly with the advent of composite resins for the restoration of anterior teeth. However, this cement warrants some discussion because it possesses anticariogenic properties and the mechanism involved has been well defined. In addition, the new glass ionomer system is based to a certain extent upon that of silicate cement.

SILICATE CEMENT

Composition and Chemistry The cement is a powder-liquid system. The powder is a finely ground ceramic that is essentially an acid soluble glass. Natural and synthetic ceramic materials are analogous to metallic alloys in that they may contain a number of constituents. The structure of such substances is likely to be quite complex, as is indicated in the next chapter. However, the silicate cement powders consist primarily of silica (SiO_2) in the range of 40 per cent, alumina (Al_2O_3) (approximately 30 per cent), and either sodium fluoride (NaF), calcium fluoride (CaF_2), or cryolite (Na_3AlF_6) (19 per cent) or combinations thereof.[1, 2] They also may contain a calcium phosphate, such as $Ca(H_2PO_4)_2 \cdot H_2O$, or in some instances lime (CaO).

The ingredients are fused at approximately 1400° C (2550° F). The fluoride salts melt at a lower temperature than the other ingredients and act as fusing agents. Such substances are known as ceramic fluxes. Aluminum phosphate may also be used as a flux. In addition to serving as a flux, it furnishes additional aluminum to the glass.

The fused mass is an acid soluble glass. The principal glass phase consists of an aluminosilicate network, SiO_4^- and AlO_4^- tetrahedrons, with cations of Al^{+++}, Ca^{++}, and Na^+ that balance the negative charge on the lattice. The secondary phase, dispersed as fine droplets in the main phase, is primarily fluoride and is responsible for the opacity of the glass. A powder is then prepared from this glass.

The compositions of liquids for the silicate cements are not greatly different from those of the zinc phosphate cements, except that zinc and sometimes magnesium phosphate are used as buffering agents in the silicate cement liquids in addition to the usual aluminum phosphate. Also, the silicate cement liquids generally contain more water (approximately 40 per cent by weight) than do the zinc phosphate cement liquids. Although innumerable powder and liquid modifications have been studied, none has been found to appreciably improve the physical properties.

When the powder and liquid are mixed together the chemical reaction is that of an acid and a base. The hydrogen ions of the phosphoric acid attack the glass, displacing Al^{+++} and other ions such as Na^+ and Ca^{++} along with F^- ions. (The silicon is not removed, nor do the phosphates transfer to the glass.) The displaced ions collect in the semiliquid phase, together with phosphate and other metal ions contained in the cement liquid.[3] As the pH of the liquid phase rises, the metal ions precipitate as phosphates and fluorides.

The principal constituent of the matrix is a hydrated aluminum phosphate. The matrix primarily is amorphous in structure, with some crystals of $Al_2(OH)_3PO_4$. Calcium fluoride also has been identified in the matrix.[4] The surface layer of the powder particles from which most of the metal and fluoride ions have been extracted remains as a hydrated aluminosilicate gel. The hydrated silaceous gel is bonded to the glass core by Si-O-Al bonding and to the hydrated aluminum phosphate matrix via hydrogen-bonded water molecules (water is essential to this cement formation).

The set cement is thereby in essence a composite material consisting of an aggregate of particles bonded in a continuous matrix.

Properties The property values representative of commercial brands of silicate cement are given in Table 30–1. Although the properties of individual brands may vary to some degree, the cements will fall into these ranges when properly manipulated.

As with any restorative material the setting must be controlled so as to

Table 30–1. *Some Properties of Silicate and Glass Ionomer Cements*

		SILICATE	GLASS IONOMER
Setting time (minutes)		3–8	4–5
Compressive strength	(MPa)	180	140
(24 hour)	(psi)	26,000	20,000
Diametral tensile			
strength	(MPa)	3.5	2.7
(24 hour)	(psi)	500	400
Hardness	(KHN)	70	60
Solubility — 24 hour H_2O (per cent)		0.7	0.4
Pulp response		Severe	Mild
Anticariogenic		Yes	Probably

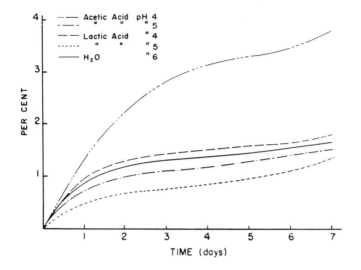

Figure 30-1 Solubility of a typical silicate cement in various solutions which were changed daily.

allow sufficient time for mixing and placement in the cavity, but once inserted in the cavity, the cement should harden as rapidly as possible. The setting time of an acceptable silicate is from 3 to 8 minutes.

Silicate is the strongest of the dental cements. When properly mixed the compressive strength is at least 167 MPa (24,200 psi). As with all cements, it is considerably weaker when tested in tension. Just as with zinc phosphate cement, the strength properties are sensitive to the powder/liquid ratio. The higher the P/L ratio, within practical limits, the higher is the strength. Any change in water content of the liquid, either increase or decrease, will impair all of the properties, including strength and solubility.

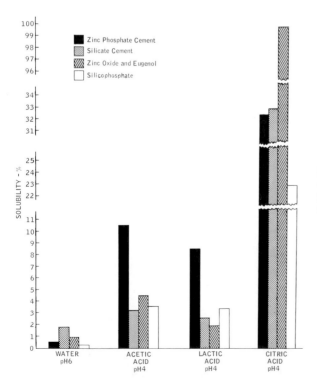

Figure 30-2 Comparison of the solubility of various cementing mediums in different solutions after immersion for seven days. The solutions were changed daily.

Table 30–2.   *Changes in Fluoride Content and Acid Solubility of Enamel Induced by Cements*

Cement	% Change in F Content	% Change in Acid Solubility
A. Silicate (without F)	0	+20
B. Silicate (with F)	+3500	−40
C. Zinc silicophosphate	+3000	−50
D. Glass ionomer	+5000	−30

Values encompassed by the straight line are not significantly different from each other.

The hardness of silicate cement is around 70 KHN, placing it in the same range as dentin.

The maximum allowable solubility and disintegration of silicate, by the American Dental Association specification, when immersed in water for 24 hours is 1.0 per cent. However, as was noted in Chapter 29, this test is only useful for comparing the disintegration and solubility of one silicate cement with another. Despite the fact that silicate cement has greater solubility by the 24 hour test in water than does zinc phosphate cement (1 per cent as compared to 0.2 per cent), it has greater durability than does zinc phosphate cement when evaluated in vivo.[5]

The solubility and disintegration of silicate cement in organic acids and water is plotted over a 7 day period in Figure 30–1. It will be noted that the rate of solubility of the cement during the first 24 to 48 hour period is quite high but after that time it decreases. The high initial solubility (24 hour) is attributed to the rather long time required for the setting reaction to go to completion. The materials leached from the cement at the early time period are primarily intermediate reaction products and include sodium and phosphate, plus fluoride. As the cement ages, the amount of the ions, particularly phosphate, leached from the cement decreases.[6, 7] As with all cements, silicate cement is attacked by organic acids, such as acetic and lactic, with the greatest destruction produced by citric acid (Fig. 30–2).

The coefficient of thermal expansion is much lower than that of resin restoratives, particularly unfilled acrylic resin (Table 3–2). Silicate changes dimension only about 0.7 as compared with the tooth. Thus from this standpoint the cement is superior to most other restorative materials.

Biological Properties   Silicate cement has a pH of less than 3.0 at the time of insertion in the cavity, and the pH remains well below 7 even after 1 month. As shown in Table 29–4, it is more acidic than either zinc phosphate or silicophosphate cement. Thus in terms of pulpal response, it is classified as a severe irritant. Just as zinc oxide–eugenol cement serves as the standard of comparison for materials that are kind to the pulp, silicate serves as the reference for those that elicit a more severe reaction. Thus in testing new materials with respect to pulpal irritation they usually are classified on the comparative behavior to the two extremes, zinc oxide–eugenol and silicate cements.

Some means of protecting the pulp from the acid cement must be employed. The protection can be in the form of a layer of a zinc oxide–eugenol or calcium hydroxide cement placed on the pulpal floor, or by coating the walls of the cavity with varnish. When a cavity varnish is used the varnish should be confined to the dentin, in order that fluoride uptake by the enamel from the cement is not impaired.

Anticariogenic Properties (Fluoride) Most commercial silicate cement powders contain fluoride salts up to 15 per cent. The exact composition of fluoride compound present in the set cement is not entirely understood. However, the clinical significance of the fluoride is extremely important.

It is commonly recognized that the incidence of secondary caries is markedly less around the silicate cement restoration than that associated with all other filling materials. For example, a survey of some 20,000 existing restorations noted a 12 per cent incidence of secondary caries occurring in time around amalgam restorations. The incidence was only 3 per cent for silicate cement restorations.[8] Also, the incidence of contact caries is less with silicate cement restorations than with amalgam restorations.[9] Contact caries is a term that has been applied to the caries occurring on the proximal surface of the tooth adjacent to the restoration. Thus, although the silicate cement has many weaknesses, it is unique from the standpoint of its anticariogenic characteristics. This behavior is somewhat surprising when one examines the gross leakage that occurs at the margins of, and even through, the silicate restoration. Few, if any, dental restorative materials show greater leakage.

The anticariogenic potential has been attributed to the fluorine present in the cement. Laboratory studies have shown fluoride to be released from silicate specimens into the aqueous medium in small but significant amounts over periods ranging from 3 months up to 1 year.[6, 10] It is probable that the leaching of fluoride continues throughout the life of the restoration. The fluoride leached from the cement probably acts through at least two mechanisms in its role as an anticariogenic agent.

A logical explanation for this unique effect, and one for which there is much scientific substantiation, is that the fluoride ions released during the setting and subsequent dissolution of the silicate cement react with the adjacent tooth to form a structure that is more resistant to acid decalcification.[11, 12] Thus, in effect, the mechanism is analogous to that of topically applied fluoride solutions.

The increase in the fluoride content of the surface layer of enamel adjacent to a fluoride containing silicate restoration and the reduction in the enamel acid solubility can be seen in Table 30–2. Measurements of fluoride in the enamel before and after restoration of teeth with silicate also show the fluoride content of surface enamel to be increased at sites on the tooth well removed from the restoration.[13] It is interesting that when similar experiments were performed with a silicate cement prepared with a non-fluoride flux there was no appreciable change in fluoride content of the enamel; the enamel solubility actually increased.

It also has been postulated that silicate cement might behave as an antibacterial agent. However, studies indicate that microbial growth is inhibited for only a short period, the first 24 to 48 hours. This initial inhibitory effect has been attributed to the phosphoric acid.

However, recent research suggests that fluorine, even in small quantities, may act as an enzyme inhibitor and thus prevent the metabolism of carbohydrates. This finding indicates a second viable mechanism through which silicate could function as an anticariogenic agent. In fact, chemical analyses of plaque collected at the margins of resin, amalgam, and cast gold restorations reveal a difference in composition, as compared with the plaque accumulated at the margins of silicate cement restorations.[14] Plaque associated with silicate cement has an appreciably higher carbohydrate/nitrogen ratio than does the plaque taken from the margins of all other types of restorations. Since protein nitrogen serves as an index to the bacterial content of the plaque, these data imply either that the metabolism of carbohydrate present in the plaque associated with silicate restorations is inhibited to a certain extent or that there are fewer microorganisms present. When comparable tests were conducted on plaque taken from restorations of a silicate prepared with a nonfluoride flux, the plaque composition was similar in composition to that found at the margins of other types of restorations.

Thus, it appears that silicate cement may inhibit caries via at least two mechanisms, both of which are related to the presence and release of fluoride from the material. Since there is evidence that the fluoride ions are slowly released throughout the life of the restoration, the protective mechanism is undoubtedly a continuous one.

Fluoride is also incorporated as a ceramic flux in the preparation of silicophosphate and glass ionomer cement powders. As can be seen in Table 30–2, both of these cements increase the fluoride content of enamel and decrease its rate of solubility in acid.[12, 13, 15]

The clarification of the anticariogenic mechanism of silicate cement has led to numerous investigations to determine the feasibility of imparting anticariogenic properties to other materials by the discrete addition of fluoride compounds. These material include resins, amalgam, zinc phosphate cement, zinc oxide–eugenol, resin pit and fissure sealants, and cavity varnishes. These studies have shown that in some cases (i.e., resins and amalgam), sufficient fluoride is initially available to reduce the acid solubility of the enamel surface. However, after a day or so, fluoride is no longer released in measurable amounts. Thus it remains to be determined whether such short-term release of fluoride is effective in combating caries.

The addition of fluoride compounds in concentrations that would act effectively as anticariogenic agents also can influence the desirable properties of the material. For example, the leaching of the fluoride makes the amalgam restoration more susceptible to corrosion and can increase the solubility of a zinc phosphate cement. When these compounds are added to cavity varnishes, holes may develop in the film and reduce the ability of the varnish to protect the underlying tooth structure.

Although the concept of adding fluorides to restorative materials in order to capture the anticariogenic potential of a silicate cement is worthy of further investigation, it is obvious that a number of problems are involved. The formulation of such materials requires research on the topical effect of the fluoride on the enamel, on the length of time that the fluoride leaches, and on the effect of the added fluoride on the properties of the material; adequate clinical evaluation of its efficacy is also necessary. Suffice to say that although the properties of silicate cement are far from ideal, its ability to resist secondary caries still makes it the material of choice in certain situations, at least in the minds of some dentists — e.g., the mouth of a child patient with rampant caries. Undoubtedly its use will continue to decrease as the anticariogenic mechanism is incorporated into other systems, such as the glass ionomer cement, to be discussed next.

Manipulation   The care of the liquid, to prevent changes in the acid/water ratio, is the same as for zinc phosphate cement. The mix should be made on a cool slab to slow the setting reaction and to ensure maximum incorporation of powder into the mix. The surface of the slab should be dry, and the liquid should not be dispensed until just prior to mixing in order to preserve the acid-water balance.

The powder is introduced into the liquid in two or three large increments, each being rapidly spatulated using only a small area of the slab. The mix should be completed within one minute and the consistency should be that of thick putty. However, the surface of the mix should have a shiny appearance.

A text on operative dentistry should be consulted concerning the details of placement and finish. Briefly, the mix is immediately inserted into the cavity and a matrix strip pulled. Upon hardening, the matrix is removed, but only the gross excess cement should be removed from the margins at that time. The restoration is then coated with a cavity varnish to protect it from contact with oral fluids. Final finish should be delayed for several days. Use of the varnish and the delay of final finish is necessary because of the slow setting reaction.

Exposure of the cement to water prior to formation of the final reaction products results in increased solubility and in a poor surface, while early finish could disturb or fracture the margins before maximum properties are attained.

Silicate cements are subject to dehydration throughout their lifetime. When exposed to air, such as during subsequent operative procedures, they rapidly lose water and the surface becomes chalky and crazed. Although they again imbibe water when re-exposed to the oral environment, much of the damage may be permanent. Therefore, silicate restorations should be protected from the air by a coat of varnish or silicone grease during subsequent dental operations. Also for this reason silicate cement restorations should never be used in mouth breathers.

GLASS IONOMER CEMENT

Because of its translucency and potential for adhesion, the glass ionomer cement initially was developed for the esthetic restoration of anterior teeth. As discussed in Chapter 29, one version of the cement (Type I) is also designed for use as a luting agent. The cement designed for use as a restorative material is classified as Type II.

The cement is recommended for restoring Class V and III lesions. It is particularly useful for the restoration of cervical eroded areas in a conservative mode. Since it is polyacrylic acid based, the potential for adhesion is comparable to that of a polycarboxylate cement, permitting the placement of the restoration without need of mechanical retention via a cavity preparation.[15, 16] Thus it has one distinct advantage over composite resins when used for this purpose. The resins must rely on acid etching for retention, and, of course, this is effective only on margins that are located in enamel. The use of resin in the restoration of such lesions was discussed in Chapter 14.

The glass ionomer cement is not recommended for Class IV restorations, since current formulations lack toughness and appear to be less resistant to wear by enamel than are the composite resins. The cement also has been used to a certain extent as a pit and fissure sealant.[17-19]

Composition and Chemistry   The cement liquid is an aqueous solution (about 50 per cent by weight) of polyacrylic acid or is a copolymer of acrylic and itaconic acid. The copolymer may also be freeze-dried and incorporated into the powder, as was described for the polycarboxylate cements. In addition to the acrylic acid–itaconic acid copolymer, it also contains a small amount of tartaric

Table 30–3.   *Composition of a Glass Ionomer Cement Powder*

	PER CENT*
SiO_2	29.0
Al_2O_3	16.6
CaF_2	34.3
AlF_3	7.3
NaF	3.0
$AlPO_4$	9.9

*Percentage by weight.
(From Wilson, AD, and Kent, BE: *Br. Pat No.* 1,316,129, 1973.)

acid, in the range of 5 per cent. The itaconic acid reduces the viscosity of the liquid and also makes it more resistant to gelation. If gelation occurs the liquid becomes extremely viscous, to the point of being unusable. The tartaric acid improves the working and setting characteristics.[20]

The powder is an aluminosilicate glass prepared with fluoride fluxes. The powder of the filling material formulation is coarser than that of the luting cement, ranging in size from 20 to 50 μm. It contains a higher Al_2O_3/SiO_2 ratio and hence is more basic than the glass used for silicate cement powders. The composition of a representative glass ionomer cement powder is shown in Table 30–3.

The setting reaction resembles that of silicate cement. When the powder and liquid are mixed to form a paste, the glass is attacked by the acid and Al^{+++}, Ca^{++}, and Na^+ ions are liberated, as is fluoride, probably in the form of complexes. Calcium and, eventually, aluminum polysalts form, which cross-link the polyanion chains. The salts hydrate to form a gel matrix, and just as with silicate the unreacted glass particle is sheathed by silica gel that arises from removal of the cations from the surface of the particles.[21, 22]

Thus the set cement consists of an agglomeration of unreacted powder particles surrounded by a silica gel which is held together in an amorphous matrix of hydrated calcium and aluminum polysalts (Fig. 30–3). The mechanism of adhesion to enamel and dentin is through reaction of the carboxyl groups of the polyacrylic with the calcium in the tooth structure and perhaps the collagen of the dentin (Figs. 29–12 and 30–3).

Properties   The pertinent properties of the glass ionomer cement are listed in Table 30–1. The compressive strength is somewhat less than that of silicate, as is the tensile strength. The hardness is also lower. The 24-hour solubility in water is similar to that of silicate cement. Like silicate, the initial solubility is probably due to the leaching of intermediate products.[23] However, when tested in vitro the glass ionomer cement tends to be more resistant to attack by acids.[22] One in vivo study showed less loss of material from glass ionomer cement specimens than from specimens of other types of cement.[24]

As with other types of cements, reduction in the powder/liquid ratio produces a decrease in physical properties.

Biological and Anticariogenic Properties   As was discussed in Chapter 29 with respect to its use as a luting agent, the glass ionomer cement is a biocompatible material. Thus no pulp protective agent is required except in the case of an actual exposure.

Although long term clinical evidence is lacking, there is every indication

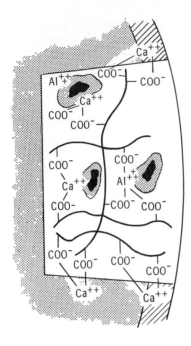

Figure 30–3 Diagram depicting the structure of the glass ionomer cement. The solid black particles represent unreacted glass particles surrounded by the gel (dotted structure) that form when Al^{+++} and Ca^{++} ions are leached from the glass as a result of attack by the polyacrylic acid. The Ca^{++} and Al^{+++} form poly salts with the COO^- groups of the polyacrylic acid to form a cross-linked structure. The carboxyl groups react with the calcium of the enamel and dentin.

that glass ionomer cement should possess the same anticariogenic properties as silicate. As can be seen in Table 30–2, the acid solubility of enamel is reduced by contact with the cement. The increase in the fluoride content of enamel adjacent to glass ionomer restorations is comparable to that of enamel in contact with silicate restorations. Similarly, the fluoride content of the enamel in more remote areas of the tooth is also increased.

Manipulation and Placement The cavity preparation must be clean and free of proteinaceous debris if bonding to the tooth is to be realized. In the conservative restoration of cervical erosion lesions, the tooth structure may be cleaned by rubbing it for 30 seconds with a cotton pledget saturated with 50 per cent citric acid. The treatment with the acid is followed by thorough rinsing with water and drying. Also, the tooth surface can be cleansed effectively with a slurry of pumice and water. Citric acid should not be applied to *cut* dentin, so if the cement is to be inserted into a prepared cavity, then the pumice slurry is the only acceptable cleaning method. It is also indicated whenever the tooth is particularly sensitive.

The glass ionomer cement liquid is somewhat less viscous than the polycarboxylate liquid. Furthermore, the acrylic acid–itaconic acid copolymer does not tend to thicken with age. The powder/liquid ratio used for the restorative materials is usually in the range of 3 gm of powder to 1 gm of liquid. Lower powder/liquid ratios result in a mix that is more difficult to handle and a restoration that is weaker and more susceptible to attack by moisture.

The mixing procedure for the restorative material is similar to that described in Chapter 29 for the luting cement. The slab should be cooled to prolong the working time. The liquid is not dispensed onto the slab until just prior to mixing, in order to avoid loss of water to the atmosphere. The powder is divided into two or three large increments which are introduced, one at a time, into the liquid with rapid spatulation. The recommended total mixing time generally is a maximum of 45 seconds.

Upon completion of the mix, the cement is immediately "packed" into the cavity or it can be injected from a syringe. At the time of insertion the surface of the cement should have a glossy appearance, as was described in Chapter 29 for polycarboxylate cement. If placement is delayed until the surface of the cement is dull in appearance, the setting reaction has progressed to such an extent that the cement may not wet the cavity walls and an insufficient number of free carboxyl groups remain to react with the calcium of the tooth. Use of such a mix will result in little or no adhesion of the restoration of the tooth.

Immediately after placement, a preshaped matrix is applied. As would be anticipated from the chemistry, this system is very sensitive to premature exposure to air or loss of water before the setting reactions have been completed. The matrix provides that initial protection. It is left in place for approximately 5 minutes.

Upon removal, the surface is covered with the water insoluble varnish supplied. This is necessary to protect the cement from dehydration during the moderate finishing procedure. Only the gross excess is removed at this time, with final finishing and polishing done at least 24 hours later. Care must be exercised during this initial finishing, since the cement is relatively soft and "ditching" may occur.

After removal of the excess cement the restoration is once again coated with the varnish in order to provide protection to the marginal areas where the varnish has been removed during finishing.

Chalky or crazed surfaces on such restorations can usually be associated with improper manipulation, e.g., low P/L ratio, or failure to provide protection against the environment by use of the matrix and/or varnish.

Clinical Considerations   Since the glass ionomer cements are new materials as compared with other anterior restorative materials, e.g., direct filling resins and silicate cement, information with respect to their clinical performance is much less extensive.

Nevertheless, several studies have been conducted to examine the clinical behavior of glass ionomer cement restorations.[25, 26] Particular emphasis has been placed upon the use of the cement in the repair of cervical erosion lesions without the use of a cavity preparation. These studies have reported a reduced incidence of sensitivity following such restoration of the areas. Retention rates vary, ranging from 70 to 90 per cent retention. One investigator reports 95 per cent retention after 6 years.[27] All investigators agree that when the loss of material does occur it is within a few weeks after placement.

Initially, the cement was suggested for restoration of small Class III cavities, but for esthetic reasons it was not recommended for use in large cavities, since the cement was somewhat lacking in translucence. However, newer formulations are considerably improved over the earlier versions.

At this time the role that the glass ionomer cements may ultimately fulfill in restorative dentistry is not known. As has been discussed, the cement has a number of characteristics that are attractive, such as adhesion to tooth structure, biocompatibility, and potential anticariogenicity. Likewise, improvements have been made in handling characteristics and properties since the materials were first introduced. The eventual scope of useful applications is dependent upon future improvement in formulations and a more complete definition of its clinical performance.

CAVITY VARNISHES, LINERS AND BASES

Prior to placement of the restoration, the dental pulp may have undergone irritation or damage from a variety of sources, such as caries and cavity preparation. Furthermore, the physical and chemical properties of the permanent restorative materials are such that the restoration itself can invoke irritation or add to that which already exists.

Irritation induced by restorative materials may stem from one or more sources. The metallic restorations are excellent thermal conductors, therefore sensitivity due to thermal shock may occur with the intake of hot and cold foods or beverages. The phosphoric acid containing cements (i.e., zinc phosphate, silicate, and zinc silicophosphate) and the direct filling resins can produce chemical irritation. Also, microleakage, such as that which occurs initially with the newly placed amalgam restoration, may be an additional source of irritation.

Cavity varnishes, liners, and insulating bases are designed to be used as adjuncts to the restorative materials in order to protect the pulp against these types of insult. In addition to serving as barriers against thermal change, irritants within the material, and marginal leakage, certain of these agents in themselves have beneficial effects upon the tooth. For example, zinc oxide–eugenol compounds have a palliative effect upon the pulp and can aid in reducing sensitivity. Calcium hydroxide is particularly beneficial, since it accelerates the formation of reparative dentin and is employed as a pulp capping agent. Thus, in any situation where there exists the slightest possibility of a microscopic pulp exposure, a layer of calcium hydroxide is applied to the pulpal wall regardless of the type of restorative material that is to be employed.

Cavity Varnishes and Liners   Technically both the varnishes and liners could be classified as cavity lining agents, since both are used for coating the freshly cut tooth structure of the prepared cavity. However, such materials usually are classified into two groups. The typical cavity *varnish* is principally a natural gum, such as copal, rosin, or a synthetic resin dissolved in an organic solvent, such as acetone, chloroform, or an ether. The second type, usually referred to as a cavity *liner,* is a liquid in which calcium hydroxide, and occasionally some zinc oxide, is suspended in a solution of natural or synthetic resins. Both varnish and liner materials are formulated to provide a fluid substance that is readily painted onto the surfaces of the prepared cavity. The solvent evaporates, leaving a film that protects the underlying tooth structure.

Cavity Varnishes

A film of varnish placed under a metallic restoration is not an effective thermal insulator. Although these varnishes exhibit a low thermal conductivity, they are not generally applied in a sufficiently thick film to provide the thickness required for thermal insulation. Even an unusually thick layer of varnish does not provide any thermal insulation when heat is applied to the surface of the dental amalgam specimen, as is illustrated in Figure 30–4.

In this experiment a constant source of heat was applied to one surface of an amalgam test specimen and the increase in the temperature of the opposite

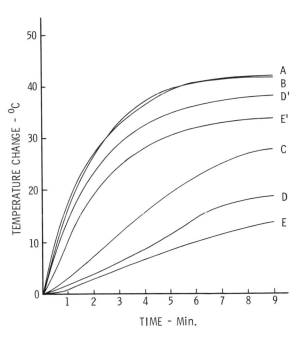

Figure 30–4 Rate of thermal diffusion through model amalgam restorations as influenced by the presence of a cavity varnish and bases. A constant heat source was applied to the surface of the amalgam and the change in temperature on the undersurface of the specimen (cavity floor) with time was monitored. A, Amalgam control; B, Amalgam plus cavity varnish; C, Zinc phosphate cement base, 1.5 mm thick; D, Calcium hydroxide base, 1.5 mm thick; D', Calcium hydroxide base, 0.15 mm thick; E, zinc oxide-eugenol base, 1.5 mm thick; E', zinc oxide-eugenol base, 0.15 mm thick.

surface (cavity floor) was measured as a function of elapsed time. Curves A and B respectively depict the thermal diffusion through the control amalgam specimen as compared with an amalgam specimen underlaid with a "heavy" coat of cavity varnish. There is no difference in rate of heat transfer through the control and the amalgam-varnish specimen.

It is true that a varnish may aid in reducing postoperative sensitivity when the permanent metallic restoration is subjected to sudden temperature changes from hot or cold fluids or foods taken into the oral cavity. However, its effectiveness in this connection probably is more closely related to its tendency to minimize marginal leakage around the restoration. In this respect, the behavior of the varnish when used in conjunction with the amalgam restoration is of special interest.

Effect on Leakage   As previously described, radioactive isotope tracers may be used as a measure of the potential for infiltration of liquids or microorganisms between the walls of the prepared cavity and the dental restoration. When this method is used, the leakage that occurs around an amalgam restoration during the first few days or weeks can be described as severe. Such leakage cannot be appreciably reduced by altering the composition of the alloy or the manipulative or condensation techniques. The postoperative sensitivity that occurs following insertion of the amalgam restoration may partially be related to the fluids and debris that penetrate the margins. These deleterious agents may act as a continuing source of irritation to the pulp, especially in the deep cavity where only a thin layer of dentin separates the restoration and the pulp, as has been discussed previously on several occasions.

The penetration of fluids is reduced around an amalgam restoration when a cavity varnish is used, as indicated in Figure 30–5.

This observation suggests that if varnishes reduce tooth sensitivity, as previously noted, the effect may be attributed to the reduced infiltration of irritating fluids. A similar effect on marginal leakage may result when a

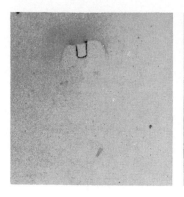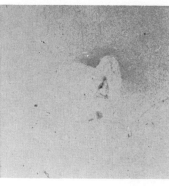

Figure 30–5 Radioautographs showing leakage around amalgam restorations. The dark line surrounding the restoration at left shows severe penetration of the ^{45}Ca. No leakage occurred in the restoration at the right in which a cavity varnish was applied before inserting the restoration.

varnish is employed with certain other restorative materials, such as gold foil.

Effect on Acid Penetration   As previously discussed, the irritational behavior of zinc phosphate and silicate cements is associated with their acidity (Table 29–4). The penetration of acid from these cements through dentin and into the pulp is a major problem in preserving the health of the pulp.

In order to study the protective effect of cavity varnishes, silicate cement restorations prepared with liquids containing radioactive phosphoric acid were placed in extracted teeth and in the teeth of monkeys.[28] The penetration of the acid from the cement into tooth structure in both lined and unlined cavity preparations was determined by measuring the radioactivity on sections of dentin underlying the restoration. The results of these experiments are shown in Figure 30–6. The protective effect of the varnish is evidenced by the marked reduction in the radioactive counts of the underlying dentin in B where the cavity walls were coated with a varnish as compared with A where the cavity was unlined. Comparable results are obtained when other phosphoric acid cements, i.e., zinc phosphate and silicophosphate, are employed.

In addition to preventing the penetration of acid, the varnish acts as a barrier to other substances. In the case of the amalgam restoration, the

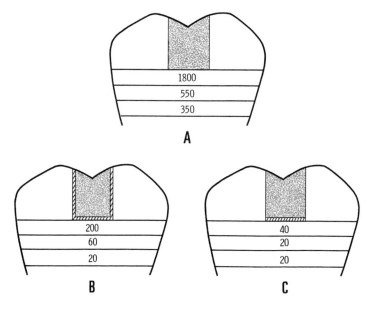

Figure 30–6 Penetration of radioactive phosphoric acid liquid into dentin from silicate cement restorations. The numbers represent the radioactive counts made on three 0.5 mm sections of dentin underlying the restoration. Obviously, the higher the number, the greater is the acid penetration. A, Silicate cement — cavity unprotected. B, Restoration placed over a cavity varnish. C, Restoration over a 0.2 mm thick layer of either a zinc oxide–eugenol or calcium hydroxide cement.

varnish can prevent penetration of corrosion products into the dentinal tubules. Thereby the unsightly tooth discoloration often associated with amalgam restorations is minimized.

Application of the Varnish   Selection of the brand of varnish should be based on individual preferences in characteristics of handling, such as flow and ability to be readily seen when applied on the surface of the prepared cavity. There are no significant differences in the inherent properties of various products.

It is of greatest importance to attain a uniform and continuous coating on all surfaces of the prepared cavity. If the coating is uneven or if voids are present, the results are erratic. Several thin layers should be applied. When the first layer dries, small pinholes usually develop. A second or third application fills in most of these voids and thereby produces a more continuous coating. The varnish may be applied by using a brush, a wire loop, or a small pledget of cotton.

It should be emphasized that the varnish should be applied in a thin consistency. If the varnish is too viscous, it will not wet the cavity wall and does not effectively inhibit marginal leakage. If the varnish becomes thick upon storage or usage, it should be thinned with an appropriate solvent.

There is no evidence that it is necessary to remove the varnish from the margins of the prepared cavity before placing an amalgam restoration, for example. The solubility of dental varnishes is low; they are virtually insoluble in distilled water. Thus, if there is a *thin* layer of varnish at the marginal area of the amalgam restoration, no apparent deterioration of the varnish in the normal oral environment occurs. However, if the varnish is left on the margin, it must be a small amount because an excess prevents proper finishing of the margins of the restoration.

However, any film of varnish should always be removed from the enamel margins before placing a silicate or silicophosphate cement restoration. The varnish inhibits the penetration of fluoride into enamel. Extreme care should be exercised in removing the varnish at the margins. It must not be inadvertently peeled from the cavity walls. Proper protection is afforded only when all of the cavity surfaces are completely covered.

Conventional cavity varnishes generally should not be employed under direct resin filling materials. The solvent in the varnish may react with or soften the resin. Also, the varnish prevents proper wetting of the prepared cavity by the resin.

Cavity Liners

The basic component of cavity liners is calcium hydroxide. The calcium hydroxide is dispersed in aqueous or resin solutions so that the liner can be applied to the cavity in relatively thin films. The solvent evaporates, leaving a layer of calcium hydroxide on the cavity walls.

As with a varnish, the thickness of these films is not sufficient to provide thermal insulation. Undoubtedly these materials were developed primarily in order to incorporate the beneficial effects of calcium hydroxide into a liner-type material. As has been noted previously, calcium hydroxide accelerates the formation of a reparative dentin. In addition, a film of calcium hydroxide beneath a phosphoric acid containing cement appears capable of neutralizing or reacting with acid. Calcium hydroxide liners have a pH in excess of 11.

It is mandatory that the margins of the cavity preparation be kept free of this type of liner. The calcium hydroxide is very soluble in oral fluids and eventually dissolves. If the carrier is a resin, once the calcium hydroxide is dissolved all that remains is a porous resin film that permits marginal leakage.

The Cement Base

The function of the layer of cement, called the *base,* that is placed under the permanent restoration is to encourage recovery of the injured pulp and to protect it against the numerous types of insult to which it may be subjected. That insult may come from thermal shock when the tooth is restored with metal and, depending upon the particular restorative material, from chemical irritation. The base in essence serves as a replacement or substitute for the protective dentin that has been destroyed by caries and/or cavity preparation.

There are a variety of materials that have been and that can be employed as bases. Zinc phosphate cement has been used for this purpose for many years, as have numerous zinc oxide–eugenol formulations. A commercial zinc oxide–eugenol, shown in Figure 30–7, is of an extremely free flowing formulation designed particularly for this purpose.

Also there are a series of two paste calcium hydroxide formulations that will harden or set when mixed together. The composition of these materials is quite complicated and they contain six or seven ingredients in addition to the calcium hydroxide.[29, 30] These so-called "hard setting" calcium hydroxides can

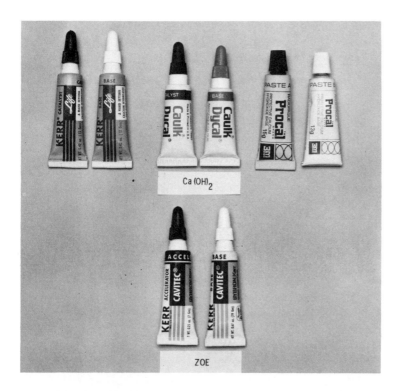

Figure 30–7 Representative commercial brands of "hard setting" calcium hydroxide materials, and a zinc oxide–eugenol formulation, for use as bases.

be built-up to the considerable thickness required for thermal insulation. Commercial products representative of this type are shown in Figure 30–7. In addition, both zinc polycarboxylate and glass ionomer cements have properties which recommend their use as bases.

Thermal Properties The relative thermal insulating characteristics of various types of bases, as indicated by the rates of heat conduction through specimens composed of amalgam placed over 1.5 mm thick bases, are shown in Figure 30–4. The test procedure was exactly the same as was employed for evaluating the thermal insulating ability of the cavity varnishes. A constant heat source was applied to the surface of the amalgam, and the temperature change induced on the undersurface of the base (cavity floor) was monitored.

The reduction in the rate of temperature change of amalgam plus base specimens as compared with the control is indicative of the thermal insulating properties of the bases. It is apparent that the rate of heat transfer through the amalgam specimen (A) is rapid in comparison with that through the amalgam-zinc phosphate (C), the amalgam-calcium hydroxide (D), and the amalgam-zinc oxide–eugenol (E) specimens.

Although data are not available with respect to the thermal diffusivity of zinc polycarboxylate and glass ionomer cements, the chemical makeup of these materials would indicate that they also would serve effectively as thermal insulators.

Clinical experience has shown that temperature changes in the mouth have a more acute affect on the pulp when the amalgam restoration is not insulated by a base. Although there are some differences in the rate of thermal diffusion through base materials, the thickness of the base is of greater significance than its composition. As was discussed in Chapter 3, thermal diffusion through a material is, of course, dependent not only upon the coefficient of thermal conductivity and diffusivity of the substance but also upon its thickness. Thus, even though a cement base material may inherently have a low coefficient of thermal conductivity, a certain minimal thickness is necessary to provide adequate thermal insulation.

As stated previously, the thickness of the bases used in obtaining the data for Curves C, D, and E in Figure 30–4 was 1.5 mm. When the layer of calcium hydroxide and zinc oxide–eugenol cement was reduced to 0.15 mm (Curves D' and E'), the temperature change on the floor of the cavity was much greater.

As yet, the minimal thickness required for adequate thermal insulation has not been determined for the base materials, but there is evidence to suggest that something in the order of 0.75 millimeter is probably required.[31, 32] For example, in vivo measurements of thermal diffusion made by placing thermal couples on the floor of Class V cavities restored with amalgam revealed that within 2 seconds after application of a thermal stimulus the temperature on the cavity floor was only 20 per cent less than that of the surface of the restoration. When a 0.5 mm base was present, the temperature was reduced by approximately one-half and to about one-third when the base was 1 mm thick. Certainly, a thin wash of the cement applied to the floor of the prepared cavity would not offer protection against the thermal changes conducted through the metallic restoration.

Protection Against Chemical Insult As would be expected, bases of calcium hydroxide and zinc oxide–eugenol provide effective barriers against the penetration of irritating constituents from the restorative materials. The hard setting calcium hydroxide and the zinc oxide–eugenols designed for this purpose flow readily and therefore can be applied to the cavity floor in a relatively thin layer. As shown in Figure 30–6, there is little or no penetration of the tooth by phosphoric acid from the cements. Thus when thermal insulation is not required, such as with direct filling resin, a thin layer of a hard setting calcium hydroxide base may be placed over the pulpal wall to prevent chemical insult to the pulp, and, when needed, to stimulate formation of reparative dentin.

With restorative materials other than resin, zinc oxide–eugenol cements are also used for this purpose. When these calcium hydroxide and zinc oxide–eugenol materials are used in this manner, the function of the materials is more analogous to that of a cavity liner than to that of a base.

Undoubtedly bases of polycarboxylate and glass ionomer cements can also serve as chemical barriers. On the other hand, if zinc phosphate cement is employed for thermal insulation, then pulp protection must be provided by use of a biocompatible varnish or liner.

Strength   The cement must have sufficient strength to withstand the forces of condensation so that the base is not fractured during insertion of the restoration. Fracture or displacement of the base can permit the amalgam to penetrate the base, contact the dentin, and thus eliminate the thermal protection provided by the base. Likewise, in a deep cavity a cement base of a low strength might even permit the amalgam to be forced into the pulp through microscopic exposures in the dentin. The base should also resist fracture or distortion under any masticatory stresses transmitted to it through the permanent restoration.

In Table 30–4 the compressive strength of representative zinc oxide–eugenol and calcium hydroxide base materials is compared with that of a zinc phosphate cement at intervals of 7 minutes, 30 minutes, and 24 hours. Materials A, B, and C are proprietary zinc oxide–eugenol cements. Material A is designed primarily for use as a base, and is furnished in paste form. A conventional zinc oxide–eugenol mix, utilizing zinc acetate as an accelerator, is also included. The calcium hydroxide materials, D and E, are hard setting systems.

The compressive strength at 7 minutes is of particular interest. This represents the time of the *initial set* of most of these materials, under the conditions of the test. Although initial set of these materials occurs more

Table 30–4.   *Compressive Strength of Cement Base Materials*

MATERIAL	7 MINUTES		30 MINUTES		24 HOURS	
	MPa	(psi)	MPa	(psi)	MPa	(psi)
Zinc oxide–eugenol						
A	2.8	400	3.5	500	5.2	750
B	15.9	2300	20.7	3000	24.1	3500
C	6.2	900	6.9	1000	12.4	1800
U.S.P. zinc oxide (+ zinc acetate)–eugenol	4.1	600	8.6	1250	8.3	1200
Calcium hydroxide						
D	7.6	1100	6.2	900	8.3	1200
E	3.8	550	4.8	700	10.3	1500
Zinc phosphate						
F	6.9	1000	86.9	12,600	119.3	17,300

rapidly in the mouth (approximately 3 minutes), the strength of a material should be the same at initial set regardless of whether it requires 3 or 7 minutes to achieve that state. Therefore the 7-minute strengths are analogous to the strength of the material at the time when amalgam condensation pressures would be exerted on the base clinically.

Although zinc phosphate cement has a considerably higher 30-minute and 24-hour compressive strength than do the other types of cements, its strength at initial set (7 minutes) is within the range of the others. In fact, at 7 minutes, zinc oxide–eugenol cement B is approximately twice as strong as is zinc phosphate cement.

In order to determine if the strength of the base materials in Table 30–4 was adequate, these materials were placed in uniform thicknesses over the proximal walls and pulpal floors of Class II cavities prepared in extracted human teeth. Dental amalgam restorations were immediately condensed over the bases. Subsequent sections of the teeth showed that the strength of the bases was adequate, as illustrated in Figure 30–8. None of the bases listed in Table 30–4 was distorted or fractured.

In order to obtain information relative to the minimum strength required to support amalgam condensation, bases were placed with experimental zinc oxide–eugenol materials of lower compressive strengths. Bases of a material with a compressive strength of only 1.2 MPa (170 psi) withstood amalgam condensation without detectable damage but bases with strengths of 0.5 MPa (70 psi) were either fractured or displaced, as shown in Figure 30–9. Thus the minimum strength requirement lies somewhere between 0.5 and 1.2 MPa.

Similar tests conducted with direct gold indicate that bases of greater strength, and perhaps with somewhat different properties, are required in order to resist the stress developed during condensation.[33] For example, material A (Table 30–4) was sometimes displaced when gold foil was con-

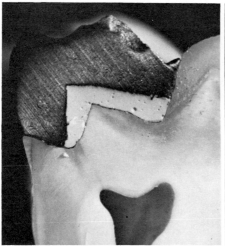 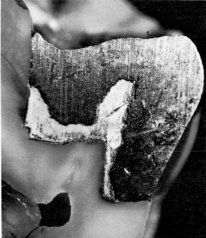

Figure 30–8   **Figure 30–9**

Figure 30–8 Section through an amalgam restoration condensed with a heavy condensation force against a base having 7-minute compressive strength of 2.8 MPa (400 psi).

Figure 30–9 Section through an amalgam restoration condensed with the same technique used in Figure 30–8, but against a base having a 7-minute compressive strength of 0.5 MPa (70 psi).

densed against it. The surfaces of bases prepared from materials A and D also flaked off and the particles were incorporated into the body of the restoration. Zinc phosphate and the stronger zinc oxide–eugenol cements, such as B, supported the condensation of the gold foil.

There is no reason to suppose that zinc polycarboxylate or glass ionomer cement would not also support condensation of direct filling golds.

The exact strength required to resist masticatory forces has not been determined. Unquestionably, the design of the cavity is a factor. In the simple Class I preparation where the base is supported on all sides by the tooth structure, less strength may be necessary than in the Class II preparation, for example. In the latter case, when a deep depression or an angle is restored, perhaps a greater resistance to biting stresses is needed. Actually, there are few clinical data on this subject. A report involving over 350 amalgam restorations that were condensed against bases of a hard setting calcium hydroxide reported no unusual incidence of failure.[34]

Clinical Considerations   Thus the selection of a base is governed to an extent by the design of the cavity, the type of permanent restorative material used, and the proximity of the pulp in relation to the cavity wall. With amalgam, one of the hard setting calcium hydroxide materials or a zinc oxide–eugenol formulation may usually serve effectively as the sole base. In other situations, such as with a direct filling gold, it may be necessary to use a stronger material for the base, i.e., zinc phosphate, polycarboxylate, or a glass ionomer cement. Thus, in those cases when it is desirable to place a calcium hydroxide or zinc oxide–eugenol preparation on the floor of the cavity, the preparation should be overlaid with a stronger cement. With respect to resin restorations, calcium hydroxide is always the material of choice, since zinc oxide–eugenol may interfere with polymerization, as does the traditional cavity varnish.

It should be emphasized that use of a base in conjunction with amalgam or gold foil does not alleviate the need for a varnish as an aid in sealing the cavity margins against leakage. However, the type of base governs the respective order of application of the varnish and the base. If a zinc phosphate cement base is to be used, then obviously the cavity varnish should be applied to the cavity walls prior to placement of the base. On the other hand, if a biocompatible agent, e.g., a calcium hydroxide or zinc oxide–eugenol, base is employed, then these should be placed directly against the dentin and the varnish should not be applied until the base material has hardened.

In summary, cavity varnishes and cement bases generally serve somewhat different functions, as has been described. In the deep cavity where maximum protection against all types of insult is required, both a varnish and a base should be used.

TEMPORARY RESTORATIONS

Temporary restorations are often required before the placement of the permanent crown or bridge. At one time gutta-percha, a thermoplastic natural gum sometimes referred to as "temporary stopping," was used extensively for this purpose. The material is softened by heating and inserted into the cavity where it hardens upon cooling. Easy to manipulate, gutta-percha is convenient to use for temporary restorations, but it is rarely employed today for that purpose. It does not seal the cavity preparation, and the microleakage is severe. Thus, teeth restored with this material are often sensitive. Gutta-percha is, however, frequently used to fill the root canals of teeth during endodontic procedures, in conjunction with a ZOE sealant.

Because of its excellent initial sealing ability and kind pulpal response, zinc oxide–eugenol is the cement of choice for temporary restorations. This material is particularly useful when a sedative treatment is required until the pulp has healed to the point where the permanent restoration can be placed. However, the relatively low mechanical properties of the zinc oxide–eugenol cement do not permit it to be used in situations in which it would be subject to high stress, such as interim coverage of a crown cavity preparation. Therefore, as was discussed in Chapter 29, in those cases a temporary resin or preformed metal crown is cemented by means of a zinc oxide–eugenol cement. The Type I zinc oxide–eugenol cements, which have strengths of 35 MPa (4500 psi) or less are employed for sedative treatments, temporary coverage, and temporary cementation.

INTERMEDIATE RESTORATIONS

The need sometimes arises for what is referred to as an "intermediate" or "holding type" of restoration, particularly in pedodontics. For example, in cases of rampant caries it is desirable to remove all of the gross caries quickly in order to change the oral flora and thus arrest the caries process. Once the initial "clean-up" has been accomplished, the dentist can then proceed with placement of the permanent restorations. The interval between removal of the caries and completion of the restorative work may be a matter of several months or longer. During that time the teeth must be protected by some type of a durable restoration.

Materials that have been used in the past for these intermediate restorations include zinc silicophosphate cement and zinc phosphate cement, with and without additives, such as amalgam alloy filings, to improve resistance to abrasion. Although such materials generally perform satisfactorily in terms of physical properties, all are irritating to the pulp.

As zinc oxide–eugenol cement is recognized as a biologically compatible material, research has centered on the development of this type of system for an intermediate restorative material. The conventional zinc oxide–eugenol cements described for use as temporary restorations are deficient in toughness and have inadequate strength and abrasion resistance to serve for any extended period of time. Several commercial products have been introduced in which the longevity of the intermediate restoration has been extended for periods of one year or longer.[35] Zinc oxide–eugenol cements for intermediate restorations are classified as Type IV. At least one is based on a polymer reinforcement of the material. The powder is composed of zinc oxide and finely divided polymer particles in the amount of 20 to 40 per cent by weight.[36] In addition, the zinc oxide powder is surface treated by an aliphatic monocarboxylic acid, such as proprionic. The liquids are eugenol.

This combination of surface treatment and polymer reinforcement results in a cement that has good strength and markedly improved abrasion resistance. In particular, the formulation results in a marked improvement in toughness. Clinical experience with this type of material indicates that it can serve effectively as a restorative material for at least one year. In order to achieve the properties necessary for this use, sufficient powder must be added to achieve a stiff puttylike or filling consistency.

The zinc silicophosphate cements were discussed in Chapter 29 relative to their use as a luting agent. As noted there, these materials are a combination of powders of silicate cement, zinc oxide, and magnesium oxide, while the composition of the liquid is comparable to that of silicate cement. The mixing procedure is similar to that employed for silicate cement. Type II cements are those designed for intermediate restorations, while Type III cements are also recommended for use as a luting agent.

The strength and solubility requirements for zinc silicophosphate cements marketed as temporary restoratives are the same as for silicate cement. However, greater latitude is permitted with respect to opacity, since the zinc silicophosphate cements are more opaque than silicate cements.

Although the 24-hour solubility of the zinc silicophosphate cements in distilled water is greater than that of the zinc phosphate cement, the solubility in other media (see Fig. 30–2) tends to be lower. Their durability in the oral cavity is as least comparable to that of zinc phosphate cement. Also, since the cement is largely a silicate cement, it contains appreciable amounts of fluoride. Since the fluoride mechanism is essentially that of a silicate cement, it may be anticipated that some anticariogenic protection would be afforded to the tooth (see Table 30–2).

References

1. Pulver JC and Rossington DR: Solubility of a silicate cement. J Dent Res 49:1530, 1970.
2. Paffenbarger GC: Dental cements, direct filling resins, composite and adhesive restorative materials: A resume. J Biomed Mater Res 6:363, 1972.
3. Kent BE, Fletcher KE, and Wilson AD: Dental silicate cements. XI. Electron probe studies. J Dent Res. 49:86, 1970.
4. Wilson AD, Kent BE, and Mesley RJ: Formation of dental silicate cement. Nature (London) 225:272, 1970.
5. Norman RD, Swartz ML, Phillips RW, and Virmani R: A comparison of the intraoral disintegration of three dental cements. J Am Dent Assoc 78:777, 1969.
6. Wilson AD and Batchelor RF: Dental silicate cements. I. The chemistry of erosion. J Dent Res 46:1075, 1967.
7. Wilson AD: Specification test for the solubility and disintegration of dental cements: A critical evaluation of its meaning. J Dent Res 55:721, 1976.
8. Laswell HR: A prevalence study of secondary caries occurring in a young adult male population. IADR Program and Abstracts, No. 426, 1967.
9. Lind V, Wennerholm G, and Nystrom S: Contact caries in connection with silver amalgam, copper amalgam and silicate cement fillings. Acta Odontol Scand 22:333, 1964.
10. DeFreitas JF: The long-term solubility of silicate cement. Aust Dent J 13:129, 1968.
11. Norman RD, Phillips RW, and Swartz ML: Fluoride uptake by enamel from certain dental materials. J Dent Res 39:11, 1960.
12. Phillips RW and Swartz ML: Effect of certain restorative materials on solubility of enamel. J Am Dent Assoc 54:623, 1957.
13. Swartz ML, Phillips RW, Clark HE, Norman RD, and Potter R: Fluoride distribution in teeth using a silicate model. J Dent Res 59:1596, 1980.
14. Norman RD, Mehra RV, Swartz ML, and Phillips RW: Effects of restorative materials on plaque composition. J Dent Res 51:1596, 1972.
15. Wilson AD: Adhesion of glass ionomer cements. In Allen, KW, ed: Aspects of Adhesion. London, Transcriptor Books, 1975, p. 145.

16. Maldonado A, Swartz ML, and Phillips RW: An in vitro study of certain properties of a glass ionomer cement. J Am Dent Assoc 96:785, 1978.
17. Council on Dental Materials and Devices: Status report on the glass ionomer cements. J Am Dent Assoc 99:221, 1979.
18. McLean JW and Wilson AD: The clinical development of the glass ionomer cement. III. The erosion lesion. Aust Dent J 22:190, 1977.
19. McLean JW and Wilson AD: The clinical development of the glass ionomer cement. II. Some clinical applications. Aust Dent J 22:120, 1977.
20. Crisp S, Ferner AJ, Lewis BG, and Wilson AD: Properties of improved glass ionomer cement formulations. J Dent 3:125, 1975.
21. Wilson AD and Crisp S: Ionomer cements. Br Poly J 7:279, 1975.
22. McLean JW and Wilson AD: The clinical development of the glass ionomer cements. I. Formulations and properties. Aust. Dent J 22:31, 1977.
23. Crisp S, Lewis BG, and Wilson AD: Glass ionomer cements: Chemistry of erosion. J Dent Res 55:1032, 1976.
24. Mitchum JC and Gronas DG: Clinical evaluation of cement solubility. J Prosthet Dent 40:453, 1978.
25. Low T: The treatment of hypersensitive cervical abrasion cavities using ASPA cement. J Oral Rehabil 8:81, 1981.
26. Mount GJ and Makinson OF: Clinical characteristics of a glass ionomer cement. Br Dent J 145:67, 1978.
27. Mount GJ: Personal communication.
28. Swartz ML, Niblack BF, Alter EA, Norman RD, and Phillips RW: In vivo studies on the penetration of dentin by constituents of silicate cement. J Am Dent Assoc 76:573, 1968.
29. Dougherty EW: United States Patent No. 3,047,408, July 31, 1962.
30. Prosser HJ, Stuart B, and Wilson AD: An infrared spectroscopic study of the setting reactions of a calcium hydroxide dental cement. J Mater Sc 14:2894, 1979.
31. Harper RH, Schnell RJ, Swartz ML, and Phillips RW: In vivo measurements of thermal diffusion through restorations of various materials. J Prosthet Dent 43:180, 1980.
32. Braden M: Heat conduction in teeth and the effect of lining materials. J Dent Res 43:315, 1964.
33. Virmani R, Phillips RW, and Swartz ML: Displacement of cement bases by condensation of direct gold. J Am Acad Gold Foil Oper 13:39, 1970.
34. Delaney JM and Seyler AE: Hard set calcium hydroxide as a sole base in pulp protection. J Dent Child 33:13, 1966.
35. Jendresen MD and Phillips RW: A comparative study of four zinc oxide and eugenol formulations as restorative materials. II. J Prosthet Dent 21:300, 1969.
36. Dougherty EW: U.S. Patent No. 3,509,089, April, 1970.

31 DENTAL PORCELAIN

Dental porcelain may be classified into three types, depending on its use. One type is employed for the construction of artificial teeth; a second type is used for the fabrication of jacket crowns and inlays; and a third type, more properly designated as an enamel, is used as a veneer over cast metal crowns. Although the principles of composition, chemistry, and technique are essentially the same for all three types, more attention will be given to the second and third types, which are employed by the dentist and laboratory technician.

Dental porcelains are in part crystalline minerals (e.g., feldspar, silica, alumina) in a glass matrix. The glass phase consists of finely ground powders which, when compacted and fired or *sintered* at high temperatures, fuse together to form a translucent, toothlike material. Dental porcelain is our most durable esthetic restorative material and, when correctly glazed, is easily cleansed of stain or plaque. Its primary defects are brittleness, a high degree of shrinkage upon firing, and problems in matching the exact color and texture of natural teeth.

Classification by Fusing Temperature Dental porcelain may be classified according to its maturing or fusion temperature. Three types of dental porcelain are generally recognized:

High-fusing	1288–1371° C (2350–2500° F)
Medium-fusing	1093–1260° C (2000–2300° F)
Low-fusing	871–1066° C (1600–1950° F)

Compositions of Restorative Porcelain High-fusing porcelain is used by commercial manufacturers in the construction of artificial denture teeth but is rarely used in the fabrication of individual porcelain restorations. These materials may contain 75 to 85 per cent feldspar, 12 to 22 per cent quartz, and up to 4 per cent kaolin. The feldspar provides a glassy phase and serves as a matrix for the quartz, which remains in suspension after firing.

Quartz (SiO_2) is used in porcelain as a strengthener. At normal firing temperatures it is structurally unchanged and serves to stabilize the mass at high temperatures.

Feldspars used in the manufacting of dental porcelain are mixtures of potassium aluminum silicate, $K_2O \cdot Al_2O_3 \cdot 6 SiO_2$, and albite, $Na_2O \cdot Al_2O_3 \cdot 6 SiO_2$. Natural feldspar is never pure and the ratio of potash (K_2O) to soda (Na_2O) may vary. When feldspar is melted at approximately 1250 to 1500° C

(2280°–2730° F), it fuses to become a glass with a free crystalline silica phase.

The soda form of feldspar tends to lower the fusion temperature, while the potash form increases the viscosity of the molten glass, causing less slump or pyroplastic flow of the porcelain to occur during firing. This is a desirable property because it prevents the rounding of margins, the loss of tooth form, and the obliteration of surface markings, which contribute to a lifelike appearance.

Kaolin is a hydrated aluminum silicate ($Al_2O_3 \cdot 2\,SiO_2 \cdot 2H_2O$) that acts as a binder to increase the moldability of the unfired porcelain. Because of its opaqueness, it is present in only very small amounts, if at all.

Although many restorative porcelains contain a free crystalline phase of quartz, they should be described as glasses, and the high-fusing porcelains could more accurately be termed "feldspathic glasses."

In medium- and low-fusing porcelains, the manufacturer mixes the components, fuses them, and then quenches the mass in water. Quenching results in internal stresses that produce considerable cracking and fracturing throughout the glass. This process is known as *fritting,* and the product is called a *frit.* The resultant brittle structure can then be readily ground to a fine powder for use by the ceramist.

During prefusing of the porcelain, the pyrochemical reaction between the ingredients has occurred and much of the shrinkage associated with this reaction has taken place. During subsequent firing in the dental laboratory, the powders are fused together to form the restoration. The fusion temperature depends upon the composition of the glass and must be carefully controlled to minimize pyroplastic flow. Compositions of typical glasses that have been employed in dental porcelain are given in Table 31–1.

The alkalis (potash and soda) are introduced either as carbonates or as naturally occurring minerals (e.g., feldspar). In the latter case, some silica and alumina are added. Boron can be present as borax or boric acid. Lime, when used, can be added as calcium carbonate which reverts to CaO during fritting.

Special Types of Porcelains   The principal reason for choosing porcelain as a restorative material is that high esthetic qualities can be attained in matching the adjacent tooth structure in translucency, color, and intensity. In order to accomplish this, various special types of porcelain are used.

Color frits are added to dental porcelain to obtain the various shades needed to simulate natural teeth. These coloring pigments are produced by fusing metallic oxides together with fine glass and feldspar and then regrinding to a powder. These various powders are blended with the unpigmented powdered frit to provide the proper hue and shade. Examples of metallic oxides and their respective color renditions are: iron or nickel oxide, brown; copper oxide, green; titanium oxide, yellowish brown; manganese oxide, lavender; and cobalt oxide, blue. Opacity may be achieved by the addition of zirconium, titanium, or tin oxides.

Stains are supplied in kits and are made in the same way as the concentrated color frits. They are employed as surface colorants or to replicate enamel check lines, hypocalcification areas, or other defects in the body of a porcelain restoration. Stains are often made from low-fusing glasses so that they can be applied at temperatures below the maturing temperature of the restoration.

Table 31–1. Chemical Composition of Some Dental Porcelains

| | High-Fire Porcelain | | Medium-Fire Porcelain | | Low-Fire Atmospheric | | Low-Fire Vacuum | | | Metal-Bonded Porcelain A | | Metal-Bonded Porcelain B |
| | | | | | | | Aluminous Core | | | | | |
	D	E	D	E	D	E		D	E	D	E	
SiO_2	72.9	65.1	63.1	64.3	68.1	67.6	35.0	66.5	64.7	59.2	63.5	66.2
Al_2O_3	15.9	19.4	19.8	19.1	8.8	9.7	53.8	13.5	13.9	18.5	18.9	14.5
CaO					3.5	3.7	1.12		1.78			1.4
Na_2O	1.68	2.4	2.0	2.4	4.7	4.5	2.8	4.2	4.8	4.8	5.0	6.1
K_2O	9.8	12.8	7.9	8.4	8.4	8.1	4.2	7.1	7.5	11.8	12.3	10.2
B_2O_3		0.15	6.8	5.2	6.4	6.3	3.2	6.6	7.3	4.6	0.12	
ZnO			0.25	0.25						0.58	0.11	
ZrO_2										0.39	0.13	
Firing temp. (C)	1300	1300	1100	1100	960	960	980	980	950	900	900	940

Chemical composition in percentages.
D = dentin; E = enamel.
(From Yamada, H, and Grenoble, P: Dental Porcelain — The State of the Art, University of Southern California Proceedings, 1977, p. 26.)

Overglazes are ceramic powders that may be added to a porcelain restoration after it has been fired. A transparent, glossy layer forms over the surface of the porcelain restoration at a maturing temperature lower than that of the body porcelain. The result is a glossy or semi-glossy surface that is nonporous.

The coefficient of thermal expansion of the overglaze should be slightly lower than that of the porcelain body to which it is applied. If the overglaze has a higher coefficient than the body, it cools under radial tension. The stresses resulting may cause a crazing of the surface. The greater the stressed condition, the finer is the crazing network produced. Conversely, if the coefficient of the overglaze is considerably lower than that of the body porcelain, compressive stresses may cause cracks in the glaze, known as "peeling."

In either case, an erosion of the overglaze may occur in the mouth. A smooth surface on the porcelain is essential in order to minimize plaque retention and soft tissue response. Thus loss of the glaze exposes the rough and sometimes porous surface of the body porcelain. Also, the strength is reduced.

If all the constituents in a dental porcelain frit are completely fused to form a single phase glass, such a porcelain can be easily "self-glazed." Because each grain of porcelain (glass) melts at the same temperature, the self-glazing can be accomplished by extending the maturing time of the porcelain, as will be discussed later.

Uses of Dental Porcelain   The porcelain *jacket crown* is constructed from several layers of porcelain. Each layer must be oversize to compensate for firing shrinkage. Generally, the medium-fusing or low-fusing porcelains are used and firing is done in a partial vacuum.

Regardless of the fusion temperature, there are three types of porcelains used in the fabrication of these restorations. An opaque porcelain is used to mask the color of the cement used in placing the restoration and thus is loaded with opacifiers such as zirconium or titanium oxides. The body, or dentin, porcelain is a feldspathic glass with high color saturation. It is used for the main build-up of the gingival or body areas of the crown. The third type, an enamel porcelain, is also a feldspathic glass and is used to cover the body porcelain in order to produce the characteristic translucency inherent in the incisal aspect of natural teeth.

The *aluminous porcelain crown* consists of a body or core porcelain containing 40 to 50 per cent alumina crystals in a low-fusing glass.[1] The structure is seen in Figure 31–1. Body porcelain of the usual glass type is fired over the luminous core, and enamel porcelain is also applied. The placement of these porcelains is illustrated in Figure 31–2. The rationale behind the aluminous porcelain crown is as follows.

The alumina particles (Al_2O_3) are much stronger, with a higher modulus of elasticity, than quartz and are more effective in interrupting crack propagation. The glass selected for the matrix should have the same coefficient of thermal expansion as the alumina. In this case, the crack is propagated through the alumina particles, as shown in Figure 31–3. Inasmuch as the alumina particles are more difficult to fracture than the glass, the energy required for crack propagation is greater than through the glass alone. Thus, the alumina bears a larger proportion of any load applied, and the strength of the alumina-glass composite is enhanced with increasing alumina content. A

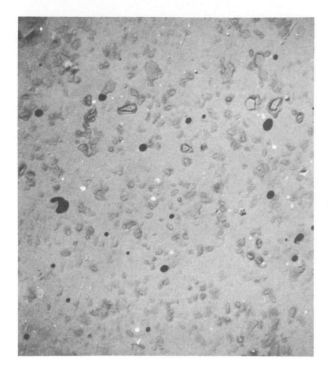

Figure 31–1 Photomicrograph of aluminous core porcelain illustrating alumina crystals (dark gray) surrounded by a matrix (light gray) of glass phase. (×200).

50 per cent by weight alumina-glass may have twice the strength of the glass phase alone.

A photomicrograph showing the propagation through an aluminous porcelain is presented in Figure 31–4. However, if the coefficients of thermal

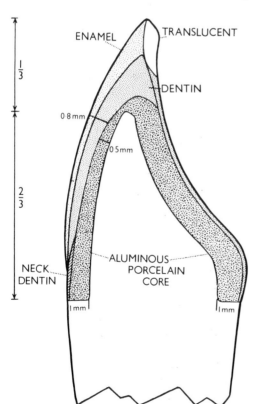

ENAMEL   TRANSLUCENT

$\frac{1}{3}$

DENTIN

0·8 mm

0·5 mm

$\frac{2}{3}$

Figure 31–2 Diagram illustrating the correct placement of the aluminous porcelain core and enamel porcelain in a jacket crown. (From McLean JW, The alumina reinforced porcelain jacket crown. J Am Dent Assoc 75:621, 1967.)

ALUMINOUS PORCELAIN CORE

NECK DENTIN

1 mm   1 mm

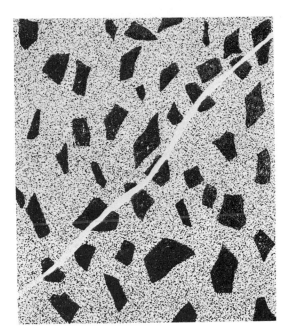

Figure 31–3   Diagram illustrating a fracture path in a two-phase alumina-glass system in which coefficients of thermal expansion of both phases are equal. (From McLean and Hughes, Br Dent J, Sept, 21, 1965.)

expansion of the two phases are different, the crack is propagated intergranularly and the strength is reduced (Fig. 31–5). The irregular path is the result of the stresses that exist around the alumina particles.

An even greater strength can be attained in the restoration by using a high purity alumina, generally in excess of 97 per cent, as a backing for the translucent porcelain. The usual translucent dental porcelain is fused as a veneer over the alumina. However, the fusing temperature of the alumina is much higher than what can be attained with the usual dental laboratory equipment. Consequently, preformed aluminous backings are supplied. These preformed high-alumina reinforcements may be used to construct bridge pontics, post crowns, or small fixed bridges.[2, 3]

The metal-reinforced porcelain crown, more correctly called the *metal-ceramic crown,* is now the most widely used restoration in dental ceramics. It

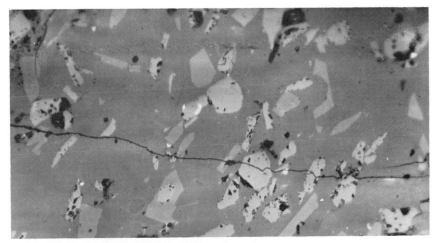

Figure 31–4   Photomicrograph of the fracture path in a two-phase system of dental porcelain reinforced with recrystallized alumina. (Courtesy of J. W. McLean.)

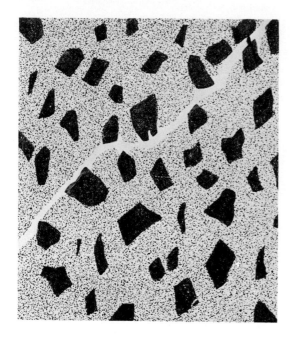

Figure 31–5 Diagram illustrating the fracture path in a two-phase alumina-glass system in which the coefficients of thermal expansion are different. (From McLean and Hughes, Br Dent J, Sept 21, 1965.)

consists of a cast metal coping onto which a porcelain veneer is fired, as diagrammed in Figure 31–6. If a strong bond is effected between the porcelain veneer and the metal, there is minimal chance for leakage at the interface. Thus, with proper design of the coping, combined with compatible physical properties of the porcelain and metal, the porcelain is so reinforced that brittle fracture is greatly minimized or eliminated. It will be recalled that the metallic ceramic restoration was previously discussed (Chapter 24) in relationship to the noble metal alloys used for the casting.

The metallic reinforcement has, therefore, permitted the use of dental porcelain in fixed bridge construction and in areas where tensile and shear forces are present. This type of restoration will be discussed in further detail later in this chapter.

Briefly, in this technique opaque porcelain is fused against the casting to mask the metal (Fig. 31–6). The opaque is heavily loaded with metallic oxide opacifiers and may be applied in thicknesses of 0.1 to 0.2 mm. Since the opaque

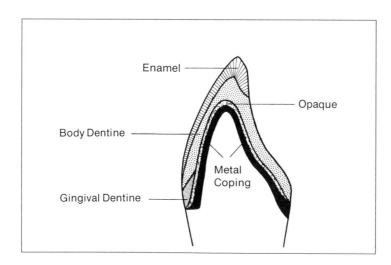

Figure 31–6 Porcelains used in the construction of a metal-ceramic crown. (McLean JW: The Science and Art of Dental Ceramics, Volume II, Quintessence Publ. Co., Chicago, 1980, p. 30.)

porcelain is reflective, it must be covered with at least 1 mm of veneer porcelain if reasonable esthetics are to be achieved.

Structure   As noted in Chapter 2, glasses are noncrystalline although they exhibit a short range order in atomic arrangement. As in most ceramic materials, the atoms are primary bonded. In silica glass, for example, the bond is both ionic and covalent with a tetrahedral arrangement of the atoms, as discussed in the previous chapter. There are no free electrons. Consequently, the ceramic materials are poor thermal and electrical conductors.

As compared with metals, the atomic arrangements are complex. Because of the great strength of the bonds and the complexity of their structures, the ceramic reactions are sluggish, if they exist. The dental porcelains are almost inert. During cooling, glass, for example, may be cooled very slowly, but the rate of atomic diffusion is so slow that the glass solidifies with a liquid structure instead of a crystalline structure. Although the internal energy of the super-cooled liquid or noncrystalline structure is greater than that of the crystalline arrangement, nevertheless the former is apparently the stable form. Such a structure is called *vitreous* and the process of forming it is known as *vitrification*. In ceramic terms, vitrification is the development of a liquid phase, by reaction or melting which, on cooling, provides the glassy phase.

The principal ion present in all glasses is oxygen, which forms very stable bonds with small multivalent atoms such as silicon, boron, germanium, or phosphorus. These structural units, such as the SiO_4 tetrahedra or the BO_3 triangles, form the random network in glass. Thus, these elements are termed *glass formers*.

Dental porcelains use the basic silicon-oxygen network as the glass-forming matrix, but additional properties, such as low fusing temperature, high viscosity, and resistance to devitrification, are built in by the addition of other oxides to the glass-forming SiO_4 lattice. These oxides generally consist of potassium, sodium, calcium, aluminum, and boric oxides.

Potassium, sodium, and calcium oxides are used as *glass modifiers;* that is, they interrupt the integrity of the SiO_4 network and act as *fluxes*. The purpose of a flux is to lower the softening temperature of a glass by reducing the amount of cross-linking between the oxygen and glass-forming elements. For example, sodium can supply an electron to an oxygen atom in the tetrahedron. Thus, the oxygen atom becomes part of only one tetrahedron instead of being shared with other tetrahedrons. In other words, the tetrahedrons become separated.

Other metallic ions can also be introduced as indicated in Table 31–1. The result is that the Si-O bonds become fewer and the fused mass becomes less viscous; a lower maturing temperature also results. If too many tetrahedrons are disrupted, the glass may crystallize or *devitrify*. However, this is not likely to occur with dental porcelains because, in most cases, the silica content is much more than half the entire mass (Table 31–1).

By contrast, although boric oxide (B_2O_3) can act as a flux, it also forms its own glass network. Because the boric oxide forms a twin lattice with silica, it may still interrupt the more rigid silica network and cause a lowering of the softening point of the glass. However, the role of Al_2O_3 in glass formation is complicated. It cannot be considered a true glass former by itself because of the dimensions of the ion and the O:Al ratio. Nevertheless, it can take part in the glass network to alter the softening point and viscosity.

Oxides like Al_2O_3 may react either way, depending on other factors, such as composition. These oxides are called *intermediates*. Generally Al_2O_3 is used in glass formation to increase the hardness and viscosity. However, B_2O_3 also prevents thermal expansion increases, thereby allowing an increase in alkali content to lower the firing temperature even further.

Mechanical Behavior Because of its structure, glass is completely non-ductile after vitrification. Dislocations and slip cannot occur. When it breaks, a *brittle fracture* occurs. Its compressive strength is high and, theoretically, its tensile strength is also high. The shear strength is low. As noted in a previous chapter, a glass fiber may have a tensile strength of approximately 1,000,000 psi.

However, in practice, the tensile strength of a ceramic is very low because of surface irregularities. Whereas in the glass fiber, which is formed by stretching the glass in its viscous condition at a high temperature, a fairly uniform surface structure is present. In the ordinary ceramic body surface defects such as minute cracks, porosities and unevenness occur, as shown in Figure 31–7.

The cracks or surface irregularities may be extremely minute as indicated in Figure 31–8. Surface irregularities may cause the cracks to deviate from a straight line as shown in Figure 31–9. Such cracks result in the concentration of stresses. In metals, these stresses can be relieved by plastic deformation, but, because glasses are nonductile, stress relief is not possible. If the structure is under tensile stress, the concentrated stress can easily exceed the strength of

Figure 31–7

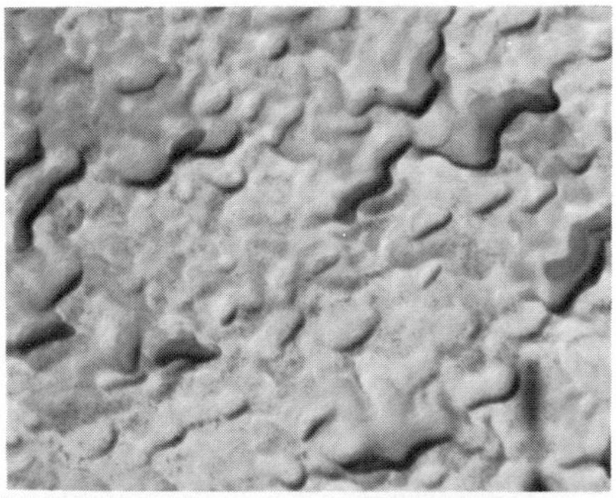

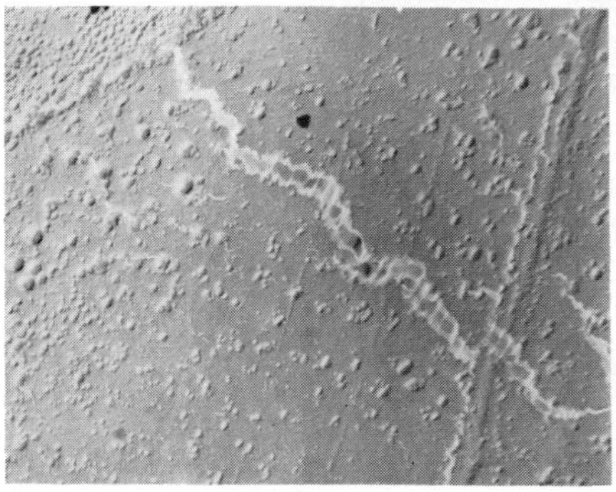

Figure 31–8 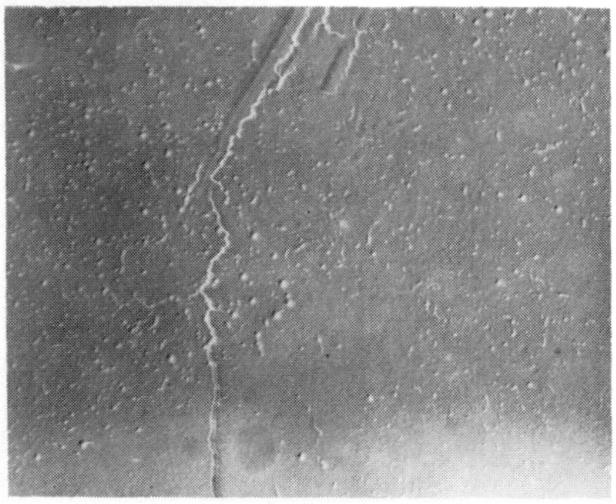   **Figure 31–9**

Figure 31–7 Electron micrograph of a surface of a dental porcelain showing flaws and discontinuities. × 30,000. (Courtesy of J. W. McLean and T. H. Hughes, Warren Spring Laboratory, England. Crown copyright reserved.)

Figure 31–8 Electron micrograph of a microcrack in dental porcelain, 0.1 μm wide. × 10,000. (Courtesy of J. W. McLean. Crown copyright reserved.)

Figure 31–9 Electron micrograph of a microcrack showing change in direction due to a surface fault. ×5000. (Courtesy of J. W. McLean and T. H. Hughes. Crown copyright reserved.)

the ceramic body, and the depth of the crack increases. The deeper the crack, the greater is the concentration of stress, and a brittle fracture occurs rapidly. This theory may account for the almost explosive fracture of ceramic bodies that commonly occurs. On the other hand, under a compressive stress, the crack is not self-propagating and the stress is resisted more successfully.

The cracks are believed to form during cooling of the ceramic after maturing. Regardless of the rate of cooling, the outside layer or "skin" cools more rapidly than the interior. Consequently, the "skin" is under compression and the interior contains tensile stresses because its thermal contraction may be partially prevented by the rigid skin which has already solidified. This differential dimensional change may possibly fracture or rupture the "skin" and produce minute cracks when the opposing stresses try to neutralize each other in this region.

This factor can be taken advantage of by purposely increasing the thickness of the "skin" by a process known as "tempering."* In this process, the glass is heated to a temperature that allows stress relaxation and then is cooled rapidly. The "skin" is sufficiently thick after such a treatment so that the interior tensile stresses are not sufficient to overcome the compressive stresses in the surface and the cracks cannot grow. Consequently, the overall strength of the glass is increased. This procedure can be applied to dental ceramic structures, but it is more effective when it is applied to flat surfaces, such as glass doors and similar structures in which the glass is not supported by a frame.

A significant clinical factor in the weakening of glass surfaces is the effect of moisture contamination. Water plays a vital part in the static fatigue of glass and produces a time-dependent reduction in strength. The process has been described as a replacement of the alkali ions in glass by hydrogen ions, which attract water molecules into the spaces originally occupied by the alkali.[4]

This water (saliva) could act as a type of network modifier in weakening the glass. Undamaged glass is weakened by wet storage and shows delayed fracture when stressed at constant load under wet conditions.[5] It is highly probable that surface weakening of dental porcelain may also occur in the mouth. Also, loads on the occlusal surfaces that would not normally fracture the material might overstress the flaw system once static fatigue is initiated.

This may explain why the metal-bonded porcelains are much stronger, since the porcelain interface is shielded from the effects of microcracks and static fatigue in water. The thickness of metal also plays a major part in this reinforcement but, as explained, the metal bonding probably accounts for the improvement in the strength of the platinum bonded alumina crown, for example.

Methods of Strengthening Dental Porcelain In order to strengthen dental porcelain, it is essential that a mechanism exist to prevent crack propagation under low tensile stresses. In the case of the metal-ceramic crown, this can be achieved in several ways. The inner surface can be reinforced with a metal (Fig. 31–6) or a high strength ceramic or, alternatively, the surface of the porcelain can be treated through ion exchange to improve its strength.

---

*The term is a misnomer; the tempering of steel, for example, is a different type of heat treatment. (See Chapter 37.)

Once a stronger material is used as an inner skin for the porcelain crown, then cracks can only develop when the stronger material is deformed or broken. This presupposes, of course, that the porcelain is firmly bonded to the reinforcing substrate.

Factors Influencing Color   The principal reason for a choice of porcelain as a restorative material is its esthetic qualities in matching the adjacent tooth structure in translucence, color, and intensity. (It will be recalled that the color phenomenon and terminology associated with it were discussed in Chapter 3.) Complete matching is extremely difficult, if not impossible. The structure of the tooth will influence its color. Dentin is more opaque than enamel and will reflect light. The enamel is a crystalline layer over the dentin and is composed of tiny prisms or rods cemented together by an organic substance. The indices of refraction of the rods and the cementing substance are different. Consequently, a light ray is diffused by reflection and refraction to produce a translucent effect and a sensation of depth as the scattered light ray reaches the eye. As the light ray strikes the tooth surface, part of it is reflected and the remainder penetrates the enamel and is diffused. Any light reaching the dentin is either absorbed or reflected to be again diffused in the enamel. If dentin is not present, as in the tip of an incisor, some of the light ray may be absorbed in the dark oral cavity. Consequently, this area may appear to be more translucent than that toward the gingival area.

In addition to the reflection and refraction, there may also be some dispersion, giving a color or shade that varies in different teeth. The dispersion can vary with the wave length of the light. Therefore, the appearance of the teeth may vary according to whether they are viewed in direct sunlight, reflected daylight, or tungsten or fluorescent light (the phenomenon of metamerism). It is, of course, impossible to imitate such an optical system perfectly. The dentist can, however, approach the esthetic characteristics sufficiently that the difference is conspicuous only to the trained eye.

Dental porcelains are pigmented by including oxides in the frit to provide desired colors as discussed earlier. Specimens of each shade (called a *shade guide)* are provided for the dentist who, in turn, can match the tooth color as nearly as possible (Fig. 3–15). Often, the dental ceramist will further blend the powders supplied to provide a more exact matching. A similar blending process is employed for the acrylic resin and silicate cement powders.

The production of color sensation with a pigment is a physically different phenomenon from that obtained by optical reflection, refraction, and dispersion. The color of a pigment is determined by selective absorption and selective reflection. For example, if white light is reflected from a red surface, all of the light with a wave length different from that of red is absorbed. Only the red light is reflected. It follows, then, that if a red hue is part of the blend in the porcelain jacket crown, but the red wave length is not present in the light beam, the tooth appears to be a different shade.

In practice, the dentist usually matches the tooth with the shade guide in the northern light from a blue sky, because this light usually contains all the primary colors. If the sky is cloudy, the shade may appear to be grayer than if reflected sunlight is present. If the light is reflected from a red brick wall, for example, the shade takes on a pink hue. Thus, if possible, the color matching should be done under two or more different light sources, as was noted in Chapter 3. At least one should be northern exposure daylight, and the matching should be done during the middle portion of a day that is slightly overcast if this is possible. In any event, porcelain restorations exhibit the best esthetic qualities in an illumination of the same wave length as that employed for the original color matching.

Another factor that is important to the esthetic qualities is the cementing medium. For example, an opaque material, such as zinc phosphate cement, can change the shade of a jacket crown because of its light absorption and color. Thus silicophosphate and, more recently, the glass ionomer cements are used for such restorations.

One method for overcoming the influence of the cement is to apply a first layer of opaque porcelain and cover it with translucent porcelain of the proper shade.

There are many other ramifications of such techniques. The coloring of the porcelain restoration is, in the last analysis, an art, not a science. Many of the factors involved are psychological rather than physical and cannot be specified exactly.

Condensation   The porcelain used to construct the jacket crown or metal-ceramic crown must be shaped to proper tooth form before it is fired. The complete details of how such restorations are fabricated is beyond the scope of this text and the reader is referred to excellent books in this field.[6, 7] Briefly, the chosen shade of porcelain powder is mixed to a paste with distilled water or a special liquid and applied to a platinum matrix or metal-ceramic framework. It is mandatory that the porcelain particles be packed together as closely as possible in order to minimize shrinkage during the firing process. This packing or *condensation* may be achieved by various methods, including the vibration, spatulation, and brush techniques.

The first method utilizes mild vibration to densely pack the wet powder upon the underlying framework. The excess water is blotted away with a clean tissue. In the second method, a small spatula is used to apply and smooth the wet porcelain. The smoothing action brings the excess water to the surface where it is removed. The third method utilizes the addition of dry porcelain powder to the surface in order to absorb the water. The dry powder is placed by a brush to the side opposite from an increment of wet porcelain. As the water is drawn toward the dry powder, the wet particles are pulled together. Whichever method is used, it is important to remember that the surface tension is the driving force in condensation and that the porcelain must never be allowed to dry out.

Firing Procedure   After the condensation is completed, the porcelain restoration is placed on a fire-clay slab or tray and inserted in the muffle of a porcelain furnace. The porcelain should never be allowed to contact the muffle walls or floor. At high temperatures, the porcelain melts and some of the ingredients may fuse into the heating element. Such a contamination renders the heating element extremely brittle, and it may fracture during cooling or subsequent heating. This precaution is particularly important when a platinum-wound muffle is used.

The thermochemical reactions between the ingredients are virtually completed in most cases during the original fritting process. Therefore, the purpose of the firing by the ceramist is simply to fuse the particles of powder together properly, a process called sintering, as will be recalled.

The condensed porcelain mass is placed in front of the muffle of a preheated furnace (approximately 650° C [1200° F]). This permits the remain-

COURSE
+ 120 MESH

Temp. °F   2150   2200   2250   2300   2350

FINE
- 325 MESH

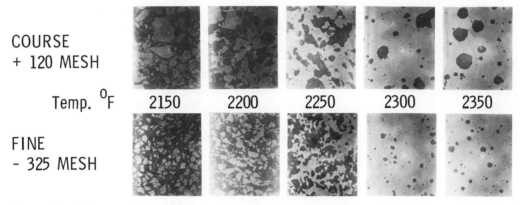

Figure 31–10 Progressive vitrification of coarse- and fine-grained porcelain. Top row: diameter of powder particles is greater than 125 μm. Bottom row: diameter of particles is less than 44 μm. Cross section of porcelain teeth fired on a 15-minute cycle to the temperatures indicated. Orig. mag. × 200. (From Vines and Semmelman, J Dent Res, Dec., 1957.)

ing water vapor to dissipate. Placement of the condensed mass directly into even a moderately warm furnace will result in a rapid production of steam, thereby introducing voids or fracturing large sections of the veneer. After preheating for approximately 5 minutes, the porcelain is placed into the furnace and the firing cycle initiated.

Not only does the size of the powder particles influence the degree of condensation of the porcelain but it also influences the soundness or apparent density of the final product. The progressive changes that occur during the firing of porcelain powders of coarse and fine particle sizes respectively are shown in Figure 31–10. The upper row of photomicrographs represents the structure of a porcelain during firing at the temperatures indicated with particles greater than 125 μm in diameter, and the lower row the same vitrification changes for particles 44 μm or less in diameter.

Regardless of the particle size, the white areas at 1177° C (2150° F) are the powder particles. The areas between are the voids. At this temperature the voids are occupied by the atmosphere of the furnace. As fusion begins, the particles unite at their points of contact (2200° F, Fig. 31–10). As the temperature is raised the fused glass gradually flows to fill up the air spaces, but the air becomes trapped in the form of bubbles because the fused mass is too viscous to allow all of it to escape.

Stages in Firing   At least three stages are generally recognized in the firing of dental porcelain. The temperature at which each occurs depends upon the type of porcelain employed. The lower the fusing temperature of the porcelain, the lower is the temperature of each firing stage.

A *low bisque** firing is recognized as the stage when the glass grains have softened and have started to flow. The fired article exhibits rigidity, but it is very porous. The powder particles lack complete cohesion. A negligible amount of firing shrinkage occurs.

A *medium bisque* firing is characterized by the fact that the glass grains have flowed to the extent that the powder particles exhibit complete cohesion; the article is still porous, and at this stage there is a definite shrinkage.

After a *high bisque* firing, the shrinkage is complete, and the mass

*Sometimes called "low biscuit," "medium biscuit," and "high biscuit."

exhibits a smoother surface. Slight porosity may be visible, but the body does not appear glazed.

The work can be removed from the furnace and cooled at any of these stages, so that additions can be made. However, the fewer the firing cycles to which the restoration is exposed, the higher will be the strength and the better the esthetics. Too frequent refiring results in a lifeless and overly translucent porcelain. The greatest changes occur in the value and chroma of air-fired porcelain; lesser deviations occur in vacuum-fired restorations.[8] The porcelains used in metal-ceramics are particularly vulnerable to repeated firings.

It should also be noted that additions of porcelain at the low bisque stage can cause layering and cloudiness in the porcelain. Owing to contamination of the surface, low bisque surfaces should *never* be ground.

Glazing   The surface of the crown or inlay should be completely smooth when the restoration is placed in the mouth. Otherwise food and other débris may cling to it.

Air-fired porcelain cannot be polished. There are always sufficient blebs and porosities present to prevent obtaining a smooth, polished surface. Lack of ductility prevents flowing or burnishing the surface. Such surface defects can be masked only by a surface glaze.

An overglaze can be applied to the surface as described in a preceding section, or the body itself can be glazed by a separate firing. If the body, previously fired to a high bisque, is heated rapidly (10 to 15 minutes) to its fusion temperature, and maintained at that temperature for approximately 5 minutes before it is cooled, the glass grains flow over the surface to form a vitreous layer, which is a glaze.

Cooling   The production of submicroscopic surface cracks during cooling has already been discussed. Because of the low thermal conductivity of the porcelain, the differential between the thermal dimensional change of the outside and inside can introduce stresses which embrittle the porcelain.

Thermal Shock   Stressing of a ceramic crown by thermal shock is not uncommon. This may be caused by uneven dimensional change upon cooling. For example, the surface of a crown may expand or contract more rapidly than the interior, depending upon the heating and cooling cycle. All ceramics are stronger under compression than under tension, as previously discussed. When a crown is removed from the furnace and cooled in air, the surface will be losing heat more rapidly than the interior. The crown surface will contract faster than the interior but generally will be placed in compression by the balancing tensile stresses developed either in the core porcelain or metal coping as a result of their higher thermal expansions.

Also, a crown that is moved into the furnace rapidly, prior to glazing, will receive the full force of the radiant heat through the muffle. The surface of the crown will tend to expand faster than the interior and the latter surface can be placed in such tension that thermal cracks could develop from the inner surface and break through the outer skin. Thermal shock is generally more severe during reheating or glazing of a crown than when cooling it.

Shrinkage   The cause of shrinkage during the firing of dental porcelain is loss of water and densification through sintering.

From a practical standpoint, composition has little effect on the volume

Table 31–2. *Influence of Condensation Method on the Physical Properties of Dental Porcelain*

METHOD OF CONDENSATION	FIRING SHRINKAGE, VOLUMETRIC *(per cent)*	APPARENT SPECIFIC GRAVITY	MODULUS OF RUPTURE	
			MPa	*(psi)*
Vibration	38.1	2.35	48.3	7000
Spatulation	38.4	2.34	49.6	7200
Brush application	40.5	2.36	36.5	5300
No condensation	41.5	2.36	33.8	4900

shrinkage of a dental porcelain, nor does the method of condensation as indicated in Table 31–2. Even when no condensation is employed and water is withdrawn only with a paper tissue, the difference in volume shrinkage is negligible in comparison to the shrinkage obtained with the conventional methods. These results again indicate that the most important property is surface tension which, in such a wet slurry, draws the powder particles closer together. The effect of condensation method on the modulus of rupture is seen in Table 31–2. However, the strength is influenced more by composition, the firing cycle, and integrity of the glazed surface.

The effect of the firing temperature on the shrinkage is demonstrated in Table 31–3. Small specimens of a high temperature maturing porcelain were fired to the temperatures indicated in 15 minutes, and held at those temperatures for 30 minutes before cooling. As can be noted, the volume shrinkage did not change to any extent after the firing temperature (1175° C) was attained.

The immediate cause for the shrinkage is the contraction of the body as the powder particles melt and fuse together as indicated in Figure 31–10. A surface tension action by the fused mass draws any unfused portions toward the center and into the voids or interstices. The final structure may be cored with the quartz crystalline phases, the glass phase forming the matrix (Fig. 31–11).

Porosity　As previously described, the bubbles, or voids, in the photomicrographs on the right in Figure 31–10 are due to the inclusion of air during fusion, although there is evidence that in the case of some of the high temperature maturing porcelains they may appear also as a by-product of the vitrification of the feldspar.

As might be expected, bubbles reduce the translucence and strength of the dental porcelain. As can be noted from Figure 31–10 the bubbles formed with the larger size porcelain powders, although larger, are not as numerous as are the smaller bubbles formed with the smaller size particles. Because of the

Table 31–3. *Effect of the Firing Temperature on the Physical Properties of a Dental Porcelain*

TEMPERATURE (°C)	(°F)	FIRING SHRINKAGE BY VOLUME *(per cent)*	APPARENT SPECIFIC GRAVITY	MODULUS OF RUPTURE MPa	*(psi)*
1040	1900	16.0	1.73	12.9	1870
1100	2000	......	2.14	33.1	4800
1150	2100	27.7	2.35	55.2	8000
1175	2150	35.4	2.37	65.9	9560
1200	2200	34.5	2.33	58.1	8430

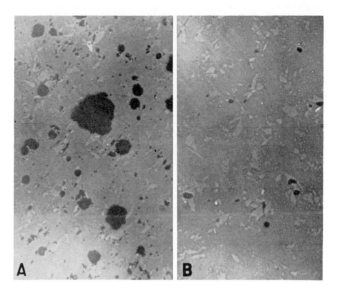

Figure 31–11 *A,* Air-fired porcelain. *B,* Vacuum-fired porcelain. The cored structure is crystalline quartz. (From Vines and Semmelman, J Dent Res, Dec. 1957.)

difference in indices of refraction between the porcelain body and the entrapped gas, the porcelain with the larger particle sizes with fewer bubbles is more translucent than that fired with the smaller particle size. When the bubbles are fewer or are eliminated, the finer size porcelain produces the more translucent body.

These bubbles or blebs seldom appear on the surface of a ceramic tooth or crown because the entrapped gases near the surface can be released. Also, gas bubbles are not as numerous in high temperature maturing porcelains as in low temperature maturing ones. The viscosity of the glass phase in the former porcelains is sufficiently low to allow some escape of the air during vitrification.

Three methods for the reduction or elimination of such voids have been suggested.[9]

1. The porcelain is fired in a partial vacuum so that the air is removed before it is entrapped. Vacuum firing is by far the most common method used for producing dental restorations.
2. A diffusible gas is substituted for the ordinary furnace atmosphere. The air is then driven out of the interstices during the firing and the diffusible gas is substituted. During fusion, such entrapped gases diffuse outward through the porcelain or are dissolved in the porcelain.
3. If the fused porcelain is cooled under pressure, the air bubbles can be compressed in size so that their effect is negligible.

The reduction in number and size of the air voids by vacuum firing is shown in Figure 31–11. Not all of the air can be evacuated from the furnace. Therefore, a few bubbles are present in *B* but they are in contrast to the bubbles obtained with the usual air firing method shown in *A*.

The diffusible gases that can be introduced into the furnace during vitrification are helium, hydrogen, or steam. As previously noted, when these gases are trapped in the voids they diffuse into the porcelain body. The structure of the final product resembles that of the vacuum fired porcelain shown in Figure 31–11*B*.

The structure shown in Figure 31–11 was obtained with a high bisque firing. When the porcelain is self-glazed by reheating, the diffusible gas method is somewhat superior to the others because further gas diffusion takes place and the bubbles virtually disappear. When the vacuum fired porcelain is reheated, the bubbles are unchanged.

If the porcelain is fired in air, the bubbles can be reduced by increasing the air pressure to 10 atmospheres, for example; the bubbles are reduced to a size comparable to that obtained with the other two methods. The pressure is, of course, maintained until the porcelain has cooled to rigidity.

The pressure method offers a disadvantage in that the porcelain cannot be refired or glazed at atmospheric pressure without the bubbles being restored to their original size by the compressed gas.

Physical Properties   The strength of the porcelain restoration is probably the most important mechanical property. As previously noted, the compressive strength of ceramic bodies is greater than either their tensile or their shear strength. The tensile strength is low because of the unavoidable surface defects. The shear strength is low because of the lack of ductility or ability to shear, caused by the complex structure of the glass ceramic materials.

Usually, the strength of a dental porcelain is measured by a cross-bend test which indicates its flexure strength or modulus of rupture. As previously discussed in Chapter 3, this test is a measure of both compressive and tensile stresses as well as shear. The tensile strength of porcelain is less than its compressive strength; it follows that the lower surface of the specimen is weaker and should fracture first. Therefore, the measurement is possibly more indicative of tensile strength than of compressive strength.

The strength of the porcelain is greatly dependent on its composition, surface integrity, and internal structure. The presence of voids and blebs can affect its strength, as illustrated in Figure 31–12. The load required to fracture

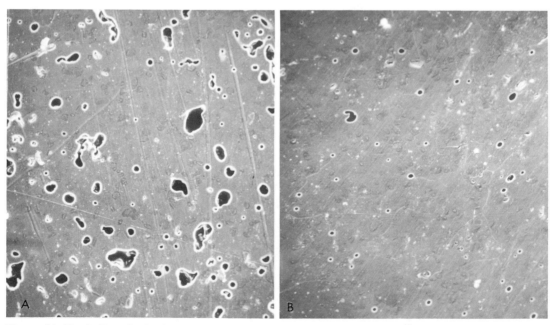

Figure 31–12   A, Porosity in the core porcelain of a jacket crown that failed under an incisal load of 94 kilograms. B, Porosity in the core porcelain of a jacket crown that failed under an incisal load of 160 kilograms. 200 ×.

the crown with the lesser porosity was almost twice that at which the more porous crown broke. The firing temperature is also important (Table 31–3). Unless the vitrification is complete, the structure is weak. Also, if the ceramic is overfired, its strength decreases because more of the core is dissolved in the flux and the core network is weakened. However, this effect is more deleterious to the esthetic qualities. Overfiring causes the material to become more transparent and to appear "glassy."

As previously noted, a too rapid cooling increases the surface cracks and weakens the porcelain. Glazed porcelain is much stronger than the unglazed variety, as can be noted in Table 31–4. As previously stated, the glaze is effective in reducing crack propagation. If the glaze is removed by grinding, the transverse strength may be only half that with the glaze present (Table 31–4). The same effect as in glazing is achieved with a "tempered" porcelain.

This observation is of clinical importance. After the porcelain restoration is cemented in the mouth, it is common practice for the dentist to make a final adjustment of the occlusion by grinding the surface of the porcelain. Unfortunately, this procedure weakens the porcelain markedly if the glaze is removed.

Vacuum firing has little effect on the transverse strength of porcelain (Table 31–4). The reason is probably that surface crack formation is not related to the atmosphere during firing. Apparently, so far as transverse strength is concerned, this factor is of greater importance than is the weakening effects of the voids.

It is interesting to note that the modulus of rupture of aluminous porcelain is the same whether the porcelain is glazed or unglazed (Table 31–4). Apparently, the strengthening effect of the alumina core is sufficient to counteract to some extent the weakening effect of the surface discontinuities. The strengthening effect of using sintered alumina also as a backing for translucent porcelain is considerable, as indicated by its modulus of rupture (Table 31–4.)

The method of firing also affects the strength (Table 31–3). A firing schedule that employs a lower temperature and a longer time is superior, so far as strength is concerned, to a shorter firing period at a higher temperature. Also, the sharp edges and angles are better preserved at the lower firing temperatures.

Table 31–4. *Modulus of Rupture of Various Dental Porcelains**

CLASSIFICATION	FIRING ATMOSPHERE	SURFACE CONDITION	MODULUS OF RUPTURE MPa	psi
Porcelain†	Air	Ground	75.8	11,000
		Glazed	141.1	20,465
	Vacuum	Ground	79.6	11,547
		Glazed	132.3	19,187
Aluminous porcelain	Air	Ground	135.9	19,709
		Glazed	138.9	20,142
Fused alumina			519.3	75,310

*Adapted from McLean and Hughes, Br Dent J, Sept. 21, 1965.
†A dental porcelain. Both porcelains are the medium temperature maturing variety and fused in air.

Evidently, sufficient time at the proper temperature should be allotted for the viscous melt to flow completely through the unmelted parts and weld them together. As the temperature rises, the viscosity of the molten phase decreases and it flows more easily, but perhaps too much of the material is fused at the higher temperature, with the result that the strength is decreased. As with similar materials, an optimal ratio between the matrix and the core should be maintained for the maximal strength.

Sintering Time and Strength of Aluminous Porcelain   It is essential that chemical bonding occur between the glass matrix and the alumina crystals so that maximum strength can be achieved in aluminous porcelain. This system is most effective in inhibiting fracture when cracks can pass indiscriminately through both the glass and alumina crystal phases, thus allowing the crystals to bear a greater proportion of any stress applied to the porcelain.

It is advisable to utilize a prolonged sintering time when firing low-fusing aluminous core porcelains, in order to permit efficient wetting of the crystals by the glass.[10] The additional sintering, for a time approximately 15 minutes beyond that recommended by the manufacturer, should be done in a normal atmosphere.

Strengthening Via Ion Exchange   It was previously noted that porcelain can also be strengthened by ion exchange. When dental porcelains possessing sufficient soda (Na_2O) content are immersed in a potassium nitrate salt bath, potassium ions will replace some of the sodium ions located close to the surface layers. A crowding of atoms occurs as the larger potassium ions displace the sodium ions, and a stressed surface layer is produced. This surface compression results in increased strength of the porcelain.[6, 11]

The clinical significance of strengthening crowns by ion exchange, or other such concepts,[12] has yet to be established but this area of research merits further exploration.

Specific Gravity   When the specific gravity or the density of a dental porcelain is discussed, a distinction must be made between the *apparent specific gravity* and the *true specific gravity*. The values for the specific gravity given in Tables 31–2 and 31–3 were obtained from fired specimens of dental porcelain. Any blebs or other internal voids in the porcelain reduce the specific gravity. Consequently, the figures represent the specific gravity of the specimens and not necessarily that of the porcelain itself.

On the other hand, if the porcelain specimens are ground to a fine powder so that the effect of the flaws is eliminated, the specific gravity of the powder indicates the true or actual specific gravity of the porcelain. The true specific gravity of the porcelain used to obtain the data in Tables 31–2 and 31–3 is 2.42. Consequently, because none of the values for specific gravity in either table is as high as the true specific gravity, it can be concluded that the fired porcelain is not free from internal voids and similar flaws, regardless of the method of condensation or firing.

It is apparent that the specific gravity of the porcelain is not greatly affected by the method of condensation (Table 31–2).

The compressive strength of dental porcelain is approximately 331 MPa (48,000 psi). Its coefficient of thermal expansion is 6.4 to 7.8 $\times$ 10^{-6} per degree centigrade, a value which is close to that of the human tooth (Table 3–2).

General Considerations   The construction of a porcelain restoration that functions properly requires considerable skill and knowledge on the part of the dentist. The shear and tensile strength of the fired porcelain is so low that the slightest imperfection in the preparation of the cavity in the tooth may cause the jacket crown to fracture in service.

On the other hand, the porcelain restoration possesses excellent esthetic qualities, is completely insoluble in the oral fluids, and is dimensionally stable after it has been fired. It is doubtful, however, that a porcelain inlay or crown can be constructed with sufficient accuracy that the margins are completely sealed because of the unavoidable errors resulting from the firing shrinkage.

The restoration is usually cemented in position with a luting agent such as silicophosphate, polycarboxylate, or a glass ionomer cement, as noted earlier. All of these cements are subject to erosion in oral fluids (Chapters 29 and 30). If the erosion is severe, the crevice left becomes stained, to take on a bluish hue beneath a jacket crown for example.

The porcelain restoration is compatible with the soft tissues, and is resistant to abrasion. When all factors are considered, dental porcelain is probably the most serviceable of the tooth restorative materials that possess good esthetic qualities.

METAL-CERAMICS

As frequently noted in previous sections, the chief objection to the use of an all porcelain restoration in fixed prosthodontics is its lack of strength, particularly tensile and shear strength. Although it can resist compressive stress with reasonable success, the necessary design factors usually do not permit shapes in which the compressive stress is the principal force. It may either not be a factor or be a factor of minor importance, as on the incisal edges of the anterior teeth during function.

A method by which this disadvantage may be minimized is to fuse the porcelain directly to a casting that fits the prepared tooth. If a strong bond is effected between the porcelain veneer and the metal, there is no chance for leakage at the interface. Furthermore, with proper design and physical properties of the porcelain and metal, the porcelain is reinforced so that brittle fracture can be avoided or at least minimized. This is often referred to as a *porcelain fused to metal* restoration. A more proper term is a *metal-ceramic* restoration, as was noted in Chapter 24 and earlier in this chapter.

The components in, and fabrication of, a metal-ceramic restoration were covered previously in this chapter, in Figure 31–6, and originally in Chapter 24 in conjunction with the noble metal alloys used in its construction. The final enamel-veneered structure is then cemented on the prepared tooth as usual. The opaque metal and ceramic enamel prevent any color alteration by the cementing medium.

Physical Requirements   The alloys used for the construction of metal-ceramic restorations have a number of rather stringent requirements that must be met. The desired characteristics have been discussed both in Chapter 24 and in this chapter. To summarize, for example, both the metal and ceramic must have coefficients of thermal expansion that are closely matched if undesirable tensile stresses at the interface are to be avoided.

Another equally important property is that the alloy should have high proportional limit, and, particularly, a high modulus of elasticity. Alloys with a high modulus will also reduce stress on the porcelain. However, if the modulus is unduly high, the stresses developed in the porcelain during cooling cannot be easily relieved by metal deformation, resulting in more serious cracking problems.

The metal framework must not melt during firing of the porcelain and must also resist thermally induced stresses which can produce creep or "sag." Heat treatment is another way of improving resistance to creep at high temperatures (Chapter 24).

In regard to tarnish and corrosion resistance and similar properties, the alloy should be equal to any other successful alloy used in the oral cavity.

Composition of Alloys   The composition of the noble metal alloys used in metal-ceramics was discussed in Chapter 24. The reader is referred to that description of these systems, and of the effects and purposes of the constituent metals, as well as to other texts.[6]

The compositions of the base metal alloys used in metal-ceramic restorations can be found in Chapter 34, which is devoted to these basic systems. Certain differences in fabrication and performance, as compared with the noble metal alloys, are also covered in that chapter.

Composition of the Ceramic   The composition of the ceramic generally corresponds to that of the glasses in Table 31–1 except for an increased alkali content. The addition of greater quantities of soda and potash is necessary in order to increase the thermal expansion to a level compatible with the metal coping.

The opaque porcelains contain relatively large amounts of metallic oxide opacifiers in order to conceal the underlying metal and to minimize the thickness of the opaque layer.

It is important to note that the high-expansion porcelains used in metal-ceramics have an increased tendency to devitrify because of their alkali content. These porcelains should not be subjected to repeated firings, as this will increase the risk of producing a cloudiness within the porcelain.

Thus it is obvious that a proper meshing of the properties of the alloy and porcelain is imperative to success. Criteria and test methods for determining that compatibility have been suggested.[13] They include measurements of the compatibility of coefficients of thermal expansion, thermal conductivity (to determine resistance to thermal shock), and the nature and strength of the bond, which will now be discussed.

Enamel-Metal Bonds   The nature of the bond between noble metal alloys and dental porcelain has been the subject of considerable discussion. This is appropriate, since the success of a metal-ceramic crown depends upon the firmness of the bond between the metal and ceramic veneer. Earlier workers considered that "wetting bonds" in one instance, and van der Waal's forces in the other, could adequately explain the observed strengths of metal-ceramic bonds.[14, 15] However, current research in this field tends to disregard the part played by van der Waal's forces, since such forces are small and can be subject to misinterpretation.[16]

Therefore, the nature of the gold-porcelain bond has become better defined and probably can be divided into three main components: mechanical, compressive, and chemical, as diagrammed in Figure 31–13.

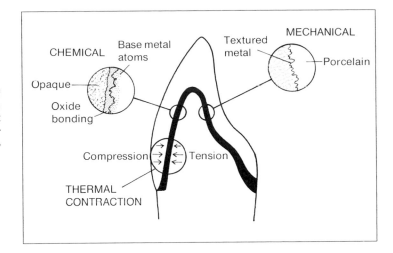

Figure 31–13 Components of metal-ceramic bond. (From McLean, JW: The Science and Art of Dental Ceramics, Vol. I, Quintessence Publ. Co., Chicago, 1979, p. 72.).

Mechanical Retention If close contact on rough surfaces is to be achieved, mechanical retention is very dependent upon good wetting of the metal or metal oxide surface by the porcelain. Mechanical retention is improved by a textured surface, as illustrated in Figure 31–13.

A microsection of a gold-porcelain bond (Fig. 31–14) indicates the effectiveness of the wetting of the metal by the porcelain. This was typical of all the gold alloy specimens examined in this particular study. In view of the fact that the porcelain has entered what might appear to be re-entrant angles and no significant amounts of porosity were detectable at the interface, it is reasonable to conclude that some form of *mechanical interlocking* has taken place. Such a mechanical "bond" must contribute something to the resistance of the porcelain to shear stresses.

A rough surface may enhance the bond resistance against induced shear stresses, especially for base-metal alloy systems.[17] Suggested advantages of an air-abraded surface over a smooth surface for noble metal and base metal alloys are (1) enhancement of wettability of the metal substrate by porcelain, (2) some additive bond strength because of mechanical interlocking of porcelain under compression, and (3) increased surface area for porcelain chemical bonding.

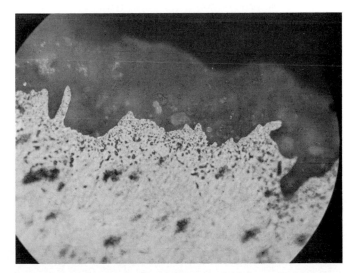

Figure 31–14 Oblique section through gold alloy — porcelain bond showing internal oxide near the surface of the metal and the effective wetting by the porcelain. ×700. (Courtesy of Sced, IR, Hopkins BE, and McLean JW. Report on the Strength of Metal to Porcelain Fused Bonds as Used in Dental Restorations, National Physical Laboratory, Crown copyright.)

Suggested disadvantages of an air-abraded surface over a smooth surface are (1) excessive roughness resulting in stress concentration at the metal-ceramic interface, and (2) steep interface angles that may not allow complete wetting and therefore result in air entrapment and voids at the metal-ceramic interface.

Compressive Stresses   Compressive stresses set up during the cooling of the sintered porcelain veneer will also play a part in improving the bond strength. Ceramo-metallic systems are deliberately designed with a very small degree of thermal mismatch in order to leave the porcelain in a state of compression.

Chemical Bonding   The evidence is considerably stronger for some form of chemical bonding. Electron microprobe examination of the metal-ceramic interface indicates that indium or tin migrates to the alloy surface to form indium or tin oxide, which combines with the porcelain during firing.[18-20]

Further evidence of chemical bonding is that cleansing of the metal with hydrofluoric acid reduces the bond strength.[16] This indicates that the oxide film does contribute to the bonding mechanism. When dental porcelain is fired onto a metal with a definite oxide layer, the oxygen surface of the molten glass (porcelain) diffuses with the oxygen surface on the metal to reduce the number of bridging oxygens, and thus improves the screening of the cations at the interface.[21] If the glass is not saturated with the particular oxide, it dissolves the oxygen with its metallic cations. The glass at the glass-oxide interface then becomes saturated with oxide. This glass remains constant in composition (at constant temperature) and is in thermodynamic equilibrium with the oxide, resulting in a balance of bond energies and a chemical bond.

The critical requirement for maintaining saturation at the oxygen-glass interface is that the rate of solution of the oxide at the interface is higher than the rate of diffusion of the dissolved oxide away from the interface.

As noted in Chapter 2, the first requisite for a strong adhesive bond is that the adhesive must wet the adherend. In the present case, the enamel is treated as the adhesive because it flows onto the alloy during firing. Again, as described in Chapter 2, the wettability of the adhesive can be measured by its contact angle. Obviously, the contact angle of the ceramic enamel is determined while it is a liquid above the fusion temperature, but its adhesion can be measured at room temperature because the same thermodynamic conditions of stress persist after solidification.

The contact angles of various commercial enamels for dental use are given in Table 31–5. Special casting alloys which have been matched with each

Table 31–5.   *Contact Angles (Degrees) for Enamels on Various Metals Used in Dental Restoration**

Enamel	Without Bonding Agent	With Bonding Agent	On Platinum†	On Palladium†	Temperature °C	°F
A	40	50	54	52	1040	1900
B	53	39	64	60	1040	1900
C	59	70	97	95	1040	1900
D	102	92	102	108	1150	2100
E	52	28	48	46	1040	1900

*Adapted from O'Brien and Ryge, J Prosthet Dent, Nov.–Dec., 1965.
†Without bonding agent.

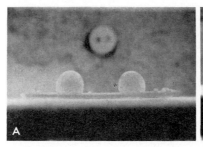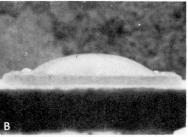

Figure 31–15 *A,* Poor wetting by enamel D (Table 31–6) with large contact angle. *B,* Good wetting by enamel A (Table 31–6) with small contact angle. (From O'Brien and Ryge, J Prosthet Dent, Nov.–Dec., 1965.)

enamel are supplied. Also, bonding agents are usually supplied with each enamel and are applied to the adherend metal. Two types of bonding agents are used. One type makes use of a ceramic material that fuses to the metal; the second is a paste of powdered gold.

As previously noted, the less the contact angle, the better is the wetting ability of the enamel. Any contact angle greater than 90 degrees indicates a lack of wetting and, of course, adhesion. Apparently, enamel D does not adhere to any of the metals or alloys. Enamel A appears to exhibit the best wetting properties regardless of the adherend, with enamels B and E being compara ble. It is evident that the bonding agent is generally ineffective in reducing the contact angle, with the exception of enamels B and E. It is also evident from the changes in contact angle when the enamels are applied to platinum and palladium that the composition of the metal adherend is important. The difference between poor wetting and good wetting by the enamel is illustrated in Figure 31–15.

As previously mentioned, in Chapter 2, the adhesion between two surfaces may be stronger than the strength of either the adhesive or adherend. This is the case in the adhesion between the enamel and alloy under tensile stress. The fracture generally occurs in the enamel.[22]

Another very important requisite is that the enamel and metal have compatible linear coefficients of thermal expansion. The effect is the same as for added porcelain glaze. If the expansion coefficients are not essentially equal, radial stresses may occur that weaken the enamel as well as the bond. For example, a difference in the coefficients of thermal expansion of only 3×10^{-6} per degree Fahrenheit can produce a shear stress of 280 MPa (39,800 psi) in a gold-enamel interface when the temperature changes from 954° C (1750° F) to room temperature. The shear resistance to failure is not greater than approximately 73 MPa (10,300 psi) as shown in Table 31–6. Therefore, these thermal stresses would probably cause a spontaneous rupture of the bond.

Even with good quality control, the order of residual stress has been calculated to be in the order of 21 MPa (3000 psi).[23] The occlusal stresses upon the restoration would, of course, be added to these residual thermal stresses. However, fracture is unlikely to occur except in cases of extreme stress concentration or an incorrect occlusal relationship.[16]

Bond Strength   A variety of tests have been advocated for measuring the strength of the metal-ceramic system. None can be regarded as providing an exact measure of the adhesion of porcelain to metal except in cases in which the metal-porcelain couple is so exactly matched thermally as to be totally

Table 31–6.   *Shear Strengths of Enamel-Metal Bonds* *

METAL	SURFACE CONDITION	SHEAR STRENGTH	
		MPa	*psi*
Gold alloy A	Polished	25	3,560
Platinum-palladium alloy A	Polished	27	3,800
	Roughened longitudinally	28	3,900
	Roughened transversely	26	3,700
Platinum-palladium alloy B†	Polished	50	7,160
Gold alloy B†	Polished	69	9,810
	Roughened longitudinally	70	9,980
	Roughened transversely	70	9,900
	Polished, bonding agent used	72	10,220
	Polished, vacuum fired	73	10,280

*Adapted from Shell and Nielsen, J Dent Res, Nov.–Dec., 1962.
†Modifiers added.

stress free, a situation virtually impossible to attain.[16] Even then, the adhesive strength would have to be lower than the strength of the porcelain itself.

Another approach has been suggested as more realistic than that used to secure the data shown in Table 31–6, which involved a shear test.[24, 25] This is to assess the type of fracture in which failure occurs, either through the porcelain (cohesive) or a mixture of cohesive and adhesive failure, i.e., part interfacial and part through the porcelain. In the absence of tensile failure through the porcelain, as in the gold alloy system, McLean states that the "clinical safety of any metal-ceramic system must be suspect since the maximum possible strength is not being achieved and is likely to be variable depending on the precise conditions of preparation of the restoration."[26]

A study of the interfacial separation following fracture is necessary in order to determine the weakest layer. A classification has been made of the various types of porcelain-metal failures, as seen in Figure 31–16. Obviously failure can occur cohesively within the porcelain or metal or at the various oxide interfaces.

Bonding Using Tin Oxide Coatings   Another method of bonding porcelain to metal using tin oxide coatings has also.been developed, with the objective of an improvement in the esthetics of metal-ceramic crowns. By a reduction in the thickness of the metal coping, a sufficiently esthetic layer of porcelain may be achieved without excessively cutting the tooth or overcontouring the artificial crown. Another objective is the reduction of light reflectivity from the metal-opaque porcelain. The light-gray color of tin oxide-coated platinum is said to be a more suitable background than dark metal oxides for the application of opaque porcelain.[27]

The method consists of bonding aluminous porcelain to platinum foil copings. Attachment of the porcelain is secured by electroplating the platinum foil with a thin layer of tin and then oxidizing it in a furnace to provide a continuous film of tin-oxide for porcelain bonding. It was considered that combining a high strength aluminous porcelain with a crack-free metal surface might result in a composite that possessed the optimum properties of both materials. The bonded foil acts as an inner skin on the fit surface, reducing subsurface porosity and microcracks in the porcelain and increasing the strength of the unit. The mechanism apparently involves a chemical interaction involving diffusion and dissolution of tin oxide into the glass phase

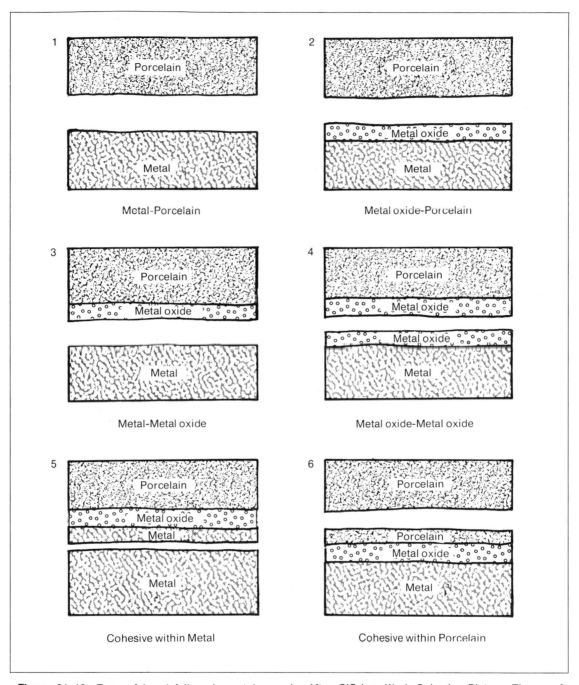

Figure 31–16 Type of bond failure in metal-ceramic. After *O'Brien, W. J.* Cohesive Plateau Theory of Porcelain-Alloy Bonding. Conference Proceeding. University of Southern California. 1977. Dental Porcelain. State of the Art. (From McLean JW: The Science and Art of Dental Ceramics, Vol. I, Quintessence Publ. Co., Chicago, 1979, p. 84.)

of the porcelain and a better wetting of the tin plated substrate by the porcelain.[28]

Technical Considerations for Metal-Ceramic Restorations   The appliance is generally fabricated by a dental technician. The casting procedures are similar to those described for the casting of inlays and crowns.

Because of the high melting temperature of the alloys, gypsum-bonded investments cannot be used. A phosphate (Chapter 26) or silicate binder (Chapter 35) is used. The investment thermal expansion method for shrinkage compensation is used. A gas-oxygen flame is generally employed for melting the alloy.

The casting should be carefully cleaned to insure a strong bond to the enamel. The casting, in some cases, is heated in the porcelain furnace to a temperature of 980° C (1800° F) to burn off any remaining impurities and to degas it. The need for a clean metal surface cannot be overemphasized. Degassing is necessary for all gold-porcelain systems. The number of bubbles formed at the interface decreases as the time and temperature of degassing are increased.[29] Oil from the fingers can also be a possible contaminant. The surface may be cleansed adequately by finishing with ceramic bonded stones or sintered diamonds, which are used exclusively for finishing. Final texturing with an alumina air-brasive will insure that the porcelain is bonded to a mechanically receptive surface.

Opaque enamel is condensed with a thickness of approximately 0.1 to 0.2 mm. It is then fired to its maturing temperature. The translucent enamel is then applied and the tooth form built. The unit is again fired. In fact, several firings may be necessary. A final glaze is then obtained as with the porcelain jacket crown.

The enamel powder is applied by the condensation methods previously described.

Creep   Unfortunately, some flow or creep of the gold alloy occurs when it approaches 980° C (1800° F). The creep can be reduced if the metal has the proper composition so that a dispersion strengthening effect occurs at the high temperature. The effect is similar to that in the dispersion strengthening of amalgam at room temperature.

When the gold alloy is heated to 980° C, ideally a second phase is precipitated which can produce a hardening or strengthening of the alloy.[30] Such creep has been reduced in some of the commercial alloys, but it apparently cannot be eliminated.

General Considerations   A clinical evaluation of the metal-ceramic restoration is difficult to make. The properly made crown is stronger and more durable than the ordinary porcelain jacket crown. However, a long-span bridge of this type may be subject to bending strains and the enamel may craze or fracture because it is nonductile. These difficulties can be partly overcome with the proper design factors. One factor is to avoid sharp angles and corners in the gold alloy castings because discontinuities produce stress concentrations that weaken the enamel. Proper occlusal relationships are most important for this type of restoration.

The most outstanding advantage is probably the permanent esthetic quality of the properly designed reinforced ceramic unit. Unlike similar acrylic resin veneered structures, there are almost no losses by abrasion or change in color because of leakage between the veneer and the metal.

On the other hand, the fit of veneered crowns may not be adequate. The castings fit the dies before the enamel is applied. After firing, a lack of adaptation may occur, undoubtedly as a result of high temperature creep or too great a difference in the coefficient of thermal expansion between the alloy and the enamel. Because the enamel and alloy have similar coefficients of thermal expansion, it does not seem likely that the distortion can be primarily caused by the enamel per se.

Another problem is that more tooth structure may need to be removed to provide the proper bulk for the crown than with the all-porcelain restoration. As previously noted, almost complete rigidity of the structure is needed to prevent fracture of the enamel. Although the modulus of elasticity of the enamel is high, its low tensile and shear strengths indicate a low maximal flexibility because, in brittle fracture, the breaking strength and proportional limit coincide. Consequently, only limited elastic deformation of the enamel can be allowed. It follows, therefore, that even with a high modulus of elasticity a considerable bulk of metal is also necessary to provide the proper rigidity. The bulk of the crown cannot be conspicuously out of line with the adjacent teeth. Therefore, the bulk of the natural tooth may need to be sacrificed to provide adequate space.

In spite of these disadvantages, metal-ceramic restorations are the most widely used material in fixed prosthodontics today.

References

1. McLean JW and Hughes TH: The reinforcement of dental porcelain with ceramic oxides. Br Dent J 119:251, 1965.
2. McLean JW: The alumina tube post crown. Br Dent J 123:87, 1967.
3. McLean JW: High-alumina ceramics for bridge pontic construction. Br Dent J 123:571, 1967.
4. Wang F and Tooley FV: Influence of reaction products on reaction between water and soda-lime-silica glass. J Am Ceram Soc 41:521, 1958. Ref. cited in Chem Abst 53:3625e, 1959.
5. Gurney C: Source of weakness in glass. Proc Roy Soc A 192,537, 1964.
6. McLean JW: The Science and Art of Dental Ceramics, Volume I, Quintessence Publ. Co., Chicago, 1979.
7. McLean JW: The Science and Art of Dental Ceramics, Volume II, Quintessence Publ. Co., Chicago, 1980.
8. Barghi N and Goldberg J: Porcelain shade stability after repeated firing. J Prosthet Dent 37:173, 1977.
9. Vines RF, Semmelman JO, Lee PW, and Fonvielle FD: Mechanisms involved in securing dense, vitrified ceramics from preshaped partly crystalline bodies. J Am Ceram Soc 41:304, 1958.
10. Jones DW, Jones PA, and Wilson HJ: The relationship between transverse strength and testing methods for dental ceramics. J Dent 1:85, 1972.
11. Southan DE: The physical properties of dental porcelain. Ph.D. Thesis, University of Sydney, Australia, 1968.
12. Pameijer CH, Grossman D, and Adair PJ: Physical properties of a castable ceramic dental restorative material. IADR Program and Abstracts, No. 827, 1980.
13. Council on Dental Materials, Instruments and Equipment: Porcelain-metal alloy compatibility: criteria and test methods. J Am Dent Assoc 102:71, 1981.
14. O'Brien WJ and Ryge G: Relation between molecular force calculations and observed strengths of enamel-metal interfaces. J Am Ceram Soc 47:5, 1964.
15. Ryge G: Current American research on porcelain-fused-to-metal restorations. Int Dent J 15:385, 1965.
16. Sced IR, Hopkins BE, and McLean JW: Report on the Strengths of Metal to Porcelain Fused Bonds as Used in Dental Restorations. National Physical Laboratory, England, October, 1970.
17. Carpenter MA and Goodkind RJ: Effect of varying surface texture on bond strength of one semi-precious and one non-precious alloy. J Prosthet Dent 42:86, 1979.
18. Nally JN: Chemico-physical analysis and mechanical tests of the ceramo-metallic complex. Int Dent J 18:309, 1968.

19. Nally JN, Monnier D, and Meyer JM: Distribution topographique de certains elements de alliage ed de la porcelaine an niveau de la liaison ceramo-metallique. Schweiz Monatsschr Zahnheilkd 78:868, 1968.
20. Szantho von Radnoth M and Lautenschlager EP: Metal surface changes during porcelain firing. J Dent Res 48:321, 1969.
21. Cascone PJ: The theory of bonding for porcelain-to-metal systems. In: Dental Porcelain. The State of the Art, Proceedings of the University of S. California. Eds. Yamada, H, and Grenoble, P, 1977, pp. 109–117.
22. Shell JS and Nielsen JP: Study of the bond between gold alloys and porcelain. J Dent Res 41:1424, 1962.
23. Nielsen JP and Tuccillo JJ: Interfacial stress in porcelain bodies bonded to metal prosthetic restorations. J Biomed Mater Res Symp 2:395, 1972.
24. McLean JW and Sced IR: Bonding of dental porcelain to metal. II. The base-metal alloy porcelain bond. Trans Brit Ceram Soc 72:237, 1973.
25. O'Brien WJ: Cohesive plateau theory of porcelain-alloy bonding. In: Dental Porcelain. The State of the Art, Proceedings of the University of S. California. Eds. Yamada, H, and Grenoble, P, 1977, pp. 137–161.
26. McLean JW: The Science and Art of Dental Ceramics, Volume I, Quintessence Publ. Co., Chicago, 1979, p. 82.
27. McLean JW and Sced, IR: The bonded alumina crown. 1. The bonding of platinum to aluminous dental porcelain using tin oxide coatings. Aust Dent J 21:119, 1976.
28. Sakar NK and Jeansonne EE: Strengthening mechanism of bonded alumina crowns. J. Prosthet Dent 45:95, 1981.
29. Jarvis RH and Mumford G: A study of the factors effecting discontinuities at the porcelain-metal interface of porcelain fused to metal restorations. IADR Program and Abstracts, No. 323, 1968.
30. Tuccillo JJ and Nielsen JP: Creep and sag properties of a porcelain-gold alloy. J Dent Res 46:579, 1967.

32 WROUGHT GOLD ALLOYS

In modern dentistry, wire is the principal form in which wrought gold alloy is used. Gold alloy wires are occasionally employed in the construction of removable partial denture clasps. They are also used in the construction of orthodontic appliances and as retention pins for restorations. In the fabrication of certain appliances, a casting alloy is cast directly to the wire, e.g., a wire clasp on a cast gold partial denture, a wire connector between two castings, or retention pins.

Composition Many gold wires resemble the type IV gold casting alloys in composition, but typically they contain less gold. The composition limits of some dental gold alloy wires are given in Table 32–1. As the gold content decreases to 30 per cent or less, the plantinum and palladium content increases, and the composition is similar to that of the "white gold" alloys.

Two types of gold wire are recognized in American Dental Association Specification no. 7. Type I, high precious metal alloys, must contain at least 75 per cent gold and platinum group metals, and Type II, low precious metal alloys, must contain at least 65 per cent of the same metals.

The P-G-P wires, because of their high fusion temperature, and therefore high recrystallization temperatures, are especially useful as wires to be cast against, and obviously meet the composition requirements for an American Dental Association Type I wire. Some of them also satisfy the mechanical requirements (Table 32–2) for a Type I wire, even though they are not age hardenable (the mechanical properties listed are for the wire in the quenched condition).

The palladium-silver-copper alloy wires (P-S-C) are neither Type I nor Type II gold wires, but their mechanical properties would meet the requirements for an American Dental Association Type I or II wire.

Corrosion resistance of palladium-silver or even silver-palladium dental alloys, both in cast and wrought form, in the oral environment is generally very satisfactory.

General Effects of the Constituents As with casting alloys, extensive data on the composition and physical properties of gold alloy wires have been published so that empirical relationships can be obtained between the chemical composition of the alloy and its chemical and physical properties.[1]

The contributions of the individual metals are essentially the same as for

531

Table 32–1. *Composition Limits of Some High Strength Wires Used in Dentistry*

	GOLD	PLATINUM	PALLADIUM	SILVER	COPPER	NICKEL	ZINC
ADA Type I	54–63	7–18	0– 8	9–12	10–15	0–2	0–0.6*
ADA Type II	60–67	0– 7	0–10	8–21	10–20	0–6	0–1.7*
P-G-P	25–30	40–50	25–30				†
P-S-C		0– 1	42–44	38–41	16–17	0	†

*Dentists Desk Reference: Materials, Instruments and Equipment, 1st ed., Metals and Alloys: Precious Metal Wrought Wire. American Dental Association, Chicago, 1981.

†Lyman T, Metals Handbook, 8th ed., Vol. I, Properties and Selection of Metals. American Society for Metals, Metal Park, Ohio, 1964.

the casting gold alloys. The increased palladium and platinum content insures that the wire will not melt or recrystallize during soldering procedures. Also, these two metals insure a fine grain structure.

Copper contributes to the ability of the alloy to age harden. When copper is present, silver may be added to balance the color.

Nickel is sometimes included in small amounts as a strengthener of the alloy, although it tends to reduce the ductility.[2] The presence of a large quantity of nickel tends to decrease the alloy's tarnish resistance[3] and to change its response to age hardening.[4] In the amounts represented in Table 32–1, any deleterious effects are not likely to be present.

Zinc is added as a scavenger agent to obtain oxide-free ingots from which the wires are drawn.

Fusion Temperature The minimum fusion temperatures are established to insure that the wires do not melt or lose their wrought structure during normal soldering procedures. According to American Dental Association Specification no. 7 for a Type I wire, this temperature is 955° C (1751° F); for the Type II wire the minimum fusion temperature is 871° C (1600° F).

Mechanical Properties A wire of a given composition is generally superior in mechanical properties to a casting of the same composition. The casting contains unavoidable porosity which has a weakening effect. When the cast ingot is drawn into a wire, the small pores and blebs may be collapsed, and welding may occur so that such defects disappear. Any defects of this type that are not eliminated will weaken the wire.

Table 32–2. *Physical Properties of Some Wires Used in Dentistry*

TYPE	YIELD STRENGTH Oven-Cooled Min. (MPa)	(1000 psi)	TENSILE STRENGTH Oven-Cooled Min. (MPa)	(1000 psi)	ELONGATION Quenched Min. %	Oven-Cooled Min. %	FUSION TEMPERATURE Min. °C	°F
ADA I	862	125	931	135	15	4	955	1750*
ADA II	690	100	862	125	15	2	871	1600*

	PROPORTIONAL LIMIT Range		Range		Range	Range	Range	
P-G-P	552–1034	80–150□	862–1241	125–180□	14–15		1500–1530	2730–2790†
P-S-C	690– 793	100–115△	965–1070	140–155△	16–24	8–15	1050–1080	1910–1970†

□ = Quenched—Alloy does not age harden. △ = Hardened.

*Dentists Desk Reference: Materials, Instruments and Equipment, 1st ed., Metals and Alloys: Precious Metal Wrought Wire. American Dental Association, Chicago, 1981.

†Lyman T, Metals Handbook, 8th ed., Vol. I, Properties and Selection of Metals. American Society for Metals, Metal Park, Ohio, 1964.

Some of the mechanical properties of the alloys shown in Table 32–1 are indicated in Table 32–2.

The relationship between the Brinell hardness number and the proportional limit or tensile strength of gold alloy wires is the same as described for the casting gold alloys. Also, there appears to be a relationship between the proportional limit and the strength of these alloys when they are tested under tension. As a rule, the value for the proportional limit is approximately two-thirds that of the tensile strength.[5]

The modulus of elasticity of wrought gold wires is in the range of 96,500 to 117,200 MPa (14,000,000 to 17,000,000 psi), which is slightly higher than that for the gold casting alloys. It increases approximately 5 per cent following a hardening heat treatment.

Heat Treatment   Both types of gold alloy wires that contain copper are heat treatable in the same manner as described for the casting gold alloys. The considerations for solution heat treatment and age hardening are also the same.

Microstructure   The microstructural appearance of cold-worked or wrought alloys is fibrous with very elongated crystals. It results from the deformation of the grains during the drawing operation to form the wire. Such a structure generally exhibits enhanced mechanical properties as compared with a corresponding cast structure. Specifically, the wrought material possesses increased tensile strength and hardness.

There is a tendency for wrought alloys to recrystallize during heating operations. The extent of recrystallization is related directly to the duration of heating, to the temperature employed, and to the cold work or strain energy imparted to the alloy when the wire was drawn. Recrystallization is inversely related to the fusion temperature of the wire when heating temperature and time are constant. Since there is a concomitant decrease in the mechanical properties of the alloy as recrystallization increases, sufficient platinum and palladium should be present to increase the fusion temperature of the wrought gold alloy wire. Therefore, of those wires listed, the P-G-P are the most resistant to recrystallization.

This is especially important when casting an alloy against the wire. The wire may be held at the mold burnout temperature for an extended period of time, and the temperature of the molten casting alloy is greater than that of a gold solder, especially if the casting alloy is one to which porcelain is to be fused.

References

1. Souder W and Paffenbarger GC: Physical Properties of Dental Materials. National Bureau of Standards Circular C433, Washington, D.C., U.S. Government Printing Office, 1942, pp. 38, 60.
2. Souder W: Nickel in dental alloys. Metals and Alloys 6:194, 1935.
3. DeWald LN: Nickel in precious metal alloys. Metals and Alloys 6:331, 1935.
4. Paffenbarger GC, Sweeney WT, and Isaacs A: Wrought gold wire alloys: Physical properties and a specification. J Am Dent Assoc 19:2061, 1932.
5. Bush SH, Taylor DF, and Peyton FA: Comparison of the mechanical properties, chemical composition, and microstructures of dental gold wires. J Prosthet Dent 1:777, 1951.

33 GOLD ALLOY SOLDERS. SOLDERING PROCEDURES

Soldering is the oldest known metallurgical joining method. It is vital to dentistry for joining parts of an assembly, as in assembling a bridge, and for building up or adding to the bulk of certain structures, such as the establishment of proper contact areas on inlays and crowns with adjacent teeth. Solder used for the latter purpose is sometimes known as a *building solder*. Solder is also used for joining parts of orthodontic appliances, for fastening attachments to fixed and removable partial dentures, and for repairing metal dental appliances.

Definition *Soldering* is the joining of metals by the use of a filler metal which has a substantially lower fusion temperature than that of the metal parts being joined. The process involves the melting and flowing of the filler metal, or solder, via capillary action between and around the parts to be joined. The solder depends upon wetting for the bond formation and neither diffusion nor melting of the metal assembly is required to achieve primary metallic bonding.

Before proceeding, it may be advisable to summarize the events that occur during soldering. First, a flux is applied to the metal surfaces to be united. Upon heating, the molten flux displaces the atmospheric gas layer on the metal surfaces and removes tarnish films. The solder then displaces the molten flux, wets the metal, and forms an interface, thus bonding and establishing a metallic continuity through the joint.

Fluxes The Latin word "flux" means flow. In soldering, fluxes are used to dissolve surface impurities and protect the surface from oxidation while heating. Tarnish films react chemically with the flux by either (1) combining with a component of the flux to form a third compound which is soluble in the flux, or (2) being reduced to a tarnish-free alloy.

Several high melting salts, notably borax, or boric acid, can be used individually as fluxes. However, because each chemical of this type exhibits certain fluxing characteristics of its own, they are usually combined so that a superior flux can be produced with the good characteristics of each of the ingredients. A formula for an efficient soldering flux is:

Borax glass	55 parts
Boric acid	35 parts
Silica	10 parts

The ingredients may be fused together and then ground to a fine powder.

Borax glass, or sodium pyroborate ($Na_2B_4O_7$), is preferable to ordinary borax, or sodium tetraborate ($Na_2B_4O_7 \cdot 10\ H_2O$), for fluxing purposes. Borax effloresces when it is heated on the work as its water of crystallization is driven off, and, as a result, a part of the surface may be exposed and a pit may result.

The boric acid reduces the fusion point of the flux so that it flows smoothly over the work at a low temperature. The silica contributes a viscosity or toughness to the film after fusion so that it stays on the work.

The flux can be employed in a powdered form or as a paste. If it is used as a paste, alcohol should be used as the liquid agent rather than water. A paste formed by mixing fused borax in water results in a hydration of the sodium pyroborate to common borax, and the efflorescence is troublesome.

One method for forming a paste that has been highly successful is to mix the powdered flux with an inert grease or plastic gel such as petrolatum. The grease protects the flux from the air, and when the organic petrolatum is fused on the metal with the flux, it carbonizes and is eliminated into the air or flame.

An *antiflux* is any material that is placed on the work, before the soldering flux is applied, to confine the flow of the molten solder. If the soldering temperature is not too high, the area can be marked off with a lead pencil. The molten solder does not flow across the graphite line, unless a temperature is reached at which the carbon combines with the oxygen and thus is removed from the surface. Another effective means for the production of a barrier is to paint the work with a suspension of iron rouge or whiting in alcohol.

Requisites for a Dental Solder   Dental solders are classified metallurgically as *hard solders* in contrast to the low melting *soft solders* used by plumbers and tinsmiths. The hard solders are generally high fusing, more resistant to tarnish, and stronger than the soft solders.

The following general properties may be listed as being important in a hard dental solder:

1. The first requirement to be met by a dental solder is resistance to tarnish and corrosion in the oral fluids. Not only must it inherently be tarnish resistant but also it must not be susceptible to electrolytic tarnish by anodic action upon the metal to which it is fused.

The exact minimal gold and platinum group metal content necessary in the solder to resist corrosion is unknown. There is little evidence to indicate that solders of extremely high fineness are more resistant to discoloration and corrosion. The enhanced mechanical properties of lower fineness solders (650 to 680) may be more important than any modest improvement in tarnish resistance.

2. The fusion range of the solder must be lower than that of the parts to be soldered so that the parts do not melt, and in order that the solder may be "easy

flowing" over the work when it is fused. This factor is controlled by the composition of the solder. The fusion temperature of the solder is often at least 100° C (180° F) below the fusion temperature of the work, although technicians expert in the art often join parts with solders possessing a fusion temperature 50° C (90° F) or less below that of the work.

3. The composition of the solder should be such that it is "free-flowing," that is, it flows freely after it melts. The term covers certain characteristics of the solder which are related to its fluidity and surface tension as well as its ability to adhere to the work to be soldered. For example, if the solder adheres too readily to the metal to be soldered, it may "soak in" instead of flowing along the surface. A freely flowing solder spreads easily and quickly over clean metal surfaces; it penetrates small openings, and follows points of contact by capillary action.

The fluidity and adhesion of the solder to the metal are extremely important. Without true adhesion there is no actual soldering action, but only an interlocking with surface irregularities. The molten solder adheres when it leaves a continuous permanent film on the surface of the alloy instead of merely rolling over it. The minimal temperature for adhesion does not always correspond exactly with the liquidus of the particular solder.[1] Adhesion is thus a complex property related to the composition of the solder, its melting range, and the thermal conductivity of the metal being soldered.

4. The solder should not cause pitting of the soldered joint. Unfortunately, pitting is one of the most prevalent flaws encountered in soldering procedures, and it is usually the result of improper technique. However, pits may be more prevalent when solder is used that contains a considerable amount of base metal. On overheating, the base metals volatilize and the vapor creates pits.

Pitting is also related to the distance, or gap, between the parts to be soldered.[2-4]

5. The strength of the solder should be at least as great as that of the parts to be soldered. The hardness and strength of the gold alloy solders increase as the gold content or fineness of the solder decreases. Solders above 650 fine should not be used when considerable stress is involved.

6. The color of the solder should match that of the parts to be soldered. However, after a soldered joint has been polished, it usually is not noticeable, even though there may be considerable difference in color between the solder and the work, provided that the proper soldering technique has been employed.

Composition   The basic composition of a gold solder is similar to that of a casting alloy, namely, gold, silver, and copper (Table 33–1). Zinc and tin are added to reduce the fusion temperature of the solders because the addition of

Table 33–1.   *Composition of Dental Gold Solders**

SOLDER No.	GOLD (%)	SILVER (%)	COPPER (%)	ZINC (%)	TIN (%)
A	65.4	15.4	12.4	3.9	3.1
B	66.1	12.4	16.4	3.4	2.0
C	65.0	16.3	13.1	3.9	1.7
D	72.9	12.1	10.0	3.0	2.0
E	80.9	8.1	6.8	2.1	2.0

*From Coleman, R. L., National Bureau of Standards Research Paper No. 32

copper is not sufficient for this purpose. Because of its toxicity and possible release from the solder during electrochemical corrosion, cadmium should not be used.[5]

In addition to the base metals, phosphorus may be added in a small amount as a deoxidizer to improve the resistance of the solder to oxidation while it is fused.

If a "white" colored solder is required, nickel is added to replace the copper. The copper and silver content can be varied, with the gold and base metal content held constant, to modify the color of the solder from a rich gold color contributed by the copper to a light gold color contributed by the silver.

The higher the silver content, the more narrow is the melting range, the greater is the adherence of the solder to the metal, and the more free-flowing is the solder. Conversely, when a considerable amount of copper is added at the expense of the silver, the fusion range is increased to such a degree that only partial melting of the solder may occur and the solder penetrates the part to be soldered instead of flowing. As a result, the composition of both the solder and the part may be changed.

Solders used to join metal-ceramic restorations are significantly different in composition. Generally, the gold casting alloys used in this technique (Chapter 24) contain at least 80 per cent gold and platinum group metals. The balance is silver and base elements such as iron, tin, and indium. The solder composition is normally comparable to the casting gold alloy except additional metals, such as zinc, are added to reduce the melting range by approximately 56° C (133° F). Since the solder is usually used prior to firing the porcelain, the melting range is generally above 1090° C (2000° F).

The gold composition of the solder is properly designated by its fineness, as it has been designated in the previous discussion. Gold manufacturers, however, may designate their solders as "14-karat," "18-karat," etc. Such a designation does not indicate the gold content of the solder, but rather the karat of the gold alloy on which the solder is intended to be used. For example, an 18-karat solder does not contain 18 parts in 24 parts of pure gold; rather it is a solder to be used with a gold alloy of 18 karat. In Table 33–1, solders A, B, and C are 18-karat solders, and the other two solders are 20 karat. With modern dental alloys, which may contain platinum and palladium in addition to the gold, such a designation is meaningless because the melting point and other properties are altered by the additions.

Fusion Temperature   As a general rule, the greater the gold content of the solder, the higher is its fusion temperature. This condition does not necessarily follow, however, by merely increasing the gold content. For example, although the gold content of solders D and E in Table 33–1 is progressively higher than that of the first three solders tested, their fusion temperatures (Table 33–2) are not appreciably different from those of the lower gold-content solders, A, B, and C.

It is desirable that the fusion temperatures of different solders vary progressively from a low temperature to a high temperature. Occasionally, in the construction of complicated dental appliances it is necessary to solder a part of the appliance to another part that has already been soldered. Then, a solder with a lower fusion temperature than the first one used is necessary. A third soldering procedure may be required, and a solder with a still lower fusion temperature must be used, and so on. It is possible to formulate

Table 33–2. *Melting Ranges of Dental Gold Solders**

	MELTING RANGE	
SOLDER No.†	(°C)	(°F)
A	745–785	1375–1445
B	750–805	1385–1480
C	765–800	1410–1470
D	755–835	1390–1535
E	745–870	1375–1595

*Coleman, R. L., National Bureau of Standards Research Paper No. 32.
†Compositions given in Table 33–1.

satisfactory dental solders with graded fusion temperatures if the proper proportions of the constituent metals are employed.[6]

Heat Treatment and Mechanical Properties   The mechanical properties of the solders with the compositions given in Table 33–1 are seen in Table 33–3. The heat treatment designated as "softened" consists of quenching the alloy in water from a temperature of 700° C (1292° F) and, when the alloy is "hardened," it is age hardened by cooling it slowly from 450° C (840° F).

The proportional limit and tensile strength of the solders (Table 33–3) are similar to those of a Type II or Type III cast gold alloy (Table 24–5), but they are generally less in magnitude than the similar properties of a gold alloy wire (Table 32–2). It is axiomatic, therefore, that a soldered joint should not be introduced into a wire appliance at a point of great stress.

The values for the elongation of the solders are definitely lower than those for any of the other types of gold alloy.

The gold solders are generally amenable to age hardening, although solder E in the accompanying tables is an exception. Often, the solders age harden radically, and the values for the elongation may be so low after such a heat treatment that the soldered joint is brittle.

Thus the minimal information required in the selection of a dental gold alloy solder would include:

1. The lower limit of the melting range of the alloy being soldered, or the recrystallization temperature if the alloy is in wrought form.

2. The upper and lower limits of the melting range of the solder.

3. The fineness of the solder.

Table 33–3. *Tensile Properties of Gold Solders**

SOLDER No.†	HEAT TREATMENT	PROPORTIONAL LIMIT (MPa)	(psi)	TENSILE STRENGTH (MPa)	(psi)	ELONGATION (%)
A	Softened	186	27,000	293	42,500	14
	Hardened	379	55,000	434	63,000	1
B	Softened	203	29,500	307	44,500	12
	Hardened	534	77,500	576	83,500	< 1
C	Softened	207	30,000	303	44,000	9
	Hardened	531	77,000	634	92,000	< 1
D	Softened	165	24,000	248	36,000	7
	Hardened	424	61,500	483	70,000	< 1
E‡	Softened	141	20,500	259	37,500	18

*From Coleman, R. L., National Bureau of Standards Research Paper No. 32.
†Compositions given in Table 33–1.
‡Not appreciably affected by age hardening.

The melting range limits provide an indication of the Ag/Cu ratio and whether the solder will flow and wet well or just build up and penetrate the parent alloy. The fineness, as previously stated, influences the corrosion resistance and strength of the alloy.

INVESTMENT SOLDERING

Investment soldering is commonly used in the assembly of bridgework or partial dentures where precise alignment of the parts is essential.

In brief, the technique is as follows: After the parts are thoroughly cleaned the bridge is usually assembled on a master cast. It may be fastened together with sticky wax, and the assembly then carefully lifted from the master cast and imbedded in a soldering type of investment with only the joints exposed. More commonly, a plaster or resin labial or occlusal index is utilized as an aid in transferring the units of the bridge from the master cast or the mouth to the soldering investment. The wax is then eliminated with boiling water. The investment is heated and the parts are brought to the soldering temperature in an oven or with a gas-air flame and the soldering is completed.

Gap Distance   The correct gauging of the distance between the parts to be soldered is important to prevent warpage.

Theoretically, the distance between the parts should be related to three factors: the thermal expansion of the investment during heating, the thermal expansion of the parts, and the shrinkage of the solder during solidification. During heating, the thermal expansion of the investment causes the parts to move farther apart, but the thermal expansion of the metal parts themselves tends to close this gap and partially or totally neutralize the expansion effect of the investment. The shrinkage of the solder during solidification is presumably of the same magnitude as the casting shrinkage of a casting gold alloy.

Unfortunately, these relationships have not been subjected to detailed analyses, as has been done with the inlay casting procedure. If the parts are in contact before heating, the joint strength will be low[3] and the distortion high.[4] In one investigation it was demonstrated that the parts should be separated at least 0.13 mm (0.005 inch) in order to prevent warpage.[4] An excessive gap will increase distortion, but not decrease strength.[3]

Excessive gap width is not well defined, but falls somewhere between 0.25 mm (0.010 inch) and 0.75 mm (0.030 inch). Figure 33–1, which shows a solder joint after being pulled apart, illustrates the porosity resulting from a gap width that is too narrow.

Soldering Investment   The composition of the soldering investment is similar to that of a quartz casting investment. In fact, the stronger casting

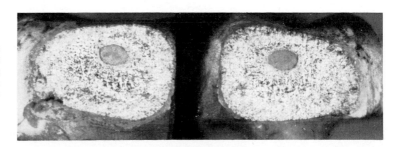

Figure 33–1 Proximal surfaces of two bridge units which were soldered together. The two units were in contact in the area where no solder is present. (Courtesy of G. Ryge.)

investments can sometimes be used as soldering investments. An investment containing quartz is preferable to a cristobalite investment because of the lower thermal expansion of the former.

Furthermore, an investment with a low normal setting expansion is preferred to one with a high setting expansion. The setting expansion tends to change the spacing of the parts and may even cause a warpage. Under no circumstances should the investment come in contact with water during setting because this causes a hygroscopic setting expansion.

A third requisite of a soldering investment is that it withstand the heat of the flame during soldering without cracking.

Microstructure of the Soldered Joint   The union of the solder with the work is the result of adhesion by primary (metallic) bonding. However, overheating or prolonged heating may lead to diffusion of the solder and the formation of new alloys at the solder-work interface.[4, 7] Such a process would contribute to the chemical inhomogeneity of the materials and a reduction in the strength and quality of the joint.

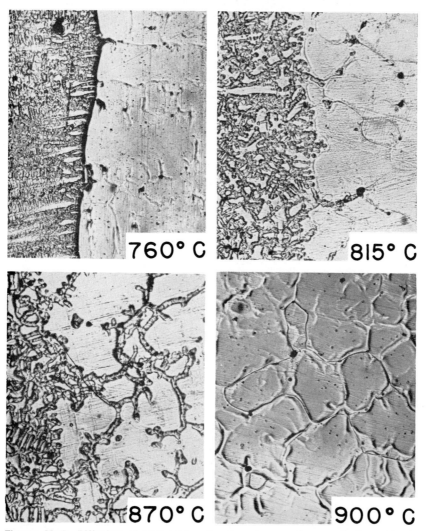

Figure 33–2   Diffusion of gold solder at various temperatures as indicated in the lower right corner of each photomicrograph. (From Ryge, Dent Clin N Amer, Nov., 1958.)

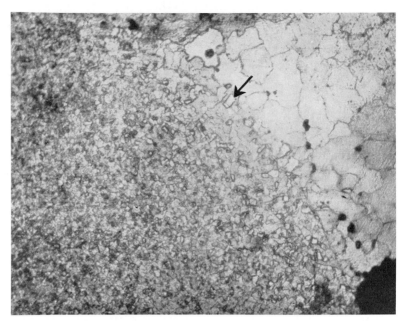

Figure 33–3 Cross section through a wire on which solder has been flowed (solder structure at right). The arrow indicates a grain in the wire which may have been a nucleus of crystallization for the solder. Note the banded wire structure in cross section. × 200. (Courtesy of R. L. Coleman.)

An illustration of the diffusion process is presented in Figure 33–2. The proper fusion temperature of the solder employed for the joints is 760° C (1400° F). The metallographic structure of a correctly soldered joint is depicted by the upper left photomicrograph. The dendritic structure of the solder is evident adjacent to the cast structure, with no visible diffusion between the two. When the solder is overheated to a temperature of 815° C (1500° F), the diffusion of the solder into the grain boundaries of the bridge unit becomes evident, as does a tendency for the diffusion of the cast structure into the solder. As the soldering temperature increases, the atomic diffusion continues until, at 900° C (1650° F), the solder and casting alloy completely fuse with one another.

Examination of electron photomicrographs confirms that no diffusion of the solder into the alloy occurs in the properly heated joint and that there is a well-defined boundary between solder and soldered parts.[8]

The same effect, diffusion of the solder, can occur at lower temperatures, although not as readily, if the heating time is prolonged.[7] Therefore, soldering should be accomplished at the lowest temperature and in the least time possible.

Maximum strength is attained if the appliance is cooled slowly in the investment for 5 to 7 minutes before it is quenched. If it is allowed to cool slowly to room temperature, there is a tendency for excessive brittleness to develop in the joint.

It is possible that the grains in the soldered part may act as nuclei of crystallization for the solder. Thus, the microstructure of the solder will tend to match that of the casting with which it is in contact during solidification. This is advantageous in that a more homogeneous microstructure is created for the joint. Also when fine grain castings are soldered together, the physical properties and corrosion resistance of the joint may be improved as the solder assumes a fine grain structure.[9]

The grain indicated by the arrow in Figure 33–3 is evidence for such a theory.

Strength of Soldered Joints   Probably the factor having the greatest effect on the strength of a soldered joint is the presence of porosity in the solder after solidification. Improper cleaning, fluxing, spacing of the parts, or application of the flame may cause porosity, as does overheating. In addition to the porosity caused by volatilization of base metals, the borax flux may fuse with the metal and prevent the solder from flowing over the surface. Placing the solder in the joint before heating will produce more porosity than if the solder is applied after heating the work.

Corrosion   The general lack of compositional homogeneity between the solder and the parts tends to produce electrolytic couples and promotes discoloration and corrosion. A highly polished surface on the soldered joint improves its resistance to tarnish and corrosion.

Distortion   The distortion occurring during investment soldering of the assembled units is greater than that caused by the indexing or investing procedures.[10] Also, the greater the number of soldered joints united in the final assembly, the greater will be the distortion.[11]

Laser Welding   A method of eliminating distortion during assemblage of the appliance is the use of laser welding to join the cast units. The claimed advantages, in addition to superior fit of the appliance, are that the welding can be made directly on the master stone cast without damage to the cast or adjacent resin or porcelain and the rapidity of the procedure.[12, 13]

The tensile strength of laser-welded cast gold alloy joints has been found to be comparable to that of soldered joints. The ability of the alloy to age harden is not significantly altered by the rapid heating and cooling during the laser welding. However, occasionally, microcracking does appear in the center of the fusion zone.

Further evaluation of the properties of joints made using laser energy and refinement of the instrumentation are needed.

JOINING OF METAL-CERAMIC UNITS

Metal-ceramic alloy units may be joined by soldering either before or after the application of the porcelain veneer.[2, 3] The terms "preceramic" soldering or "presoldering" and "postceramic" soldering or "postsoldering" are used to designate one or the other of these two procedures.

In the presoldering procedure the high fusing gold alloy or the palladium-silver alloy units are invested in a phosphate-bonded investment using only water as the liquid. The appropriate or matching high fusing solder may have a liquidus temperature within 28° C (50° F) to 56° C (100° F) of the solidus temperature of the casting alloy units. Therefore, a single orifice gas-oxygen torch is required for heating the joint and melting the solder. A flux as well as an oven pre-heat may or may not be used, depending upon the user's preference.

For postsoldering, either a phosphate-bonded or a gypsum-bonded soldering investment, preferably carbon free, may be used; the phosphate-bonded investment is more likely to stain the procelain. In any case, neither the investment nor the flux should be allowed to contact the porcelain. A 650 to 615 fine gold solder is suitable for the yellow high gold content alloys, but special matching solders may be preferred when other alloys are being postsoldered.

The joint may be melted and the solder heated with a gas-air torch, applying the flame from the lingual so as not to torch the porcelain. Or the heat may be supplied by an oven. If the porcelain veneer has been vacuum fired, a vacuum atmosphere may be preferred. In either case, the regular soldering flux is used sparingly.

When a base metal alloy is the substrate for the porcelain, presoldering is avoided by unit casting of short span bridges. Longer spans are made by postsoldering together two or more shorter sections.

SOLDERING METAL WROUGHT WIRE

Although most of the principles described for investment soldering apply equally well to orthodontic appliances or to clasps, the use of wrought metal structures complicates the situation because of the danger of weakening the joint by recrystallization and grain growth of the wires during heating.

Microstructure of the Soldered Joint   As in investment soldering, a properly soldered joint should show no evidence of diffusion of the solder into the wires, nor should the characteristic band structure of the latter be altered. A correctly soldered joint is shown in Figure 33–4.

With overheating, not only does a solution of the solder and parts occur but also the wrought structure can recrystallize with an accompanying loss of physical properties. An example of grain growth occurring in a wire is shown in Figure 33–5.

A prolonged heating time can also cause a solution of the wire in the solder, as indicated in Figure 33–6. The reduction in area of the wire decreases

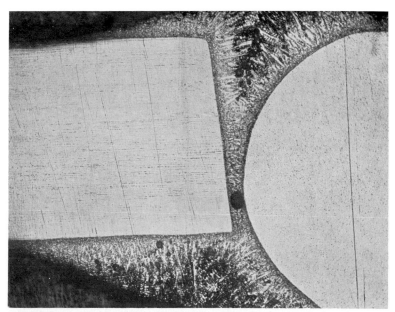

Figure 33–4   Cross section through an orthodontic arch wire and finger spring which had given good service. The solder has not diffused into the wire, nor has the structure of the wire been changed. The two blebs are gas inclusions. (Courtesy of R. L. Coleman.)

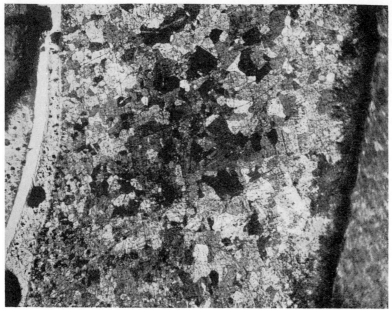

Figure 33-5 Microstructure of a wire which broke in service. The grain growth indicates that the wire was heated to a high temperature for too long during soldering. × 100. (Courtesy of R. L. Coleman.)

the mechanical properties of the joint substantially. Excessive overheating may produce the structure shown in Figure 33-7, in which the solder and gold alloy wire have fused together and a dendritic structure has appeared.

Heat Treatment   Whenever possible, the soldered joint should be quenched immediately to provide a solution heat treatment. The resulting increased ductility of the solder allows the wire to be bent close to the joint and provides additional insurance against fracture in service.

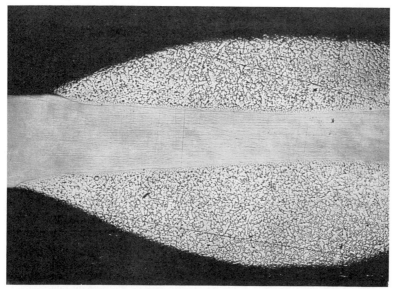

Figure 33-6   Solder was flowed onto a wire and kept molten for 45 seconds before the flame was removed. × 30. (Courtesy of R. L. Coleman.)

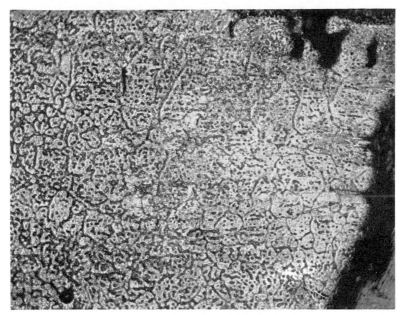

Figure 33–7 Microstructure of a wire which broke in service near the soldered joint. The solder has dissolved in the wire and a dendritic structure has replaced the characteristic banded structure. × 500. (Courtesy of R. L. Coleman.)

Casting to Embedded Alloy Wires A technique employed in the construction of partial dentures involves casting directly to wrought gold wires, eliminating the soldering procedure.

The wrought wire to be incorporated into a casting should be a high fusing alloy, commonly called P-G-P wire because of its composition (wire P-G-P, Table 32–1), with a fusion temperature greater than 1480° C (2700° F). This reduces the possibility of grain growth and, hence, embrittlement during burnout and casting. The technique may be used when casting either gold or American Dental Association Type II base metal alloys.

When base metal alloys are utilized, microprobe studies have indicated that there is a definite diffusion of platinum and gold from the wire, across the interface, and into the cast structure.[15] Likewise, chromium is diffused into the interface, indicating that the union is more than a simple mechanical bond.

References

1. O'Brien WJ, Hirthe WM, and Ryge G: Wetting characteristics of dental gold solders. J Dent Res 42:675, 1963.
2. Rasmussen EJ, Goodkind RJ, and Gerberich WW: An investigation of tensile strength of dental solder joints. J Prosthet Dent 41:418, 1979.
3. Stade EH, Reisbick MH, and Preston JD: Preceramic and postceramic solder joints. J Prosthet Dent 34:527, 1975.
4. Ryge G: Dental soldering procedures. Dent Clin North Am, Nov., 1958, pp. 747–757.
5. Bergman B, Bergman M, and Söremark R: Dissolution and uptake of cadmium from dental gold solder alloy implants. Scand J Dent Res 85:623, 1977.
6. Taylor NO, and Teamer CK: Gold solders for dental use. J Dent Res 28:219, 1949.
7. Bergman M: Combinations of gold alloys in soldered joints. Swed Dent J 1:99, 1977.

8. El-Ebrashi M, Asgar K, and Bigelow W: Electron microscopy of gold soldered joints. J Dent Res 47:5, 1968.

9. Saito T, and Santos JFF: Studies on microstructure of gold soldered joints. J Dent Res 58:1108, 1979.

10. Stackhouse JA: Assembly of dental units by soldering. J Prosthet Dent 18:131, 1967.

11. Fusayama T, Wakumoto S, and Hosada H: Accuracy of fixed partial dentures made by various soldering techniques and one-piece casting. J Prosthet Dent 14:334, 1964.

12. Gordon TE and Smith DL: Laser welding of prosthesis — an initial report. J Prosthet Dent 24:472, 1970.

13. Huling JS and Clark RE: Comparative distortion in three-unit fixed prostheses joined by laser welding, conventional soldering, or casting in one piece. J Dent Res 56:128, 1977.

14. Smith DL, Burnett AP, and Gordon TE: Laser welding of gold alloys. J Dent Res 51:161, 1972.

15. Davidson TJ, Sweeney WT, Love LD, and Fischer TE: Failures of Wrought Wire Clasp and Cast Chromium Cobalt Alloy. IADR Program and Abstracts, No. 226, 1972.

34 BASE METAL ALLOYS FOR DENTAL CASTINGS

The pressures of economics, as well as a search for improved mechanical properties, have led to the development of base metal alloys for the construction of dental prosthetic devices. For reasons of historical development and because of differences that exist in required properties to meet clinical applications, this discussion will be divided into two parts. First will be a description of the base metal alloys developed to cast bases and frameworks for removable appliances (dentures). Then will follow a more recent development, that of base metal alloys for small castings and fixed bridgework.

BASE METAL CASTING ALLOYS FOR REMOVABLE PROSTHETICS

Since their introduction in the 1930's, the chromium-cobalt-nickel base alloys have become the alloys of choice for the fabrication of partial denture frameworks.

The advantages of using these alloys for dental castings are that they are lighter in weight and are likely to possess better mechanical properties, although exceptions to this statement can be found. They are as corrosion resistant as the gold alloys because of the passivating effect of the chromium. They are, of course, less expensive than the gold alloys. For these reasons such alloys have largely replaced the precious metal alloys for partial dentures.

A disadvantage of this type of alloy is the complexity in the production of dental appliances. The high fusing temperature precludes the use of the usual gas-air flame for casting. Its extreme hardness requires the use of special equipment for cleaning and smoothing the work after casting. These and similar procedures not usually adaptable to a laboratory in a dental office have generally limited the fabrication of such castings to the commercial dental laboratory. Consequently, only those factors will be discussed in detail that are of importance to the dentist in evaluating and directing the work of the technician.

Composition The chromium-cobalt-nickel base alloys are covered by American Dental Association Specification no. 14. A minimum of 85 per cent by weight of chromium, cobalt, and nickel is required. Thus, the iron base

Table 34–1. *Composition (w %) of Chromium-Containing Base Metal Alloys*

					ELEMENTS						
ALLOY	Cr	Co	Ni	Fe	Mo	W	Mn	Si	C	Al	Be
A (Co-Cr)	30	62.5	—	1	5	—	0.5	0.5	0.3	—	—
B (Ni-Cr)	17	—	67	—	5	—	5	0.5	Trace	5	1
C (Co-Cr-Ni)	26	54	14	0.1	4	—	0.8	0.6	0.2	—	—
D (Fe-Cr)	24	6	4	63	2.5	—	—	—	Trace	—	—
HS 21	27	62.6	2	1	6	—	0.6	0.6	0.2	—	—
HS 31	23	57.6	10	1	—	7	0.6	0.6	0.4	—	—

A, B, C, and D from Morris, Asgar, Rowe, and Nasjleti: J Prosthet Dent 41:388, 1979; HS 21, HS 31 from *Metals Handbook*, 1948.

corrosion-resistant alloys (the stainless steels to be discussed in Chapter 37 as well as the iron-chromium casting alloys) are excluded.

The early versions of this type of alloy system were composed largely of chromium and cobalt. In some products nickel was used as a replacement for a certain amount of cobalt. These alloys became known as Haynes stellites, after Elwood Haynes who patented such an alloy for industrial uses in automobile manufacturing. They are often referred to as *stellite* alloys. Materials and techniques for casting appliances in one of the Haynes stellites were developed in 1929. The now commonly known name of Vitallium has been given to that alloy. A number of such products are now available.

The compositions of five chromium-cobalt-nickel alloys and one iron base alloy are shown in Table 34–1. Alloys A, B, C, and D are partial denture alloys while HS 21 and HS 31 are industrial alloys. The similarity between HS 21 and the Co-Cr alloy A is quite apparent. Alloy A is the nickel-free Vitallium which, as previously mentioned, has been used in dentistry for 50 years for the casting of partial dentures. This type of alloy has also been used extensively in dentistry and medicine as an implant material.

Effect of Alloy Constituents   In the cobalt-chromium system, cobalt is the basic element in what can be considered as essentially a solid solution of 70 per cent cobalt and 30 per cent chromium.[1] Chromium, by its passivating effect, insures corrosion resistance of the alloy. Along with other elements it also acts in solid solution hardening. Thirty per cent chromium is considered the upper limit for attaining maximum mechanical properties.

Cobalt and nickel are somewhat interchangeable. As nickel replaces cobalt, strength, hardness, modulus of elasticity, and fusion temperature tend to decrease while the ductility may increase.

However, the effect of the other elements on the physical properties of the alloy is more significant than the relative chromium-cobalt-nickel concentration. For example, molybdenum and tungsten are very effective solid solution hardeners. Molybdenum is preferred because it reduces ductility to a lesser extent.

Iron, copper, beryllium, and other elements in small quantities doubtlessly also aid in solid solution hardening. Although manganese and silicon are hardeners, they are present primarily as oxide scavengers to prevent oxidation of other elements during melting. Generally the deoxidizers tend to cause increased brittleness in a cobalt base alloy.

Boron also acts as a deoxidizer and hardener but reduces ductility and markedly increases the hardness of the nickel-chromium alloy. It widens the melting range, primarily by reducing the solidus temperature.

As nickel replaces chromium, the deoxidizer content (manganese, silicon and boron) can go up. Silicon, up to 3.5 per cent, can increase ductility of a nickel-chromium alloy.

Although beryllium is a hardener and grain structure refiner, it is generally added in order to reduce the fusion temperature. In addition to furnishing some solid solution strengthening, aluminum forms a nickel-aluminum compound (Ni_3Al) to effect precipitation hardening in the alloys that are principally nickel based.

Of all the constituents, the carbon content is the most critical. Small variations have a pronounced effect on the strength, hardness, and ductility of the alloy. Carbon can form carbides with any of the metallic constituents. Carbide precipitation is a very important factor in strengthening these alloys, but in excess it can produce severe brittleness. Thus, as will be seen, control of the carbon content in the alloy during casting is important.

Control of the carbon content is difficult during both the manufacture and casting procedures. Either a carburizing oxyacetylene flame or a carbon arc will add carbon during melting of the alloy. Thus, modest differences in the relative concentration of these various elements can play a major role in altering certain physical properties, as will be discussed later.

Microstructure Compared with a gold casting alloy, the grains are large. The grain boundaries may be obscured by a prominent dendritic structure, with intergranular and interdendritic carbides clearly visible.

In a cobalt-chromium alloy the boundary *carbide* formation may be either *continuous* or *discontinuous,* with the discontinuous formation being either *nodular* or *lamellar.* The extent and nature of the carbide formation will depend upon the composition and thermal treatment during and after casting. In general, the higher the fusion temperature and the faster the cooling, the more likely is the formation of a discontinuous carbide formation.[2]

Unfortunately, a high melt temperature promotes the reaction between the alloy and the mold and thus a deterioration of the surface texture of the casting.[3]

The carbides provide slip interference and thus increase the strength properties and decrease the ductility of the alloy, especially when the carbide precipitation is continuous.

The microstructure of a nickel-chromium alloy is likely to be more complex than that of the cobalt-chromium alloy because of the presence of aluminum (or titanium) and the formation of the Ni_3Al precipitate within the matrix.

As in the Co-Cr alloys, the carbides with the Ni-Cr system are primarily interdendritic and intergranular. In addition, an appropriate etch will disclose an almost continuous band of isolated particles of Ni_3Al on either side of the interdendritic boundaries.[4]

Physical Properties The tensile strength of both the cobalt-chromium and the nickel-chromium alloys may exceed 700 MPa (100,000 psi). The elastic modulus of the cobalt-chromium alloys is approximately 225×10^3 MPa (33×10^6 psi), that of the nickel-chromium alloys approximates 185×10^3 MPa (27×10^6 psi). The percentage elongation may vary from less than 1 per cent to as high as 12 per cent, depending upon the composition, the rate of cooling, and, even more important, the fusion and mold temperatures employed. The

Table 34–2. *Mechanical Properties of Partial Denture Alloys*

Alloy	Yield Strength MPa (psi × 10^3)	Tensile Strength MPa (psi × 10^3)	Elongation %	Hardness VHN	Modulus of Elasticity MPa × 10^3 (psi × 10^6)
A (Co-Cr)*	710 (103)	870 (126)	1.6	432	223.5 (32.4)
B (Ni-Cr)*	690 (100)	800 (116)	3.8	300	182 (26.4)
C (Co-Cr-Ni)*	470 (68)	685 (99)	8	264	198 (28.7)
D (Fe-Cr)*	703 (102)	841 (122)	9	309	202 (29.3)
Type IV Gold Alloy†	493 (71.5)	776 (112.5)	7	264	90 (13)

*Bench cooled in the investment after casting.
†Age hardened.
A, B, C, and D from Morris, Asgar, Rowe, and Nasjleti: J Prosthet Dent 41:388, 1979.

physical properties of some of these alloys can be seen in Table 34–2. For comparison, the properties of a Type IV gold alloy are included.

The relatively low ductility of these alloys is considered to be a major deficiency when they are used for partial denture castings. Certain handling procedures can increase ductility but will also produce undesirable effects. For example, increasing the melting temperature of a cobalt base alloy will increase ductility,[2] but it will also result in a rougher surface on the casting.[3]

Although a 15 minute heat treatment at 870 to 1200° C (1600 to 2200° F) can markedly increase the ductility of a nickel base alloy, yield and ultimate tensile strength will be reduced by as much as 50 per cent. The properties of a cobalt base alloy are much less susceptible to the same heat treatment. In general, the most desirable combination of mechanical properties is present in the "as cast" alloys, bench cooled in the investment, rather than in the alloys following heat treatment for 15 minutes at temperatures between 700° C (1300° F) and 1200° C (2200° F).[5] At the highest temperatures, a non-oxidizing atmosphere is highly desirable in order to prevent oxidation of the alloy components.

The fusion temperature of the Cr-Co-Ni alloys is considerably higher than that of the Type IV casting gold alloys (minimum of 870° C [1600° F]). American Dental Association Specification no. 14 divides the alloys into two types on the basis of fusion temperature, which is defined as the liquidus temperature. Type I (high fusing) alloys have a liquidus temperature greater than 1300° C (2372° F); the maximum fusion temperature for Type II alloys (low fusing) is 1300° C. An early version of alloy B in Table 34–2 had a fusion temperature between 1275 and 1290° C (2327 and 2354° F). The cobalt containing alloys in Table 34–1 have fusion temperatures in the 1400–1500° C (2552–2732° F) range, as have almost all other cobalt base metal partial denture alloys.

These alloys cannot be melted with a gas-air torch. A mixture of oxygen and acetylene gases is usually employed as a fuel although other types of fuel can be used as well. Electrical sources of melting are often used to advantage, such as carbon arcs, argon arcs, high-frequency induction, or silicon-carbide resistance furnaces. In some instances, sophisticated electronic equipment is used to control the temperature, casting time, and similar variables in order to regulate the grain formation and carbide precipitation.

The carburizing section of the oxygen-acetylene flame can add carbon to the alloy.[6] The extra carbon changes not only the microstructure but also the mechanical properties.[7] In general, hardness and yield strength increase, whereas ductility decreases. Therefore, when melting the alloy with an oxygen-acetylene torch, the proportion of the two gases, the length of the flame, and the distance of the torch tip from the alloy should be standardized.

The density of the cobalt-chromium alloys is between 8 and 9 gm/cm^3, a value which is less than half that of the gold alloys.

These alloys are harder than most gold alloys even though the latter are age hardened. Most are very difficult to cut, grind, or finish. As far as dental finishing processes are concerned, special hard, high-speed finishing tools are generally necessary for cutting, smoothing, or trimming such alloys. However, some of the newer, more ductile and softer alloys are easier to cut and polish.

All dental stellites work harden very easily. Consequently, regardless of the percentage elongation in the "as cast" condition, as indicated for the less ductile alloys shown in Table 34–2, the adjustment of clasp arms is difficult, within a certain factor of safety. Even though the clasp arm may not be fractured during the actual adjustment, it may later fail in service because of the strain hardening received. Even a slight increase in the original ductility of the alloy may prevent such a failure. Inasmuch as the strength of these alloys is so great, a moderate sacrifice of this property can be tolerated in order to enhance the ductility. In general, the percentage elongation of the dental stellites is comparable to that of a Type IV gold alloy after age hardening. The minimum value for the percentage elongation is 1.5 per cent in American Dental Association Specification no. 14.

The modulus of elasticity of these alloys is greater than that of the gold alloys. The modulus of the nickel-chromium base alloys is somewhat lower than that of the cobalt-chromium base alloys, although it may vary considerably according to the exact composition.[8] In either case it is approximately twice that of the Type IV casting gold alloys.

Consequently, it can be expected that the stellite dental appliances may be stiffer than those made with gold alloys. Actually, however, advantage can be taken of this to decrease the thickness of the stellite appliance and thus decrease its weight. Also less undercut is used for the retentive arm of the clasp than when gold alloys are used.

Such a change in design should be done conservatively, however, because the proportional limit (and the strength) of the stellite may be less than that of a comparable age hardened gold-base alloy. As a result, the modulus of resilience of the structure may be reduced to the extent that its resistance to impact may be lowered in comparison with that of a gold alloy.

According to the current American Dental Association Specification no. 14, the tensile strength of a dental stellite should be greater than 620 MPa (90,000 psi).

Casting Shrinkage   As with cast gold alloys, a casting shrinkage occurs for the same reasons during solidification. As might be expected, because of their high fusion temperatures, the casting shrinkage of the dental stellites is greater than that of the gold casting alloys. Values of 2.3 per cent for the cobalt-chromium base alloys and approximately 2.0 per cent for the nickel-chromium base alloys are representative.[9]

Investment   The properties of the investment employed for casting these alloys are similar to those for casting gold alloys, except that the binder in the former must be able to withstand the much higher temperature of the molten stellite alloy.

The refractory in the investment is either quartz or cristobalite, and the expansion at the inversion temperatures of the two forms of silica is expected to provide part of the mold compensation as in the gypsum investments for gold castings. The chief differences in composition between the types of investment are in the binder employed.

Gypsum-Bonded Investments   As with other dental investments, α-hemihydrate can be used as a binder if the fusion temperature of the alloy is sufficiently low. The primary objection to the use of a gypsum binder is the danger of embrittlement of the casting from the sulfur dioxide evolved by the breakdown of the gypsum in contact with the molten stellite. When a gypsum binder is used with the lower fusing stellites, this objection can be minimized by the incorporation of an oxalate in the investment.[10] During heating, the oxalate decomposes to form carbon dioxide in the mold, which protects the molten metal from the sulfur dioxide.

The manufacturer of alloy B, Table 34-1, recommends the use of such a gypsum-bonded investment. This is quite satisfactory when the temperature of the melt and the mold is carefully controlled. A melt temperature 150° C in excess of that recommended will result in investment decomposition, especially around the thicker areas of the casting. Sulfur contamination and surface roughness of the alloy result.[11]

Phosphate-Bonded Investments   These investments are described in Chapter 26. When a base metal partial denture alloy is to be cast, a carbon-free investment is generally selected. The mix that is used for making the refractory cast is made with the special liquid to provide maximum expansion. The total linear expansion can exceed 2 per cent.

The waxed refractory cast is commonly invested in a mix made with water, in part to provide an increase in mold permeability. Burnout is not done for at least two hours after investing. Slow burnout is desirable to insure against cracking of the mold. The burnout temperature is generally higher than that used with a gypsum-bonded investment. A commonly recommended temperature range is 732 to 982° C (1350 to 1800° F). Burnout time will depend upon temperature, oven size, and number and size of molds in the oven. A heat soak is generally not less than one hour at maximum temperature.

Silica-Bonded Investments   In this case the binder is a silica gel which reverts to silica (cristobalite) on heating. Several methods may be used to produce the silica or silicic acid gel binders.[12] When the pH of sodium silicate is lowered by the addition of an acid or an acid salt such as mono-ammonium phosphate, a bonding silicic acid gel forms. The addition of magnesium oxide will strengthen the gel.[13] Or an aqueous suspension of colloidal silica can be made to gel by the addition of an accelerator, such as ammonium chloride.

Another system for binder formation begins with ethyl silicate. A colloidal silicic acid is first formed by hydrolyzing ethyl silicate in the presence of hydrochloric acid, ethyl alcohol, and water. In its simplest form, the reaction can be expressed as:

$$Si(OC_2H_5)_4 + 4H_2O \rightarrow Si(OH)_4 + 4C_2H_5OH$$

Because a polymerized form of ethyl silicate is actually used, a colloidal sol of polysilicic acids is to be expected instead of the simpler silicic acid sol shown in the reaction.

The sol is then mixed with the quartz or cristobalite to which is added a small amount of finely powdered magnesium oxide to render the mixture alkaline. A coherent gel of polysilicic acid then forms accompanied by a *setting shrinkage*. This soft gel is dried at a temperature below 168° C (334° F). During the drying, the gel loses alcohol and water to form a concentrated, hard gel. As might be expected, a volumetric contraction accompanies the drying, which reduces the size of the mold. This contraction is known as "green shrinkage" and it occurs in addition to the setting shrinkage.

This gelation process is apt to be slow and time-consuming. An alternative and faster method for the production of the silica gel can be employed. Certain types of amines can be added to the solution of ethyl silicate so that hydrolysis and gelation occur simultaneously.

It follows that with an investment of this type the mold enlargement before casting must compensate not only for the casting shrinkage of the metal, but also for the "green shrinkage" and the setting shrinkage of the investment.

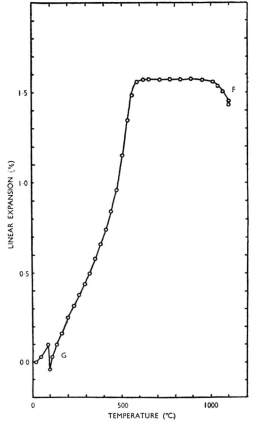

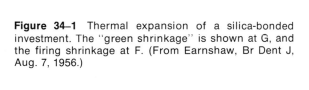

Figure 34–1 Thermal expansion of a silica-bonded investment. The "green shrinkage" is shown at G, and the firing shrinkage at F. (From Earnshaw, Br Dent J, Aug. 7, 1956.)

As can be noted from Figure 34–1, the thermal expansion of such an investment is likely to be considerable because both the binder and the refractory are forms of silica which can invert during heating. The "green shrinkage" is shown at G and a third shrinkage is shown at F. This shrinkage occurs at the temperature at which the polysilicic acid gel is changed to silica (above 675° C). Generally there is not a great deal to be gained by heating the mold much above 700 to 800° C (1292 to 1472° F), at which temperature sufficient mold compensation can be obtained for most dental appliances. As with other investments, the thermal expansion can be controlled by the amount, particle size, and type of silica filler employed.

Silica-bonded investments, being more refractory than phosphate-bonded investments, can tolerate a higher burnout or mold-casting temperature. Temperatures between 1090 and 1180° C (2000 and 2150° F) are commonly recommended when the higher fusing chromium-containing alloys are being cast.[14]

Laboratory Procedures   Although the general procedure for waxing, spruing, investing, and casting is the same as for a gold alloy, modifications are required because of differences in certain physical properties of gold and the base metal alloys. The consequences of varying the elastic modulus of the alloy, for example, have been noted earlier. Many of the other procedural differences, such as the investment used, burnout temperature, alloy casting temperature, and heat source for melting the alloy, have also been mentioned.

After divesting and cleaning, the casting is commonly electrolytically polished in an acid bath prior to a final mechanical polishing. Two finished cast partial denture appliances are shown in Figure 34–2.

Porosity   As in small gold castings, porosities can result from solidification shrinkage and evolution of dissolved gases during solidification of the alloy. However, shrinkage and gas inclusion porosity are not distinctly separate in

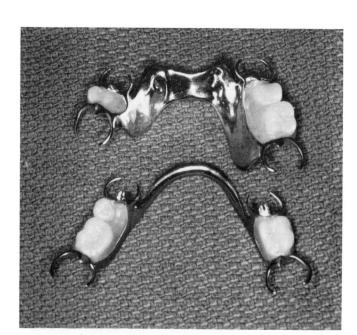

Figure 34–2 Finished partial denture appliances cast with chromium base alloy. (Courtesy of D. M. Cunningham.)

location, since both occur in those parts of the casting that are the last to solidify. Thus, in general, the porosities will most frequently be interdendritic.

In one metallographic evaluation, three types of porosities were described.[15] Two well defined voids, associated with external imperfections or cracks, were found. A second type of porous area, much more widely dispersed, was seen where there was an abrupt change in cross-sectional area of the casting. These defects appeared as relatively large central voids surrounded by an aggregation of small and apparently isolated individual cavities.

A third type of porosity was even more diffuse, being rather uniformly dispersed throughout the partial denture casting and consisting of areas of small and isolated interdendritic cavities.

Porosity is affected by the composition of the alloy and its manipulation.[16] Manipulative variables would include design of the appliance, spruing, composition of the investment, mold and alloy temperature, and technique of melting the alloy.[17-18]

Corrosion   All of the alloys listed in Table 34–1 are adequately corrosion resistant in oral fluids, the chromium content being a crucial factor.

Solutions of hypochlorite and other chlorine-containing compounds that are present in some denture cleaning agents will cause corrosion of such base metal alloys. Even the oxygenating denture cleansers will stain such alloys. Therefore, these solutions should not be used for cleaning chromium base alloy appliances.

BASE METAL ALLOYS FOR SMALL CASTINGS

The success of base metal alloys for removable prosthetic devices led to some early interest in applying these same alloys to the fabrication of small castings. However, intensive research in the characterization of such alloys for this purpose did not begin until the 1970's. At that time the rapidly escalating price of noble metals stimulated a search for the development of alternate alloy systems, as was described in Chapter 24. The established record of the chromium-cobalt-nickel alloys made them the first choice for evaluation as likely alternatives to gold based alloys.

Although the subject of fixed prostheses encompasses both all metal and metal-ceramic alloy applications, the demands of the metal-ceramic system are more restrictive, and virtually all of the commercial interest to date has been focused in that direction. Therefore, this discussion will be restricted to base metal systems designed for metal-ceramic application even though much of the discussion is also germane to the all metal restoration.

Owing to the requirements of metal-ceramic compatibility, the majority of these base metal-ceramic alloys are composed primarily of nickel and chromium, as shown in Table 34–3. The nickel content may range from 70 to 80 per cent, while the chromium may vary between 13 and 20 per cent. The similarity of these alloys to those used for partial prostheses (Table 34–1) is evident. The chromium is essential to provide passivation and corrosion resistance.

Other alloy formulations include chromium-cobalt and iron-chromium.

As is the case with base metal partial denture alloys, these alloys melt at elevated temperatures. In general, the use of phosphate or silica-bonded investments is indicated. The silica-bonded investments have just been dis-

Table 34–3. *Composition of Base Metal Alloys for Small Castings*

ELEMENT	A	B	C	D	E	F
Nickel	80.75	79.67	78.51	68.96	80.86	68.75
Chromium	12.58	13.24	19.47	16.54	11.93	19.57
Iron	0.34	0.11	0.43	0.37	0.20	0.38
Aluminum	3.42	3.87	0.21	4.15	2.95	—
Molybdenum	1.53	1.52	—	5.10	1.87	4.22
Silicon	0.29	0.30	1.10	0.83	0.18	2.72
Beryllium	0.57	0.65	—	—	1.55	—
Copper	0.15	—	—	—	0.13	1.54
Manganese	0.13	0.12	—	3.05	0.14	1.24
Cobalt	—	—	—	0.42	—	—
Tin	—	—	—	—	—	1.25

Adapted from Physical and Mechanical Properties of Gold and Base Metal Alloys, J. P. Moffa, Alternatives to Gold Alloys in Dentistry, DHEW Publication No. (NIH) 77-1227.

cussed and the phosphate-bonded materials were covered in Chapter 26. In addition, the use of high temperature heat sources are required for casting. More important is the compensation for casting shrinkage required at these elevated temperatures if a clinically acceptable fit is to be obtained.

Mechanical Properties   The clinical success of a metal-ceramic restoration is dependent in large measure on the ability of the underlying alloy substructure to resist the potentially destructive masticatory stresses. Although the esthetic fused porcelain veneer has relatively high resistance to compressive stresses, its low tensile strength and characteristic lack of ductility make this brittle material extremely susceptible to the destructive types of stresses that accompany flexure of the metal substructure. Therefore, it is imperative that the metal-ceramic restorations be formulated and designed in such a way as to maximize the rigidity of the prosthesis.

One obvious approach would be to increase the thickness of the metal substructure, since by doubling its thickness, the structure can be eight times more rigid. However, a metal-ceramic restoration is a finite structure wherein increasing the thickness of the alloy framework is limited by the minimal thickness of overlying porcelain required to achieve acceptable esthetics, occlusion, and correct physiological contour of the fixed restoration.

An examination of the mechanical properties of base metal alloys and a gold alloy (Table 34–4) shows that in general the base metal alloys have a modulus of elasticity approximately twice that of previously used gold alloys. Since elastic modulus is a measure of the stiffness or rigidity of materials, this property would enhance the application of base metal alloys for long span bridges where flexure is a major cause of failure. Given an equal thickness of precious metal alloy and base metal alloy, the base metal alloy bridge would flex only half as much as the precious alloy material under the same occlusal forces. In a similar manner, the higher modulus of elasticity may be utilized to permit the grinding of thinner castings where insufficient tooth structure has been removed to allow adequate esthetics, proper physiological contour, and occlusion.

The Vickers hardness of base metal alloys may range from approximately 175 to 360 DPH. Although certain of the base metal alloys may approach the hardness of noble metal alloy (approximately 160 DPH), the majority of these alloys are considerably harder. Because of this relatively high hardness, cutting of sprues and grinding and polishing of the prosthesis require the use

Table 34–4. *Physical and Mechanical Properties of Base Metal Alloys and a Gold Alloy*

Properties	A	B	C	D	E	F	Gold Alloy
Tensile Strength — MPa	1,142	1,139	1,355	661	540	703	490
— (psi)	(165,600)	(165,200)	(196,500)	(95,900)	(78,300)	(101,900)	(71,000)
Yield Strength — MPa	591	782	838	360	260	543	400
— (psi)	(85,700)	(113,400)	(121,500)	(52,200)	(37,700)	(78,700)	(58,000)
Modulus of Elasticity							
MPa ($\times 10^3$)	207	190	210	193	154	208	88
psi ($\times 10^6$)	30.0	27.6	30.4	28.0	22.3	30.2	12.8
Percent Elongation (%)	23.9	11.6	18.0	27.9	27.3	2.3	9.1
Vicker's Hardness (DPH)	293	348	357	211	175	316	161
Density (gm/cm^3)	8.1	8.0	7.9	8.0	8.7	8.3	18.3
Porcelain Bond — MPa	97.9	51.0	87.6	70.3	80.7	106.2	111.0
— (psi)	(14,200)	(7,400)	(12,700)	(10,200)	(11,700)	(15,400)	(16,100)

Adapted from Physical and Mechanical Properties of Gold and Base Metal Alloys, J. P. Moffa, Alternatives to Gold Alloys in Dentistry, DHEW Publication No. (NIH) 77-1227.

of high speed equipment. Clinically, it is unlikely that significant occlusal wear of the alloy will occur. Therefore, particular attention must be directed toward perfecting occlusal equilibration. The removal of defective clinical units is also more difficult than with noble metal alloys, since the high hardness results in rapid wear of carbide burs and diamond points.

There is considerable variation in the yield strength of the base metal alloys. Thus it is difficult to make generalized statements comparing the yield strengths of base metal and noble metal alloys. Although certain base metal alloy formulations have strengths that are more than twice that of comparable gold based alloys, there are others that are similar to or considerably less than the gold alloys. It is conceivable that materials with a very low yield strength would have limited application for high stress bearing areas. Similarly, alloys with high yield strengths would be desirable in these clinical circumstances; but this high resistance to deformation may limit the ability to burnish the alloy.

The ductility, as measured by the per cent elongation, of base metal alloys ranges between approximately 10 and 28 per cent. Since noble metal alloys have an elongation of approximately only 5 to 10 per cent, one might assume that base metal alloys might lend themselves to burnishing. However, it must be remembered that in order to burnish an alloy, sufficient stress must be exerted to permanently deform the alloy, i.e., exceed the yield strength. Since many of the base metal alloys have high yield strengths, achieving the full potential of the higher ductility might be unrealistic.

The density of base metal alloys is approximately 8.0 gm/cm^3, as compared with 18.39 gm/cm^3 for comparable noble metal alloys (Table 34–4). Since casting alloys are purchased on a weight basis, a lower density is indirectly reflected to the purchaser, who receives more than twice the volume of material for each unit weight acquired. Also, by composition the intrinsic value of the component elements in base metal alloys is significantly less than that of comparable noble metal alloys. Thus, on the basis of their lower density and the low intrinsic value of the component metals, the cost differential between base metal and noble metal alloys can be substantial.

In addition to the obvious economic considerations, the lower density of base metal alloys may also be a factor in producing adequate dental castings. Since most dental castings are fabricated by centrifugal casting machines, the lower density may play a role in the difficulty reported by some investigators in attaining precision castings with certain of these alloys.[19]

It will be remembered (Chapter 31) that when porcelain is first fired to the metal substructure, the alloy is subjected to considerable temperature variations and stresses induced by the shrinkage of the overlying porcelain. It is desirable that the underlying metal framework resist any deformation induced by these thermal stresses. Sag resistance is the property that has been used to describe the ability of an alloy to resist the permanent deformation or creep induced by thermal stresses. It is particularly important in long span bridges, where under the influence of its own weight, the porcelain firing temperature may cause the unsupported structure to permanently deform. Under controlled conditions, it has been found that a base metal alloy will deform less than 0.001 inch, while a noble metal alloy will deform 0.009 inch.[20] It is conceivable that the higher fusion temperature common to base metal alloys is a factor that contributes to the superior sag resistance properties of these alloys.

The question of metal-ceramic compatibility is basic to the selection of an alloy system for this type of restoration. Two requirements are implicit. The metal must not interact with the ceramic in such a way as to visibly discolor the porcelain at the interface or marginal regions. Moreover, the metal-ceramic system must form a stable bond at the interface which can withstand normal stresses in the mouth.

Evaluation of the metal-ceramic bond is complicated by the lack of an accepted laboratory test with proven clinical significance, as was discussed in Chapter 31. Different bond strength tests have resulted in widely varying results in regard to the strength of base metal-ceramic bonds. Some tests indicate that the strength of such bonds equals or exceeds that of the high noble metal alloys while other tests indicate the reverse.

However, these tests do make clear that different base metal alloys vary widely in their abilities to bond to porcelain. These differences are related to the minor constituents of the alloy. It is also clear that certain base metal-ceramic combinations are incompatible. The American Dental Association acceptance program for metal-ceramic alloys suggests certain screening tests for such compatibility. It is also apparent that the base metal alloys are much more technique sensitive than their high noble metal alloy counterparts. Fortunately, from a practical point of view, these considerations are primarily a concern for the dental laboratory and the technicians who fabricate prosthetic devices from these alloys.

Bonding Using Electrodeposition   Electrodeposition of gold has been used to provide an intermediate layer between the cast metal and the porcelain. Deposition of a layer of pure gold onto a base metal casting, followed by a short "flashing" deposition of tin, has been shown to improve the wetting of porcelain onto the metal and reduce the amount of porosity at the porcelain-metal interface.[21] The electrodeposited layer acts as a barrier to strong oxide-forming elements, such as chromium, provided that the number of firings is kept to a minimum.[22]

The gold color of the resulting oxide film is said to enhance the vitality of the porcelain, when compared with the otherwise dark oxides which require a heavy opaque layer. Also, it is suggested that the deposited layer of metal acts as a buffer zone, absorbing the stresses caused by differences in thermal coefficient of expansion between the metal casting and the porcelain as it cools from firing temperature to ambient temperature.[23] Further research is in progress to optimize the concept.

Various proprietary agents are also available that are intended for application to the metal surface prior to condensation of the opaque porcelain layer. These are applied as a thin liquid to the metal surface and fired in a manner similar to that of the opaque porcelain.

The function of these agents is twofold. They are supposed to improve metal-ceramic bonding by limiting the build-up of oxide on the base metal surface during firing. They also are claimed to improve esthetics by helping to block the color of the dark metal oxide.

Clinical Performance   On the basis of recent surveys, the use of base metal alloys by dental laboratories is rapidly increasing, at the expense of the traditional high noble metal-ceramic alloys. Laboratory personnel indicate a very high degree of satisfaction with the handling properties of base metal-ceramic alloys such as casting, finishing, and porcelain bonding. Unfortunately, at the present time long term data are not available concerning the clinical performance of restorations fabricated from these alloys. One 5-year study did indicate that performance is governed by differences in the properties of the alloys used, the length of the span, and the laboratory manipulative characteristics.[24]

Biological Considerations   Certain base-metal alloys contain beryllium (Table 34–3). This element is added to the alloy to reduce the fusion temperature, improve the casting characteristics, refine the grain structure, and possibly participate in the bonding of porcelain. It is widely recognized that beryllium is potentially toxic under uncontrolled conditions. Inhalation of the dusts and fumes of beryllium and its compounds is the main route of exposure. The diagnosis of chronic beryllium disease is difficult and requires the establishment of beryllium exposure.

To date, there have been no documented cases of beryllium toxicity of dental origin. However, it has been shown that under certain working conditions, notably the absence of adequate local exhaust ventilation, beryllium in base metal alloys can present a dental occupational health problem.[25] Therefore, in laboratory and clinical situations where grinding of beryllium-containing alloys is performed, adequate local exhaust ventilation safeguards should be employed.

In certain non-dental industrial applications and environmental conditions, nickel and its compounds have been implicated as a potential carcinogen and as a sensitizing agent. Since the nickel content of base metal alloys (Table 34–3) can exceed 80 per cent, precautions should be employed during the usage of these alloys.

There is no experimental evidence that nickel compounds are carcinogenic when administered by oral or cutaneous routes.[26] However, there is strong epidemiological evidence to indicate that occupational exposure of workers to certain nickel compounds is associated with increased incidence of specific types of cancer. Numerous studies have shown that nickel refinery workers have had an increased mortality rate from lung and nasal cancer.[27, 28] Based on this conclusion, the prudent course of action requires that precautions be taken to prevent the aspiration of nickel-containing dust produced during dental grinding operations.

In addition to its carcinogenic potential, nickel is also recognized as a potent sensitizing agent. It is maintained that nickel produces more instances of contact dermatitis than all other metals combined.[29] One study found that 9 per cent of women and 0.9 per cent of men are allergic to nickel.[30] Furthermore, it has been documented that the nickel in base metal alloys is available as an allergen and could be considered a potential sensitizer.[31]

On the basis of the available evidence, the potential risks that might be anticipated with intraoral exposure to nickel-containing alloys contraindicate their use in nickel sensitive patients.

References

1. Paffenbarger GC, Caul HJ, and Dickson G: Base metal alloys for oral restorations. J Am Dent Assoc 30:852, 1943.
2. Asgar K and Peyton FA: Effect of microstructure on the physical properties of cobalt-base alloys. J Dent Res 40:63, 1961.
3. Carter TJ and Kidd JN: The precision casting of cobalt-chromium alloy. Br Dent J 118:383 and 431, 1965.
4. Lewis AJ: Metallographic changes and phase identification in a nickel base alloy upon fusion and casting. Aust Dent J 20:378, 1975.
5. Morris HF, Asgar K, Rowe AP, and Nasjleti CE: The influence of heat treatments on several types of base-metal removable partial denture alloys. J Prosthet Dent 41:388, 1979.
6. Strandman E: Influence of different types of acetylene-oxygen flames on the carbon content of a dental Co-Cr alloy. Odont Revy 27:223, 1976.
7. Strandman E: The influence of carbon content on the mechanical properties in a cast dental Co-Cr alloy. Odont Revy 27:273, 1976.
8. Harcourt HJ, Riddibough M, and Osborne J: The properties of nickel-chromium casting alloys containing boron and silicon. Br Dent J 129:419, 1970.
9. Earnshaw RG: The casting shrinkage of cobalt-chromium alloys. Aust Dent J 3:159, 1958.
10. Earnshaw RG: The Casting Shrinkage of Some Dental Cobalt-Chromium Alloys and Its Compensation by Investment Expansion. A thesis presented to the Victoria University of Manchester (England) for the degree of Doctor of Philosophy (1957).
11. Lewis AJ: Mould-reaction with gypsum bonded refractory investments. Aust Dent J 21:172, 1976.
12. Earnshaw R: Investments for casting cobalt-chromium alloys. Br Dent J 108:389 and 429, 1960.
13. Dootz ER, Craig RC, and Peyton FA: Simplification of the chrome-cobalt partial denture casting procedure. J Prosthet Dent 17:464, 1967.
14. Mabie CP: Petrographic study of the refractory performance of high-fusing dental alloy investments: II. Silica-bonded investments. J Dent Res 52:758, 1973.
15. Lewis AJ: A metallographic evaluation of porosity occurrings in removable partial denture castings. Aust Dent J 24:408, 1979.
16. Lewis AJ: Porosity in base metal partial denture casting alloys, related industrial alloys, and pure metals. Aust Dent J 22:208, 1977.
17. Lewis AJ: The influence of the refractory investment on the development of porosity in cast structures. Aust Dent J 22:455, 1977.
18. Lewis AJ: The effect of variations in mold temperature, metal temperature and mold size on the development of internal porosity in cast structures. Aust Dent J 22:243, 1977.
19. Nitkin DA and Asgar K: Evaluation of alternative alloys to Type III gold for use in fixed prosthodontics. J Am Dent Assoc 93:622, 1979.
20. Moffa JP, Lugassy AA, Guckes AD, and Gettleman L: An evaluation of nonprecious alloys for use with porcelain veneers. Part I. Physical properties. J Prosthet Dent 30:424, 1973.
21. Rogers OW: The dental application of electroformed pure gold. I. Porcelain jacket crown technique. Aust Dent J 24:163, 1979.
22. Griffith JR: Personal communication, Dec., 1980.
23. Rogers OW: The dental application of electroformed pure gold. III. An investigation into an alternative ceramic bonding system for base metal alloys. Aust Dent J 25:205, 1980.

24. Moffa JP, Jenkins WA, and Hamilton JC: Five year clinical evaluation of two base-metal alloys. IADR Program and Abstracts, No. 380, 1981.

25. Moffa JP, Guckes AD, Okawa MA, and Lilly GE: An evaluation of nonprecious alloys for use with porcelain veneers. Part II. Industrial safety and biocompatibility. J Prosthet Dent 30:432, 1973.

26. Sunderman FM: Metal carcinogens. In Krayhill HF and Mehlman MA: Advances in Modern Toxicology, Volume 2: Environmental Cancer. New York, Halsted Press, 1977, Chapter 9, p 257.

27. Bidstrup CL and Case LAM: Carcinoma of the lung in workmen in the biochromatic producing industry in Great Britain. Br J Ind Med 13:260, 1956.

28. Dall R, Morgan LG, and Speiger FE: Cancer of the lung and nasal sinuses in nickel workers. Br J Cancer 24:623, 1970.

29. Fisher AA: Contact Dermatitis, 2nd Ed., Philadelphia, Lea & Febiger, 1973, Chapter 6.

30. Prystowsky SD, Allen AM, Smith RW, Nonomura JH, Odom RB, and Akers WA: Allergic contact hypersensitivity to nickel, neomycin, ethylenediamine and benzocaine. Arch Dermatol 115:959, 1979.

31. Moffa JP, Beck WD, and Hoke AW: Allergic response to nickel containing dental alloys. IADR Program and Abstracts, No. 107, 1977.

35 MECHANICS OF CUTTING WITH DENTAL BURS

As has been stated many times throughout this book, before any dental restoration can be placed in the mouth, the teeth or other tissues must be prepared to receive the restoration. Usually such preparation requires the cutting of tooth structure. Although hand tools, such as chisels, may be used in cutting, the present discussion will be mainly concerned with rotating cutting tools, similar to a milling cutter.

Cutting is generally understood to mean the removal of a part of a structure or surface by means of a shearing action, as with a carpenter's plane or chisel. The working edge or blade of the cutting tool is shaped to an angle as generally prescribed by the *work* or substance to be cut. The blade is not necessarily "sharp" in the sense used for a knife blade, for example. The sharpness of the blade is determined by its ability to cut the structure efficiently and smoothly.

In a cutting tool, the blade cuts through the work at a predetermined rate which is controlled by many factors. Unfortunately, studies in the cutting of tooth structure have been meager compared with those conducted in industrial cutting. Consequently, the principles of dental cutting must, to some extent, be presented as analogous to those employed in industrial cutting.

Such analogies should be made with reservation, however. In dental cutting the biologic factors are paramount. For example, the generation of excessive heat in industrial cutting is to be avoided on the basis of tool wear and possible change in the physical properties of the work. In dental cutting, the heat generation may cause irreversible injury to the dental pulp as well as severe discomfort to the patient. Temperatures involved in cutting teeth must be kept much lower than in metal cutting for this reason.

Another difference between industrial cutting and dental cutting is the method of applying the cutting tool. In metal work, the work is usually carried or *fed* to the tool at a constant rate, whereas the dentist carries the tool to the work.

A third difference is that the force applied to the dental tool is much less than is ordinarily employed in industrial cutting; less material may be removed per unit of time by the dentist.

DENTAL BURS

Dental burs are essentially miniature milling cutters as used in industry. Occasionally industrial cutters are as small as dental burs, although they usually have shanks of greater diameter.

Many shapes and sizes of dental burs are available for various purposes in the preparation and finishing of cavities and restorations. A few of the typical shapes are shown in Figure 35–1.

Composition and Manufacture   Dental burs can be classified by their composition. One type is made from hypereutectoid steel with hardening agents added in minor amount as will be described in Chapter 37. Burs of this type are generally called *carbon steel burs* or merely *steel burs. Tungsten carbide burs,* or, simply, *carbide burs,* are a second type.

The steel bur is usually cut from blank stock by a rotating cutter that cuts parallel to the axis of the bur as, for example, the straight fissure bur (Fig. 35–1). The bur is then hardened and tempered.

Regardless of the bur design, whenever a steel bur contacts tooth enamel during cutting, its edges are turned, chipped, and worn almost immediately. As long as the cutting is in dentin, the steel tool cuts effectively, but the junction of the dentin and the enamel is so irregular in reference to the tooth contour that it is difficult to cut dentin without contacting an irregular contour of enamel. The Vickers hardness number of the tempered steel bur is approximately 800, whereas that of enamel is 260 to 300.[1]

The tungsten carbide bur is a product of *powder metallurgy.* Powder metallurgy refers to a process of alloying in which complete fusion of the constituents does not occur. For example, if a tungsten carbide powder is mixed with powdered cobalt in proportion of 90 parts to 10 parts, placed under pressure in a vacuum, and heated to approximately 1350° C (2460° F), a partial alloying, or sintering, of the metals takes place. Presumably, a eutectic alloy is formed which becomes the bond, or matrix, for the particles of tungsten carbide not previously attacked.

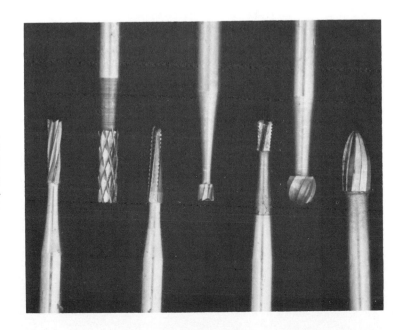

Figure 35–1 Some bur types. Left to right: Straight fissure (spiral bladed), straight fissure (double spiral bladed), tapered dome fine crosscut, inverted cone, pear-shaped fine crosscut, round, and egg-shaped bur.

A typical microstructure of such a cobalt-tungsten carbide alloy is shown in Figure 35–2. The core is formed by the tungsten carbide with the cobalt-tungsten carbide mixture as the matrix, or bond. The composition of the dental tungsten carbide bur ranges from 5 to 10 per cent cobalt with the remainder being tungsten carbide and possibly small amounts of iron (approximately 0.2 per cent), nickel (0.15 to 0.25 per cent), titanium (0.01 to 0.1 per cent), and silicon (approximately 0.1 per cent). Most of the dental tools probably contain not more than 5 to 7 per cent cobalt. The Vickers hardness number of the carbide bur is given as 1650 to 1700.[2]

A blank is formed and the tungsten carbide bur is cut with diamond tools. The cutting head is fastened to a steel shank either by soldering or (mainly) by electric butt welding; or, in some instances, the entire tool, including the shank and shaft, are constructed with the tungsten carbide alloy.

Design of Dental Burs   As previously stated, the dental bur is a small milling cutter. The possible tooth designs of such dental burs are shown in Figure 35–3.

It should be noted in the diagram that the tool is turning clockwise. The upper drawing indicates a portion of the tool with its teeth in outline. The *blade,* or *cutting edge,* is in contact with the horizontal line or work. The side of the tooth ahead of the cutting edge in the direction of rotation is known as the *tooth face;* the opposite or following surface is called the *back,* or *flank,* of the tooth.

The face of the bur tooth is at an angle to the radial line from the center to the cutting edge. This angle is known as the *rake angle.* In this instance, the face is beyond or leading the radial line in reference to the direction of rotation. The angle thus formed between the face and the radial line is called a *negative rake angle.* As can be noted immediately below the large drawing, the radial line and the face contour correspond. In this case, the rake angle is zero. In such an instance, the bur tooth is said to have a *zero* or *radial rake angle.* If the radial line leads the face so that the rake angle is on the inside of the radial

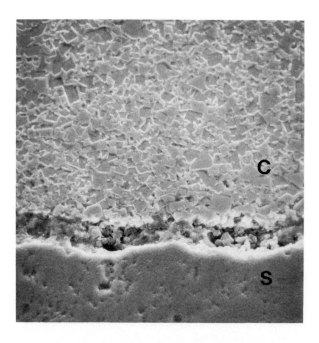

Figure 35–2 Microstructure of a cobalt-tungsten carbide alloy bur head (C), showing the weld joint to the steel shank (S). × 3000.

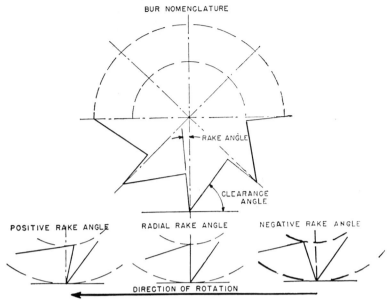

Figure 35–3 Bur tooth designs and nomenclature. (From Henry and Peyton, J Dent Res, April, 1954.)

line, the rake angle is said to be *positive*. Most commonly used hand wood cutting tools are made with positive rake angles.

The angle between the back of the tooth and the work is known as the *clearance angle* (Fig. 35–3). An outline of a possible cutter, rotating counterclockwise in this case, is shown in Figure 35–4. The plane surface immediately following the cutting edge is called the *land*, and the angle it makes with the work is known as the *primary clearance*. The angle between the back and the work is called the *secondary clearance*. Although many milling cutters are of this type, so far as is known this design is not employed with dental burs. It has been included for purposes of comparison only.

The *tooth angle* is measured between the face and the back, or, if a land is present, between the face and the land. The space between successive teeth is known as the *flute* or *chip space*.

The number of teeth in a dental bur is usually six or eight. An eight-tooth bur is shown in cross section in Figure 35–5. The burs in Figures 35–6 to 35–8 have six teeth. As a rule, dental burs are provided with negative rake angles, although the bur designs shown in Figures 35–7 and 35–8 are exceptions. In

Figure 35–4 Possible design for a dental bur. (From Osborne, Anderson, and Lammie, Br Dent J, May 1, 1951.)

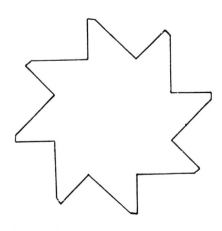

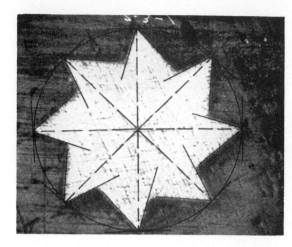

Figure 35–5 Eight-tooth bur. (From Henry and Peyton, J Dent Res, April, 1954.)

the bur cross section in Figure 35–7, the rake angle is almost zero and is possibly intended to be so by the manufacturer. The bur cross section shown in Figure 35–8 is that of a carbide bur with a radial rake angle.

The clearance angle of most burs is straight and clearly defined, as noted in Figures 35–5 and 35–6. When the back surface of the tooth is curved, the clearance is said to be *radial* as illustrated in Figures 35–7 and 35–8.

Figure 35–6

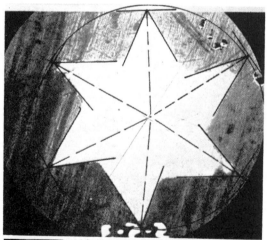

Figure 35–6 Six-tooth bur. (From Henry and Peyton, J Dent Res, April, 1954.)

Figure 35–7 Six-tooth bur with radial rake angle. (From Henry and Peyton, J Dent Res, April, 1954.)

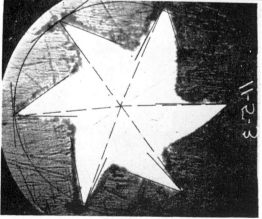

Figure 35–7

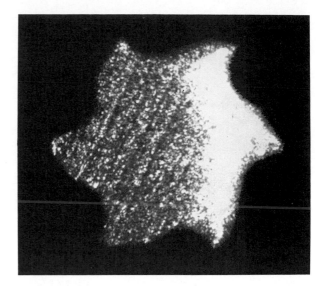

Figure 35–8 Six-tooth bur with a radial clearance.

Rake Angles In industrial cutting, a positive rake angle is used whenever possible. One advantage is that it improves the flow of the metal along the face of the tool. The smaller the positive rake angle, the greater is the resistance to cutting. This is illustrated in Figures 35–9 and 35–10. The dental bur shown in Figure 35–8 with a radial rake angle cuts more effectively in tusk ivory than do the other designs with negative rake angles under the same conditions of load and rotational speed. Tusk ivory has been shown to be equivalent to tooth dentin in its "machinability" by dental burs.[3]

When a negative rake angle is used, the chip moves directly away from the edge and is often fractured into small bits or dust. A cutting edge with a negative rake angle is shown in Figure 35–11 as it cuts tusk ivory. As can be observed, the chip is in the form of a shaving, but, instead of sliding along the face of the cutter as in Figures 35–9 and 35–10, it moves directly away from the edge in the direction of motion.[4] In more brittle enamel, the chip is always small and irregular, as shown in Figure 35–12.

There are practical objections to the use of positive rake angles in dental burs, particularly with steel burs. For example, the small tooth angles of the bur teeth in Figure 35–7 would be turned or flattened more easily in a steel bur than the teeth shown in Figures 35–5 or 35–6 because of the smaller bulk at the cutting edge in the former. A positive rake angle would reduce the bulk at the edge even more. On the basis of such an argument, it is evident that, in a steel bur, the use of a zero or negative rake is necessary and it is further desirable in all bur designs.

The design shown in Figure 35–8 can be used successfully with a tungsten carbide bur, in which the greater hardness and strength of the material allow a certain amount of sacrifice of bulk to obtain a more efficient cutting edge, based on recognized milling principles. However, the design in Figure 35–13 is more nearly the rule. The negative rake angle together with the radial clearance and short tooth height provide maximal strength to the teeth and possibly contribute to a longer bur life.

Clearance Angles The purpose of the clearance angle is, as its name implies, to provide clearance between the work and the cutting edge to prevent

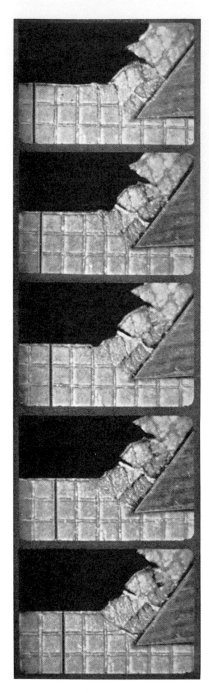 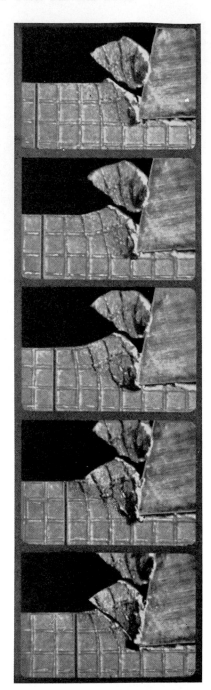

Figure 35–9   **Figure 35–10**

Figure 35–9   Steel chip formed with positive rake angle of 35 degrees. Note that the metal slides along the tool face with little discontinuity. (From A Treatise on Milling and Milling Machines, Cincinnati Milling Machine Co.)

Figure 35–10   Chip formed in steel with positive rake angle of 15 degrees. Note greater deformation of metal in cutting. (From A Treatise on Milling and Milling Machines, Cincinnati Milling Machine Co.)

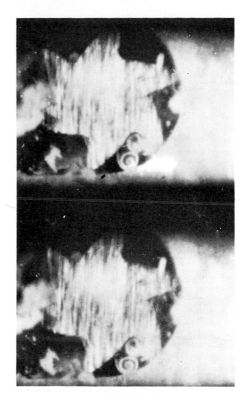

Figure 35–11 Chip formed in tusk ivory using a cutting edge with a negative rake angle.

the tool back from rubbing the work. There is always a frictional force component on any cutting edge as it rubs against the surface following the dislodgment of the chip. It logically follows that the frictional energy, or heat, is less, when the area of contact at the cutting edge is small. The clearance angle of the milling cutters in Figures 35–9 and 35–10 is very small but nevertheless evident. In Figures 35–8 and 35–13, radial clearances are provided.

Theoretically, the clearance angle should be small to provide additional bulk at the cutting edge. Not only is strength provided for the cutting edge but

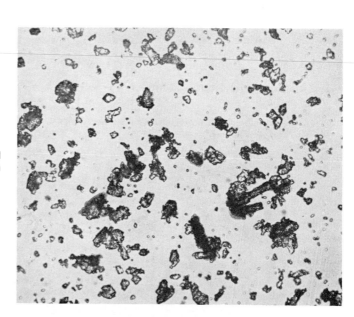

Figure 35–12 Enamel chips produced by a tungsten carbide bur. × 335. (From Lammie, Br Dent J, May 15, 1951.)

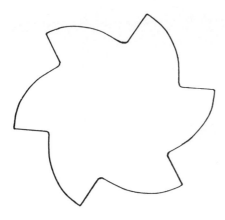

Figure 35–13 A typical cross section design of a tungsten carbide bur. (From Osborne, Anderson, and Lammie, Br Dent J, May 1, 1951.)

also more metal is present to dissipate the heat generated during cutting. However, the clearance should not be so small as to negate its original purpose, i.e., to prevent the tooth back from rubbing the work. Any dulling or flattening of the tooth edge may provide a plane surface which rubs against the surface of the work and partially negates the usefulness of the clearance.

This particular effect is likely to be very important in the dental bur. It is estimated that only about 1 μm (0.00004 inch) of the cutting edge is effective in cutting tooth dentin. The depth of the effective cutting edge in enamel is possibly reduced tenfold in comparison. It should be evident that any slight wear of the cutting edge increases the dulling perceptibly. It is possible that the large clearance angles often employed with steel burs (Figs. 35–5 to 35–7) may result in less rapid dulling on this basis.

Number of Teeth   As previously noted, the number of teeth in a dental bur is usually limited to six or eight. When it is considered that the diameter of the bur head may be 0.5 mm (0.02 inch), the dimensions of the teeth may be quite small.

The number of blades on the bur and the size of the flutes are definitely related. If too many blades are present, there is not sufficient space for chip removal, and the bur clogs. Actually, however, it has been shown by high speed photography that any dental bur is likely to clog repeatedly as it is used, but with proper flute design, it unclogs within two or three revolutions.[4]

Theoretically, a greater speed of cutting should result when more teeth are in the tool, other factors being constant. In practice, the difference in speed of cutting tusk ivory, for example, with a six-tooth, as compared with an eight-tooth, dental bur is unimportant.[5]

As might be expected, the fewer the teeth, the greater is the tendency for vibration. However, if two or more blades are in contact with the work at one time, this effect should not be of great importance, particularly as related to the difference between a six-tooth and an eight-tooth dental bur.

If the teeth are crosscut (Fig. 35–1), the general effect is to increase the number of teeth. Coarse crosscut burs are not recommended for use at ultra speeds. In this range the crosscut bur behaves as an abrading instrument rather than a milling instrument and produces a rough, irregular cut surface. It is also speculated that crosscut burs utilized at ultra speeds contribute to the problem of vibration and its potentially harmful effects on tooth structure and pulpal tissues. When employed in low speed (10,000 rpm) operations, the crosscut bur is more effective than its plain fissure counterpart.[6]

All of these factors are considered in the design of burs in order to attain maximum cutting efficiency. The American Dental Association Specification no. 23 for excavating burs includes a cutting ability test. The requirement specifies a certain maximum time for a given type of bur to cut a 0.51 mm (0.020 inch) hole in brass under standardized test conditions.

Concentricity and Runout   *Concentricity* is a static measurement of how precisely a single circle can be scribed through the cutting edges of all the blades of a bur. It is, therefore, a measurement of the symmetry of the bur head. *Runout* is a dynamic measurement of the accuracy with which the cutting edges pass through a single point as the bur turns. It is thus used to describe the eccentricity or maximal displacement of the bur head from its axis of rotation. Even the most precise bur will exhibit some runout if the head is mounted off-center on its shank, if the neck of the bur is bent, or if the chuck is eccentric, loose, or worn. If the shaft or collet attached to the bur wobbles during rotation, the effect is magnified at the bur head according to the length of the bur shank. These phenomena cause a bur to cut measurably larger holes than the head diameter would ideally produce.

The runout of a bur is also related to its efficiency in cutting. If the bur moves away from the tooth periodically, all of the blades do not cut equally. For example, a study of the motion picture frames in Figure 35–14 indicates that not all of the teeth are cutting. Rarely do all blades of a bur touch a tooth during a single rotation. As a single blade forms a chip of enamel or dentin, the resulting force causes the bur to bounce away. It may not retouch the tooth before another full rotation. On other occasions, when the excursion is less violent, two or three blades may strike the tooth before the bur again bounces.

If the dentist senses this lack of cutting, a greater force is probably being exerted on the bur. The result is, at one stage of the revolution, that the bur and tooth tend to be pushed apart only to be driven together at the next half wobble. This produces vibration, which is disagreeable to the patient.

Although the rate of removal of the tooth structure may appear to be increased during such vibration, the structure is removed by a shattering process rather than by cutting. This method of tooth removal is inefficient and inaccurate, and increases heat generation and discomfort.

Bur Life   The life, or length of use, of a bur depends upon many factors, some of which are not under the control of the dentist. The influence of the design of the bur on the preservation of its cutting edge has already been discussed. The speed of rotation is a factor which the dentist can control, but its influence on the life of the bur is not clear.

The probable life history of a dental bur during cutting is presented graphically in Figure 35–15. A dental tungsten carbide bur was arranged to cut for successive 15-second periods directly into a plate of optical glass, under water. The depth of cut during each period was noted and plotted as a function of the number of cuts.[2]

Generally, such a *life function curve* indicates a rapid decrease in cutting with distance or number of cuts as indicated by burs Nos. 2 and 3 in Figure 35–15. The cutting rate tends to become constant with further cutting.

Occasionally, a dental bur exhibits an increase in cutting rate before it begins to dull (bur No. 1, Fig. 35–15). The reason is not entirely understood. However, it might be because of an irregularity in the height of the bur teeth

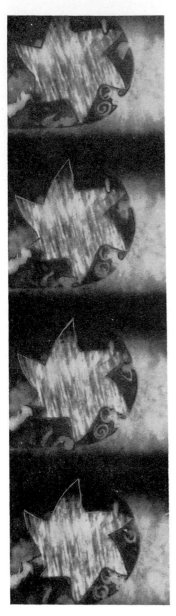

Figure 35–14   Successive motion picture frames of a six-tooth bur cutting ivory. Not all of the cutting blades are in contact with the work.

as a result of the manufacturing process. If one or two of the teeth are slightly higher than the others, it is possible that, as the blades on the higher teeth dull, more blades are brought into action, and an increased cutting rate results.

So far as is known, the life function curve is independent of the speed of rotation, but as the rotational speed increases, the rate of cutting increases also.

The durability test in American Dental Association Specification no. 23 involves the cutting of holes in plates of crystal glass which has a KHN of 450 to 510. Under a given load, the bur is held in contact with the glass for 2000 revolutions. The plate is then rotated and another hole is drilled. The total depth of five holes cut by five burs of the test sample must equal or exceed that specified.

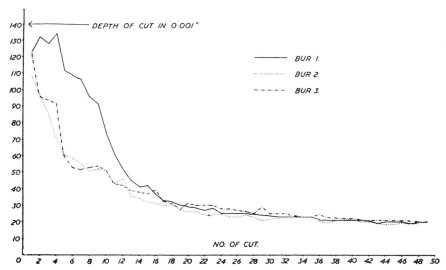

Figure 35–15   Life function curve of a tungsten carbide bur showing the relation between the depth of cut in optical glass and the number of successive cuts. (From Lammie, Dent Rec, Dec., 1952.)

Influence of Load   The force, or *load,* exerted by the dentist on a bur during cutting is related to the rotational speed of a bur of a given design. The exact amount of force generally employed is not known, but it has been estimated as being equivalent to a maximum of approximately 60 gm (2 oz). Although forces as high as 120 gm (4 oz) have been suggested, some air-driven handpieces will stall when placed under that load, especially with use of a variable speed foot control. Forces large enough to produce stalling are abusive and inefficient. A light, intermittent brushing motion should be employed to increase efficiency and decrease heat generation and vibration. Actually, the dentist operates according to his or her judgment as influenced by tactile sense, and the force exerted changes according to the variables encountered.

It should be noted that the discussion is concerned with the force, or load, exerted by the dentist on the tool head and not the pressure or stress induced in the tooth during cutting. The latter quantity is related to the force divided by the area of contact of the bur during the cutting, and this area, in turn, varies according to the type of bur employed and the material cut.

With a given load, the rate of cutting increases with the rotational speed, but the increase is not in direct proportion. The rate of increase in cutting at rotational speeds above 30,000 rpm is greater than that below this speed. However, at high speed (100,000 to 150,000 rpm) the time required for the removal of the same weight of tooth structure may not be much less than when ultra high (300,000 to 400,000 rpm) rotational speeds are used. This may be the result of the handpiece not maintaining its torque. If the torque could be maintained, the time for tooth removal must be reduced. In any case, no tests to establish the validity of this hypothesis have been reported.

There is, however, a minimal rotational speed for a given load below which the bur does not cut. The greater the load, the lower is this minimal rotational speed. The correlation between the load and the minimal rotational speed depends upon whether enamel or dentin is being cut, the design and composition of the bur, and similar factors. Here again, the tactile sense of the dentist is the controlling factor under clinical conditions of cutting.

Coolants   A coolant applied to the bur reduces the heat generated during cutting and increases its cutting rate. The chief purposes of the coolant are to reduce the temperature during cutting, to aid in the removal of debris, and, when water is used, to lubricate the rotary tool.

There are three types of coolant available to the dentist: air, water, and water spray (air and water combined). All three coolants are effective in reducing the temperature during cutting. The water stream is the most effective, water spray, second, and air blown on the bur during cutting, third.[7]

According to one investigation, when a heavy air blast is employed as a coolant, the bur tends to clog during the cutting of dentin, and the cutting rate is reduced. Also, the desiccating effect of the air may result in additional damage to the pulp. On the other hand, the presence of a water spray increases the cutting rate of the bur 10 times when cutting enamel in comparison with the cutting rate when no coolant is used. No noticeable difference in this regard could be noted when a water stream was substituted for the water spray.[7] This observation was based upon high speed, not ultra high speed, rotational handpieces. In the latter case, it has been noted that flooding the bur with water increased the cutting speed, as compared with use of a water spray.[8]

Heat Generation   During cutting, heat is generated by the internal friction of the material being deformed in the process of forming the chip, the friction between the face of the tooth and the chip as it is sheared from the work, and the friction of the blade as it moves across the work. This heat can be dissipated by conduction through the tool, by conduction through the work, by the chip itself as it is removed, and by a coolant. Although the life of the bur may be reduced markedly by the first method, the most important factor from the dental standpoint is the heat absorbed by the tooth. If the temperature of the tooth becomes too great, irreversible pulp damage may occur.

The dry cutting of tooth structure is not only potentially injurious to the pulp but also it is capable of inducing thermal stresses of sufficient magnitude to fracture the surrounding enamel. Such damage may eventually contribute to marginal failure of a restoration or to secondary caries. It has been demonstrated that dry cutting at ultra speeds can generate a temperature increase of 136° C (245° F) within two seconds in the area that lies within a 1 to 2 mm radius of the point being cut.[9] Even preparation of pin channels in dentin at relatively low speeds can produce a small temperature rise in the pulp. The magnitude of the temperature rise is related to the twist drill diameter, depth of the channel, and rotational speed.[10]

The use of a coolant greatly reduces the amount of heat generated, regardless of the rotational speed of the bur. At ultra speeds, an air-water spray is effective if a water flow rate of 35 to 50 ml per minute is maintained. A temperature rise of 20 to 30° C at the cutting site might be anticipated. An alternate procedure uses a high velocity water syringe with an output of 10 ml per minute directed on the bur head and is equally effective. Also, the reduced water flow rate contributes to increased visibility.[11]

Another important factor is the period of time the bur is applied to the tooth. Intermittent cutting at intervals of a few seconds should be the rule. Removing the bur from the tooth intermittently for even a few seconds can reduce the heat generation considerably. Even though the temperature is kept comparatively low, a sustained application may result in greater pulp damage than would result if a higher temperature were applied for a short time.

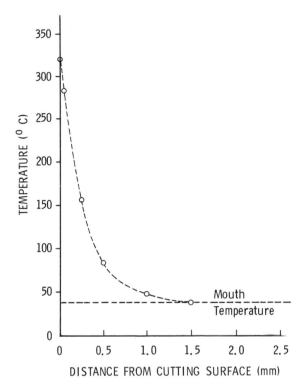

Figure 35–16 Calculated average temperature versus distance from the surface being cut in enamel without coolant for various energy-deposition rates. (Modified from Brown, WS, et al.: J Am Dent Assoc, 96:451, 1978.

Actually, the greatest protecting factor against pulp damage is the low thermal conductivity of the dentin itself. It it were not for this factor, the preparation of a tooth cavity would be a serious problem even under optimal conditions of temperature control.

MECHANICS OF CUTTING

Many of the conclusions presented in the previous discussion can be summarized and accounted for on the basis of a theory of cutting.

Let it be assumed that a dental bur is rotating as diagrammed in Figure 35–3. As one of the teeth rotates into position to contact the work, a compressive stress is first induced as the blade forces its way into the work. If cutting results, the blade essentially fractures or shears the surface; it gradually becomes parallel with the surface of the work and it pushes the material ahead along the tooth face to form the chip. The chip is subjected to compressive stress and the material behind the blade is under tension. However, the material at the cutting edge is subjected to a shearing stress predominantly as it is removed from the surface of the work.

Although the stresses are complex, nevertheless they can be categorized by analysis into the three stress types. Furthermore, both elasticity and permanent deformation of the work are involved.

For example, as the rotating bur tooth contacts the work, the first stress introduced is elastic in nature. If the force at the cutting edge is sufficient, the stress soon exceeds the proportional or elastic limit of the material, and a permanent deformation and then fracture occur.

On the other hand, if the force exerted by the blade in rotation is insufficient to cause the induced stresses to exceed the elastic limit of the material, only elastic deformation occurs as the blade moves across the work, with no cutting or chip formation. This explanation accounts for the fact that for any rotational speed there is a minimal load that need be exerted to produce cutting. When such a situation is encountered in practice, the dentist merely exerts more force on the handpiece so that cutting occurs.

It can be reasoned, therefore, that the greater the load, the more the blade "bites" into the work, and the more material is removed. There is a limit, however, to the magnitude of the load that can be exerted on a given bur tooth at a constant rotational speed. For example, the friction of the cutting edge against the work increases with the load, and excessive heat may be generated as well as a dulling and chipping of the cutting edge. Even more important, particularly with modern dental handpieces, the bur stalls because of insufficient torque, particularly at very high rotational speeds.

When the load is held constant, the rate of cutting can be increased by increasing the rotational speed. One reason is, of course, that more blades contact the work per unit of time. On the other hand, the increase in cutting rate is not necessarily directly proportional to the increase in rotational speed.

This latter effect can be explained on the basis of the rate of recovery or relaxation of the work after deformation. After the material cut has been permanently deformed, time must elapse for relaxation. If one blade follows another in cutting so rapidly that there is not sufficient time for the stressed material to recover, the amount of deformation of the work produced by the succeeding blade is less. In other words, the following blade probably contacts the work while it is permanently deformed from the previous blade so that energy need not be expended for the initial elastic deformation. Thus, the total efficiency of the cutting is increased. Consequently, the amount of material removed per tooth at the higher speeds is greater than at the lower speeds under the same conditions of loading. Therefore, the rate of cutting at the higher speeds is greater in proportion to the cutting rate at lower speeds, as previously concluded.

References

1. Osborne J, Anderson JN, and Lammie GA: Tungsten carbide and its application to the dental bur. Br Dent J 90:229, 1951.
2. Lammie GA: A study of some different tungsten carbide burs. Dent Rec 72:285, 1952.
3. Bryton B, Skinner EW, Lindenmeyer RS, and Lasater RL: The cutting effectiveness of a dental bur as related to its design. J Dent Res 33:693, 1954.
4. Skinner EW, Lasater RL, Lindenmeyer RS, and Rigas TJ: Dental Bur Research. Report to the Office of the Surgeon General, Department of the Army, 1955, p 107.
5. Ibid., p 70.
6. Skinner EW, Lasater RL, Lindenmeyer RS, and Bryton B: Dental Bur Research. Report to the Office of the Surgeon General, Department of the Army, 1954, p 64.
7. Skinner EW, Lasater RL, Lindenmeyer RS, Rigas TJ, and Rigas DJ: Dental Bur Research. Report to the Office of the Surgeon General, Department of the Army, 1957, p 114.
8. Gardella JM, SS White Co.: Personal communication, May 17, 1972.
9. Brown W, Christensen DO, and Lloyd BA: Numerical and experimental evaluation

of energy inputs, temperature gradients, and thermal stresses during restorative procedures. J Am Dent Assoc 96:451, 1978.

10. Cooley RI and Barkmeier WW: Temperature rise in the pulp chamber caused by twist drills. J Prosthet Dent 44:426, 1980.

11. Lloyd BA, Rich JA, and Brown WS: Effect of cooling techniques on temperature control and cutting rate for high-speed dental drills. J Dent Res 57:675, 1978.

36 ABRASION AND POLISHING. DENTIFRICES

Before any dental restoration or appliance is placed permanently in the mouth, it should be highly polished. Not only is a rough surface on a restoration, denture, orthodontic appliance, etc., uncomfortable but also food and other debris cling to it. Such a restoration or appliance becomes dirty and in some cases tarnish or corrosion may occur.

Rough surfaces are likely to occur unavoidably during the construction of an appliance. For example, in spite of all the care possible, an acrylic denture base may have minor surface roughnesses that need to be removed before the denture is polished.

Abrasion The term *abrasion* in the strict sense of the word denotes a wearing of one surface against another by friction. Such abrasion is destructive and is to be avoided. The type of abrasion under consideration is useful in order to smooth a roughened surface in preparation for *polishing*. It is actually a cutting action. However, in a "cutting tool," e.g., a dental bur, the blades or cutting edges are regularly arranged. The pattern of removal of material by the tool corresponds to the regular arrangements of the cutting blades. This can be seen in a photograph of a tooth surface cut by a dental bur (Fig. 36–1).

In contrast to cutting instruments, abrasive tools have many abrasive points which generally are not arranged in an ordered pattern. For example, a grinding wheel or a diamond rotary instrument may contain thousands of sharp abrasive points which pass over the work during each revolution of the instrument. Each point acts as an individual blade and removes a chip or shaving from the material. Since these many cutting blades are randomly arranged, innumerable scratches are produced on the surface, as illustrated in Figure 36–2, which shows a tooth surface cut by a diamond instrument.

Rough nodules on a denture base can be removed with an abrasive. They can be removed with sandpaper, an emery arbor, or a grinding wheel. In each case, the blades formed by the abrasive particles can remove the rough spots as they move over the surface. Abrasives are available in varying particle size. Coarse abrasives leave scratches in the surface, which must be removed with finer abrasives. Finally, the abrasive can be so fine that a surface results that

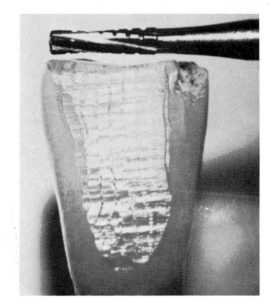

Figure 36–1 Tooth cut by a bur. Note the regular pattern of removal of tooth structure, which corresponds to the regular arrangement of the blades of the cutting tool (bur).

is so smooth that it reflects light regularly, and the surface is said to be *polished.*

The abrasives used in dentistry are applied to the work by means of a number of abrasive tools. The abrasive particles may be glued onto paper or plastic disks that can be attached to a dental handpiece. In the case of diamond rotary instruments the diamond chips are attached to steel wheels, disks, and cylinders. With grinding wheels and dental stones the abrasive particles are mixed with a bonding agent or matrix material that holds the particles together. Prior to hardening, the matrix material containing the abrasive is molded to form tools of the desired size and shape, examples of which are shown in Figure 36–3.

Abrasives can also be mixed with water, glycerine, or some other medium

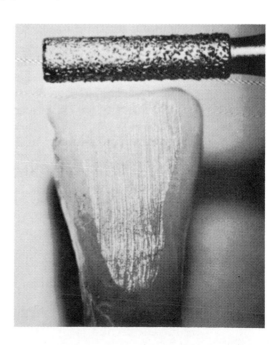

Figure 36–2 Tooth cut by a diamond instrument. Note random pattern of tooth removal, which corresponds to the irregular arrangement of the cutting edges on the abrasive tool (diamond).

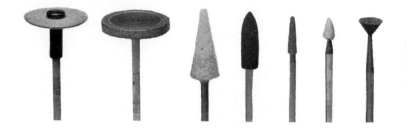

Figure 36-3 Typical dental abrasive tools, some of which are designed for use in the oral cavity and others for use in the laboratory.

to produce pastes or slurries. The slurry is then rubbed over the surface of the material with a cloth or felt wheel, rubber cup, or brush. This means of applying an abrasive is particularly useful in finishing and polishing irregular surfaces, such as dentures and restorations, and for prophylaxis of teeth.

Types of Abrasives   There are many abrading and polishing agents available, but only those which can be used in dentistry will be discussed.

EMERY   Emery consists primarily of a natural oxide of aluminum, called *corundum.* There are various impurities present, such as iron oxide, which may also act as abrasives.

ALUMINUM OXIDE   Pure aluminum oxide is manufactured from *bauxite,* an impure aluminum oxide. It can be produced in various grain sizes, and has partially replaced emery for abrasive purposes.

Extremely fine particles of aluminum oxide can be obtained by a water flotation process. In this form it is known as *levigated alumina* and it is used extensively for polishing metallographic specimens.

GARNET   This term includes a number of different minerals which possess similar physical properties and crystalline form. The minerals comprise the silicates of any combinations of aluminum, cobalt, magnesium, iron, and manganese. Garnet is usually coated on paper or cloth with glue or a similar binder. It is one of the common abrasives used in denture abrasive disks which are operated with the dental handpiece.

PUMICE   Pumice is a highly siliceous material of volcanic origin, and it is suitable for use either as an abrasive or as a polishing agent, according to its particle size. It is used in dentistry for many operations, from the smoothing of denture bases to the polishing of teeth in the mouth.

KIESELGUHR   Kieselguhr is composed of the siliceous remains of minute aquatic plants known as *diatoms.* The coarser form is called "diatomaceous earth," which is used as a filler in many dental materials, such as the hydrocolloid impression materials. It is excellent as a mild abrasive and polishing agent.

TRIPOLI   This mild abrasive and polishing agent is often confused with kieselguhr, which is often substituted for it. True tripoli originates from certain porous rocks, first found in northern Africa near Tripoli, for which it was named.

ROUGE   Rouge is a fine red powder composed of iron oxide. It is usually employed in cake form. It may be impregnated on paper or cloth, known as "crocus cloth." It is an excellent polishing agent for gold and noble metal alloys, but it is likely to be dirty to handle.

TIN OXIDE   Tin oxide, or "putty powder," is used extensively as a polishing agent for teeth and metallic restorations in the mouth. It is mixed with water, alcohol, or glycerin and used as a paste.

CHALK   Chalk is calcium carbonate prepared by a precipitation method. There are various grades and physical forms of calcium carbonate available for different polishing techniques. Calcium carbonate is sometimes employed as one of the polishing agents in commercial dentifrices.

CHROMIC OXIDE   Chromic oxide (Cr_2O_3) is a relatively hard abrasive which is capable of polishing a variety of metals. It is often used as a polishing agent for stainless steel.

SAND   Sand as well as other forms of quartz is used as an abrasive agent. Its use in sandpaper is a common example. It is also used as a powder in sandblasting equipment.

CARBIDES   Various carbides, such as silicon carbide (SiC) and boron carbide (B_4C), are employed effectively as abrading agents. Both of these products are manufactured by heating silicon and boron at a very high temperature to effect their union with the carbon. The silicon carbide is sintered, or pressed with a binder, into grinding wheels or disks. Most of the stone burs employed for the cutting of tooth structure are made of silicon carbide.

DIAMOND   The hardest and most effective abrasive for tooth enamel is composed of diamond chips. The chips are impregnated in a binder or plated onto a metal shank to form the diamond "stones" and disks so popular with the dental profession.

ZIRCONIUM SILICATE   Occurring in nature as zircon, this material is ground to various particle sizes and used as a polishing agent. Zirconium silicate is frequently used as a constituent of dental prophylactic pastes and in abrasive-impregnated polishing strips and disks.

Abrasive Action   The action of the abrasive as it moves over a surface is essentially a cutting action. Each tiny abrasive particle presents a sharp edge that cuts through the surface in a manner similar to a sharp pointed chisel. A shaving is formed which immediately crushes to a fine powder and often clogs the abrasive tool so that frequent cleaning is necessary. The theory of the cutting involved is similar to that discussed in the previous chapter for the cutting of dental burs.

In the abrading of metals, the crystalline structure of the surface is disturbed, sometimes to a depth of 10 μm. The grains become disoriented and strain hardening may occur. The more abrasion there is, the greater is the disorientation. Strain hardening accompanies the disorientation, and the superficial hardness of the surface is increased.

Some of the crystals fracture and the minute powder-like particles may remain in the surface. Many of these minute particles may be removed by washing the work with soap and water; such a cleansing should always be done before a polishing operation.

The surface effect varies with different metals. For example, in a ductile metal, such as gold, less of the surface may be removed by the abrasive than in a brittle metal. In a ductile metal, the scratch left by the abrasive may display a ridge of metal on either side, like the soil on either side of a plowed furrow. In other words, the abrasive particle has merely "plowed" through the surface, without actually removing much of it. As a result, many of the hard gold alloys may be less resistant to abrasion than are some of the softer alloys.

The surface disturbance of a resin, as in a denture base, undoubtedly includes the introduction of surface stresses which may cause a distortion if the abrasion is too rigorous. The generation of heat during the abrasion partially relieves such stresses, but if it is too great it may relieve processing stresses so that a general warpage results, as well as an actual melting of the surface of the resin.

Desirable Characteristics of an Abrasive   In the first place, the abrasive should be irregular in shape, so that it presents a sharp edge. Round, smooth particles of sand, such as are found on the seashore, possess poor abrasive properties. Also, sandpaper impregnated with cubical particles, which always present a flat face to the work, is not as effective in abrasion as is paper impregnated with irregular jagged particles.

Secondly, the abrasive should be harder than the work it abrades. If the abrasive cannot indent the surface to be abraded, it cannot cut it. In such a case, the abrasive dulls or wears. The KHN of five abrasives are presented in Table 36–1.

A third desirable property of an abrasive is that it possess a high impact strength or *body strength*. For example, when a grinding wheel is applied against a metal, the abrasive particle strikes the work suddenly as it moves along the circumference of the wheel. If it shatters the instant it contacts the work, it is ineffective. On the other hand, if it never fractures, its edge may become dull, and the efficiency of the abrasive is reduced. Ideally, the abrasive should fracture rather than dull, so that a sharp edge is always present. Fracture of the abrasive is also helpful in shedding the debris accumulated from the work. Although diamond burs cut almost any type of tooth structure or restorative material, the diamond particles do not fracture; rather they lose substance at the tip. Furthermore, they are likely to become clogged when ductile or soft substances are abraded. They are most effective when they are used on the very hard and brittle tooth enamel.

The rating of the body strength of the abrasives listed in Table 36–1 is in the same order as their hardness.

A fourth desirable quality of an abrasive is that it possess *attrition resistance* so that it does not wear. An example of attrition is the normal wear of chalk on a blackboard or a pencil on paper. Attrition or dulling is not always

Table 36–1.   *Knoop Hardness Numbers of Abrasives**

ABRASIVE	KHN
Sand	800
Emery	2000
Silicon carbide	2500
Boron carbide	2800
Diamond	> 7000

*Wayner, Welding Engineer, Nov., 1950.

the result of wear, however. The abrasive may be "dissolved" or impregnated into the work by a chemical action. For example, silicon carbide dulls more rapidly on steel than does aluminum oxide because it is soluble in steel.

Grading of Abrasive and Polishing Agents   Abrasives are graded on the basis of the fineness of the standard sieve through which they can pass. For example, an abrasive graded as number 8 can pass through a sieve with 8 meshes to the inch, but it cannot pass through a finer sieve. Different types of abrasives are graded differently. For example, a silicon carbide abrasive is graded as 8, 10, 12, 14, 16, 20, 24, 30, 36, 46, 60, 70, 80, 90, 100, 120, 150, 180, 220, 240, and so on. Finer abrasives are designated as powders or flours and are graded in increasing fineness as F, FF, FFF, etc., or, in the case of impregnated papers, as 0, 00, 000, etc.

Binder   As previously noted, in abrasive wheels and disks, the abrasive particles are held together by a binder. For example, ceramic bonding may be used for silicon carbide or corundum in a mounted abrasive point. Electroplating with a nickel base matrix is often used to bind the diamond chips in diamond rotary instruments. For "soft grade" disks, rubber or shellac may be used. The latter types, as might be expected, wear rapidly, but they are useful in some dental operations in which delicate abrasion is required.

The type of binder is intimately related to the life of the tool in use. In most abrasives, the binder is impregnated throughout with an abrasive of a certain grade so that, as a particle is wrenched from the binder during use, another takes its place as the binder wears. Furthermore, the abrasive should be so distributed that the surface of the tool wears evenly, particularly if the disk or wheel is used for cutting along its periphery.

Diamond Burs   Either natural or synthetic diamond chips are employed for dental rotary instruments. There are sintered diamond abrasive instruments for use in the dental laboratory, which do have diamonds impregnated throughout the matrix. However, since diamond chips are relatively expensive, they are usually applied as a coating. Diamonds dull less rapidly than do other abrasives. One manufacturer's idea for placing the diamond chips on a dental tool is shown in Figure 36–4. The arrangements in A and B provide for smooth cutting with little tool vibration. In C, the points protrude farther from the binder and are more widely spaced. This tool cuts faster but the scratches on the surface are deeper. It is intended for coarse cutting. The wide spaces between the points provide room for the debris from the cutting with less chance for packing or clogging.

The heterogeneous arrangment of the diamond chips in D provides a rough contour to the tool surface. Not only is there a greater chance that the chips will be removed from the binder during use but also the tool may vibrate, or "chatter," causing excessive heat generation and generally inefficient cutting. Furthermore, the control of cutting by the operator is more difficult. The surface contour of such a diamond tool can be seen in Figure 36–5A in contrast to the regular outline of the tool at the right, Figure 36–5B.

The cutting efficiency of diamond rotary instruments depends on whether natural or synthetic diamonds are used, the grit size, the distribution, and the extent of plating that attaches the particles to the instrument shank. Overplating can reduce cutting efficiency by less exposure of cutting edges, while underplating may result in detachment of diamond particles.[1]

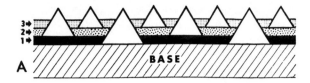

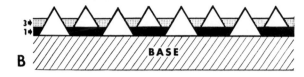

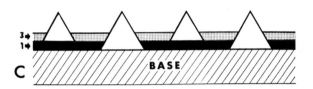

Figure 36–4 Diagrammatic arrangement of diamond chips on a dental abrasive tool in cross section. *A,* A sturdy three-layer construction using three grades of diamond chips attached with a ceramic binder to a metal base. *B,* A thinner arrangement with two grades of chips. *C,* A coarse cutting tool with two grades of chips. *D,* Miscellaneous chip sizes and shapes in one layer of binder. (Courtesy of Densco, Inc.)

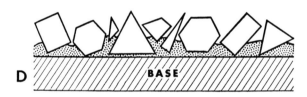

Adequate water spray is essential not only to minimize heat but also to reduce clogging of diamond rotary instruments when used to prepare teeth.

Factors Affecting the Rate of Abrasion   Assuming that the abrasive possesses the proper characteristics as outlined in the previous section, the size of the abrasive particle is an important factor in the rate at which the surface

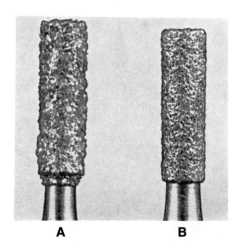

Figure 36–5   Two dental diamond burs enlarged to show the effect of irregularly arranged chips (*A*) in comparison to the regular arrangement (*B*). (Courtesy of Densco, Inc.)

is abraded. The larger the particle, the deeper the scratches in the surface, and the faster the surface is worn away.

The choice of the size of an abrasive is largely a matter of judgment. If there are many large nodules and similar coarse rough spots on the surface of the work, the use of a coarse abrasive is indicated. However, a coarse abrasive introduces deep scratches which must subsequently be removed by progressively finer abrasives. On the other hand, it would be a waste of time and material to start with a fine abrasive on a very rough surface, simply to avoid the deep scratches.

A second factor to be considered is the pressure of the work against the abrasive. This factor is best illustrated in a grinding wheel or an abrading tool that the dentist might use with a dental handpiece. If the work is pressed tightly against the grinding wheel, the scratches are deeper and the abrasion is more rapid. Such an observation does not, however, take into account the force on the abrasive particle. As the particle passes over the work, the back pressure of the work tends to dislodge or fracture the abrasive. Obviously, the greater the pressure of the work on the wheel, the deeper is the scratch, and the greater is the tendency for the abrasive particle to be dislodged or fractured. The efficiency of the abrasive operation is greatly reduced under such circumstances, and the grinding wheel is worn away.

A third and very important factor in the control of the rate of the abrasion is the speed at which the particle travels across the work. The faster the wheel turns, the more times per unit of time the particle contacts the surface. Increasing the speed of the wheel is the logical method for increasing the rate of abrasion with a given abrasive without wearing away the abrasive tool. With many particles of abrasive passing across the work at a rapid rate, the pressure of the work against the wheel can be decreased without a decrease in the rate of abrasion.

If too great a load or pressure is applied, the fracture or wear of the abrasive is more rapid than at lower rotational speeds. Furthermore, the head of the silicon carbide or diamond tool may be broken from the shank. The same observations apply to the use of the steel and, particularly, the carbide bur.

Rotational Speed and Linear Speed The speed at which the particle passes over the work is its *linear speed*. The linear speed of an abrasive wheel or bur is related to its rotational speed, according to its size. For example, if the abrasive particle is on the circumference of the wheel, when the wheel turns around once, the particle travels the length of the circumference, which is, of course, π times the diameter of the wheel. If the wheel turns at the rate of n revolutions per minute, the linear speed of the particle is given by the mathematical relation:

$$v = \pi\, dn$$
$$\text{Where } d = \text{diameter of the wheel}$$
$$\text{and } n = \text{revolutions per minute (rpm)}$$
$$v = \text{linear speed}$$

The unit generally employed for the linear speed is feet per minute.

Different abrasives require different speeds for their maximal efficiency, and such optimal speeds are determined largely by experience. Assume a linear speed of 5000 feet per minute to be an average value for the optimal speed. On such a basis, the motor speed of a lathe should be 6300 rpm for an abrasive wheel 3 inches in diameter. Because most dental lathes operate at two rotational speeds, 1750 and 3400 rpm, such abrasive wheels cannot be operated at their optimal speeds under such circumstances.

Assuming the optimal linear speed to be 5000 feet per minute as before, it can be calculated from the formula that an inverted silicon carbide cone bur 3/16 inch in diameter should turn at a rotational speed of 120,000 rpm for greatest efficiency. At slower speeds, the silicon carbide bur wears and dulls considerably faster. Such speeds are well within the range of dental practice.

It is evident from these calculations that the abrasive wheels and rotating tools used in dentistry should be specially constructed if they are to be efficient in dental operations. Unfortunately, many of the dental abrasive tools are not efficient, and they wear rapidly. The use of the diamond abrasive tool has greatly improved the effectiveness of cutting or abrading tooth enamel. The diamond particle is so hard, strong, and resistant to attrition that practically the only way in which such a tool can wear is for the diamond to be pulled from the binder.

Polishing   Metallographically speaking, polishing denotes the production of a smooth, mirror-like surface on a metal without the use of a film. A surface can be made to "shine" with a wax, for example, but such a method of "polishing" is not a true polish and it is not included in the present discussion. A metallographic polish is accomplished by producing a virtually scratch-free surface.

As described previously, the finer the abrasive, the smaller are the particles that are removed or cut from the surface and the finer are the scratches that are formed.

If the particle size of the abrasive is reduced sufficiently, the scratches finally become extremely fine and may disappear entirely. The surface then acquires a smooth shiny layer known as a *polish*. Such a layer is thought to be composed of minute crystals and is said to have a *microcrystalline* structure. Although the process is not completely understood, the most recent theory suggests that polishing agents actually remove material from the surface, molecule by molecule, and thus produce very smooth surfaces. In the process, fine scratches and irregularities are filled in by the powdered particulate being removed from the surface. This microcrystalline layer is referred to as the *polish layer* or *Beilby layer*. (A scientist named Beilby first noted the presence of such a surface layer after polishing.)

Photomicrographs of the surface of a gold casting during three stages of the polishing procedure are shown in Figure 36–6. The coarse abrasive used initially to remove gross surface irregularities produced deep scratches (Fig. 36–6*A*). When finer abrasives were used the deep scratches were removed and replaced by finer scratches (Fig. 36–6*B*). Finally, a polishing agent was employed. It will be noted (Fig. 36–6*C*) that the polishing agent obliterated or eliminated almost all the fine scratches, leaving a smooth finish.

The difference between an abrasive agent and a polishing agent is somewhat difficult to define. In practice, the terms are generally used interchangeably. This is often justified because a given agent having a large particle size may act as an abrasive, producing scratches. The same abrasive with a smaller particle size may leave a polish layer on the surface.

Polishing agents differ in the amount of material that they will remove from the surface during polishing. Some may produce a high surface polish yet at the same time remove a considerable amount of material. Although such an

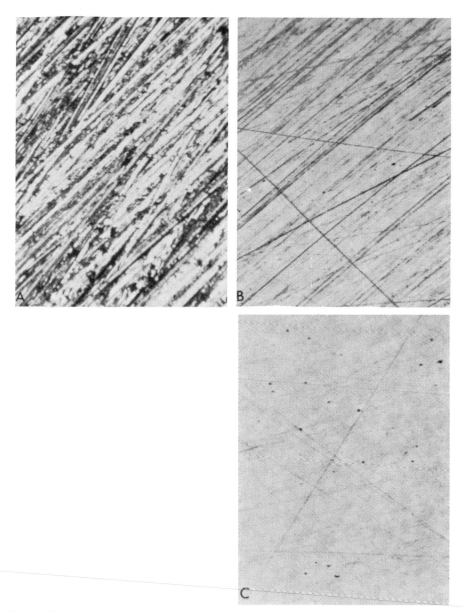

Figure 36–6 Photomicrographs of the surface of a gold casting at three stages during the polishing operation. *A,* Scratches produced by the coarse abrasive used for the initial finishing. *B,* Coarse scratches are obliterated and replaced by smaller scraches as the result of the use of a finer abrasive. *C,* Scratches are virtually eliminated by action of the polishing agent. (From Phillips RW, Elements of Dental Materials, 3rd ed., Philadelphia, W. B. Saunders Co., 1977.)

agent might have a small particle size, it may cut very rapidly because of the sharpness and hardness of the particles. In such a case the rate at which particulate material would be removed from a surface would depend to a considerable degree upon the properties of the material being polished.

Therefore, one agent may be better suited than another for polishing one substance. For example, levigated alumina is often used for polishing metal. It produces an excellent polish layer without removing an undue amount of metal. Although levigated alumina imparts a very high polish to tooth enamel and dentin, it wears away tooth structure very rapidly. Its use in dentistry is confined to the polishing of metals, and it should never be used for polishing teeth.

The optimal speeds for polishing are somewhat higher than for abrading. Linear speeds as high as 10,000 feet per minute may be used. The optimal linear speed varies with different polishing agents, but the average speed is approximately 7500 feet per minute. Very little of the surface is removed during polishing, not more than 0.005 mm (0.0002 inch).

Burnishing   Burnishing is somewhat related to polishing in that the surface is drawn or moved. However, instead of using many tiny particles only one large smooth point is employed. If a round steel point is rubbed over the margin of a gold inlay (Type I or II gold alloy), the metal may be moved so that any small discrepancy between the inlay and the tooth can be closed. The dentist may use this method, or he may employ a special bur revolving at high speed.

It is important that the burnishing instrument not be of such material that it adheres to or dissolves in the surface of the burnished metal. The use of a brass instrument would undoubtedly impregnate copper atoms into the surface of the gold inlay. The reverse practice is sometimes used commercially for "gold plating." For example, a gold layer can be placed on a brass or copper surface by burnishing it with a rapidly revolving gold-wire brush.

Technical Considerations   The techniques to be described are to be used in the dental laboratory on large pieces. Those for use in the mouth are best considered in the dental technique courses. The general principles of the two techniques are fundamentally the same.

The first smoothing of the work can be done with a coarse abrasive or a bur, both of which leave large scratches, as illustrated in Figure 36–6. These scratches are removed with a finer abrasive, but the difference in fineness should not be too great. The use of too fine an abrasive after a relatively coarse abrasive is not economical in time, and it is likely to cause an appearance of streaking or a formation resembling fish tails in the final surface.

After changing to a finer abrasive, the direction of the abrasion should be changed each time if possible, so that the new scratches appear at right angles to the coarser scratches. A more uniform abrasion thus results.

When the scratches are no longer visible to the eye, the preliminary polishing can be accomplished with a pumice flour applied with a canvas buff wheel. Such a procedure is especially valuable in polishing a resin denture.

The work is cleansed thoroughly with soap and water to remove all traces of abrasive and as many of the particles of the material removed by the abrasive as possible. The bench should be cleaned as well.

A paste is formed by mixing the pumice with water to a sticky "muddy" consistency. As water evaporates or is otherwise lost, it should be replenished. The buff wheel should turn at a high speed toward the operator from its top side. The work is grasped firmly in one hand, and some of the pumice paste is applied to the work with the other. The work is then carried into the revolving wheel at its bottom side, and immediately removed. The process is repeated again and again, over the entire surface to be polished, until the surface appears bright and reasonably well polished. It should be stressed that the paste is applied to the work and not to the wheel. The wheel does not hold the pumice. As it revolves, the water and pumice are thrown off by the rotational forces involved.

The work should again be cleansed thoroughly. One grain of abrasive remaining at this stage may roughen the surface to the extent that the entire polishing procedure may need to be repeated. The canvas wheel is replaced with a felt or cotton flannel buff wheel. The wheel should rotate as before at the highest speed available. A polishing agent in cake form, with a grease as a binder, can be used. The cake is held against the wheel until the latter is thoroughly impregnated. The grease aids in holding the polishing agent on the wheel, and at the same time it cushions the action of the polishing agent so that a more uniform finish and luster are attained. The work is held against the wheel and turned so that all of the surfaces are polished uniformly. A light pressure should be used in contacting the work with the wheel so that too much heat is not generated. Such a precaution should be observed especially when a resin denture is polished.

There are a number of reasons for obtaining a high polish on teeth, appliances, and restorations, aside from cosmetic considerations. For example, laboratory studies indicate that smooth enamel and acrylic surfaces are less receptive to bacterial colonization and dental plaque formation.[2, 3] Similarly, a retardation in the formation of dental calculus on smooth enamel surfaces has been reported.[4] Although it has been shown[5] that the use of a high-polish dentifrice significantly increases enamel luster, or smoothness, in children, the clinical impact upon plaque and calculus formation remains to be completely documented. However, without doubt, smooth surfaces are desirable.

Perhaps even more important, the polished layer on metals aids in preventing tarnish and corrosion. Since the entire surface is protected by a homogeneous polish layer, there is less likelihood of electrolytic and similar corrosive actions, as was discussed in Chapter 19. In addition, an appliance or restoration with an extremely rough surface is uncomfortable for the patient.

There is evidence that a Beilby layer may be obtained on enamel surfaces as well as on metal surfaces.[6] In such a case, it might be expected that a highly polished tooth will be more resistant to cariogenic action than one that is not polished. For example, it has been shown that a polished tooth surface is approximately 15 per cent less soluble in acid than one with a rough surface. Such a consideration stresses the importance of a thorough prophylaxis and adequate dental hygiene by the patient.

DENTIFRICES

No discussion of the action of abrasives or polishing agents in dentistry would be complete without mentioning the effect of dentifrices on tooth surfaces.

The primary function of a dentifrice is to assist the toothbrush in cleansing the accessible surfaces of the teeth of stain and debris. Unquestionably, the dentifrice plays an important role in this cleansing procedure. While it is generally recognized that a dentifrice may not be necessary for the removal of debris and superficial portions of dental plaque, it is also accepted that a dentifrice is essential for the removal of stained pellicle. There can be no doubt that some dentifrices are more effective than others in this regard and that the choice of dentifrice should be influenced by the patient's needs.

However, the results of clinical studies comparing the cleaning and polishing properties of dentifrices are rarely published, and manufacturers periodically change the abrasive systems in their formulations, for a variety of reasons. Thus, the effectiveness of dentifrices with regard to cleaning and polishing remains a controversial subject obscured by the lack of published data and the desire of manufacturers to protect commercial interests. The subject of dentifrices as a dental material is discussed only from the physical science viewpoint. A discussion of fluorides and bactericides in dentifrices is not included.

Composition Historically dentifrices have been of three types, dependent upon their general composition: pastes, powders, and liquids. Liquid dentifrices contain no abrasive and are no longer marketed owing to their deficiencies in cleaning, cited earlier. In terms of usage and commercial sales, more than 98 per cent of the dentifrices used today in the United States are in a paste form. The composition of dentifrice pastes and powders is presented in Table 36–2.

Certain basic ingredients are common to all dentifrices, regardless of whether they are pastes or powders. These basic ingredients are a flavoring agent, a detergent, and an abrasive or polishing agent.

Discounting any claims for the therapeutic value of the dentifrice, most people tend to choose a dentifrice on the basis of taste. Thus, the flavoring agent, although directly unimportant to the function, is a major consideration of the manufacturer. For the most part, the flavoring agents are complex mixtures of bland synthetic extracts and essential oils. Artificial sweeteners are employed because the presence of fermentable carbohydrate might have a deleterious effect on tooth structure. Coloring agents are sometimes added to accentuate the flavor and promote consumer acceptance.

The detergent decreases the surface tension of the dentifrice and aids in removing debris from the tooth surface, just as a detergent aids in removing soil from any surface. Examples of dentifrice detergents are sodium lauroyl sulfate and sodium N-lauroyl sarcosinate.

From a functional standpoint the abrasive is the most important ingredient of dentifrices, since it is essential for adequate cleaning. Ideally, a dentifrice should be sufficiently abrasive to remove stain but it should not cut or wear away the tooth structure unduly. The result should be a clean, polished surface. Dentifrice abrasives are insoluble powders that are generally prepared synthetically using carefully controlled conditions to maintain uniformity of particle size and configuration. Commonly used dentifrice abrasives are dibasic calcium phosphate (dihydrate and anhydrous), calcium carbonate, calcium pyrophosphate, insoluble sodium metaphosphate, hydrated silica, alumina (trihydrate and anhydrous), magnesium oxide, and tricalcium phos-

Table 36–2. *Typical Composition of Dentifrices**

TYPE OF CONSTITUENT	PASTE-TYPE DENTIFRICES	POWDER-TYPE DENTIFRICES
Abrasive	20–55%	90–98%
Water	15–25%	0
Humectants	20–35%	0
Detergents	1–2%	1–6%
Binders	1–3%	0
Color and flavor	1–2%	<3%
Therapeutic agents	0–1%	0

*Courtesy of G. Stookey.

phate. In many instances a dentifrice is prepared using a blend of two or more types of abrasives, each of which is selected for a specific purpose.

Typical paste-type dentifrices contain 20 to 30 per cent water. This ingredient gives the formulation the desired consistency and also may serve as a solvent for some of the minor constituents, such as the coloring agent or the fluoride additive.

In order to retard or prevent a paste-type dentifrice from drying out (such as when the cap is not replaced on the tube after use) and to improve the appearance and consistency of the product, a so-called humectant is included. The most commonly used humectants are glycerine, sorbitol, and propylene glycol.

Binders are included in paste-type formulations to prevent the separation of the liquid and solid components and to help maintain the consistency of the dentifrice. Historically, various natural gums have been used for this purpose. In recent times, however, synthetic materials such as carboxymethylcellulose are generally used.

Although an evaluation of the possible therapeutic properties of dentifrices is beyond the scope of this discussion, it should be noted that many formulations contain compounds that may impart additional beneficial characteristics to the dentifrice. In particular, a number of dentifrices contain fluoride, provided as sodium fluoride, stannous fluoride, or sodium monofluorophosphate, to contribute to the control of dental caries. Other formulations contain strontium chloride and other agents which may reduce the sensitivity of exposed dentin or cementum.

It should be emphasized that the mere presence of fluoride, or other potentially therapeutic additives, should not be construed as an indication of effectiveness. Indeed, many instances of a lack of compatibility of dentifrice constituents and therapeutic additives are well known; for example, sodium fluoride is not compatible with many abrasives such as calcium carbonate and dicalcium phosphate. Such incompatibilities obliterate any possible therapeutic benefits of the additive. Thus it is essential that therapeutic benefits be documented through controlled clinical investigations.

From the foregoing overview, it should be apparent that the exact composition of dentifrices is quite variable. Furthermore, it appears that only those dentifrices that are developed, tested, and marketed for their therapeutic properties have a constant composition. The other non-therapeutic dentifrices are in a constant state of formulation modification in an attempt to appeal to other factors that may influence the product selection by the public.

Measurement of Abrasiveness   There is no relationship between the abrasive action of the agent and its ability to produce a smooth tooth surface. For example, as discussed earlier, levigated alumina is effective in producing a highly polished surface yet it is so abrasive that it cannot be used alone in a dentifrice.

Various techniques have been employed for measuring dentifrice and dentifrice ingredient abrasiveness, such as dimensional change and weight loss measurements on tooth structure. Because of the inherent variables in individual tooth surfaces, various metals have been tried as substitutes for the tooth structure itself. The weight loss or dimensional change of blocks of antimony, copper, and silver after brushing with dentifrices has been measured. Although antimony shows the most promise, there is adequate evidence that there is no good correlation between the amount of abrasion on metal plates and that produced on enamel. To date the best method for determining abrasiveness of a dentifrice is on tooth structure itself.

A shadowgraphic method has been used for measuring dentin wear. This study shows that the abrasion of exposed cementum is greater than that of either dentin or enamel when the teeth are brushed at an angle perpendicular to the long axis of the tooth rather than parallel to it.[7] The cervical erosion that is often observed clinically may be owing in part to the abrasive effect of the dentifrice and brush. Dentin abrades approximately 25 times faster than enamel, and cementum 35 times more rapidly than enamel. Also using teeth, other investigators have demonstrated the deleterious effects of certain impurities that may be present in the dentifrice.[8] For example, small amounts of silica greatly increase the abrasiveness of calcium carbonate.

In view of the pronounced effect of impurities that could be present in dentifrices, a qualitative test has been devised to determine the presence of small percentages of highly abrasive particles.[9] The dentifrice is placed on a clean glass slide and rubbed with a metal instrument comparable to a five-cent coin. If a dentifrice powder is used, distilled water is added to produce a slurry. The instrument is rubbed over the slide for 100 double strokes under a given load. A lubricant control, such as glycerol, is used on an adjacent part of the slide. The glass is cleaned with acid to remove any metal particles and the residue is viewed in both transmitted and reflected light. If the test shows greater scratching when the dentifrice is used as compared to the lubricant control, the dentifrice is considered unduly abrasive.

Although this test is not designed to determine quantitatively the relative abrasiveness of commercial products, it is useful in detecting the presence of traces of highly abrasive materials. As little as 0.0156 per cent flour of pumice or 0.0037 per cent silica can be detected in this manner.

During the 1970's, a collaborative research program was initiated by the American Dental Association to identify, refine, and adopt standard procedures for determining the abrasivity of dentifrices to dentin. Although a number of methods were considered, this work ultimately focused upon a profilometric procedure and a radiotracer procedure.[10-12] The latter procedure, with some modifications,[13] has since been identified as the preferred means of determining abrasivity. In essence, this method involves the controlled irradiation of dentin specimens, brushing the radioactive dentin with slurries of a reference abrasive or the dentifrice of interest, and the determination of the radioactivity present in the slurry as a result of dentin abrasion during the brushing period. The degree of abrasivity is then calculated as a ratio relative to that of the reference abrasive.

Abrasion and Polishing of Tooth Structure   The relative abrasive action of several common abrasive and polishing agents on tooth enamel is shown in Table 36–3. By means of specially designed equipment using water slurries of specific concentrations of abrasives, abrasiveness was measured in terms of the thickness of enamel removed from teeth during brushing. It is interesting to note that flour of pumice, which is sometimes used during prophylactic treatment, is highly abrasive and causes as much loss of enamel as does levigated alumina. It is obvious that daily use of such highly abrasive agents is contraindicated and that abrasives such as pumice are totally unsuitable for a dentifrice.

The majority of commercially available dentifrices are very similar with regard to their abrasivity to dentin. In fact, nearly all current dentifrices are

Table 36–3.   *Relative Abrasiveness of Various Compounds on Tooth Enamel* *

ABRASIVE	ABRASION LOSS *(mm)*
Calcium carbonate (extra dense)	0.012
Light chalk (USP)	0.103
Flour of pumice	0.300
Levigated alumina	0.300
Dibasic calcium phosphate, dihydrate	0.001
Dibasic calcium phosphate, anhydrous	0.021
Tribasic calcium phosphate	0.001
Calcium pyrophosphate	0.005
Insoluble sodium metaphosphate and dibasic calcium phosphate (equal parts)	0.001

*From Gershon S, Cosmet Sci Technol, 15:296, 1957.

considered to be within a moderate abrasivity range that is commonly recognized to be without clinically detectable damage to exposed dentin. Even though small differences in abrasivity between products can be observed in vitro, the clinical significance of these observations is doubtful.[14]

The fact that a correlation does not necessarily exist between cutting action and polishing ability can be readily illustrated. Both calcium carbonate and insoluble sodium metaphosphate produced only a slight weight loss; however, there is a vast difference in the degree of polish imparted to the enamel by these two agents. Calcium carbonate yields a dull surface, whereas the insoluble sodium metaphosphate polishes the tooth. The difference in the effects of these two agents on the tooth surface can be seen in Figure 36–7. The

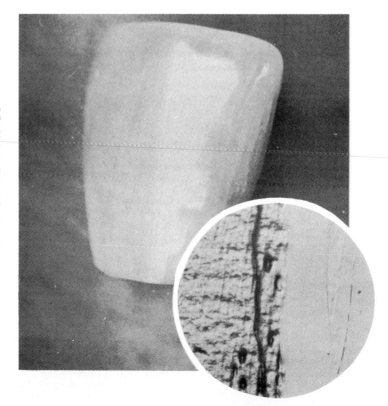

Figure 36–7   The left half of the tooth was brushed with a slurry of calcium carbonate and the right half with a slurry of sodium metaphosphate. The superior polish produced on the right side of the tooth by the sodium metaphosphate is obvious. The microscopic difference in the character of the surfaces can be seen in the insert. (From Phillips RW, Elements of Dental Materials, 3rd ed., Philadelphia, W. B. Saunders Co., 1977.)

left side of the tooth, which is dull, was brushed with the slurry of calcium carbonate, and the right side was brushed with insoluble sodium metaphosphate. The difference in the surfaces is even more pronounced in the insert.

A wide variety of these and other abrasives are used alone and in combination in commercial dentifrices. Therefore, the effect of the various products on the teeth differs with respect to both the abrasion and the character of the surface produced. A group of commercial dentifrices and their principal abrasives are listed in Table 36–4.

These products have been evaluated from the standpoint of their abrasive and polishing characteristics.[15] The abrasion was determined by measuring the amount of tooth structure removed during a given period of brushing. In this particular study the teeth had been placed in an atomic pile in order to make them radioactive. After the teeth were brushed, the slurries of the dentifrices were examined to determine the amount of radioactivity. Thus, the greater the radioactivity of the slurry, the greater is the amount of tooth structure removed and the more abrasive is the dentifrice (Table 36–4, third column). The degree of polish imparted to the enamel was determined by measuring the amount of light reflected from the tooth surface (fourth column). The higher the reading, the greater is the degree of polish.

The data shown in Table 36–4 reveal that there is a difference in the action not only of products that employ different abrasive agents but also between products that contain the same abrasive agent. For example, in both dentifrices A and B insoluble sodium metaphosphate is the principal abrasive. However, dentifrice A produced markedly greater loss of tooth structure and did not polish enamel quite as well as did dentifrice B. The two calcium carbonate dentifrices, C and D, also differed in their behavior.

There are a number of interrelated factors that may assist in explaining these observations. As has been noted, abrasion is a physical process, and the two major physical characteristics that influence the amount of abrasion are the relative hardness of the materials and the particle size of the abrasive. In general, the greater the hardness of the polishing agent as compared with that of enamel or dentin, the greater is the amount of abrasion that may be expected. Table 36–5 shows the relative hardness of some selected materials, and it may be seen, for example, that calcium carbonate exists in two different

Table 36–4. *Abrasion and Polish of Tooth Structure by Commercial Dentifrices**

Brand	Abrasive	Abrasion Dentin	Abrasion Enamel	Polish Enamel
A	Insoluble sodium metaphosphate	194.0	37.6	1.0
B	Insoluble sodium metaphosphate	446.5	3.7	1.2
C	Calcium carbonate	179.0	17.2	0.9
D	Calcium carbonate	433.0	11.3	0.1
E	Calcium pyrophosphate	217.0	20.2	1.2
F	Dicalcium phosphate dihydrate and anhydrous calcium phosphate	83.0	7.6	1.2
G	Dicalcium phosphate dihydrate and anhydrous calcium phosphate	180.0	8.6	0.8

The teeth used for this study were activated in an atomic pile. The degree of abrasion was based upon the radioactivity (^{32}P) of the dentifrice slurry. The higher the count, the greater is the amount of tooth structure removed by the dentifrice. Polish (last column) was assessed by measuring the light reflected off the enamel surface. The higher the value, the greater is the polish.

*From Stookey GK and Muhler JC, J Dent Res, 47:524, 1968.

Table 36–5. *Comparative Hardness of Selected Materials*

SUBSTANCE	KNOOP HARDNESS NUMBER (KHN)
Dentin	65–70
Calcite ($CaCO_3$)	135
Aragonite ($CaCO_3$)	200–260
Enamel	300
Apatite	430
Feldspar	650

crystal forms, calcite and aragonite, which differ appreciably in their relative hardness. Further, the aragonite form more closely approximates the hardness of enamel and may therefore be expected to be more abrasive to enamel than the softer calcite crystal structure.

Concerning the role of particle size in abrasion, it is recognized that the larger the particles of a particular polishing agent are, the greater is the amount of abrasion. Thus, it is quite probable that the explanation for the observed differences between the two calcium carbonate dentifrices reported in Table 36–4 is related to differences in the particle size of the polishing agent and the crystal type of calcium carbonate utilized.

It is recognized that, to be an efficient polishing agent, the particles must be small and have a physical hardness approaching that of the surface being polished. Thus, the generally inferior enamel-polishing abilities of the calcium carbonate dentifrices may be explained, at least in part, on the basis that the polishing agent is softer than enamel and/or has a particle size larger than desired to produce maximum polish.

In addition to these considerations of hardness and particle size, the action of a given abrasive may be modified considerably when it is used in conjunction with other abrasives or incorporated in a paste. For example, paste and powder forms of dentifrices containing the same abrasive do not abrade or polish tooth structure to the same degree. Invariably, the powder has a greater effect. Factors such as the lubricating effect upon the particles of the abrasion by the vehicle used to make the paste contribute to the reduced action.

With everything else equal, a dentifrice that produces a highly polished surface affords certain advantages over one that leaves a scratched or abraded structure. A highly polished tooth surface reflects light and is thereby esthetically superior to that of a dull, abraded tooth surface. Aside from the cosmetic effect, bacteria accumulate more rapidly on a rough abraded enamel surface than upon one which is highly polished. Furthermore, the bacteria are retained in greater numbers by the rough surfaces, even after vigorous brushing.[16] It can be assumed that this would be true of other types of debris, such as foodstuffs or dental plaque.

Thus, it appears that a dentifrice which produces a smooth surface is clinically advantageous. Such a surface looks better and stays cleaner for a longer period of time.

Effect of the Toothbrush The toothbrush itself, whether it be nylon or natural bristle, has no abrasive effect on enamel or dentin. Abrasion of tooth structure is independent of the stiffness or composition of the bristle. It depends almost entirely on the properties of the dentifrice used in conjunction with the toothbrush.

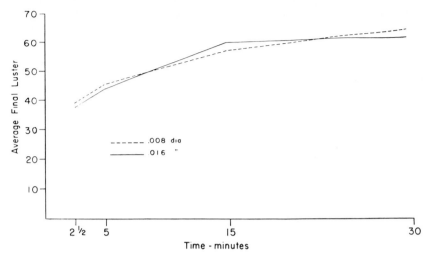

Figure 36–8 Effect of two different diameter nylon toothbrushes on surface luster (arbitrary units) of enamel. Although the same dentifrice was employed, no difference is evident.

The diameter of the bristle does not influence the effect that a given dentifrice produces on the enamel surface. This is demonstrated in Figure 36–8, in which two nylon brushes of widely varying bristle diameters were used in conjunction with a dentifrice which tends to polish the enamel surface.[17] The change in luster varies little with either brush. Furthermore, the effect of the polishing agent is neither impaired nor enhanced by the wetness of the bristle.

An epidemiologic study has been reported in which an attempt was made to relate various factors, including toothbrushes and dentifrices, to clinical dentin abrasion.[18] The results of that investigation indicated that the most important factors associated with clinical abrasion were the frequency and manner of toothbrushing. Contributing factors of lesser importance were dentifrice abrasivity and the hardness of the toothbrush.

References

1. Pines M, Schulman A, and Vaidyanathan JK: SEM evaluation of commercial diamond stones. IADR Program and Abstracts, No. 509, 1981.
2. Swartz ML and Phillips RW: Comparison of bacterial accumulations on rough and smooth enamel surfaces. J Periodontol 28:304, 1957.
3. Wickliffe TJ, Liu KT, and Katz S: Enamel polishing and its effects on bacterial adhesion. IADR Program and Abstracts, No. 790, 1971.
4. Barnes GP, Stookey GK, and Muhler JC: In vitro studies of the calculus-inhibiting properties of tooth surfaces, polishing agents and chelating agents. J Dent Res 50:966, 1971.
5. Sturzenberger OP, Beiswanger BB, and King JD: Method for the clinical evaluation of enamel polish. J Dent Res 54:931, 1975.
6. Skinner EW, Osborne J, Copeland PL, and Fiegel LJ: Surface structure of enamel and apatite — a progress report. IADR Program and Abstracts, No. 70, 1957.
7. Manly RS: Factors influencing tests on the abrasion of dentin by brushing with dentifrices. J Dent Res 23:59, 1944.
8. Tainter ML and Epstein S: A standard procedure for determining abrasion by dentifrices. J Am Coll Dent 9:353, 1942.

9. Souder W and Schoonover IC: A specification for toothpaste. J Am Dent Assoc 24:1817, 1937.
10. Ashmore H, van Abbe NJ, and Wilson SJ: The measurement in vitro of dentine abrasion by toothpaste. Br Dent J 133:60, 1972.
11. Davis WB and Winter PJ: Measurement in vitro of enamel abrasion by dentifrice. J Dent Res 55:970, 1976.
12. Grabenstetter RJ, Broge RW, Jackson FL, and Radike AW: The measurement of the abrasion of human teeth by dentifrice abrasives: A test utilizing radioactive teeth. J Dent Res 37:1060, 1958.
13. Hefferren JJ: A laboratory method for assessment of dentifrice abrasivity. J Dent Res 55:563, 1976.
14. Volpe AR, Mooney R, Zumbrunnen C, Stahl D, and Goldman HM: A long term clinical study evaluating the effect of two dentifrices on oral tissues. J Periodontol 46:113, 1975.
15. Stookey GK and Muhler JC: Laboratory studies concerning the enamel and dentin abrasion properties of common dentifrice polishing agents. J Dent Res 47:524, 1968.
16. Swartz ML and Phillips RW: Comparison of bacterial accumulations on rough and smooth enamel surfaces. J Periodontol 28:304, 1957.
17. Phillips RW and Swartz ML: Effects of diameter of nylon bristles on enamel surface. J Am Dent Assoc 47:20, 1953.
18. Bergstrom J and Lavstedt S: An epidemiologic approach to toothbrushing and dentin abrasion. Community Dent Oral Epidemiol 7:57, 1979.

37 WROUGHT BASE METAL ALLOYS

A number of wrought base metal alloys are used in dentistry, mainly as wires for orthodontic treatment. The metallography of these alloys is extremely complex and only applications of practical interest will be discussed. The primary alloy used for orthodontic wire is stainless steel, an iron-chromium-nickel alloy. Other major systems for this application include cobalt-chromium-nickel, nickel-titanium, and beta titanium alloys. Before considering each of these systems in detail, a brief discussion of their application in orthodontics is appropriate.

PROPERTIES OF ORTHODONTIC WIRES

Orthodontic wires are formed into various configurations or appliances in order to apply forces to teeth and move them into a more desirable alignment. The force system is determined by the appliance design and the material properties of the wire. For a given design and deflection, the force applied to the tooth is proportional to the wire's modulus of elasticity. Low, constant forces are biologically desirable,[1] although a threshold force level is necessary for tooth movement. Large elastic deflections are clinically desirable, since they produce a more constant force during the time of tooth movement and allow for greater activation or "working range". The maximum elastic deflection of an orthodontic wire is proportional to its ratio of yield strength to modulus of elasticity. The maximum force that can be applied is a function of the yield strength.

Other material properties are also important in orthodontic treatment. A ductile wire can be formed into various shapes, although there are applications which do not require permanent bends. Ease of joining is important, and most wires can be either soldered or welded together. Finally, the wire must demonstrate corrosion resistance, stability in the oral environment, and biocompatibility.

As has been pointed out, the stainless steels constitute the major alloy system used in orthodontics. However, the metallurgy and terminology of these alloys are intimately connected to that of the simpler binary iron-carbon alloy system and the ordinary carbon steel alloys. Therefore this discussion will begin with a brief outline of the metallurgy of the iron-carbon system.

CARBON STEEL

An understanding of the complex metallurgy of *carbon steel* begins with the equilibrium phase diagram for the iron-carbon system. Note in Figure 37–1 that, following tradition, the two components on the composition axis are iron and the metastable iron carbide (Fe_3C), which is referred to as *cementite*. The decomposition rate of iron carbide to form iron and carbon (graphite) is so low that this is quite reasonable.

The carbon atom is too small to form a substitutional solid solution with iron. However, the atom is too large to allow for extensive interstitial solid solution formation.

Pure iron at room temperature has a body-centered cubic (BCC) structure and is referred to as α-iron or *ferrite*. This phase is stable up to 912° C (1674° F). The spaces between atoms in the BCC structure (interstices) are small and oblate, hence carbon has a very low solubility in ferrite (0.02 weight per cent maximum).

At temperatures between 912° C (1674° F) and 1394° C (2541° F) the stable form of iron is a face-centered cubic (FCC) structure called γ-iron or *austenite*. The interstices (holes) in the FCC lattice are larger than in the BCC structure. However, the size of the carbon atom is such that the resulting lattice strain still limits the maximum carbon solubility to 2.11 weight per cent. Since, by definition, steel is an alloy of iron containing less than 1.2 per cent carbon, the carbon in steel is entirely soluble in the solid state at elevated temperatures.

As can be seen in Figure 37–1, iron-carbon alloys containing carbon in excess of the solubility limit must form the second phase iron carbide. Iron

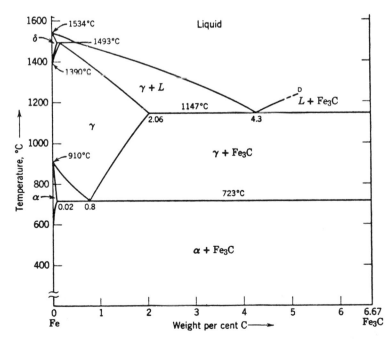

Figure 37–1 Phase diagram of the iron-carbon system. (Modified from Moffatt, et al, Structure and Properties of Materials, Vol. 1, New York, John Wiley & Sons, 1964.)

carbide is a hard, brittle material. The ferritic or austenitic forms of iron are soft and ductile. The combination of a soft, ductile matrix with a hard, brittle filler forms a *composite* material in analogy to the composite resins studied in Chapter 14. The ability to alter the proportion of filler to matrix (and hence the mechanical properties) by small changes in the carbon content is one of the reasons for the prominent role of steel as an engineering material.

Considering the portion of the equilibrium phase diagram that contains compositions corresponding to steel alloys (C < 1.2 per cent), an invariant transformation is seen to occur at a carbon concentration of 0.77 per cent and a temperature of 727° C (1341° F).

This transformation on cooling is the decomposition of austenite to form ferrite and iron carbide. Schematically this can be written

$$\gamma \rightarrow \alpha + Fe_3C$$

This is referred to as the *eutectoid* reaction and is the solid state analog of the eutectic transformation described in Chapter 17. Solid state diffusion is required to produce the carbon-poor ferrite and the carbon-rich carbide. The resulting microstructure is a lamellar composition with alternate layers of ferrite and carbide similar to that shown in the eutectic lead-tin alloy in Figure 17–7. This microstructure is called *pearlite*. Steel alloys having compositions above or below the eutectoid composition would form areas of primary carbide or ferrite, respectively, in addition to pearlite, on cooling, in analogy to the situation described in Chapter 17 for hyper- and hypoeutectic alloys.

Because the eutectoid decomposition of austenite is a solid state reaction and requires solid state diffusion of carbon atoms, the microstructure of the two phase system will be extremely dependent on rate of cooling through and below the transformation temperature. In principle, if instantaneous cooling could be achieved, the non-equilibrium austenite could be retained at room temperature just as non-equilibrium phases were obtained by rapid cooling (quenching) of certain dental alloys, described in Chapter 18. However, austenitic iron-carbon alloys will undergo a spontaneous transformation at low temperatures (120–220° C) to form a single non-equilibrium phase, not shown in Figure 37–1.

This phase is called *martensite* and is formed by a simultaneous shearing of the entire FCC austenite lattice to form a body-centered tetragonal (BCT) structure. This transformation does not require diffusion and occurs very rapidly. The resulting BCT structure is highly distorted and the large amounts of trapped strain result in a very hard, strong, brittle alloy.

The formation of martensite is an important strengthening mechanism for carbon steels. The cutting edges of carbon steel instruments are ordinarily martensitic, since the extreme hardness allows for grinding a sharp edge that will be retained in use. Martensite will decompose to form ferrite and carbide. This process can be accelerated by appropriate heat treatment and reduces the hardness but increases the toughness. Such a heat treatment is called *tempering*.

Hardness of Steel   The two factors that are of primary importance in determining the hardness of a steel are the carbon content and the per cent of austenite which transforms to martensite during cooling.[2] The hardness will increase with carbon content and with an increase in the per cent transformation to martensite.

If cooling is more rapid than the *critical cooling rate* for any particular alloy, only martensite will be formed from austenite. A slower cooling rate will produce a structure containing some or all ferrite plus carbide. The lower the critical cooling rate — i.e., the greater the time required for the formation of ferrite plus cementite at a particular temperature — the greater is the hardness of the steel. The critical cooling rate, and thus the hardness, depends upon composition.

Of all the common alloying elements added to steel only cobalt decreases the hardness. This element increases both the rate of nucleation and the rate of growth of pearlite. Other alloying elements decrease the rate of diffusion of the carbon. In a steel high in alloying elements (with the exception of cobalt), pearlite formation will be so delayed that martensite will form at even rather slow cooling rates.

The various alloying elements also depress the temperature at which martensite formation begins and ends. Carbon is by far the most effective element in this respect. In austenitic stainless steel the alloying elements, especially the chromium and nickel, make the diffusion rate of carbon so low that austenite cannot decompose to pearlite, and the temperature is too low to allow the formation of martensite. Therefore, austenite is retained at room temperature and below.

STAINLESS STEEL

Chromium Steels   When the chromium content of a steel exceeds 11 per cent (generally in the 12 to 30 per cent range), the alloy is commonly defined as *stainless steel*. Elements other than iron, carbon, and chromium may also be present, resulting in a wide variation in composition and properties of the stainless steels. Room temperature yield strengths may range from 211 MPa (30,000 psi) to over 1760 MPa (250,000 psi), for example.

These steels resist tarnish and corrosion primarily because of the passivating effect of the chromium. Simply stated, a very thin, transparent but tough and impervious oxide layer forms on the surface of the alloy when it is subjected to an oxidizing atmosphere as mild as clean air. This protective oxide layer prevents further tarnish and corrosion. If the oxide layer is ruptured by mechanical or chemical means, a loss of protection against corrosion results.

There are essentially three types of stainless steels. This classification, with approximate compositions, is seen in Table 37–1.

Surgical and cutting instruments would be made from the martensitic alloy for greater strength and hardness. If corrosion resistance is more important than strength or hardness, an austenitic stainless steel would be used. Dental applications include sterilizing equipment, autoclaves, instrument cabinets, operating table tops, and orthodontic bands and wires.

Table 37–1.   *Composition (Percentages) of the Three Basic Types of Stainless Steel*

Type (space lattice)	Cr	Ni	C
Ferritic (bcc)	11.5–27	0	0.2 max.
Austenitic (fcc)	16–26	7–22	0.25 max.
Martensitic (bct)	11.5–17	0–2.5	0.15–1.20

Si, P, S, Mn, Ta, Ti, and Nb may also be present in small amounts. The balance is iron.

One austenitic stainless steel is also popular as an implant and splinting material.

The ferritic alloys provide good corrosion resistance at lower cost, provided strength is not required.

Ferritic Stainless Steels (AISI* series 400. This series number is shared with the martensitic alloys.) The essential composition of *ferritic* stainless steel is shown in Table 37–1. The high chromium and low carbon content results in the austenite region shrinking to nonexistence. The higher the Cr/C ratio, the more extensive and stable is the ferrite phase.

Since temperature change induces no phase change in the solid state, the alloy is not hardenable by heat treatment. Also, ferritic stainless steel is not readily work hardenable. Corrosion resistance, even at high temperature, is good.

Martensitic Stainless Steels As noted, these martensitic stainless steel alloys share the type 400 designation with the ferritic alloys. They can be heat treated in the same manner as plain carbon steels, with similar results. Since the chromium content is 11.5 to 18 per cent, atomic diffusion is retarded and hardness is high.

If the chromium content of the alloy exceeds 18 per cent, austenite cannot exist at any temperature. Since martensite is formed from a thermal transformation of austenite, a martensitic stainless steel is limited to an 18 per cent chromium content. A ferritic stainless alloy is not so restricted, since it is body-centered at all temperatures. Were it not for the fact that carbon and nickel act to expand the austenitic region, the chromium content of the martensitic stainless steel would be even more limited than it is. Except for a higher carbon content, the composition of a martensitic and ferritic stainless steel could be essentially the same.

The nickel content of a martensitic stainless steel is also limited. Nickel, along with the chromium that is necessary to make the steel corrosion resistant, depresses the martensite formation temperature and slows atomic diffusion.

Yield strength of a high carbon martensitic stainless steel may range from 492 MPa (70,000 psi) in the annealed condition up to 1898 MPa (270,000 psi) in the hardened (quenched and tempered) state. The corresponding BHN range would be 230 to 600.

Corrosion resistance of the martensitic stainless steel is less than that of the other types and is reduced following a hardening heat treatment. As usual, when the strength and hardness increase, ductility decreases. It may go as low as 2 per cent elongation for a high carbon martensitic stainless steel.

Austenitic Stainless Steels The *austenitic* stainless steel alloys are the most corrosion resistant of the stainless steels. AISI 302 is the basic type, containing 18 per cent chromium, 8 per cent nickel, and 0.15 per cent carbon. Type 304 has a similar composition, the chief difference being that the carbon content is limited to 0.08 per cent. Both 302 and 304 may be designated as *18–8 stainless steel* and are the types most commonly used by the orthodontist in the form of bands and wires. Type 316L (0.03 per cent maximum carbon) is the type ordinarily employed for implants.

---

*American Iron & Steel Institute.

Transformation of austenite to ferrite can be induced at elevated temperatures by the removal of chromium from the solid solution through the formation of chromium carbide complexes or the precipitation of chromium-rich intermetallic compounds. This loss of chromium from the solid solution will also reduce the corrosion resistance of the alloy. This loss of corrosion resistance of an austenitic stainless steel by removal of chromium from the gamma solid solution is termed *sensitization* and will be discussed further in a subsequent section. Conversely, methods employed to retain the chromium in the solid solution are called *stabilization*.

Cold working can also bring about a transformation of some austenite to a body-centered lattice.

The high chromium and nickel content not only reduces the rate of transformation of austenite to ferrite but also depresses the martensite start temperature so much that the austenite does not transform to martensite.

The net result of inhibiting transformation of austenite to either ferrite or martensite provides a stable austenitic structure down to the temperature of liquid nitrogen. Thus, this 300 series of steels cannot be hardened by heat treatment. However, they are readily hardened by cold working.

Generally, austenitic stainless steel is preferable to the ferritic alloys because of[3]:

1. Greater ductility and ability to undergo more cold work without breaking.
2. Substantial strengthening during cold working (some transformation to a body-centered lattice).
3. Greater ease of welding.
4. Fairly readily overcome sensitization.
5. Less critical grain growth.
6. Comparative ease in forming.

Sensitization The 18–8 stainless steel may lose its resistance to corrosion if it is heated between 400° and 900° C (752° and 1652° F), the exact temperature depending upon its carbon content. Such temperatures are definitely within the range used by the orthodontist in soldering and welding; therefore, this effect merits further discussion.

The reason for a decrease in corrosion resistance is the precipitation of chromium carbide at the grain boundaries at the high temperatures. The small, rapidly diffusing carbon atoms migrate to the grain boundaries from all parts of the crystal to combine with the large, slowly diffusing chromium atoms at the periphery of the grain where the energy is highest. The formation of Cr_3C is most rapid at 650° C (1202° F). Below that temperature the diffusion rate is less while above it a decomposition of Cr_3C begins. When the chromium combines with the carbon in this manner, its passivating qualities are lost, and, as a consequence, the corrosion resistance of the steel is reduced. Because that portion of the grain adjacent to the grain boundary is the portion generally "robbed" of chromium to produce the carbide, an intergranular corrosion occurs, and a partial disintegration of the metal may result with a general weakening of the structure.

There are several methods by which this condition can be minimized. An obvious method from a theoretical standpoint would be to reduce the carbon content of the steel to an extent that such carbide precipitation cannot occur. However, in general, this remedy is not economically feasible.

If the stainless steel is severely cold worked, the carbides precipitate along the slip planes. As a result, the distribution of the areas deficient in chromium is less localized, or, in other words, the carbides are more uniformly distributed so that the resistance to corrosion is greater than when only the grain boundaries are involved. Such a method is presumably relied upon in orthodontic stainless steel wires.

Stabilization   The method employed most successfully is the introduction of some element that precipitates as a carbide in preference to chromium. Titanium is often used for this purpose. If titanium is introduced, in amount approximately six times the carbon content, the precipitation of chromium carbide can be inhibited for a short time at the temperatures ordinarily encountered in soldering procedures. Stainless steels that have been treated in this manner are said to be *stabilized*. Unfortunately, very few, if any, of the stainless steels used in orthodontics are so stabilized.

General Causes of Corrosion   As previously noted, the function of the chromium is to prevent corrosion by oxidation. The situation in respect to the prevention of electrolytic corrosion is somewhat analogous to that of dental amalgam discussed in Chapter 19.

Any surface inhomogeneity is a potential source of tarnish or corrosion. Severe strain hardening may produce localized electric couples in the presence of an electrolyte such as saliva. Any surface roughness or unevenness may allow corrosion cells to form. The stainless steel orthodontic appliance should be polished not only for the comfort of the patient but also so that it remains cleaner and freer from tarnish or corrosion during use.

A common cause of the corrosion of a stainless steel is the incorporation of bits of carbon steel or similar metal in its surface. For example, if the stainless steel wire is manipulated carelessly with carbon steel pliers, it is conceivable that some of the steel from the pliers may become embedded in the stainless steel. Or if the stainless steel appliance is abraded or cut with a carbon steel bur or similar steel tool, some of the steel from the tool may also become embedded in the stainless steel. Such a situation results in an electric couple that may cause considerable corrosion.

Solder joints in orthodontic appliances also lead to a galvanic couple. In addition, austenitic stainless steels are susceptible to attack by solutions containing chlorine. Chlorine containing cleansers should not be used to clean removable appliances fabricated from stainless steel.

Mechanical Properties   The general range of the mechanical properties of 18–8 stainless steel is presented in Table 37–2. In orthodontic wires, strength and hardness may increase with a decrease in the diameter because of the amount of cold working in forming the wire. Tensile strengths of 2100 MPa (300,000 psi), yield strengths of 1400 MPa (200,000 psi), and Knoop hardness values of 600 may be expected. Regardless of their treatment, the austenitic stainless steels are definitely not so strong or hard as many of the carbon steels. Cold working during the fabrication of stainless steel orthodontic wires contributes a substantial proportion to the strength values shown in Table 37–2.

The property of being readily strain hardened is a characteristic of austenitic stainless steel. Part of this increase in hardness is ordinary strain hardening, but a considerable amount is the result of phase change from a face-centered to a body-centered lattice. This phase change can be readily

Table 37–2. *Mechanical Properties of Orthodontic Wires*

Alloy	Modulus of Elasticity 10³ MPa (10⁶ psi)	0.2% Offset Yield Strength MPa (10³ psi)	Ultimate Tensile Strength MPa (10³ psi)	Number of 90° Cold Bends without Fracture*
Stainless steel	179 (26.0)	1579 (229)	2117 (307)	5
Chromium-cobalt-nickel	184 (26.7)	1413 (205)	1682 (244)	8
Nickel-titanium	41.4 (6.0)	427 (62)	1489 (216)	2
Beta titanium	71.7 (10.4)	931 (135)	1276 (185)	4

*ADA Specification no. 32 for Orthodontic Wires, 0.432 × 0.635 mm (0.017 × 0.025 inch) wires.

demonstrated, since the body-centered lattices (ferrite and martensite) are ferromagnetic at room temperature; austenite is nonmagnetic. Unfortunately, after strain hardening, a stainless steel wire can become fully annealed in a few seconds at a temperature of 700 to 800° C (1292 to 1472° F). After such an annealing, it has lost much of the range of elasticity or working range so necessary to a satisfactory orthodontic appliance. Because the annealing temperatures involved are in the soldering and welding temperature ranges normally employed, an unavoidable softening of the wire during normal heating operations is a decided disadvantage unless the wire can be subsequently strain hardened.

This disadvantage can be minimized by using low-fusing solders and by confining the time for soldering and welding procedures to a minimum. Any softening that occurs under such conditions of heating can be remedied considerably by the strain hardening incurred in subsequent operations, such as contouring and polishing.

Braided and Twisted Wires Very small diameter stainless steel wires can be braided or twisted together by the manufacturer to form wires for clinical orthodontics. The separate strands may be as small as 0.178 mm (0.007 inch), but the final intertwined wires may be either round or rectangular in shape and between 0.406 mm (0.016 inch) and 0.635 mm (0.025 inch) in overall cross section. Figure 37–2 shows a magnified cross section of two such wires.

Braided or twisted wires are able to sustain large elastic deflections in bending. Because of their low "apparent" modulus in bending, these wires

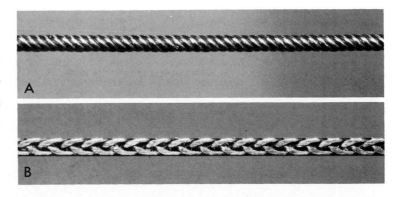

Figure 37–2 Multistranded stainless steel wires for orthodontic application. *A,* Twisted form with an overall diameter of 0.44 mm (.0175 inch). *B,* Braided form with overall dimensions of 0.44 × 0.63 mm (.017 × .025 inch). (Courtesy of JY Morton and J Goldberg.)

apply low forces for a given deflection when compared with solid stainless steel wire.

Solders for Stainless Steel   It is important that the stainless steel wire not be heated to too high a temperature, in order to minimize carbide precipitation and to prevent an excessive softening of the wire so that its usefulness is lost. The requirement of a low temperature soldering technique generally rules out of consideration any of the gold solders normally employed with gold alloy wires because their melting points are generally too high. In order for a gold solder to be sufficiently low melting for the soldering of stainless steel, a fineness of approximately 250 (10-karat solder) is necessary. With such a low corrosion resistance, it makes little difference in this respect from a practical standpoint whether such a gold solder or a silver solder is used.

Silver solders are essentially alloys of silver, copper, and zinc to which elements such as tin and indium may be added to lower fusion temperatures and improve solderability.

Although such solders definitely corrode in use because they are anodic to the stainless steel, in orthodontic appliances such a condition is not too objectionable. The appliance is a temporary structure, not usually worn in the mouth for more than 6 to 30 months, and frequent inspections by the orthodontist are necessary.

The soldering temperatures for orthodontic silver solders are in the range of 620 to 665° C (1150–1250° F). The solidus-liquidus ranges of the solders should be small. This is an important characteristic of the solder for free-hand soldering as normally practiced by the orthodontist. In free-hand soldering, the solder should harden promptly when the work is removed from the flame. Otherwise, the operator tires and unavoidably moves the work before the solder has completely solidified, and the joint is thus weakened.

Fluxes   In addition to the usual reducing and cleaning agents incorporated in a flux, a flux used for soldering stainless steel also contains a fluoride to dissolve the passivating film supplied by the chromium. The solder will not wet the metal when such a film is present. Potassium fluoride is one of the most active chemicals in this respect.[4]

The flux is similar to that recommended for gold soldering, with the exception of the addition of the potassium fluoride. The boric acid is used in a greater ratio to the borax than in the flux for gold soldering because it lowers the fusion temperature.

Technical Considerations   The free-hand soldering operation with stainless steel is not greatly different from that of gold soldering described in Chapter 33.

A needle-like, nonluminous, gas-air flame may be used. The thinner the diameter of the flame, the less the metal surrounding the joint is annealed. The work should be held about 3 mm (⅛ inch) beyond the tip of the blue cone, in the reducing zone of the flame. The soldering should be observed in a shadow, against a black background, so that the temperature can be judged by the color of the work. The color should never exceed a dull red.

If possible, prior to soldering, the parts should be tack welded together to hold them in alignment during the soldering procecure. Then flux should be applied and the heavier gauge part should be heated first. Flux must cover all of the areas to be soldered before heat is applied. As soon as the flux fuses, solder should be added and heating continued until the solder flows around the joint. After the solder has flowed, the work should be immediately removed from the heat and quenched in water. Based on the previous discussion of the metallurgy of the austenitic stainless steels, it should be evident that the objective during soldering is to use as little heat as possible, for as short a time as possible.

In addition to the conventional gas-air blowpipe a number of other techniques can be used to supply the heat for soldering. These include a hydrogen-oxygen torch, electric resistance heating of the solder, and indirect heating using a brass wire intermediary. The direct heating techniques have been shown to produce comparable joints in terms of strength. In particular, the gas-air and hydrogen-oxygen torches produce very similar results.[5]

A photomicrograph of a cross section of stainless steel wire-silver solder junction is shown in Figure 37–3. Although intimate contact between the metals is seen, present evidence indicates that no measurable amount of atomic diffusion occurs at the interface and that the bond is strictly mechanical.[6] The tensile strength of a good silver solder joint can exceed that of the bulk silver solder. Interfacial constraint between the thin layer of solder and the harder wire could conceivably account for the higher strength of the joint.[7, 8]

WELDING

Although soldering of orthodontic wires is not uncommon, flat structures such as bands and brackets are usually joined by welding. The electric spot welding apparatus produces a large electric current which is forced to flow through a limited area (spot) on the overlapped materials that are to be welded. The

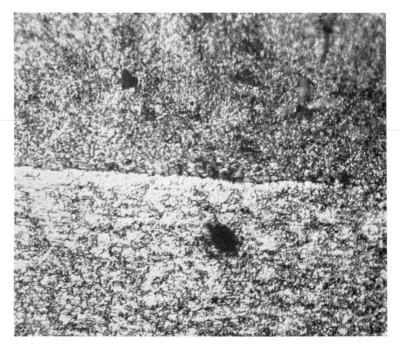

Figure 37–3 Photomicrograph of a soldered joint between a stainless steel orthodontic wire and a silver solder. × 800.

resistance of the material to the flow of current produces intense localized heating and actual fusion of the overlapped metals. No solder is employed. Ideally, the melting is confined to the junction area and can be observed metallographically in cross section as a *nugget* of resolidified cast structure. The grain structure of the surrounding alloy should not be affected.

The strength of the welded joint is decreased with increasing recrystallization of the wrought structure. The strength becomes greater by an increase in the weld area.[9]

Corrosion   The weld joint area becomes susceptible to corrosion, primarily because of chromium carbide precipitation and consequent loss of passivation.

WROUGHT COBALT-CHROMIUM-NICKEL ALLOYS

Cobalt-chromium-nickel alloys drawn into wire can be used successfully in orthodontic appliances. These alloys were originally developed for use as watch springs (Elgiloy), but their properties are also excellent for orthodontic purposes.

The wires are furnished to the orthodontist in different gauges and cross-sectional shapes with differing physical properties as well. Their resistance to corrosion and tarnish in the mouth is excellent. Furthermore, they can be subjected to the same welding and soldering procedures as described for the stainless steel orthodontic wires.

Composition   A representative composition for such an alloy is: Co, 40 per cent; Cr, 20 per cent; Ni, 15 per cent; Mo, 7 per cent; Mn, 2 per cent; C, 0.15 per cent; Be, 0.04 per cent; and Fe, 15.8 per cent.

Heat Treatment   A cobalt-chromium-nickel alloy may be softened by heat soaking at 1100 to 1200° C (2012 to 2192° F), followed by a rapid quench. The age-hardening temperature range is 260 to 650° C (500 to 1202° F), e.g., holding at 482° C (900° F) for five hours as recommended by the manufacturer of Elgiloy.

Ordinarily the wires are heat treated before being supplied to the user and may be ordered in several degrees of hardness (soft, ductile, semispring temper, and spring temper). The orthodontist can, in addition, heat treat the wires either in an oven or by passing an electric current through the wire by using certain types of spot welders. A typical cycle would be 482° C (900° F) for 7 to 12 minutes. This heat treatment would increase the yield strength and decrease the ductility.

Wires made from this alloy should not be annealed. The resulting softening cannot be reversed by subsequent heat treatment. Moreover, if only a portion of a wire is annealed, severe enbrittlement of adjacent sections may occur.

Physical Properties   Tarnish and corrosion resistance is excellent. Hardness, yield, and tensile strength are much the same as those of 18–8 stainless steel. Typical mechanical properties are shown in Table 37–2. Ductility in the softened condition is greater than that of the 18–8 stainless steel alloys, and less in the hardened condition.

RECOVERY HEAT TREATMENT

An increase in the *measured* elastic properties of a wire can be effected by heating it to comparatively low temperatures (370–480° C [690–896° F]) after it has been cold worked. This *stress relief heat treatment* removes residual stresses during recovery without pronounced alteration in mechanical properties. Such a treatment also stabilizes the shape of the appliance.

For an 18–8 stainless steel wire, the apparent effect is a slight increase in the modulus of elasticity, a somewhat greater increase in the yield strength, and a considerable increase in the modulus of resilience.

If the wire is bent into tight loops of 180°, or a spiral of small radius, the measured increase in elastic strength may be as great as 50 per cent. Phase change during the heat treatment (in the temperature range of 370–480° C) cannot account for this strength increase. Release of residual stress is the explanation generally given.

When a force is applied to a wire in bending, tension, or torsion the total stresses that are present are the sum of the residual stresses and those induced by the load. Thus, when a wire has been bent sharply or coiled, the residual stresses are much higher and more concentrated than in a straight piece of wire. Therefore, less additional stress from the external force is required to produce plastic deformation than is required in a straight wire. Also the measured increase in the yield strength after a stress relief heat treatment is greater for the formed appliance.

Cobalt-chromium-nickel wires are more responsive than the 18–8 stainless wires to the low temperature heat treatment. A reduction in ductility accompanies the increase in yield strength. A phase change as well as stress relief is probably responsible. As has been noted, caution must be used to avoid excessive enbrittlement.

Although the optimum temperature range for the stress relief heat treatment is most often reported as 370 to 480° C, there appears to be no reason to exceed the low temperature limit of 370° C when the wire is a nonstabilized grade of austenitic stainless steel. Eleven minutes at approximately 370° C results in a maximum proportional limit for a severely cold-worked appliance.[10] This temperature is also below the lower limit (425° C [797° F]) of the sensitization temperature range.

A stress relief heat treatment not only improves the working elastic properties of a wire appliance but also can reduce failure due to corrosion, which may occur in areas of high localized stress.[10]

NICKEL-TITANIUM ALLOYS

The alloys previously discussed in this chapter have, in general, similar mechanical properties. Although processing, stress relieving, and heat treating allow for small product differences, those wrought base metals have elastic moduli in the range of 152 to 200 × 10³ MPa (22–29 × 10⁶ psi), while yield strengths range between 1170 and 2070 MPa (169 and 300 × 10³ psi). The wires with lower strength usually have superior formability. The nickel-titanium alloy (Nitinol) represented the first significant change in properties for base metal orthodontic wires.[11]

Mechanical Properties   The modulus of elasticity of Nitinol is 41.4×10^3 MPa (6.0×10^6 psi), the yield strength is 427 MPa (62,000 psi), and the ultimate tensile strength is 1489 MPa (216,000 psi). These properties result in very low orthodontic forces when compared with similarly constructed and activated stainless steel appliances (Table 37–2). The low stiffness in combination with moderately high strength account for this wire's large elastic deflections, or working range. The alloy has limited formability.

Composition and "Shape Memory"   The original Nitinol alloy contained 55 per cent Ni and 45 per cent Ti, which resulted in a one-to-one atomic ratio of its two components. The most unique feature of the alloy is the "memory" phenomenon, which is a result of temperature induced crystallographic transformations.[12] After establishing a shape at temperatures near 482° C (900° F), the cooled wire can be permanently deformed. Subsequent heating through a lower transition temperature causes the wire to return to its original shape. The orthodontic Nitinol wire contains 1.6 per cent cobalt to bring the lower transition temperature near 37° C (98° F). The memory principle is not used clinically, although research in this area is continuing. Nevertheless, the mechanical properties of Nitinol still make it an advantageous orthodontic wire for certain clinical situations.

Nitinol wires have to be joined by mechanical crimps, since the alloy can be neither soldered nor welded.

BETA TITANIUM ALLOYS

Crystallographic Forms   Like stainless steel and Nitinol, pure titanium has different crystallographic forms at high and low temperatures. At temperatures below 885° C (1625° F) the hexagonal close-packed (HCP) or alpha lattice is stable, while at higher temperatures the metal rearranges into a body-centered cubic (BCC) or beta crystal. The hexagonal close-packed lattice has room-temperature modulus and yield strength values of 110×10^3 MPa (16×10^6 psi) and 379 MPa (55×10^3 psi), respectively.

Ti-6 per cent Al-4 per cent V, a representative commercial alloy based on the HCP lattice, can have a yield strength as high as 965 MPa (140,000 psi). These properties in a wrought wire, however, do not result in improved springback characteristics when compared with austenitic stainless steel, so that alpha titanium has not been used in orthodontic applications,

Through the addition of alloying elements like molybdenum, the beta form of titanium can be stabilized down to room temperature. An alloy with the composition Ti-11 per cent Mo-6 per cent Zr-4 per cent Sn is produced in wrought wire form for orthodontic application.[13]

Mechanical Properties   Wrought beta titanium orthodontic wire has a modulus of elasticity of 71.7×10^3 MPa (10.4×10^6 psi) and a yield strength between 860 and 1170 MPa (125 and 170×10^3 psi). These properties produce several clinically desirable characteristics. The low modulus allows for low forces even with large deflections. The high ratio of yield strength to modulus produces orthodontic appliances that can sustain large elastic activations when compared with stainless steel devices of the same geometry.

Beta titanium can be highly cold worked. The wrought wire can be bent into various orthodontic configurations and has formability comparable to austenitic stainless steel.

The mechanical properties of many titanium alloys can be altered to heat

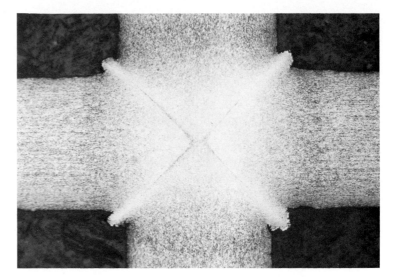

Figure 37–4 Photomicrograph of a weld joint between two 0.43 × 0.63 mm (.017 × .025 inch) beta titanium orthodontic wires showing minimum distortion of the original cold-worked microstructure. (Courtesy of TC Labenski and J Goldberg.)

treatments which utilize the alpha to beta transition. However, heat treatment of the current orthodontic beta titanium wire is not recommended.

Welding   Clinically satisfactory joints can be made by electrical resistance welding of beta titanium.[14] Such joints need not be reinforced with solder. A weld made with insufficient heat will fail at the interface between the wires, whereas overheating may cause a failure adjacent to the weld joint. Figure 37–4 is a cross section of a welded beta titanium joint, showing minimum distortion of the original cold-worked structure.

Corrosion Resistance   Both forms of titanium have excellent corrosion resistance and environmental stability. These features have stimulated the use of titanium alloys in chemical processing, as well as biological applications including heart valves, hip implants, and orthodontic appliances.

References

1. Burstone CJ: Application of bioengineering to clinical orthodontics. *In* Graber TM and Swain BF (Eds): Current Orthodontic Concepts and Techniques. 2nd ed, Philadelphia, W. B. Saunders Co., 1975, Vol 1, pp 230–258.
2. Reed RE and Hill D: Physical Metallurgy Principles. Princeton, N. J., Van Nostrand Company, Inc., 1964, pp 448, 501, and 515.
3. Parr JG and Hanson A: An Introduction to Stainless Steel. Metals Park, Ohio, American Society for Metals, 1965, p 52.
4. Subcommittee on Brazing: Brazing, Silver Brazing, Copper-Hydrogen Brazing and Related Joining Methods. *In* Lyman T: Metals Handbook, 6th edition, Cleveland, American Society for Metals, 1948, pp 78–81.
5. Brown T, Mitchell R, and Barenie J: Evaluation of Five Silver Soldering Techniques. IADR Program and Abstracts, No 1267, 1981.
6. Rogers O: A metallographic evalution of the stainless steel-silver solder joint. Aust Dent J 24:13, 1979.
7. Lautenschlager E, Marker B, Moore K, and Wildes R: Strength mechanisms of dental solder joints. J Dent Res 53:1361, 1974.
8. Hayden HW, Moffatt WG, and Wulff J: The Structure and Properties of Materials. New York, John Wiley & Sons, 1965, Vol III, pp 137–138.
9. Vassar RJ: A Metallographic Study of the Welded Bond Between Two Pieces of

Stainless Steel Band Material. Thesis, Northwestern University Dental School, 1957.

10. Marcotte MR: Optimal Time and Temperature for Maximum Moment and Spring-back and Residual Stress Relief of Stainless Steel Wire. Thesis, Indiana University School of Dentistry, 1970.

11. Andreasen GF and Hilleman TB: An evaluation of 55 cobalt substituted Nitinol wire for use in orthodontics. J Am Dent Assoc 82:1373, 1971.

12. Buehler WJ and Wang FE: A summary of recent research on the Nitinol alloys and their potential applications in ocean engineering. Ocean Eng 1:105, 1968.

13. Goldberg AJ and Burstone CJ: An evaluation of beta titanium alloys for use in orthodontic appliances. J Dent Res 58:593, 1978.

14. Burstone CJ and Goldberg AJ: Beta titanium: a new orthodontic alloy. Am J Orthod 77:121, 1980.

APPENDIX OF CONVERSION FACTORS

To Convert From	To	Multiply By
Force		
kilograms force	pounds	2.2046
kilograms force	newtons	9.807
pounds	kilograms force	0.4536
pounds	newtons	4.448
newtons	kilograms force	0.1020
newtons	pounds	0.2248
Force per unit area		
psi	MPa(MN/m^2)	0.006895
psi	kg/cm^2	0.0703
kg/cm^2	MPa(MN/m^2)	0.09807
kg/cm^2	psi	14.2233
MN/m^2	psi	145.0
MN/m^2	kg/cm^2	10.1968

SI Units

N   — newton
MN — meganewton
Pa   — pascal
MPa — megapascal

INDEX

Note: In this Index, page numbers in *Italics* refer to illustrations; page numbers followed by "t" refer to tables.

615